Congenital Abnormalities and Preterm Birth Related to Maternal Illnesses During Pregnancy

Nándor Ács · Ferenc G. Bánhidy ·
Andrew E. Czeizel

Congenital Abnormalities and Preterm Birth Related to Maternal Illnesses During Pregnancy

Springer

Nándor Ács, MD, PhD
Semmelweis University
Second Department of Obstetrics
and Gynecology
Budapest 1082, Üllői út 78/a
Hungary
acs01@axelero.hu

Ferenc G. Bánhidy, MD, PhD
Semmelweis University
Second Department of Obstetrics
and Gynecology
Budapest 1082, Üllői út 78/a
Hungary
banhidyferenc@hotmail.hu

Andrew E. Czeizel, MD, PhD, DSci
Foundation of the Community Control
of Hereditary Diseases
Budapest 1026
Törökvész lejtő 32
Hungary
czeizel@interware.hu

ISBN 978-90-481-8619-8 e-ISBN 978-90-481-8620-4
DOI 10.1007/978-90-481-8620-4
Springer Dordrecht Heidelberg London New York

Library of Congress Control Number: 2010922898

Printed on acid-free paper

Springer is part of Springer Science+Business Media (www.springer.com)

Contents

Part II Results of Studies and Their Interpretation

Introduction

The major objective of our studies in the last decade was a systematic analysis of maternal diseases during pregnancy to reveal their possible adverse effects on birth outcomes. The two most important factors of infant mortality were particularly analyzed: structural birth defects, known as *congenital abnormalities* (CAs) and *preterm birth* (PB).

In general the objectives of scientific studies might be either to test a new hypothesis or to confirm or confront previously published results. However, less frequently the authors/scientists have personal motivations determined by their professional activities. The authors of this book are practicing physicians and genetic epidemiologist who are mainly interested in the following three practical questions:

1. *The possible adverse effects of pharmaceutical products*. The possible teratogenic potential of about 170 drugs has been evaluated very thoroughly using the data set of the *Hungarian Case-Control Surveillance of Congenital Abnormalities* (HCCSCA) in the last 50 years. These drugs were used to treat maternal diseases and the findings of our population-based case-control studies will be cited in this book and are shown in the Appendix at the end of the book.

   However, our long experiences showed two problems in the drug teratology. In general the evaluation of clinical doses of these drugs is a particularly difficult challenge due to the modification effects of confounders. This problem motivated one of the authors to establish a new model of disaster epidemiology. This new model is based on self-poisoning pregnant women (see Appendix), where pregnant women used extremely large doses of drugs for suicide attempt making it possible to check the dose-dependent teratogenic effect of the applied drugs. The findings of disaster epidemiological studies confirmed our clinical experience implying that possible teratogenic or fetotoxic risk of drugs has been exaggerated. Another experience was that the underlying diseases, the so-called indications of these drugs, are frequently neglected.
2. Therefore, in the 1990s we started to evaluate the *possible associations between maternal diseases during pregnancy and adverse birth outcomes*. Our analyses in this field, again, resulted in a great surprise. On the one hand, some maternal diseases have been studied frequently and thoroughly in terms of possible risks

for the expectant mothers while the possible adverse effects of these diseases on fetal development were only considered as a minor factor. On the other hand, we were all surprised to see that there are "favored maternal diseases" like diabetes mellitus, epilepsy, thrombosis but many other common – though not that severe – maternal conditions, such as infectious diarrhea, viral genital warts, migraine, peptic ulcer, constipation, varicosities, hemorrhoids, etc have not even been evaluated in controlled epidemiological studies. Additionally, the methodological standard of these studies was rather weak in several occasions because new methodological recommendations have not yet been utilized.

Our concept is based on the Koch's rule: the public health importance of a disease is determined by the number of victims and the severity of that particular disease. Thus, we present the available data of each maternal disease separately in the HCCSCA. To our best knowledge our book is the first attempt to evaluate all recorded maternal diseases during pregnancy in a population-based material.

3. Third, in 1980 one of us established a *population-based surveillance of cases with CA and controls*. At present time to our best knowledge HCCSCA represents the largest case-control database in the topic of CAs related to maternal diseases from all over the world. Though the data of the HCCSCA have been available for medical doctors and scientists for decades, these data were not used frequently for research. The founder of the HCCSCA is turning 75 year old in 2010 and he was afraid that the product ("child") of his life would remain unused. Therefore, it made him particularly delighted when two middle aged obstetricians wanted to utilize the data of the HCCSCA. This fruitful collaboration has lead to many publications and finally to this unique book.

The results of different studies were published in international periodicals to face the opinions/comments/suggestions of reviewers and international experts of this topic. This preliminary work and feedback helped us to present our results in its present form. And here we would like to express our gratitude for all the reviewers and critics for improving the quality of our published data.

The merit of the HCCSCA is not only limited to its size but it has an excellent quality of data as well. The surveillance is population-based (the population of Hungary is about 10 million), and the validity of CAs is good due to obligatory hospitalization for delivery. In Hungary all deliveries take place in obstetrical inpatients clinics therefore birth weight and gestational age is always medically recorded. All infant deaths are autopsied. In addition, the diagnoses of CAs were reported by medical doctors and underwent several checking procedures by experts in the HCCSCA. Each case with CA has at least two matched controls without CA. In general, the diagnoses of maternal diseases are also scientifically accurate due to mandatory prenatal care in Hungary. Most maternal diseases were recorded prospectively by medical doctors in the prenatal maternity logbook. When analyzing teratogenic exposure we did not use the old-fashion and unscientific first trimester concept, in addition we did our best to use modern statistical analyses to evaluate our data set.

The authors equally shared the work among themselves. Andrew E. Czeizel, MD, PhD, DoctSci prepared the data of the HCCSCA for the analyses with the help of his computer expert: Erika Varga. Nándor Ács, MD, PhD and Ferenc Bánhidy, MD, PhD checked the validity of diagnoses of the different maternal diseases and pregnancy complications including applied drug treatments. They also reviewed the recent international literature on CAs and pharmaceutical side effects of drugs in pregnancy. These two authors analysed the effects of maternal diseases on CAs and pregnancy outcomes. The statistical analyses were done by Erzsébet Horváth-Puhó. The previous papers were written in collaboration of the above mentioned three physicians and the biostatistician of the project.

This book follows the concept of O. P. Heinonen et al.' (1977) monograph entitled "Birth Defects and Drugs in Pregnancy" (PSG Publishing Company, Inc., Littleton, MA). In their publication all drugs used in the Collaborative Perinatal Project in the USA were evaluated.

Our book includes three parts. In the first part (Part I including Chapter 1) Dr. Czeizel describes the Hungarian Congenital Abnormality Registry and the Hungarian Case-Control Surveillance of Congenital Abnormalities, the source of data for the analyses of CAs and PB. The first part of the book is also completed by a short summary about the principles of terato-epidemiological studies.

In the second part (Part II including Chapter 2–18) Dr Ács and Dr. Bánhidy summarize the most important findings and recommendations of their studies. The authors followed the same design for each disease. First, the definition of the disease, the diagnostic criteria and related drug therapy is described. This is followed by the results of studies presented in two different aspects. First, cases with CA have been evaluated in case-control analysis by Dr Ács, while PB and low birthweight (LBW) as indicator of intrauterine fetal growth retardation were analyzed in the cohort of the so-called controls (i.e. babies without CA) by Dr Bánhidy. In the latter approach only controls will be presented in the book because CAs may have a more drastic effect on gestational age at delivery and birth weight than the studied maternal disease itself. Finally, the authors attempt to summarize the most important available knowledge of adverse effects of maternal diseases on birth outcomes, particularly on CAs, PB and LBW from the international literature. At the end of different chapters of Part B, authors are discussing the similarity or discrepancy between international and own findings.

In the third part (Part III including Chapters 19–21) of the book the authors attempt to summarize the most important findings of their studies and try to draw conclusions on the basis of their own research and international literature to define recommendations for medical practice.

The greatest merit of our studies is that by analyzing our data we managed to identify some new previously unknown associations between maternal diseases and adverse birth outcomes. However, when interpreting new findings in our studies we must remind our readers of the phrase written by Heinonen et al in their book: "None of the associations presented in this book should be regarded as anything more than hypotheses requiring independent confirmation."

We are aware of the fact that our unique data set have some limitations and these problems will be thoroughly discussed later in the book. Here we only mention the fact that different populations have different genetic background, lifestyle, and health care. Nevertheless, we discuss our Hungarian findings within the international literature to clarify the differences and to draw attention to particular problems.

Budapest, Hungary Nándor Ács
Budapest, Hungary Ferenc G. Bánhidy
Budapest, Hungary Andrew E. Czeizel

Technical Notes

1. Different maternal diseases were evaluated separately from different aspect in the data set of the HCCSCA. Therefore, some new data cleanings have become necessary and these comparative analyses may result some minor changes in the basic numbers of cases and controls between in our previous publications and this book.
2. We did extra effort to consult with medical doctors to specify previously unspecified CAs, thus there are some minor differences in the data of previously published papers and the chapters of this book.
3. We cite our previous publications regarding to maternal diseases by roman number in the different chapters, while other references are mentioned by the name of the authors and the year of publication. Some of our recent papers have been accepted for publication, these papers are cited as in press.
4. At the evaluation of maternal diseases we have to consider related drug treatments based mainly on our previous population-based case-control studies in the data set of the HCCSCA and in the material of the Budapest Monitoring System of Self-poisoned Pregnant Women. In addition the recent breakthrough in the primary prevention of CAs by periconceptional folic acid/multivitamin supplementation is very important, and our trials based on the Hungarian Periconceptional Service contributed to this progress. These data are cited frequently in our chapters. We wanted to avoid the repetition of writing out the related own papers; therefore, we created an Appendix at the end of the book which includes all these publications. These publications are cited by their Arabic numbers in the book.
5. When evaluating maternal diseases we followed the nomenclature of the 10th revision of WHO (World Health Organization) International Classification of Diseases (ICD), (WHO, Geneva, 2007) and we will not cite it. It is available on the website of WHO.
6. From practical aspect, we use the abbreviations of the most frequently used terms, such as CA, PB, LBW, HCCSCA (mentioned in the Introduction), OR (odds ratio) and CI (confidence interval). In addition, we use the abbreviation of diseases as well introduced in their own chapters. Gestational months are mentioned by Roman numbers without "the" (thus "I gestational month" instead of the usual "the first gestational month" in order to shorten the text).

7. Our previous experiences verified that highlighting of significant associations with bold characters in the tables helps the reader to recognize easier the important findings. Therefore, we follow the same practice in this book.
8. Different associations of quantitative variables such as gestational age and birth weight were estimated by adjusted t value due to Student test, expressed in the different levels of significance with p value. In the text in general only p value is mentioned. Associations of categorical variables such as CA, PB or LBW were estimated by adjusted OR, but again – to shorten the text – only numerical figures are written e.g. (0.7, 0.4–1.1).
9. The objective of Part III is to summarize the major findings of our project and to define some recommendations for the medical practice, thus here we did not cite the previous references.
10. The data of the HCCSCA are available for further research after request.

Part I
The Study Population and Methods

Andrew E. Czeizel

The evaluation of structural birth defects, i.e. congenital abnormalities (CAs) is based on the data set of the Hungarian Congenital Abnormality Registry.

Chapter 1
The Hungarian Congenital Abnormality Registry (HCAR)

The HCAR was established in 1962 as the first national-based registry in the world (I), after the greatest tragedy of human teratology, the thalidomide-Contergan catastrophe. After a pilot period, the HCAR started to work according to the internationally recommended principles under my direction as part of the Department of Human Genetics and Teratology, *National Institute of Public Health* (NIPH) in 1980 (Fig. 1.1). The HCAR had a budget from the Ministry of Health for the salary of the staff, computer work, printing, and mailing costs. Extra projects needed special funds.

The Hungarian population size is about 10 million in a relatively small territory (92,031 km^2) with a decreasing number of births during the study period (Table 1.1).

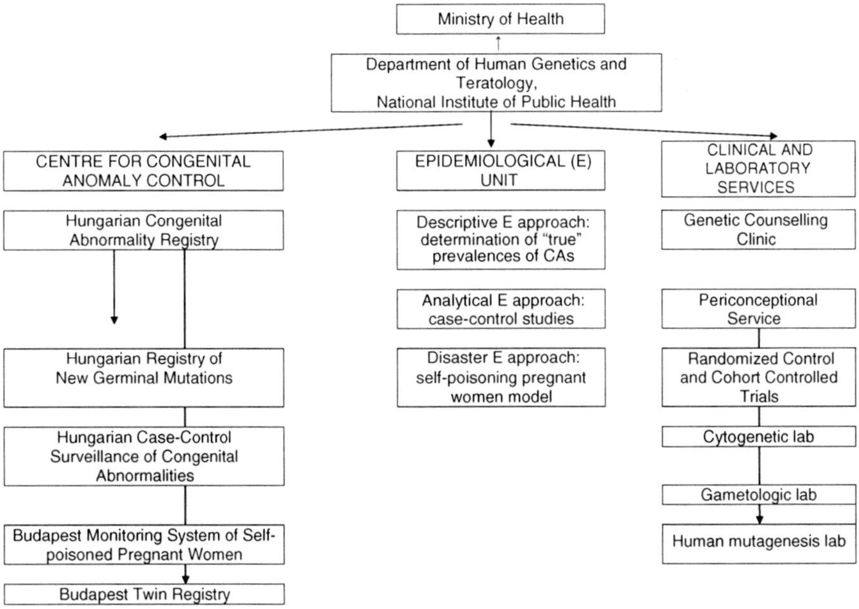

Fig. 1.1 Sructure of department of human genetics and teratology, NIHP

N. Ács et al., *Congenital Abnormalities and Preterm Birth Related to Maternal Illnesses During Pregnancy*, DOI 10.1007/978-90-481-8620-4_1,

Table 1.1 Annual number and recorded rate (per 1,000 total births) of cases with congenital abnormalities (CAs) in the HCAR between 1970 and 2008. (The number of prenatally diagnosed malformed fetuses occurring from 1984 is not included to the denominator)

	Total births	CAs			Total births	CAs	
Year	No.	No.	Rate	Year	No.	No.	Rate
1970	153,339	3,304	21.55	1990	126,378	4,295	33.99
1971	152,159	4,355	28.62	1991	128,299	3,786	29.51
1972	154,668	4,802	31.04	1992	122,233	3,227	26.40
1973	157,623	4,780	30.33	1993	117,458	3,157	26.88
1974	187,957	6,301	33.52	1994	116,006	2,897	24.97
1975	195,847	6,909	35.28	1995	112,447	2,634	23.42
1976	186,916	7,582	40.56	1996	105,669	2,206	20.88
1977	179,152	7,219	40.30	1997	100,830	2,294	22.75
1978	169,524	7,277	42.93	1998	97,857	2,416	24.69
1979	161,677	6,905	42.71	1999	95,116	2,510	26.39
1980	149,829	7,011	46.79	2000	97,597	2,722	27.89
1981	144,062	6,186	42.94	2001	97,047	2,973	30.63
1982	134,579	6,197	46.05	2002	96,804	3,322	34.32
1983	128,160	6,089	47.51	2003	94,647	3,154	33.32
1984	126,158	5,428	43.02	2004	95,137	4,545	47.77
1985	131,008	4,999	39.62	2005	97,496	5,052	51.82
1986	129,032	4,961	37.86	2006	99,871	5,231	52.38
1987	126,722	4,151	32.86	2007	97,613	4,789	49.06
1988	125,112	4,319	34.54	2008	99,580	4,704	47.24
1989	123,957	4,287	34.58	2009			

The task of the HCAR has been to determine the baseline occurrence of different CAs as reliably as possible to accomplish 3 missions: (1) to detect temporal and/or spatial increases ("clusters") of CA; (2) to help plan medical and social services for affected persons; and (3) to estimate the public health importance of different CAs so that resources can be properly allocated.

1.1 Materials and Methods

In our Hungarian public health system the input of medical doctors to the HCAR is called "notification" while the output of the HCAR for the medical community as "report". The notification of cases with CA diagnosed from the birth until the end of first postnatal year is mandatory for physicians according to the order of health minister.

There are 5 sources of notification of cases (Fig. 1.2):

(1) CAs diagnosed after birth were notified by obstetricians. In Hungary practically all deliveries took place in inpatient obstetric clinics and birth attendants were obstetricians during the study period. However, only about 25% of cases with CA were notified by the medical doctors of obstetrical institutions.

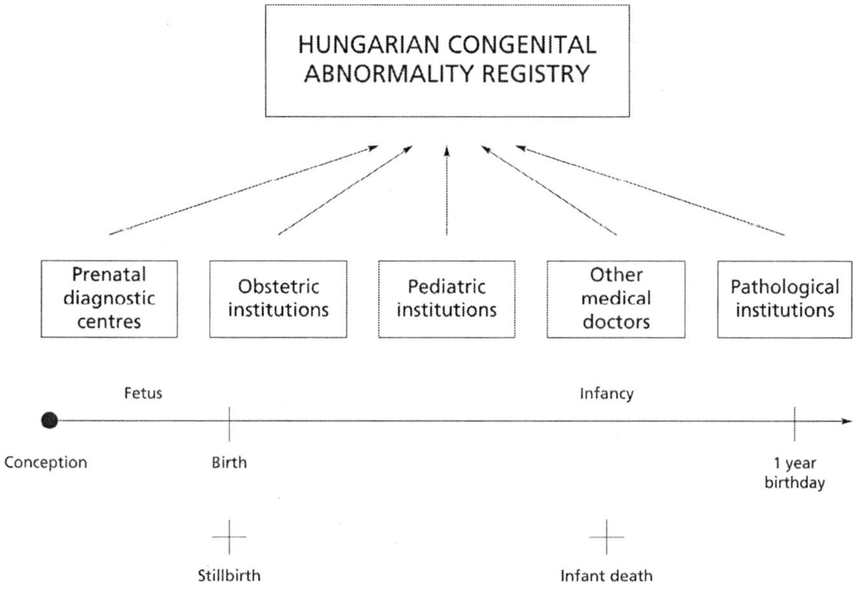

Fig. 1.2 Sources of notification of cases with CA to the Hungarian congenital abnormality registry (HCAR)

(2) The major supporters of the HCAR were pediatricians working in the neonatal units of inpatient obstetric clinics as neonatologists, and in various general and special (surgical, cardiologic, orthopedic, etc.) inpatient and outpatient pediatric clinics where malformed children were treated and cared. About 70% of cases have been notified by the medical doctors of pediatric institutions.
(3) The autopsy was obligatory for all infant deaths and was usually performed in stillborn fetuses during the study period. Pathologists sent a copy of the autopsy report to the HCAR if defects were identified in stillbirths and infants deaths.
(4) Other medical doctors, e.g. general practitioners working in non-obstetric and non-pediatric institutions.
(5) Since 1984 the prenatal diagnostic centers have also been included in the HCAR, and their experts notified affected fetuses after prenatal diagnosis mainly during the second trimester with or without termination of pregnancy.

A printed *Notification Form of Malformed Fetuses/Newborns/Infants* was filled in by medical doctors and sent to the HCAR by post in a prepaid envelop. This form included the name of mother and their newborn infant, their address, age of mother and parity of the study pregnancy, in addition the sex, singleton/twin, weight and gestational age of fetus or newborn infant. Common and moderately frequent CAs were printed in this Form thus these CAs were underlined or circled, while there was an empty column for the description of rare CAs. Finally name, address (institution), telephone number and stamp of medical doctors who notified the case with CA were asked to put down.

About 50% of cases were notified more than once (the record was 8 notifications of a case with spina bifida), duplicate registrations of cases were excluded on the basis of personal data, but the multiple notifications helped to improve the accuracy of data. About 60% of cases with CA were notified in the first month after birth or pregnancy termination and 77% of cases in the first quarter of life during the study period.

The director of the HCAR had a right to check the mandatory notification of cases with CA. The completeness of notifications was checked by the help of comparison of expected number of notifications (based on the number of deliveries in inpatient obstetric institutions and the number of patients in inpatient pediatric clinics) and observed number of notifications in the HCAR according to the different medical institutions. After the recognition of significant under notification, the director of the given institute was informed about this error of medical work. The negligence of this mandatory notification task of medical doctors sometimes led to disciplinary actions.

Cases with CA had a critical evaluation procedure in two steps. First a qualified assistant (prepared for this job) evaluated the Notification Forms, while secondly a medical doctor interested in dysmorphology of fetuses/newborns/infants classified cases with more than one CA.

The first step of CA evaluation included the following tasks:

(1) The contents of Notification Form was checked, and if cases were notified with unspecified CA and/or with incomplete data (e.g. the lack of sex), the assistant called through telephone the medical doctor asking him/her to specify CA or to complete the necessary data.
(2) The diagnostic criteria of CAs were checked, here only some CAs are mentioning with special diagnostic criteria:

    (a) The time of diagnosis is important at the diagnosis of persistent ductus arteriosus (this diagnosis is accepted only after the third postnatal week, but in PB and/or LBW newborns only after the third postnatal month) and of undescended testis (this CA is included in the HCAR if the diagnosis existed after third postnatal month).
    (b) The surgical intervention is a diagnostic criterion in cases with congenital pyloric stenosis (without it, this may be only pyloric spasm), congenital inguinal hernia, rectus diastasis and omphalocele/exomphalos (frequently confused with umbilical hernia).
    (c) The minor manifestations of certain CAs, such as mild microcephaly (based on the percentile of head conference), mild macrocephaly (based on the percentile of head conference), coronal type of hypospadias, small hemangioma (less than 2 cm), small and moderate rectus diastasis (without surgical intervention), were not included among CAs.

(3) The notified minor anomalies/morphologic variants (i.e. unusual morphologic features that are of no serious medical or cosmetic consequence to the children)

were recorded but not evaluated at the calculation of total and different rates of cases with CA in the data set of the HCAR.

The following list of minor anomalies was used in the HCAR:

Head: Larger cranium (mild macrocephaly) – Smaller cranium (mild microcephaly) – Prominent forehead – Prominent occiput – Flat occiput – Abnormal cranium configuration – Double hair whorl – Other abnormal hair pattering –Alopecia.

Eyes: Inner epicanthal fold(s) – Short palpebral fissure – Upward ("mongoloid") slant of palpebral fissures – Downward ("antimongoloid") slant of palpebral fissure – Confluent eyebrow – Hypertelorism – Hypotelorism – Ptosis.

Ear: Protruding auricle – Asymmetrical size of ears – Preauricular and/or auricular tags – Preauricular fistula – Low-set ear – Primitive shape of the ear – Cup ears – Earlobe crease.

Face and mouth: Low broad nasal bridge – Short nose – Upturn nose – Maxillary hypoplasia – Asymmetric crying facies – Small mandible – Smooth philtrum – Thin upper lip – Lip pit – Large or small oral opening – Large tongue – High arched palate – Bifid uvula – Oral (lingual) frenulum – Enamel hypoplasia – Premature eruption of teeth (Natal teeth) – Wide distance between teeth.

Extremities: Simian crease – Sydney line – Shorter 5th finger – Clinodactyly – Short fingers – Long fingers – Single flexion crease on the 5th finger – Partial syndactyly between the 2nd and 3rd toes – Wide distance between the 1st and 2nd toes – Broad hallux – Hypoplastic hallux – Dorsiflexion of the hallux – Sole crease – Prominent heel – Exostosis tibiae – Pes planus – Nail hypoplasia.

Trunk – Abdomen: Accessory nipples(s) – Wide-set nipples – Short sternum – Spina bifida occulta – Umbilical hernia – Single umbilical artery – Rectus diastasis, small and moderate.

Genital organs: Hypospadias, coronal type – Hydrocele – Shawl-like scrotal fold.

Skin: Pigmented nevus, many – Verucca – Vitiligo – Mongolian spot – Sacral dimple deep – Acromial dimples – Haemangioma (small) – Atheroma – Lipoma – Hyperpigmentation – Hypopigmentation – Café-au-lait spots – Hirsutism.

(4) The differentiation of cases with one or more notified CA. If a case had seemingly two or more CAs, this Notification Form was forwarded to the medical doctor of the HCAR for further evaluation.
(5) Coding the CA of cases according to the *International Classification of Diseases* (ICD), WHO, though we needed some corrections of this list.

The second step of CA evaluation by medical doctor of the HCAR was focused multiple CAs. Multimalformed cases notified with seemingly 2 or more CAs were differentiated into some groups and finally into two categories of CAs.

I. Cases with *isolated CA* included – beyond the so-called *single* CA (evaluated by the assistant) – 3 further groups.

   (1) The term *complex CA* (or monotopic field defect) is used if more than one CA occurs in one organ system (Opitz, 1982), e.g. two or more cardiovascular CAs (e.g. tetralogy of Fallot or ventricular + atrial septal defect), eye CAs (e.g. microphthalmos + congenital cataract), and ear CAs (e.g. microtia with absence of auditory canal), or limb deficiencies in two or more limbs (i.e. multimelic limb deficiencies), or poly- and syndactyly together (i.e. poly/syndactyly), and these complex CAs have special codes in the HCAR.
   (2) The diagnosis of *polytopic field defects* (Opitz, 1982) was accepted in the following CA-entities: holoprosencephaly with cyclopia and other CAs of brain, eyes and face; caudal dysplasia complex, i.e. renal agenesis with or without of agenesis of bladder, internal and external genital organ, and imperforatus anus; prune belly defect, i.e. abdominal muscle deficiency with urinary tract dysplasia; exstrophy of urinary bladder or cloaca with omphalocele, imperforate anus, lumbosacral spina bifida, epispadias and inguinal hernia. In these cases the primary CA is evaluated but associated CAs are recorded.
   (3) At the diagnosis of *CA-sequences*, such as spina bifida aperta/cystica (with hydrocephalus and clubfoot); CA of diaphragm (with lung a/hypoplasia and dextrocardia, in addition eventration of visceral organs to the chest cavity); Robin sequence (i.e. micrognathia with glossoptosis and U-shaped cleft palate); Potter-oligohydramnios sequence (i.e. renal a/dysgenesis with lung hypoplasia and the symptoms of fetal compression: "Potter face", deformed hand and feet due to oligohydramnios); ADAM (Amniotic Deformity, Adhesions, Mutilations) sequence (i.e. amniotic band induced asymmetric limb deficiencies , atypical anencephaly/encephalocele, and/or oral cleft and/or ectopic cordis/thoracoschisis, and/or open abdomen). In these CAs only the primary CA was evaluated though the secondary and tertiary CAs were recorded.

   The above three seemingly "multiple" CA groups were excluded from the category of multiple CAs, and were evaluted as special groups of isolated CAs.

II. The definition of *multiple CA (MCA)* is a concurrence of two or more CAs in the same person affecting at least two different organ systems (II, III). However, it is necessary to differentiate at least four groups of MCA cases:

   (1) *MCA syndromes*, i.e. "recognized patterns of CAs presumably having the same etiology and currently not interpreted as the consequence of a single localized error in morphogenesis" (Smith, 1975; Opitz, 1982; Spranger et al., 1982). MCA syndromes are caused by gene mutations, chromosomal aberration and teratogenic agents.

   In Hungary chromosomal examination was recommended in all multimalformed cases during the study period. Phenotypic manifestation and/or familial cluster of a specific MCA helped medical doctors to recognize and/or to identify MCA-syndromes caused by autosomal and X-linked gene mutations. Among teratogenic MCA-syndromes, cases with fetal rubella, varicella, hydantoin, warfarin, retinoic acid and alcohol effect, in addition diabetic embryopathy were reported to the HCAR. Cases with notified *MCA-syndromes* were recorded on the basis of notifications by medical doctors in the HCAR. The accuracy of these notified MCA-syndromes was checked in different validation studies in general with appropriate results (II).

(2) *MCA-associations*, i.e. "recognized patterns of CAs which currently are not considered to constitute MCA-syndromes" (Smith, 1975; Opitz, 1982; Spranger et al., 1982).

Cases with notified *MCA-associations* were included into the category of MCA in the HCAR. VACTERL-, MURCS- or CHARGE- associations were notified rarely to the HCAR. However, we introduced the so-called *registry diagnosis* in six well-defined MCA-associations (II): (i) *Schisis-association*, i.e. the combination of the so-called schisis-type CA such as neural-tube defects (anencephaly, encephalocele, spina bifida), orofacial clefts (cleft lip with or without cleft palate and cleft palate), diaphragmatic CAs and CAs of abdominal wall (omphalocele/exomphalos and gastroschisis) (IV), (ii) *VACTERL-association*, i.e. the combination of 3 or more VACTERL-type CAs such as V = vertebral CAs, A = anal atresia/stenosis, C = cardiovascular CAs, TE = tracheal-oesophageal atresia/stenosis, R = renal CAs, L = limb deficiency, radial type) (V), (iii) *MURCS-association*, i.e. the combination of MURCS-type CAs such as MU = Müllerian duct aplasia, R = renal a/dysgenesis, CS = cervicothoracic somite dysplasia (II), (iv) *CHARGE-association*, i.e. the combination of CHARGE-type CAs such as C = coloboma, H = heart/cardiovascular CAs, A = atresia choanae, R = retarded growth and development and/or CAs of central nervous system, G = genital anomalies, E = ear anomalies and/or deafness) (II), (v) *Postural-deformity association* i.e., the combination of 2 or more postural deformations such as congenital dislocation/dysplasia of the hip, clubfoot, torticollis and other deformations of vertebras, limbs, etc. (VI), and (vi) *GAM-association* (*g*enital *a*nomalies of *m*ales), i.e. the combination of undescended testis, hypospadias, congenital inguinal hernia and other CAs of male genitalia (VII).

(3) *Random combinations*, i.e. chance or coincidental concurrence of two or more different CAs.

(4) *Unidentified* or *unrecognized MCAs*, i.e. previously delineated MCA-syndromes or MCA-associations but not diagnosed or undelineated MCA-syndromes or MCA-associations.

Random combinations and unidentified/unrecognized MCAs cannot be differentiated in the clinical practice, therefore we use the term *unclassified MCA* (UMCA) for these MCA cases together.

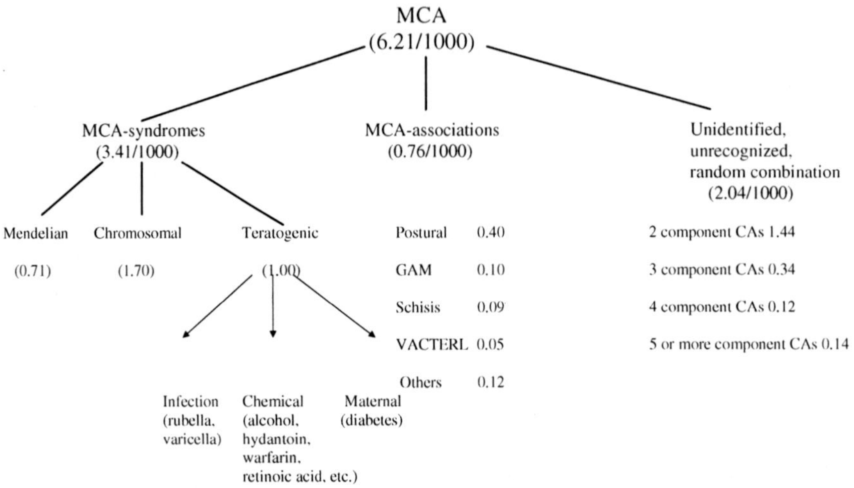

Fig. 1.3 Classification of MCA groups and their total (birth + fetal) prevalence per 1,000 births due to the results of the Hungarian MCA evaluation program in the data set of the Hungarian congenital abnormality registry, 1973–1982 (III)

Figure 1.3 illustrates the distribution of different MCA groups in the data set of the HCAR.

A new code system was introduced for the classification of MCA cases. Each specified MCA-syndrome with known origin and MCA-association without known origin had a code number while the group of UMCA cases was classified according to the number (2, 3, 4, 5 or more) of component CAs (II, VIII, IX).

The list of 45 component CAs in UMCA cases of the HCAR is shown in Table 1.2, component CAs were classified according to three criteria: severity, occurrence and validity of diagnosis (II). Thus three subgroups of component CAs were differentiated as principal, important and dubious CAs within UMCA.

In conclusion, the unit of the HCAR is the *case*, i.e. fetus/newborn/infant affected with CA (i.e. the so-called informative offspring), therefore multimalformed cases with 2 or more CA (with or without minor anomalies) are also considered as one affected subject.

The confidentiality of personal data was of growing significance and public concern in the late 1970s. Thus, since 1980 a signature for printed informed consent form has been requested from parents of cases and it has obtained in 98% of the cases by the help of the activity of the Hungarian Case-Control Surveillance of Congenital Abnormalities. The names and addresses of the remainder are deleted in the records of the HCAR (IX, X).

Table 1.2 List of 45 component CAs of UMCA cases in the HCAR

Principle CAs (in general visible and/or with good validity of diagnosis and common or moderately frequent)
AN = anencephaly
EN = encephalocele
SB = spina bifida cystica/aperta
CP = cleft palate
CL = cleft lip ± palate
OA = oesophageal atresia/stenosis with or without tracheal fistula
AA = anal/rectal canal atresia/stenosis
PY = polydactyly
SY = syndactyly
LR = limb reduction/deficiency abnormality
EX = CAs of abdominal wall: exomphalos/omphalocele and gastroschisis
Important CAs
AM = an/microphthalmia
CT = congenital cataract
HD = congenital cardiovascular malformations
DI = diaphragmatic defects
AI = atresia/stenosis of small intestine
RA = renal a/dysgenesis
CK = cystic kidney
SH = hypospadias
EG = CAs of external genitalia (No SH, UT)
Dubious CAs (heterogeneous and/or with not good validity of diagnosis)
MC = microcephaly (primary)
HY = congenital hydrocephaly
ON = other CAs of nervous system (No AN, EN, SB, MC, HY)
EY = other CAs of eyes (No AM and CT)
FS = CAs of face and skull
EA = CAs of ear
BR = branchial-cervical CAs
TC = torticollis
RS = CAs of respiratory system
PS = congenital pyloric stenosis (needed surgery)
OD = other CAs of digestive system (No OA, AA, AI, PS)
SA = spleen anomalies
US = obstructive CAs of urinary tract
OU = other CAs of urinary tract (No RA, CK, US)
UT = undescended testis (diagnosed after 3rd postnatal month)
IH = inguinal hernia (needed surgery)
CD = congenital dysplasia/dislocation of the hip
CF = clubfoot
OL = other CAs of limbs (No PY, SY, LD, CF, CD)
SK = CAs of skeletal system
MS = CAs of muscle (No DI, IH)
IM = CAs of integuement
SI = situs inversus
EO = CAs of endocrine organs
TE = teratomas and large (more than 2 cm) hemangioma

1.2 The Data Base of the HCAR

Previous Table 1.1 summarized the most important figures of HCAR. There was an obvious increase in the total rate of cases with CA between 1976 and 1984 with a maximum in 1983. A significant decrease occurred after the change in the political system in Hungary, 1989. However, recently the total rate of cases with CAs has increased again; in fact the maximum was achieved in 2006.

In the past frequently the total rate of CAs was evaluated though it is not useful from medical aspect. On the one hand it is not good to combine different CAs (as bananas and apples, though both are fruits). On the other hand in general teratogens cause specific CAs without necessarily affecting the overall rate. Finally the rate of total CA is misleading because it depends on the spectrum of CA evaluated and different studies have differences in the distribution of CAs. Thus it is necessary to define the spectrum (list) of CAs because some studies evaluate only major CAs while all notified CAs (e.g. congenital inguinal hernia in the HCAR) are recorded in other studies/systems.

Thus, the total group of CAs is not too important because comprises of different CAs with different etiology, clinical severity and public health importance, therefore it is worth evaluating CAs according to different aspects (Fig. 1.4).

Severity, CAs were classified into 3 groups in the HCAR:

(1) Lethal CAs cause stillbirth or infant death or recently associated with elective termination of pregnancy after prenatal diagnosis in more than 50% of cases.
(2) Severe CAs cause death and/or handicap without medical intervention.
(3) Mild CAs require medical intervention but life expectancy is good.

Lethal and severe CAs together constitutes the so-called "major" CAs.

Minor anomalies were also recorded and considered at the evaluation of UMCA cases, however, at the calculations the rate of different CAs were neglected.

Occurrence, four levels are differentiated in the HCAR:

(1) Common (more than 1 per 1,000 informative offspring)
(2) Moderately frequent (0.1–0.99 per 1,000 informative offspring).
(3) Rare (0.01–0.099 per 1,000 informative offspring)
(4) Very rare (less than 0.01 per 1,000 informative offspring).

There are two types of disease frequency at the evaluation of cases. *Incidence* is the rate at which a new event (i.e. fresh disorder of cases) occurs in the study population during a certain period. *Prevalence* is the rate of all cases with a defined disorder, e.g. specified CA in the study population at a given point of time or during a given period. However, the concept of incidence cannot be applied to most CAs because many malformed fetuses are selected out before birth. Thus in the past the term *prevalence at birth* (or birth prevalence) was used at the evaluation of frequency of cases with different CAs based on all live- and stillbirths. (If it was not possible to evaluate stillborn fetuses, the term live-birth prevalence was used.)

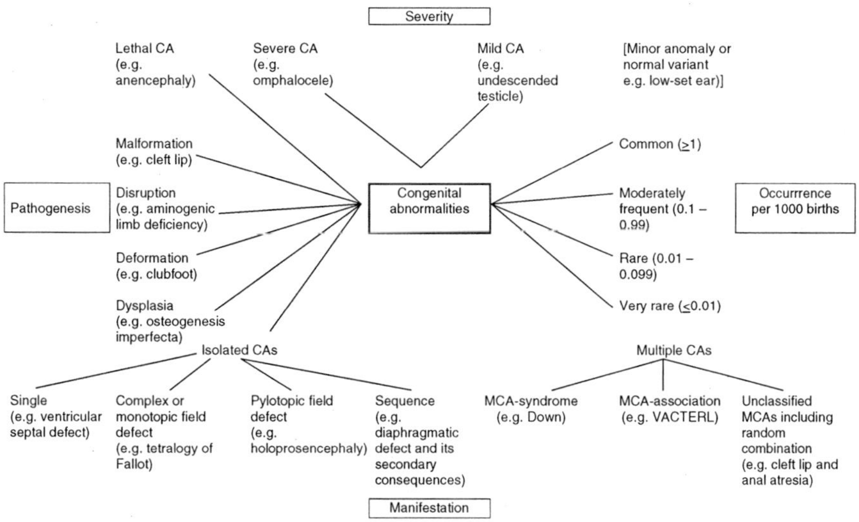

Fig. 1.4 Different classifications for congenital abnormalities (CAs)

However, recently the prenatally diagnosed malformed fetuses can also be evaluated, thus it is necessary to introduce a new term: *total (birth + fetal) prevalence* of CAs based on the informative offspring: live-born babies, stillborn fetuses and electively terminated malformed fetuses after their prenatal diagnosis.

The recorded total (birth + fetal) prevalence of cases with CA diagnosed from the second trimester of pregnancy through the age of 1 year was 35 per 1,000 informative offspring between 1980 and 1996, and about 90% of major CAs were reported to the HCAR (XI).

Pathogenesis. Four groups of CAs were recommended to differentiate (Spranger et al., 1982):

(1) Malformation: "a morphologic defect of an organ, part of an organ, or larger region of the body resulting from an intrinsically abnormal developmental process."
(2) Disruption: "a morphologic defect of an organ, part of an organ, or larger region of the body resulting from the extrinsic breakdown of, or an interference with, an originally normal developmental process."
(3) Deformation: "an abnormal form, shape, or position of a part of the body caused by mechanical forces."
(4) Dysplasia: "an abnormal organization of cells into tissues(s) and its morphologic results(s). In other words: a dysplasia is the process (and the consequence) of dyshistogenesis."

Manifestations such as isolated and multiple CAs as classification categories were shown previously. The main advantage of this classification is that helps to estimate the origin of CAs. Most isolated CAs have multifactorial (polygenic-environmental interaction because their genetic predisposition is triggered by external agents) (XII) or teratogenic (XIII) origin. Most multiple CAs are caused by chromosomal aberrations, major gene mutations and teratogens (II). In general the so-called primary teratogens induce multiple CAs, and it explains fetal rubella, varicella, alcohol etc syndromes/effects. The so-called secondary teratogens cause isolated CAs triggering the genetic predisposition of the given CA.

The data of the HCAR are reported in the *Annual Report of the HCAR* for the Ministry of Health and for all medical institutions in Hungary, in addition these data are available for further analyses and researches.

1.3 Quality Control of the HCAR

The quality of a CA-Registry is determined by the subjects studied (population or sample), completeness of notification (i.e. ascertainment of cases) and the validity of CA-diagnosis.

1.3.1 Study Populations and Samples

The measures of disease frequency, i.e. the rate of patients affected with CA, these subjects are called index patients or cases in epidemiological studies. The rate of CAs is based on a formula including cases with different CA in the nominator and all evaluated people in the denominator, therefore it is an important task to define the denominator.

Ideally all individuals of the given population can be evaluated; such programs are called population-based. The scientific advantage of a population-based design is that it avoids bias arising from the first level of selection. Frequently only random samples can be used for this purpose, this sample, i.e. a group of the given population should be represented the population at large.

In general the hospital-based designs are used in medical researches because relatively easy and inexpensive to find and/or recruit cases with CA in this approach. However, these hospital-based samples cannot represent the population at large due to the first level of selection bias of patients, i.e. special medical (e.g. higher level of medical care in university clinics) or regional/population differences.

The HCAR is population-based national registry thus the first level of selection bias is excluded.

1.3.2 Completeness of Notification

The second level of selection bias is connected with the incomplete registration of cases because a complete registration of patients is seldom reached, in addition the completeness depends on the severity of diseases. Another selection bias can occur whenever the inclusion of cases or controls into the study depends in some way on the exposure of interest, e.g. maternal diseases.

The HCAR is based of multiple sources of notifications. The recruitment of cases from multiple sources (obstetric, different pediatric and pathologic institutions) is an important chance to have as complete as possible registration of cases and a good figure for the nominator of CA-rates.

In addition there was a continuous control of notifications according to medical institutions in Hungary. The comparison on expected and observed numbers of notified cases, and the necessary action in the negligence of mandatory notification task helped to achieve a nearly complete ascertainment of cases with major CAs.

Finally another project helped to estimate the completeness of notification. The HCAR was part of the Department of Human Genetics and Teratology, NIPH and this Department had also an independent Epidemiological Unit (Fig. 1.1). Among the tasks of this Unit, one was to determine the so-called *true* birth prevalence of different CAs. These true rates of different CAs were determined by the field studies in all medical institutions connected with the CA studied. Thus the experts of our Epidemiological Unit visited all inpatients obstetric and pediatric clinics, in addition pathological institutions in the study region and they reviewed their medical records to identify cases with CAs studied and these cases were selected for further analysis (XII, XIII). These studies helped to estimate the completeness of notification in the HCAR after the comparison of recorded and true rate of different CAs.

Table 1.3 shows these data of 10 common CAs in the HCAR.

Obviously severe and visible CAs have a more complete ascertainment than less severe and internal CAs. The ascertained and non-ascertained cases with CA may have differences in the variables of mothers and cases themselves and it causes the third level of selection bias. However, it is good to know these differences in the HCAR and our validation studies helped us to estimate the above differences and to consider them at their evaluation (XIV–XVI).

In conclusion a general rule is that there is an obvious correlation between the severity of CAs and their completeness of notifications.

1.3.3 The Validity of CA-Diagnoses

Cases with CA were notified by medical doctors to the HCAR. Nevertheless the diagnosis of CAs was checked in the HCAR by an expert and if it was necessary extra information was asked from medical doctors to have more accurate diagnoses.

In addition the previously mentioned field studies performed by the experts of the Epidemiological Unit of the Department of Human Genetics and Teratology, NIPH, were appropriate to check the diagnosis of CAs notified to the HCAR.

After 1980 the recent collection of medical data of cases with CA in the Hungarian Case-Control of Surveillance of Congenital Abnormalities helped much to improve further the validity of CA-diagnoses.

The proportion of misdiagnoses in the common CAs is also shown in Table 1.3. Again these percentage figures are determined by the severity and manifestations of

Table 1.3 Main data of common CAs in Hungary between 1980 and 1996

CA category CA group	Severity	"True" prevalence per 1,000[a]	Recorded prevalence per 1,000[b]	Completeness of notification (%)	Misdiagnosis (%)
Isolated CAs					
Congenital dislocation of hip	Mild	13.61 ± 0.36	8.6	63	10
Dysplasia/dislocatable hip		13.5			
Dislocation of hip		0.1			
Congenital inguinal hernia[c]	Mild	11.04 ± 0.36	3.3	30	6
Cardiovascular CAs	Mild-Severe-Lethal	10.48 ±1.11	8.8	84	37
Common truncus		0.17			
Transposition of great vessels		0.29			
Tetralogy of Fallot		0.36			
Ventricular septal defect		1.95			
Atrial septal defect, type II.		0.89			
Endocardial cushion defect		0.28			
Aortic stenosis		0.79			
Hypoplastic left heart		0.24			
Patent ductus arteriosus		0.94			
Coarctation of aorta		0.53			
CAs of pulmonary artery		0.62			
Complex cardiovascular CAs		0.94			
Others and unspecified		2.48			
Undescended testis[d]	Mild	3.63 ± 0.60	2.1	58	5
(Only males)		6.7 ± 0.6			
Clubfoot	Mild	2.97 ± 0.08	3.2	108	48
Talipes equinovarus		1.5			
Talipes calcaneovalgus		0.7			
Metatarsus varus		0.8			

Table 1.3 (continued)

CA category CA group	Severity	"True" prevalence per 1,000[a]	Recorded prevalence per 1,000[b]	Completeness of notification (%)	Misdiagnosis (%)
Neural-tube defect	Lethal	2.80 ± 0.28	2.6	93	2
Anencephaly		1.0			
Spina bifida		1.6			
Encephalocele, occipital		0.2			
Hypospadias	Severe	2.25 ± 0.47	1.7	76	16
(Only males)		4.4 ± 0.8			
Coronal (minor anomaly)		–			
Glandular		1.2			
Penile, penoscrotal		0.9			
Scrotal, perineoscrotal		0.1			
Cong. hypertrophic pyloric stenosis[c]	Severe	1.51 ± 0.12	1.3	86	2
Cleft lip ± palate	Severe	1.03 ± 0.62	1.0	100	0
Unilateral cleft lip		0.3			
Bilateral cleft lip		0.1			
Cleft lip + cleft palate		0.6			
Multiple CA					
Down syndrome	Severe	1.17 ± 0.04 (1973–1988)	0.9	77	5
		1.71 ± 0.06 (2000–2006)	1.2		
Pure trisomy		1.10			
Robertsonian translocation		0.04			
Mosaicism		0.03			

[a]Determined in ad hoc active epidemiological studies.
[b]Recorded in the HCAR, 1980–1996.
[c]Surgical correction.
[d]Diagnosis after 3rd postnatal month.

CAs, but there are special problems in some CAs. For example medical doctors frequently could not differentiate Robin sequence and cleft palate; omphalocele and gastroschisis within the CA-group of abdominal wall; they were not able to diagnose the specific types of limb deficiencies.

Finally there was an unexpected chance for the check of the diagnosis in some CAs. Many families of cases with different CAs asked us to organize parental meetings for them to answer their questions and to help the medical and social service of their affected children. Thus we organized annual parental meetings for children with spina bifida and hydrocephalus, orofacial clefts, limb deficiencies, cardiovascular CAs, CAs of genital organs, CAs of digestive system, dwarfism and Down syndrome in different months of the year. The participation rate of these parental meetings was high resulting in an opportunity to examine these children by the expert of the HCAR personally.

The classification of CAs in the HCAR needs also some discussion. The previous classification of CAs was based on their anatomical location. The optimal classification would be an etiology-based classification but unfortunately at present a certain part of CAs has unknown etiology. Thus a compromise is a pathogenetic-oriented classification, therefore CAs are differentiated into isolated (including single, complex, polytopic field defect and sequence groups) and multiple (including MCA-syndromes, MCA-associations and unclassified multiple CAs) categories (Figs. 1.3 and 1.4).

In conclusion, the major benefits of the HCAR are the population-based system, nearly complete ascertainment of cases with major CA, the good validity of CA diagnosis and the pathogenetic-oriented classification of cases. The population-based data set is a great help to limit the first level of selection bias. The nearly complete collection of cases with major CA can reduce the second level of selection bias. The pathogenetic-oriented classification is good to evaluate the trend of etiological factors.

1.4 The Weaknesses of the HCAR

The major weakness of the HCAR is that its data set includes only CAs, though there are some other pregnancy outcomes and birth defects.

Three different levels of *pregnancy outcomes* have to consider.

I. At the evaluation of *fetal death*, three groups can be classified:

 1) Very early loss of pregnancy, i.e. the so-called chemical pregnancies (positive pregnancy test without any later clinical symptoms of pregnancy). Of 213 pregnant women who attempted suicide with very large doses of drugs in the fourth pregnancy week, 111 (52.1%) had chemical pregnancies (XVII). In general there is no chance for the examination and evaluation of zygotes and blastocysts.
 2) Miscarriages (spontaneous abortions) or early fetal deaths (until the gestational age of 20–24 weeks in different countries). In general there is no chance for the fetal examination in these embryos/fetuses because embryos

have complete destruction in the frequent so-called "missed abortion" or "blighted ova", or lost before the admittance to the hospital. Fetuses from the rare ectopic pregnancies are in general included into this group of fetal death.
3) Stillbirths or late fetal deaths. There is a good chance for the appropriate diagnosis of defects if these fetuses have autopsy.

II. There are three groups of *pregnancy termination*:

1) Termination of pregnancies due to social reasons in unwanted pregnancies. There is no chance for fetal examination after surgical interruption of pregnancy, and these pregnant women have no higher risk of CAs.
2) Termination of early pregnancy (in general until the 12th gestational week) due to medical reasons, frequently because of true or supposed teratogenic risk of maternal diseases or drugs. In general after the surgical interruption of pregnancy there is no chance to diagnose defects in these embryos. The use of abortion pills before the 9th gestational week may provide fetuses for the detection of defects.
3) The so-called elective termination of pregnancies during the second and rarely in the third trimester after the prenatal diagnosis of chromosomal aberrations, gene mutations, biochemical or structural defects in fetuses. In general these pregnancies are ended by the induction of delivery thus fetuses are available for expert examination.

III. Among *live-born newborns/infants*, three groups are worth differentiating:

1) According to gestational age at delivery: preterm, term and postterm births.
2) According to birth weight: low, medium and large birthweight.
3) According to early death: first day, early neonatal (first 6 days), neonatal (first month) and infant (first year) mortality. There is a good chance for the diagnosis of CAs if these newborns or infants have autopsy.

In general it is possible to diagnose other birth defects such as mental retardation, visual, hearing and other defects in surviving live-born babies.

However, at present CAs are evaluated only in the so-called *informative offspring* with a good chance for the correct diagnosis of CAs, and this category includes (i) live-born babies, (ii) stillborn fetuses, and (iii) malformed fetuses after termination of pregnancy followed their prenatal diagnosis.

The optimal model for the evaluation of adverse factors (e.g. maternal diseases during pregnancy) for the fetal development should consider all pregnancy outcomes.

On the other hand CAs represent only one class of birth defects, because *birth defects* or congenital anomalies comprises of all morphologic (structural-anatomic), functional and/or biochemical-molecular defects developing from conception until birth, present at birth whether detected at that time or not. Several categories can be differentiated/classified within birth defects: genetic disease with early manifestation (e.g. hypothyroidism); congenital abnormalities (i.e. structural birth defects); congenital tumours (e.g. teratomas); idiopathic intrauterine growth retardation (i.e.

newborns with small for gestational age); fetal diseases (e.g. fetal varicella disease); immunological disease (e.g. Rh maternal-fetus incompatibility); mental retardation; behavioural deviations; functional defects of sense organs, e.g. blindness, deafness, etc.

At the evaluation the fetotoxic effect of adverse agents, mainly *intrauterine growth retardation* can be considered as the most sensitive indicator of fetotoxicity (XVIII).

The development obviously does not end with gross organ development or with the end of pregnancy; the ultimate test of a fetotoxic agent depends on long-range follow-up. Some drugs, e.g. valproate (Meadow et al., 2009) can induce mental retardation with or without CA. Other studies have shown the adverse effect of intrauterine exposure to a variety of psychotropic drugs for behavioural abilities of children (Briggs et al., 2005; Shepard and Lemire, 2004; Friedman and Polifka, 2000).

The classical human teratogenic studies concentrate the occurrence of CA because teratogenic agents, e.g. drugs or maternal diseases, induce CAs. The HCAR followed this strategy, though it would be better to evaluate the whole spectrum of birth defects.

Another important weakness of CA-registries is that not able to identify the causes after the detection of clusters of specified CAs. In the history of the HCAR a cluster of cases with congenital limb deficiencies in 1975–1978 (XIX, XX) or a very significant increase of cases with Down syndrome in a small village, 1989–1990 (XXI) were detected but the available data were not appropriate to find the causes. Special field studies helped us to reveal the teratogenic agent (very high doses of estrogens used as abortifacient) associated with the cluster of limb deficiencies or to identify a mutagenic-aneugenic organophosphate insecticide: trichlorfon used by criminal action in the background of Dowen cases' cluster. The above weaknesses of the HCAR stimulated me to establish the Hungarian Case-Control Surveillance of Congenital Abnormalities in 1979.

1.5 The Hungarian Case-Control Surveillance of Congenital Abnormalities (HCCSCA)

The Hungarian Case-Control Surveillance of Congenital Abnormalities (HCCSCA) started to work officially within the Centre for Congenital Anomaly Control of the Department of Human Genetics and Teratology, NIPH in 1980 (XXII). Until now the HCCSCA has become the largest case-control data set of CA-surveillance in the world (Table 1.4).

Table 1.4 The data set of the HCCSCA, 1980–2002

Study groups	1980–1996	1997–2002	Total
Cases	22,843	7,079	29,992
Controls	38,151	14,448	52,599
Malformed controls	834	233	1,067

1.5.1 Study Groups

Cases with CA are selected from the HCAR while matched controls without CAs were chosen from the National Birth Registry of the Central Statistical Office.

There were three exclusion criteria at the selection of *cases* with CA from the HCAR for the data set of the HCCSCA.

(i) Cases reported after 3 months of birth or pregnancy termination; this subgroup included 33% of cases affected mainly with mild CA. The shorter time between birth or pregnancy termination and data collection increases the accuracy of maternal information regarding the data of study pregnancy without undue loss of power.
(ii) Three mild CAs (such as congenital dysplasia of hip, congenital inguinal hernia, and large haemangioma). The birth prevalence of these CAs is common with low completeness of notification, in addition these CAs were studied in descriptive and case-control epidemiological studies previously (XII, XIII).
(iii) MCA-syndromes caused by major mutant genes or chromosomal aberrations. These CA-syndromes had preconceptional origin and the main task of the HCCSCA has been the detection of teratogenic/fetotoxic agents in the postconception period.

Controls were ascertained from the National Birth Registry of the Central Statistical Office for the HCCSCA. Controls were defined as newborns without CA. In most years two controls were matched to every case according to sex, birth week in the year when the case was born, and district of parents' residence. We wanted to increase the number of controls therefore we selected three controls for each case between 1986 and 1992. However, unfortunately we had no financial support for the third control after 1992.

In addition a third group of *malformed/patients controls* was also used in the HCCSCA, this group included cases with Down syndrome and they were selected from the HCAR. Malformed controls were also chosen only during the first 3 months after birth or pregnancy termination and 94% were caused by non-disjunction before conception, i.e. these cases had pure trisomy 21. The explanation for the use of this malformation control group is that their mothers have similar recall for the events during pregnancy than the mothers of cases, but Down syndrome has preconceptional origin, thus teratogenic/fetotoxic agents cannot modify their manifestation.

1.5.2 Collection of Exposure and Other Data

There are three sources of data:

1. *Prospective medically recorded data*
   An explanatory letter with an informed consent form was mailed to the mothers immediately after the selection of cases, controls and malformed controls to

explain the importance of this project for the prospective pregnant women and in their future pregnancies. Mothers were asked to send us the prenatal maternity logbook and other medical records (mainly discharge summaries of their hospitalizations) concerning their diseases and related drug treatments during the study pregnancy and their child's CA. These documents were sent back within a month.

Prenatal care is mandatory for pregnant women in Hungary (if somebody does not visit prenatal care, she does not get maternity grants and leave), thus nearly 100% of pregnant women visit prenatal care with a first visit of 6–12 weeks of gestation and with an average of 7 visits. Prenatal care obstetricians are obliged to record all pregnancy complications, maternal diseases and prescribed drugs in the prenatal maternity logbook.

Discharge summaries regarding the delivery of mothers contain birth weight, gestational age and other important findings.

Finally mothers were asked to give a signature for the printed informed consent form.

2. *Retrospective self-reported maternal information*

   A printed structured questionnaire with a list of medicines and diseases were also mailed to the mothers of cases, controls and malformed controls. The questionnaire requested information on their personal characteristics (marital and employment status), medicinal product (drug and pregnancy supplement) intakes, pregnancy complications and maternal diseases during pregnancy according to gestational month, the family history of CAs and history of their previous pregnancies. To standardize the answers, mothers were asked to read the enclosed list of drugs and diseases as memory aid before they replied.

   The mean time elapsed between the end of pregnancy and return of the "information package" (including prenatal logbook, questionnaire, signed informed consent, etc.) in our prepaid envelope was 3.5 ± 1.2, 5.2 ± 2.9 and 3.3 ± 1.8 months in the case, control and malformed control groups, respectively.

3. *Supplementary data collection*

   Regional nurses were asked to visit all non-respondent case and malformed control mothers at home. Regional nurses helped mothers to fill in questionnaire and to evaluate the available medical data, in addition obtained data of fever-related disorders and lifestyles through a cross interview of mothers and fathers. Unfortunately regional nurses visited only 200 non-respondent and 600 respondent control mothers in two validation studies (XIV, XV), because the committee on ethics considered this follow-up to be disturbing to the parents of healthy children. Regional nurses used the same method in these control mothers as in non-respondent case mothers.

Overall, the necessary information was available on 96.3% of cases (84.4% from information package, 11.9% from visit), on 83.0% of controls (81.3% from information package and 1.7% from visit) and on 95.0% of malformed controls (84.9% from information package and 10.1% from visit). The informed consent form was signed by about 98% of mothers; personal identifiers were deleted from the record of the rest 2%.

The collection of data was changed in 1997 due to the new director of the HCCSCA because after 1996 all cases were visited at home by regional nurses and regional nurses selected controls from the neighborhood of cases. However, unfortunately these recent data of total material have not been validated until now. In addition one mother attacked the HCCSCA in 2002 because the regional nurse visited her at home and later mentioned the CA of her baby in other persons in the neighborhood. The activity of the HCCSCA was stopped at the start of the legal procedure in 2003 and the HCCSCA was continued again only in 2005.

These facts explain that the results of the Hungarian studies shown in this book in general are based on the period of 1980–1996 when the HCCSCA worked under my direction. This study period contained 2,147,109 total births (and within them 2,134,712 live-births) in Hungary, thus our control sample, i.e. 38,151 newborns represented 1.8% of Hungarian births. The inclusion and exclusion of cases and controls will be shown later in Fig. 1.5.

The main objective of the HCCSCA was the postmarketing evaluation of the teratogenic potential of different drugs (XXIII–XXVII), thus CAs were in the focus of the HCCSCA. There are 601 substances (of course, one substance, e.g. carbamazepine or valproate, may have several trade names) in the data set of HCCSCA, 1980–1996. Until now, of these 601 substances, 171 have been evaluated in this case-control system (see Appendix at the end of the book).

After the critical evaluation of previous methods of human teratology (XXVIII), the evaluation of cases and controls in the HCCSCA was based on the recent recommendations.

1.5.3 Classification of CA-Groups

The results of recent medical examinations of cases helped to improve further the validity of CA-diagnoses or to specify previously unspecified CAs (e.g. within the cardiovascular CA-group) in the HCCSCA.

CAs were grouped according to their occurrence and severity into 25 groups. Of these 25 groups, 24 include isolated CAs and one group comprises of cases with multiple CAs. If we found an increase in a given CA-group, we differentiated the different CAs within this group to identify the specific CA which may have an association with the possible teratogenic agent.

In addition CA-groups were differentiated into two categories from practical (frequency and good diagnostic validity) and theoretical (as homogeneous as possible from etiological aspect) aspect. Category A includes 12 CA-groups with common or moderately frequent total (birth + fetal) prevalence, good validity of diagnosis, high ascertainment and more or less similar etiological background. Category B comprises of the rest 13 CA-groups, among them cardiovascular CAs with the most common birth prevalence in the HCCSCA but relatively low ascertainment of specified types with different etiology. In addition, of 24 isolated CA-groups, one comprises of the so-called "Other isolated CAs", these CAs in general rare and cannot be classified into other specified groups (Table 1.5).

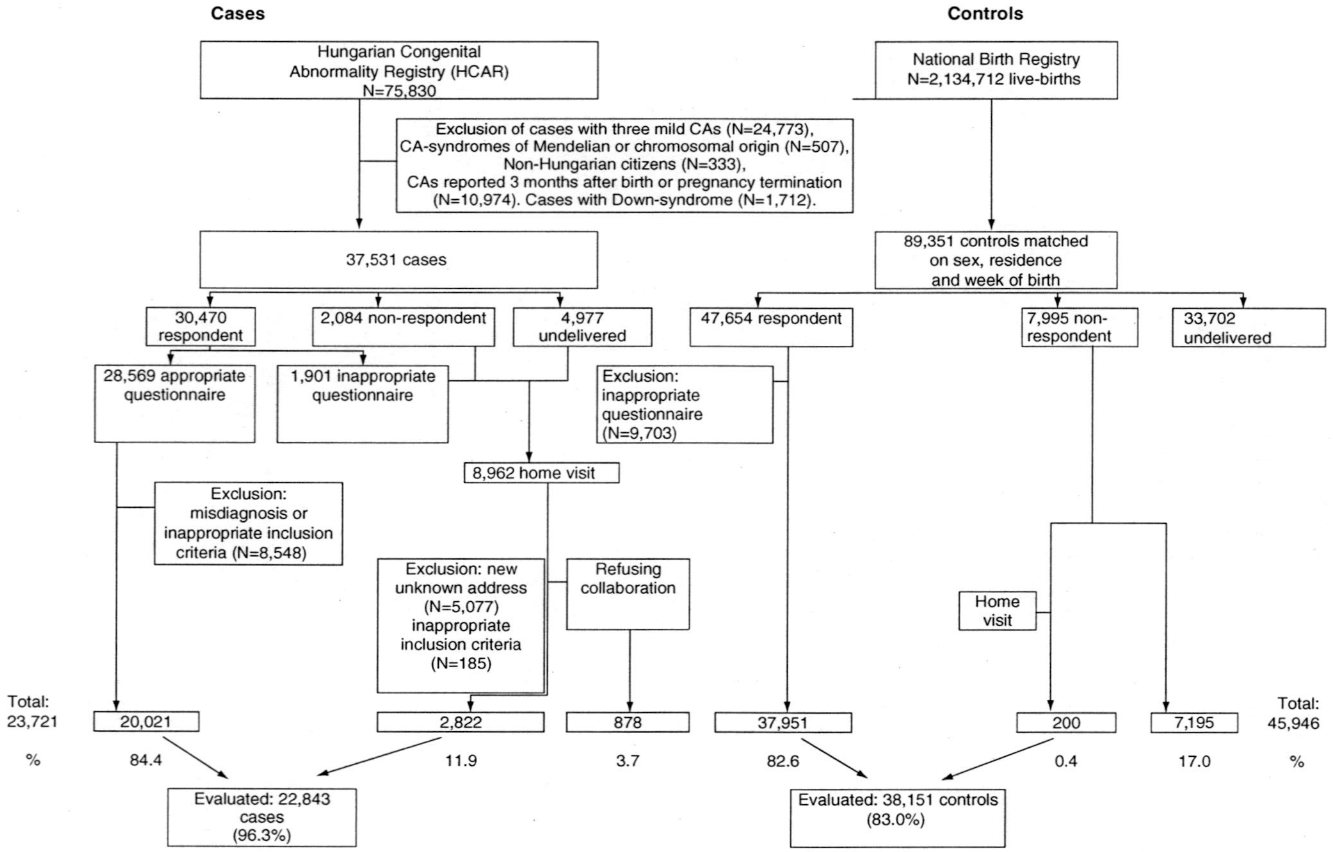

Fig. 1.5 Inclusion and exclusion of cases and controls in the data set of the HCCSCA, 1980–1996

Table 1.5 The names and components of CA groups evaluated in the HCCSCA

Category A	Total number
1. *Neural-tube defects*	1,202
Anencephalus	286
Craniorachischisis	4
Spina bifida with hydrocephalus	119
Spina bifida without hydrocephalus	610
According to localization: total and partial: cervical, thoracal, lumbar, lumbosacral, sacral spina bifida, while to clinical manifestation covered and open: meningocele and myelomeningocele are differentiated	
Encephalocele	183
According to localization occipital, parietal, frontal-anterior frontonasal and pharyngeal types are differentiated, but more than 90% belong to the occipital type. Recently some studies questioned the classification of occipital encephalocele into neural-tube defects	
The aim of the first study of cases with neural-tube defect was to determine their prevalence at birth in Hungary (2.80/1,000) and birth charateristics (XXIX), while the second study wanted to clarify the etiology of this CA-group (XXX). Later the evaluation of cases with neural-tube defects was the PhD topic of Erika Medveczky (XXXI–XXXIII)	
2. *Cleft lip with or without cleft palate*	1,375
Cleft lip (uni- or bilateral)	566
Cleft lip with cleft palate	809
3. *Cleft palate*	601
Cleft palate only	582
Robin sequence	19
It is better excluding Robin sequence due to their different etiology from this CA-group, however, nearly all studies published in the international literature included these cases to the group of cleft palate, thus we have to follow this approach	
The aims of the first Hungarian studies were to determine the prevalence at birth of these isolated CAs and understand better their etiologiocal background (XXXIV, XXXV).The evaluation of these two groups of orofacial clefts was the PhD topic of Andrea Sárközy (XXXVI–XXXIX) and partly of Erzsébet H. Puhó (XL–XLII)	
4. *Oesophageal atresia/stenosis*	217
The aim of the first Hungarian study was to clarify the possible etiological factors in cases with isolated oesophageal atresia/stenosis (XLIII). Unfortunately within *oesophageal atresia* (OA), the known 5 types according to the association with *tracheo-oesophageal fistula* (TF) cannot be differentiated on the basis of notification of this CA: (i) OA without TF, (ii) OA with proximal TF, (iii) OA with distal TF, (iv) OA with proximal and distal TF, (v) TF without OA in the HCCSCA	
5. *Congenital hypertrophic pyloric stenosis*	241
The Hungarian study showed first the higher birth weight of cases with congenital hypertrophic pyloric stenosis (XLIV) while the second family study attempted to contribute our knowledge in the etiology of this CA (XLV)	
6. *Atresia/stenosis of intestine (without rectum)*	158
Thus, atresia/stenosis of duodenum, ileum and colon are included	

Table 1.5 (continued)

Category A	Total number
7. *Atresia/stenosis of rectum and anal canal*	231
Unfortunately in general the 4 types of this CA cannot be differentiated on the basis of notification of cases with this CA: (i) congenital anal or anorectal stenosis, (ii) membranous imperforate anus or imperforate anal membrane or covered anus, (iii) anal and/or rectal agenesis, or anorectal agenesis, (iv) rectal atresia or stenosis	
8. *Renal agenesis or dysgenesis*	126
Bilateral renal agenesis is lethal CA, while unilateral renal agenesis was frequently not diagnosed in the past. However, hypoplasia or dysgenesis of kidney may have some relationship with the absence of kidney, sometimes there is renal agenesis in one side, and hypoplasia or dysgenesis of kidney in the other side, therefore these two CAs are combined	
9. *Obstructive CAs of urinary tract*	343
Obstructive CA of renal pelvis and ureter	169
Obstructive CA of urethra ad bladder neck	6
Cystic kidney disease	168
There are 4 types of cystic/polycystic kidney but polycystic type III occurs in adult people with autosomal dominant origin, while the type II is frequently unilateral without any obvious clinical symptoms after birth. The type I with neonatal-infantile manifestations is in general lethal, while type IV is caused by the obstructive CA. However, because it is difficult differentiate cases with type I and type IV on the basis of notification, these cases are classified into this CA-group	
10. *Hypospadias*	3,038
As it was mentioned previously, the so-called coronal type as minor anomaly was excluded from the HCAR, thus consequently from the HCCSCA as well. Unfortunately the other types of hypospadias such as glandular, penile, penoscrotal, scrotal, perineoscrotal were not specified in all cases, we can estimate only the proportion of mild (glandular) and severe (other types) manifestations of hypospadias as 70:30%. There was a significant increase in the prevalence at birth of cases with isolated hypospadias in Hungary during the 1970s (XLVI). Later the etiology of this CA was studied (XLVII, XLVIII) and a higher rate of pathospermic father was found (XLIX)	
11. *Undescended testis*	2,052
This diagnosis is accepted only at the existence of this CA after the third postnatal month because this CA is frequent at birth, particularly in preterm boys with a delay of descensus of testis. In the Hungarian studies the epidemiological characteristics and the etiology of cases with isolated undescended testis were described (L, LI)	
12. *CA of abdominal wall*	255
Exomphalos/omphalocele	172
Gastroschisis	83
These two groups of abdominal wall's CA have different origin, but their diagnoses sometimes are confused at their notification therefore it seemed to be better to combine them into one CA-group. On the other hand an important criterion at the differentiation of umbilical hernia as a minor anomaly and exomphalos as a severe CA the surgical intervention that occur in exomphalos. The Hungarian characteristics of this CA were decribed previously (LII)	

Table 1.5 (continued)

Category B	
13. Microcephaly, primary	111
It is important to differentiate the primary microcephaly as a real CA from the secondary microcephaly due to brain hemorrhage and other brain damages or skull CAs	
Microcephaly was the PhD topic of GMH Abdel-Salam (LIII–LVIII)	
14. *Hydrocephalus, congenital*	314
Of course, cases with secondary hydrocephalus caused by brain damage in the perinatal period are excluded from this CA-group. Unfortunately, in general the types of congenital hydrocephalus (atresia/stenosis of aquaeductus Sylvius, atresia of foramen Luschka and Magendie, etc.) were not differentiated at the notification of cases with this CA	
15. *CAs of eye*	99
Anophthalmos	5
Microphthalmos	20
Buphthalmos	11
Congenital cataract	33
Coloboma	18
Complex CAs	12
These cases were checked personally by an ophthalmologist: Gábor Vogt in the frame of his PhD work (LIX–LXIV) but he evaluated cases from the data set of the HCCSCA, 1980–2002	
16. *CAs of ear*	354
Absence/atresia of auditory canal and/or auricle	79
Accessory auricle	24
Microtia	20
Other specified CAs	50
Unspecified CAs	181
17. *Cardiovascular CAs*	4,480
Common truncus	44
Transposition of great vessels	307
Tetralogy of Fallot	223
Common ventricle	77
Ventricular septal defect	1,656
Atrial septal defect, type II	467
Endocardial cushion defects	76
Cor biloculare	10
CAs of pulmonary valve	92
Congenital tricuspid atresia/stenosis	13
Ebstein's anomaly	7
Congenital stenosis of aortic valve	57
Congenital insufficiency of aortic valve	19
Congenital mitral stenosis	11
Congenital mitral insufficiency	4
Hypoplastic left heart syndrome	76
Other specified heart CAs	37
Unspecified CAs of heart	740
Patent ductus arteriosus	181
Coarctation of aorta	113
Other CAs of aorta	37
CAs of pulmonary artery	87

Table 1.5 (continued)

Category A	Total number
CAs of great veins	3
Other CAs of peripheral vascular system	2
Other specified CAs of circulatory system	1
Complex cardiovascular CAs	84
Unspecified CAs of circulatory system	56
Absence or hypoplasia of umbilical artery is classified as minor anomaly therefore excluded from this data set. The diagnosis of cases with cardiovascular CAs was checked in the record of cardiologic, cardiologic surgical and pathological institutions by the ongoing PhD work of Melinda Szunyogh. Previously the prevalence at birth of different cardiovascular CAs were determined in Hungary, in addition epidemiological and genetic characteristics were described (LXV–LXX)	
18. *CAs of genital organs*	127
CAs of ovaries	3
CAs of fallopian tube and broad ligaments	1
Doubling of uterus	1
Other CAs of uterus	2
CAs of cervix, vagina and external female genitalia	57
Indeterminate sex and pseudohermaphroditism	51
Other specified CA of male genitalia	12
19. *Clubfoot*	2,424
Talipes equino- and calcaneovarus	2,066
Talipes calcaneovalgus	331
Metatarsus varus	27
However, in general the deformation, multifactorial, teratogenic types were not differentiated. The Hungarian characteristics of this CA-group were published previously (LXXI, LXXII)	
20. *Congenital limb deficiencies*	548
Upper limb	354
Lower limb	144
Both upper and lower limbs	50
Unfortunately this visible, thus easily diagnosed CA in general there was not specified according to the well-known types: transverse: terminal and amniogenic; longitudinal: radial-tibial, ulnar-fibular and axial: spilt hand and/or foot; intercalary, mainly phocomelia and proximal femoral a/dysplasia. In Hungary 998 cases with congenital limb deficiencies born between 1975 and 1984 were evaluated in international collaboration and the results of this project was published in several papers. Here only the monograph summarized these results (LXXIII) and a paper showing the association between terminal transverse type of congenital limb deficiencies and smoking (LXXIV) are cited	
21. *Poly/syndactyly*	1,744
Polydactyly	1,087
Syndactyly	657
The different types of polydactyly: (i) preaxial, (ii) axial, (iii) postaxial including subtype A and B, (iv) complex were not differentiated. Syndactyly has a similar location-oriented classification: (i) preaxial, (ii) axial and (iii) postaxial or etiology-oriented classification: (i) zygodactyly, (ii) synpolydactyly, (iii) ring and little finger syndactyly, (iv) complete syndactyly of all fingers, (v) syndactyly associated with metacarpal and metatarsal synostosis	

Table 1.5 (continued)

Category B	Total number
22. *CAs of musculoskeletal system*	585
Deformities of skull	16
Torticollis	315
Scoliosis and lordosis	62
Pectus excavatum (pigeon chest)	82
Pectus carinatus (funnel chest)	35
Other deformities of limb	24
Congenital genu recurvatum	12
Congenital bowing of long bones of leg	15
CAs of ribs and sternum	24
23. *CAs of diaphragm*	244
Unfortunately the types of diaphragmatic CAs: Bochdalek (posterolateral), Morgani (anterolateral), relaxation, and very rare pericardial, were rarely differentiated at the notification of these cases. About two-third of cases with this CA belonged to the Bochdalek type and most cases had no hernia, therefore the commonly used term "diaphragmatic hernia" is misleading. Previously this CA-group was also evaluated in Hungary (LXXV, LXXVI)	
24. *Other isolated CAs*	624
Reduction CA of brain, mainly arhinencephaly	8
Holoprosencephaly	12
Inien-, megalo-, poren- and lissencephaly	4
Branchial cleft, cyst and fistula	21
Pterygium colli (webbing of neck)	20
CAs of face, mainly micrognathia	30
Choanal atresia	2
CAs of nose	4
Web of larynx	5
CAs of larynx, trachea and bronchus	24
Congenital cystic lung	4
A/hypo/dysplasia of lung	23
Other CAs of respiratory system	6
CAs of tongue	19
CAs of mouth and pharynx	3
Other CAs of oesophagus	5
Congenital hiatus hernia	4
CAs of stomach	3
Meckel's diverticulum	7
Hirschsprung's disease	35
Malposition/malrotaion of intestine	53
Other CAs of intestine	10
Atresia of bile duct	31
CAs of pancreas	7
Other specified CAs of digestive system	50
Other CAs of kidney	83
Other CAs of ureter	11
Exstrophy of urinary bladder and cloacae	37
CAs of urachus	5
Other CA of bladder and urethra	5
Other CAs of upper limb and shoulder girdle	12
Other CAs of lower limb and pelvic girdle	8

Table 1.5 (continued)

Category B	Total number
Arthrogryposis multiplex congenital	4
CAs of breast	1
CAs of integument	1
CAs of spleen	8
CAs of adrenal gland	1
CAs of thyroid gland	13
Situs inversus	6
Teratoma	17
Hemangioma, large	22
25. *Unclassified multiple CAs*	1,349
2 CAs	830
3 CAs	254
4 CAs	120
5–6 CAs	117
7–9 CAs	28

Cases with multiple CA were evaluated in detail and these results were published in a monograph (II). Recently the relation between the severity (number of component CAs) and adverse birth outcomes has been evaluated (LXXVII).

Our preliminary design has not been changed later though the number of cases with torticollis exceeded the number of some specified CA-groups, however, torticollis is a mild CA and we did not want to work with more than 25 CA-groups.

1.6 The Strengths and Weaknesses of the HCCSCA

Previous human teratological studies had frequently methodological weaknesses (XXVIII), therefore we wanted to do our best to minimize these weaknesses at the evaluation of possible association of maternal diseases during pregnancy with different CAs in their offspring. Thus the following principles were followed.

1.6.1 The Maternal Disease Itself

Different maternal diseases have different causes, clinical severity and related drug treatments. Nevertheless in general cardiologic, respiratory, digestive, etc diseases were evaluated together in previous studies (Creasy et al., 2004). This so-called group-specific effect was explained by the similar modes of their action, in addition the combination of pregnant women with similar diseases can provide sufficient number of subjects for analysis, thus improves the statistical power.

On the other hand maternal diseases within specific groups may have different teratogenic/fetotoxic potential. Thus it is worth evaluating first different maternal diseases separately within the specific groups, and to combine them secondarily if the major outcomes do not show significant differences. We followed this strategy in our project.

1.6.2 Source of Exposure Information

There are two main sources of exposure data regarding maternal diseases: maternal self-reported information and medical records, in addition it is important to differentiate the time of data collection: retrospective (i.e. after the birth) and prospective (before the birth).

Major part of previous human teratological studies regarding maternal diseases was based on retrospective maternal information through personal or telephone interview, questionnaire, etc. Only one example is mentioned here. The National Birth Defects Prevention Study, Centers for Disease Control and Prevention, Atlanta, USA, obtained data through maternal interview via telephone using a standardized questionnaire and were completed no earlier than 6 weeks and no later than 24 months after the estimated date of delivery of case infants with birth defects and control infants with no major birth defects (Yoon et al., 2001). However, retrospective maternal information is burdened by recall bias, because the birth of an infant with birth defects is a serious traumatic event for most mothers who therefore try to find a causal explanation such as maternal diseases or drug uses during pregnancy for CAs of their babies. This does not occur after the birth of a healthy newborn infant. Thus recall bias might inflate an increased risk for birth defects. The data of the HCCSCA were appropriate to estimate the recall bias of drug exposures during pregnancy on the basis of comparison of prospective medically recorded and retrospective maternal information and recall bias increased the risk for CAs up to a factor of 1.9 in OR (LXXVIII).

However, there are five approaches to limit recall bias in the HCCSCA and in general. First, it is necessaty to differentiate different CAs because teratogenic agents induce specific CA, thus the increase in the total prevalence of one or few CAs is against the recall bias. Second, we evaluate maternal diseases only during the critical period of different CAs because we expect an underreporting of the maternal disease studied with related drug treatment in both the critical and non-critical periods of CAs in the control group. Third, we attempt to evaluate only prospectively and medically recorded exposure data of maternal diseases as a gold standard. Fourth, it is worth using a malformed control group with a similar recall bias. Fifth, the degree of increase in the total prevalence of a given CA is also important, because in general recall bias cannot mimic 2 or higher fold risk.

There is another bias which may arise whenever non-comparable information is obtained from the different study groups. This information bias was connected with the decision of the central Hungarian ethical committee in the HCCSCA which allowed to visit all non-respondent case mothers and malformed control mothers at home and to obtain the necessary exposure and other information but not in the mothers of control group. This problem was only partly compensated by two validation studies when the data of 800 control mothers were obtained by the similar method than in case mothers (XIV, XV).

A similar information bias is connected with non-responses which can result in skewed data and erroneous risk estimates if exceed a certain level (e.g. 30%). However, this proportion was 5% in case mothers, 16% in control mothers and 4%

in malformed control mothers in the HCCSCA. In addition the mothers of cases with CA in general have a better compliance than the mothers of controls without any defect. Again the best remedy for this bias is to use prospective and medically recorded exposure data.

1.6.3 The Time Factor

Among the criteria of human teratogenicity, the so-called time factor is very important, because the exposure of teratogenic agents can induce CA only during the organogenesis of the given organ or part of the body (Nishimura and Yamamura, 1969).

Previously this critical period of CAs was considered during the first 3 months of gestation, i.e. in the first trimester (Briggs et al., 2005; Shepard and Lemire, 2004; Friedman and Polifka, 2000). However, we calculated *gestational time/age* from the first day of the last menstrual period therefore the first month of gestation is before the organogenesis. The first 2 weeks are before conception while the third and fourth weeks comprise the pre- and implantation period of zygotes and blastocysts including omnipotent stem cells. Thus CAs cannot be induced by teratogenic agents in the first month of gestation and it explains the "all-or-nothing effect" rule, i.e. total loss or normal further development of zygotes/blastocysts. Thus the first trimester concept is misleading and unscientific (LXXIX) except at the evaluation of chronic maternal diseases with the onset before conception and continued during pregnancy.

The critical period of most major CAs is in II and III gestational months, it explains that this time window was used in the Hungarian case-control studies (LXXX). However, human teratogens may induce CAs such as cleft palate, hypospadias, undescended testis after III gestational month.

This theoretical problem would be avoided by the introduction of a new computer program based on the critical periods of different specified CAs separately (LXXXI) as Table 1.6 demonstrates.

Table 1.6 Critical period of CAs

		Fetal age		Gestational age	
Groups	CA-entities	Lunar months	Weeks (days)	Weeks (days)	Lunar months
I.	*Neural-tube defects*				
	Anencephalus	1	3 (21–26)	5 (35–41)	2
	Craniorachischisis	1	3–4	5–6	2
	Iniencephaly	1	3	5	2
	Spina bifida aperta/cystica with or without hydrocephalus	1	4 (23–28)	6 (37–42)	2
	Encephalocele, occipital	1	3–4	5–6	2
	Encephalocele, others (?)	1	3–4	5–6	2
	Subtotal	1	3–4	5–6	2
II.	*Microcephaly, primary*	3–5	10–18	12–20	3–5

Table 1.6 (continued)

		Fetal age		Gestational age	
Groups	CA-entities	Lunar months	Weeks (days)	Weeks (days)	Lunar months
III.	*Congenital hydrocephalus*	1–3	4–10	6–12	2–3
IV.	*Other CAs of nervous system*				
	Cyclopia	1	4 (23–28)	6 (37–42)	2
	Reduction CAs of brain (e.g. holoprosencephalia)	1	4 (23–28)	6 (37–42)	2
	Other specified CAs of brain (e.g. porencephaly)	1–4	4–16	6–18	2–5
	Other specified CAs of spinal cord	2–3	6–12	8–14	2–4
	Other specified CAs of nervous system	1–4	4–16	6–18	2–5
	Unspecified CAs of nervous system	1–5	3–18	5–20	2–5
	Subtotal	1–4	3–18	5–20	2–5
V.	*CAs of eye*				
	Anophthalmos Microphthalmos	1–2	4–6	6–8	2
	Buphthalmos	3–9	10–38	12–40	3–9
	Congenital cataract	2–9	6–38	8–40	3–9
	Coloboma	2–3	5–10	7–12	2–3
	Complex eye CAs	1–3	4–10	6–12	2–3
	Others	2–9	5–38	7–40	2–9
	Subtotal	2–9	4–38	6–40	2–9
VI.	*CAs of ear*				
	Absence/atresia of auditory canal	1–2	3–5 (25–29)	5–7 (39–43)	2
	Accessory auricle	2	5–8	7–10	2–3
	An/microtia	1	3–4 (24–28)	5–6 (38–42)	2
	Others	2	5–7	7–9	2–3
	Subtotal	1–2	3–8	5–10	2–3
VII.	*Branchial cyst, cleft, fistula, preauricular sinus*	2–3	8–10	10–12	3
VIII.	*CAs of face and neck*				
	Webbing of neck	2–4	8–16	10–18	3–5
	Other CAs of face and neck	2–10	8–38	10–40	3–10
	Subtotal	2–10	8–38	10–40	3–10
IX.	*Cardiovascular CAs*				
	Common truncus	1–2	4–6	6–8	2
	Transposition of great vessels	2	5–6 (34–42)	7–8 (48–56)	2
	Tetralogy of Fallot	2	5–8	7–10	2–3
	Common ventricle	2	5–6	7–8	2
	Ventricular septal defect	2–3	7–10 (43–70)	9–12 (57–84)	3
	Atrial septal defect, type II.	2	5–6	7–8	2–3
	Endocardial cushion defects	2	5–6	7–8	2
	Cor biloculare	1–2	4–6	6–8	2

Table 1.6 (continued)

Groups	CA-entities	Fetal age Lunar months	Fetal age Weeks (days)	Gestational age Weeks (days)	Gestational age Lunar months
	CAs of pulmonary valve	2–3			
	Tricuspid atresia/stenosis	2–3			
	Ebsteins' anomaly	2–3	5–12	7–14	2–4
	Cong.stenosis of aortic valve	2–3			
	Cong.insufficiency of aortic valve	2–3			
	Cong.mitral stenosis/insufficiency	2–4	5–16	7–18	2–5
	Hypoplastic left heart	2–3	5–12	7–14	2–4
	Patent ductus arteriosus	8–10	32–38	34–40	9–10
	Coarctation of aorta	2	5–8	7–10	2–3
	Other CAs of aorta	2	5–8	7–10	2–3
	CAs of pulmonary artery	2	6–8	8–10	2–3
	Complex CAs	1–2	4–8	6–10	2–3
	Others	2–10	6–38	8–40	2–10
	Unspecified	1–10	4–38	6–40	2–10
	Subtotal	1–10	4–38	6–40	2–10
X.	*CAs of respiratory system*				
	Choanal atresia	2	5–7	7–9	2–3
	CAs of nose	2	5–7	7–9	2–3
	CAs of larynx, trachea, bronchus	2	6–8	8–10	2–3
	Cong. cystic lung	2–3	6–12	8–14	2–3
	A/hypoplasia of lung	2	5–8	7–10	2–3
	Others, unspecified	2–10	6–38	8–40	2–10
	Subtotal	2–10	5–38	7–40	2–10
XI.	*Cleft palate only*	2–3	8–12 (56–84)	10–14 (70–98)	3–4
	Robin sequence	2–3	6–12	8–14	2–4
XII.	*Cleft lip ± cleft palate*				
	Cleft lip	2	5–7	7–9	2–3
	Cleft lip with palate	2	(35–49)	(49–63)	
	Subtotal	2	5–7	7–9	2–3
XIII.	*Oesophageal atresia/stenosis with or without tracheo-oesophageal fistula*	2	5–6 (30–36)	7–8 (44–50)	2
XIV.	*Congenital hypertrophic pyloric stenosis* (diagnosed after first postnatal week)	9–10	35–38	37–40	10
XV.	*Atresia/stenosis of small intestine including duodenal atresia*	2	7–8	9–10	3
XVI.	*Atresia/stenosis of rectum/anal canal*	2	5 (29–34)	7 (43–48)	2

Table 1.6 (continued)

		Fetal age		Gestational age	
Groups	CA-entities	Lunar months	Weeks (days)	Weeks (days)	Lunar months
XVII.	*Other CAs of digestive system*				
	CAs of tongue	2	6–8	8–10	2–3
	CAs of mouth/pharynx	2	6–8	8–10	2–3
	Other CAs of oesophagus	2	5–7	7–9	2–3
	Meckel's diverticulum	3	10–12	12–14	3–4
	Hirschprung's disease	4–6	13–22	15–24	4–6
	Other CAs of intestine (e.g. malrotation of gut)	3	10–12	12–14	3–4
	CAs of gallbladder, bile ducts and liver	3–4	10–16	12–18	3–5
	CAs of pancreas	2–3	6–10	8–12	2–3
	Other CAs	2–10	6–38	8–40	2–10
	Subtotal	2–10	5–38	7–40	2–10
XVIII.	*Undescended testis* (diagnosed after 3rd postnatal month)	9–10	33–38	35–40	9–10
XIX.	*Hypospadias* (without coronal type)	3–4	10–16	12–18	3–4
XX.	*Other CAs of genital organs*				
	CA of ovaries	2	5–7	7–9	2–3
	CAs of uterus and tubes	3	10–12	12–14	3–4
	CAs of cervix, vagina, external genitalia	3–10	10–38	12–40	3–10
	Indeterminate sex -pseudohermaphroditism	2–3	6–10	8–12	2–3
	Others	3–10	10–38	12–40	3–10
	Subtotal	2–10	5–38	7–40	2–10
XXI.	*Renal agenesis*	2	5–6 (29–35)	7–8 (43–49)	2
	aplasia/agenesis, hypoplasia, dysgenesis of kidney(s)	3–10	12–38	14–40	4–10
XXII.	*Cystic kidney(s) peri-neonatal*	2–3	5–12	7–14	2–4
XXIII.	*Obstructive CAs of urinary tract*				
	Obstructive CAs of renal pelvis and ureter (hydronephrosis, cong. stricture of ureteropelvic junction and ureterovesical orifice)	2–3	6–12	8–14	2–4
	Atresia/stenosis of urethra and bladder neck	2–3	5–9	7–11	2–3
	Subtotal	2–3	5–12	7–14	2–4
XXIV.	*Other CAs of urinary tract*				
	Other CAs of kidney	2–3	5–12	7–14	2–4
	Other CAs of ureter	2–3	5–12	5–14	2–4

Table 1.6 (continued)

Groups	CA-entities	Fetal age		Gestational age	
		Lunar months	Weeks (days)	Weeks (days)	Lunar months
	Exstrophy of urinary bladder, or cloaca	2	5–6 (30–42)	7–8 (44–56)	2
	Other CAs of bladder and urethra	3–4	5–12	7–14	2–4
	Unspecified	2–4	5–12	7–14	2–4
	Subtotal	2–4	5–12	7–14	2–4
XXV	*Cong. dislocation of hip*	2	5–6 (29–42)	7–8 (43–56)	2
	Cong. dysplasia of hip	6–10	26–38	28–40	7–10
XXV.	*Clubfoot*				
	Talipes calcaneovarus	2–3	7–10	9–12	3
	Talipes equinovalgus	2–3	7–10	9–12	3
	Metatarsus varus	3–4	12–16	14–18	4–5
	Deformation types	8–10	32–38	34–40	9–10
	"Clubfoot", unspecified	2–10	7–38	9–40	3–10
	Subtotal	2–10	7–38	9–40	3–10
XXVI.	*Poly/syndactyly*				
	Polydactyly	2	5–6	7–8	2
	Syndactyly (without minor anomaly)	2	5–6	7–8	2
	Subtotal	2	5–6	7–8	2
XXVII.	*Limb deficiencies*				
	Thumb aplasia	1–2	4 (22–30)	6 (36–44)	2
	Amelia of upper limb	1–2	4–5 (24–29)	6–7 (38–43)	2
	Phocomelia of upper limb	1–2	4–5 (24–33)	6–7 (38–47)	2
	Amelia of lower limb	1–2	4–5 (27–31)	6–7 (41–45)	2
	Phocomelia of lower limb	1–2	4–5 (28–33)	6–7 (42–47)	2
	Radial aplasia of upper limb	1–2	4–5 25–31)	6–7 (39–45	2
	Tibial aplasia of lower limb	2	5 (29–33)	7 (43–47)	2
	Subtotal	1–2	4–5	6–7	2
XXVIII.	*Other CAs of limbs*				
	Upper limbs	2	5 (29–35)	7 (43–49)	2
	Lower limbs	2	5–6 (34–42)	7–8 (48–56)	2
	Arthrogryposis	2	5–7	7–9	2–3
	Cong. genun recurratum, bowing of long bones of leg	4–5	13–20	15–22	4–6
	Unspecified	2–10	5–38	7–40	2–10
	Subtotal	1–10	5–38	7–40	2–10
XXIX.	*Torticollis (contracture of sternocleidomastoid muscle)*	7–10	26–38	28–40	7–10
XXX.	*CAs of skeletal system*				
	CAs of skull/face	3–5	10–18	12–20	3–5
	CAs of spine	4–5	13–20	15–22	4–6
	CAs of ribs/sternum	4–5	13–20	15–22	4–6

Table 1.6 (continued)

		Fetal age		Gestational age	
Groups	CA-entities	Lunar months	Weeks (days)	Weeks (days)	Lunar months
	Funnel/pigeon chest	4–10	13–38	15–40	4–10
	Others, unspecified	3–10	10–38	12–40	3–10
	Subtotal	3–10	10–38	12–40	3–10
XXXI.	*CAs of diaphragm*				
	Bochdalek (posterolateral)	1–2	4–7	6–9	2–3
	Morgani (anterolateral)	1	3–4	5–6	2
	Relaxation (eventration)	2–3	4–10	6–12	2–3
	Others (hiatus, pericardial, etc)	3	4–11	6–13	2–4
	Subtotal	1–2	4–11	6–13	2–4
XXXII.	*CAs of abdominal wall*				
	Exomphalos/omphalocele	3	10–12	12–14	3–4
	Gastroschisis	3–4	10–16	12–18	3–5
	Subtotal	3–4	10–16	12–18	3–4
XXXIII.	*Cong. inguinal hernia* (diagnosed in infant period)	9–10	33–38	35–40	9–10
XXXIV.	*Other CAs*				
	CAs of muscle, tendon	2–10	5–38	7–40	2–10
	CAs of integument	2–10	6–38	8–40	2–10
	CAs of spleen	2–3	6–10	8–12	2–3
	CAs of adrenal gland	2	5–8	7–10	2–3
	CAs of other endocrine glands	2–3	5–12	7–14	2–4
	Situs inversus	1–2	4–6	6–8	2
	Conjoined twins	1	1–2	3–5	1–2
	Subtotal	1–10	1–38	3–40	1–10
XXXV.	*Multiple CAs* (Mendelian and chromosomal MCA-syndromes are excluded)				
	Teratogenic MCA-syndromes				
	Rubella	1–3	3–10	5–12	2–3
	Chemical (e.g. drugs)	1–3	3–10	5–12	2–3
	Maternal (e.g. diabetes, high fever)	1–4	3–16	5–18	2–5
	Subtotal	1–4	3–16	5–18	2–5

This approach seems to be more sensitive and scientifically based approach than the use of II and/or III gestational months (LXXX).

Another problem of time factor is connected with the unreliability of gestational age based on the last menstrual period and on the maternal memory. In addition some pregnant women have some vaginal bleeding in early pregnancy or amenorrhea may occur in a female cycle before conception as well, in addition this calculation is burdened by some biological variability of females. Fortunately the introduction of ultrasound examination helps to limit this bias and it would be necessary to change the gestational age estimation from the present biased last menstrual period calculation to the more exact ultrasound measurement. Another great advantage of this new time calculation would be the suspension of the schizophrenic difference between gestational age at delivery (40 weeks) and postconception age at delivery (about 38 weeks).

Unfortunately at the planning of the HCCSCA's design the time factor was not considered appropriately, and mothers were asked to describe the time of their diseases and related drug treatments only according to gestational months. The critical period of most major CAs covers only a few days (e.g. the critical period of anencephaly is between the 21st and 24th postconception or 35th and 38th and gestational day) and the classification in whole month is too rough approach. However, the time of drug treatment was frequently given according to the days of pregnancy in the prenatal maternity logbook in the HCCSCA.

1.6.4 Confounding Factors

At the evaluation of risk for CA in the offspring of mothers affected with different diseases, we have to consider factors, the so-called confounders which can modify this association. A confounder is a factor that co-varies both with the exposure studied and the outcome. Among confounders it is worth differentiating five groups:

1.6.4.1 Related Drug Treatments

Different drugs have different chemical structure, different routes of administration, and different indications (i.e. underlying diseases) in their use. Nevertheless in general antibiotics, sulfonamides and other major classes of drugs were evaluated together in previous studies (Briggs et al., 2005; Shepard and Lemire, 2004; Friedman and Polifka, 2000).

Here only two examples are shown to demonstrate the different teratogenic effect of drugs within their specific group in the Hungarian case-control studies.

Sulfonamides cross the placenta easily to the fetus during all stages of pregnancy and inhibit the enzyme dihydropteroate synthase in the folate metabolism, therefore interfere with rapidly growing tissues. The teratogenic effect of sulfonamides as folic acid antagonists was reported (Hernandez-Diaz et al., 2000), but different sulfonamides were not differentiated. In the Hungarian case-control study 5 different products of the chemotherapeutic sulfonamides: sulfamethazine-sulfadimide, sulfathiourea, sulfamethoxypyridazine, sulfamethoxydiazine and the combination of sulfamethazine, sulfathiourea, and sulfamethoxypyridazine were evaluated separately (17). Among these 5 frequently used sulfonamides, only sulfamethoxydiazine associated with a higher risk for CAs, namely cardiovascular CAs.

Tetracyclines are on the list of proven human teratogenic drugs (Shepard and Lemire, 2004). The Hungarian case-control study confirmed the teratogenic effect of oxytetracylines beyond the well-known staining of deciduous teeth because a higher risk for a characteristic pattern of multiple CA ("oxytetracycline syndrome") was also found (8). However, the teratogenic effect of doxycycline was not detected (9).

Similar examples are known in the international literature as well, there is a specific teratogenic effect of valproate among antiepileptics (Meadow et al., 2009) or paroxetin among SSRI drugs (Briggs et al., 2005).

Thus an important rule in human teratology is that first we have to analyze the different drugs separately within the similar classes of medicines to differentiate the possible group-specific effects versus specific drug effects. However, this rule is valid maternal diseases as well.

Another important aspect is the route of drug administration. Nearly all drugs that reach significant maternal plasma levels diffuse passively through the placenta. However, the plasma level of drugs or their metabolites in pregnant women depends on the route of administration: parenteral, oral, rectal, vaginal, ophthalmic, otic, nasal, topical and inhalant medications. If a drug is poorly able to penetrate through skin, and is applied to a small surface, the low concentration of plasma levels is negligible. In general it is the case at the use of ear-, eye- and otic-drops. Drug absorption after vaginal medication is similar to skin.

It is necessary to consider that about 90% of pregnant women used medicinal products in Hungary; their mean number per pregnant women was 3.4 in the 1990s (XXV). Thus drug treatments frequently occurred parallel, we call it polytherapy, and in addition it may also indicate co-morbidity. Polytherapy related drug interaction, i.e. the combined pharmacologic effects of two or more drugs may result in additive, potentiated or antagonistic effects. The drug interaction may have adverse effect for the fetuses of pregnant women as well (45, 114).

Finally we had to consider the recall bias, particularly in the control group, therefore in general first we evaluated of the given drug treatment based on both prospective medically recorded data (mainly in prenatal maternity logbook) and retrospective self-reported maternal information (in the questionnaire) together. However, in the second step we evaluated only prospective medically recorded data of drug treatment as a golden standard.

1.6.4.2 Concomitant or Other Maternal Diseases

Pregnant women frequently are affected with two or more diseases during pregnancy. Their evaluation is easier if they occur different periods of pregnancy. However, sometimes these diseases occur parallel, i.e. concomitantly, and the separation of their effects is difficult, in addition they may have an interaction as well.

As it was mentioned previously, the information regarding maternal diseases had two sources: (i) prospective and medically recorded data in the prenatal maternity logbook, discharge summary of hospitalized pregnant women and rarely some other medical records, and (ii) retrospective maternal self-reported information in the questionnaire in the HCCSCA. The main effort of our studies was to limit or exclude recall bias therefore we decided to evaluate pregnancy complications based only on prospective medically recorded data. In addition the diagnostic characteristics of the given disease studied are determined by the source of information. If the validity of diagnosis was poor due to retrospective maternal information, only the data of medically recorded maternal disease were analyzed.

1.6.4.3 Maternal Factors

Mainly the so-called demographic factors, such as age, parity, marital and socioeconomic status, etc are considered among these counfounders. In general maternal age and parity are not distorted by maternal memory, motivation and/or well-documented. Maternal age is a particularly important confounder at the evaluation of certain CAs, e.g. Down syndrome. On the other hand the marital and socioeconomic status of mothers depends on the population studied and the social structure of society.

In the data set of the HCCSCA maternal age and parity (birth order) were based on both medically notified data in the Notification Form of the HCAR and the maternal information in the questionnaire, while pregnancy order (based on the history of previous pregnancies), marital and employment status of mothers, in addition the occurrence of CA in the mothers, fathers, and sibs were analyzed on the basis of maternal information in questionnaire.

The age and employment status of fathers were also part of the questionnaire.

1.6.4.4 Lifestyle Factors

Unfortunately lifestyle factors such as smoking, consumption of alcohol beverages and illicit drugs have adverse impacts for fetuses, therefore it is necessary to consider them as confounders at the calculation of adjusted OR for the risk of different CA. However, in general these data are unreliable.

The results of a validation study in the data set of the HCCSCA are shown here (XVI). First mothers were asked regarding their smoking habit and alcohol drinking during the study pregnancy after the birth of their child affected with isolated congenital limb deficiency through an interview in our institute. Each case had matched child without CA and a similar interview was performed in their mothers. Later these women were visited at home and the father (or the maternal grandmother) of children living together was asked through an interview on the smoking habit and alcohol drinking of mothers. There was significant discrepancy in data obtained from these persons, therefore we organized a family discussion and finally a family consensus was accepted (Table 1.7).

Table 1.7 Prevalence of cigarette smokers and alcohol drinkers among pregnant women who delivered newborn infants with *congenital limb deficiency* (CLD) and newborn infants without CA (matched controls). These data were obtained retrospectively from mothers through interview in our institure and from fathers through an independent interview in their home, and the so-called family consensus after the cross-interview of the fathers and mothers was accepted

	Cases with CLD (N = 537)					Matched controls (N = 537)				
	Maternal information		Family consensus			Maternal information		Family consensus		
Smoking during pregnancy (c/day)	No.	%	No.	%	Comparison OR (with 95% CI)	No.	%	No.	%	Comparison OR (with 95% CI)
1–10	93	17.3	106	19.7	0.8 (0.6–1.1)	69	12.8	76	14.2	0.3 (0.6-1.3)
11–20	31	5.8	59	11.0	0.4 (0.3–0.7)	23	4.3	24	4.5	0.9 (0.5–1.7)
21 or more	0	0.0	3	0.6		0	0.0	0	0.0	
Total	124	23.1	168	31.3	0.7 (0.5–0.9)	92	17.1	100	18.6	0.9 (0.7–1.2)
Drinking during study pregnancy										
Occasional	73	13.6	92	17.1	0.8 (0.5–1.0)	88	16.4	104	19.4	0.8 (0.8-1.1)
Regular	2	0.4	6	1.1	0.3 (0.0–1.2)	2	0.4	4	0.7	0.5 (0.0–2.3)
Daily	0	0.0	1	0.2		0	0.0	0	0.0	
Total	75	14.0	99	18.4	0.7 (0.5–0.9)	90	16.8	108	20.1	0.8 (0.6–1.1)

Similar investigation was conducted in the mothers of children affected with orofacial clefts and the findings were nearly the same.

These data indicated the low reliability of retrospective self-reported information of case mothers on their smoking habit during the study pregnancy, while these data of control mothers did not show significant deviation from the family consensus. The mothers of cases with CA might have a guilty feeling; therefore they did not want to confess their smoking habit. This information bias can modify the adjusted risk for adverse birth outcomes in case-control study.

The retrospective maternal information regarding alcohol drinking during the study pregnancy through interview was underreported by both case and control mothers according to the family consensus. Thus this information is also distorted significantly, particularly in case mothers.

Another validation study showed that the maternal information regarding smoking habit and alcohol drinking was more unreliable obtained by questionnaire (XVI).

Unfortunately the prospective data of smoking and alcohol drinking recorded by medical doctors or qualified nurses in the prenatal maternity logbook are also unreliable because they are based on the maternal information. This information bias was proved by laboratory test in a special sample of mothers (LXXXII).

The question is whether it is better to evaluate unreliable and biased data of lifestyle factors or it is worth omitting them among confounders at the calculation of adjusted risk. Smoking is a rather weak confounder for most CAs but it is important at the evaluation intrauterine growth retardation and the rate of LBW newborns.

1.6.4.5 Folic Acid and Folic Acid Containing Micronutrient Combination (The So-Called Multivitamin) Supplementations

There is a breakthough in the primary prevention of neural-tube defects (125, 127, 129, 131) and some other CAs such as cardiovascular CAs, CAs of urinary tract and congenital limb deficiencies after the periconceptional use of folic acid and folic acid—containing multivitamins (126, 128, 129, 131, Botto et al., 2004). Thus it is worth considering this protective effect at the calculation of adjusted risk for CA.

1.6.5 The Evaluation of Possible Risk

The first step in the detection of a possible causal association between maternal disease and CAs or other adverse pregnancy/birth outcomes is to demonstrate a statistical significant association between the exposure and outcome.

However, it is necessary to remember the old rule of epidemiology: "unexpected is expected", therefore the second step is to exclude or consider different biases, to evaluate the effect of confounders, and to estimate the effect of chance. In the HCCSCA 25 different CA-groups are studied simultaneously, and the multiple testing results in a significant association at 95% confidence interval (0.05 level of probability) in every 20th analysis due to chance. Thus it is necessary to use the Bonferroni correction (Shaffer, 1995; Perneger, 1998) depending on the number of multiple testing with a higher level of significance.

Finally a statistically significant association sometimes does not mean a real clinical importance. Later some examples will be demonstrated at the evaluation of maternal diseases. Here the results of a previous study regarding the teratogenic effect of a drug are shown here. The Hungarian case-control study based on the data set of the HCCSCA showed a significant association between medically recorded ampicillin (an antibiotic which belongs to the group of aminopenicillins) used in II and/or III gestational months and a higher risk for cleft palate (3.0, 1.2–7.6) (4). However, if this association is causal, the absolute risk is small. In Hungary the birth prevalence of cleft palate is 0.42 per 1,000 total births, and even a 3-fold increase would results in a prevalence of only 1.3 cases among 1,000 newborn babies. The proportion of pregnant women receiving ampicillin treatment during II and/or III months of gestation is about 2%. Thus among 100,000 pregnant women about 2,000 pregnant women are treated with ampicillin during this period, which could then induce approximately 2 extra cases of cleft palate yearly.

1.7 Preterm Birth and Low Birth Weight Newborns

Beyond CAs, *preterm birth* (BP) is the other leading cause of infant mortality and handicaps. The data set of the HCCSCA is appropriate for the evaluation of gestational age at delivery and birth weight, thus the rate of PB and *low birthweight* (LBW) newborns can be calculated. The gestational age specific birth weight is a sensitive indicator of intrauterine fetal growth, thus *intrauterine growth retardation* (IUGR) can be detected.

In general only controls are used as a cohort for the evaluation of gestational age at delivery and birth weight, and the rate of PB and LBW in the data set of the HCCSCA because CAs may have a more drastic effect for the fetal growth in utero than the drug or maternal disease studied. The fetotoxic effect of drugs or maternal diseases frequently induces IUGR. Here as an example the fetotoxic effect of ergotamine treatment during pregnancy is shown (86). The mean birth weight and the rate of LBW of newborn infants born to mother with or without ergotamine treatment during the different trimesters of pregnancy were compared in the data set of the HCCSCA (Table 1.8). The number of controls born to pregnant women with ergotamin treatment was 55, and the ratio of boy and girl was 37:18, while the number of untreated controls was 38,074.

Thus there was a significantly lower mean birth weight in agreement with a higher rate of LBW. This mean birth weight reducing effect (495 g) was most obvious after the ergotamine treatment in the third trimester and it resulted in 7.1-fold increase in the rate of LBW. However, an unexpected difference was found in male and female newborns, while this decrease in the mean birth weight was significant in males, this difference did not reach the level of significance in females.

Table 1.8 Mean birth weight and rate of low birthweight newborns, and within them males and females born to mothers with or without treatment of ergotamine drops in the second and third trimester of study pregnancy

	Birth weight (g)						Low birthweight				
	Treated		Untreated		Comparison		Treated		Untreated		Comparison
Study groups	Mean	S.D.	Mean	S.D.	*t*	*p*	No.	%	No.	%	OR (95%CI)
Male (M)	**3,079**	693	3,324	513	2.0	**0.03**	6	**16.2**	1,232	5.0	**3.7 (1.5–8.8)**
Female (F)	3,081	489	3,187	494	0.9	0.36	3	16.7	926	7.0	2.7 (0.8–9.2)
Together (M + F)	**3,080**	629	3,276	511	2.1	0.04	9	**16.4**	2,161	5.7	**1.9 (1.0–4.0)**
Period (trimester)											
Second	**2,961**	681	3,276	511	**0.01**	38.3	6	**19.4**	2,161	5.7	**4.0 (1.6–9.7)**
Third	**2,781**	740	3,276	511	**0.007**	37.9	6	**30.0**	2,161	5.7	**7.1 (2.7–8.4)**

In the past and present the possible teratogenic effect of drug treatments has been studied frequently (Briggs et al., 2005; Friedman and Polifka 2000; Shepard and Lemire, 2004), but in general the underlying diseases have been neglected. This unbalanced approach stimulated us to concentrate our recent activities on the possible teratogenic/fetotoxic effect of maternal diseases. Thus beyond CAs we evaluated other adverse birth outcomes such as PB and LBW as well in the data set of the HCCSCA.

1.7.1 Definitions

The definition of gestational age according to the WHO:

> The duration of gestation is measured from the first day of the last normal menstrual period. Gestational age is expressed in completed days or completed weeks (e. g. event occurring 280 and 286 days after the onset of the last normal menstrual period are considered to have occurred at 40 week of gestation).

According to the WHO definition, there is no lower limit of gestational age at delivery because at present only two categories of pregnancy outcomes are differentiated:

> Live birth is the complete expulsion or extraction from its mother of a product of conception, irrespective of the duration of the pregnancy, which, after such separation, breathes or shows any other evidence of life, such as beating of the heart, pulsation of the umbilical cord or definite movement of voluntary muscles, whether or not the umbilical cord has been cut or the placenta is attached; each product of such a birth is considered live born.
>
> Fetal death is death prior to the complete expulsion or extraction from its mother of a product of conception, irrespective of the duration of pregnancy; the death is indicated by the fact that after such separation the fetus does not breath or show any other evidence of life, such as beating of the heart, pulsation of the umbilical cord, or definite movement of voluntary muscles.

Traditionally the term spontaneous abortion (or miscarriages) was used for pregnancies ended before 28, later 24 or 20 completed weeks of gestation.

The definition of PB is any delivery, regardless of birth weight that occurs before 37 completed gestational weeks (i.e. less than 259 days). In Hungary the traditional definition of PB was followed during the study period, and about 5% of preterm births occurred at less than 28 weeks of gestation.

1.7.2 The Hungarian Data of Preterm Births

Table 1.9 shows the rate of preterm births in Hungary between 1980 and 2007.

Two broad categories of PB are worth differentiating: spontaneous and indicated.

Table 1.9 Rate of preterm births and low birthweight newborns in Hungary between 1980 and 2007

Year	Live birth No.	Preterm birth No.	Preterm birth %	Low birth weight newborns No.	Low birth weight newborns %
1980	148,673	9,791[a]	6.6	15,391	10.4
1981	142,890	9,669[a]	6.8	14,590	10.2
1982	133,559	12,564	9.4	13,258	9.9
1983	127,258	11,813	9.3	12,421	9.8
1984	125,359	13,398	10.7	12,602	10.1
1985	130,200	12,611	9.7	12,938	9.9
1986	128,204	11,879	9.3	12,606	9.8
1987	125,840	11,614	9.2	12,062	9.6
1988	124,348	11,480	9.2	11,626	9.3
1989	123,804	10,667	8.6	11,299	9.1
1990	125,679	10,986	8.7	11,654	9.3
1991	127,207	11,053	8.6	11,800	9.3
1992	121,724	10,563	8.7	10,972	9.0
1993	117,033	8,908	7.6	10,061	8.6
1994	115,598	8,895	7.7	9,961	8.6
1995	112,054	8,159	7.3	9,192	8.2
1996	105,272	8,308	7.9	8,773	8.3
1997	100,350	7,620	7.6	8,412	8.4
1998	97,301	7,220	7.4	8,091	8.3
1999	94,645	7,301	7.7	8,071	8.5
2000	97,597	7,923	8.1	8,196	8.4
2001	97,047	7,647	7.9	8,294	8.4
2002	96,804	7,795	8.1	8,226	8.5
2003	94,647	7,950	8.4	8,202	8.7
2004	95,137	8,181	8.6	7,896	8.3
2005	97,496	8,189	8.4	7,995	8.2
2006	99,871	8,389	8.4	8,289	8.3
2007	97,613	8,395	8.6	8,004	8.2

[a]Gestational age was not specified in all births.

In the latter category the causes of PB are maternal or fetal indications in which labor is either induced delivery through vaginal or the newborn is delivered by cesarean sections. In Hungary the proportion of spontaneous and indicated PB was about 75:25% during the study period, recently with an increasing proportion of indicated PB including cesarean section. In addition the category of spontaneous PB can be differentiated into two subcategories: spontaneous PB with intact membranes and preterm premature rupture of the membranes (PPROM). In the USA about 30–35% of PB is indicated and 40–45% belongs to the group of spontaneous preterm labor, while 20–25% is caused by PPROM (Goldenberg et al., 2008). In addition it is worth differentiating early PB before 32nd week and very early PB before 28th week within the total category of PB.

The definition of birth weight according to the WHO:

> The first weight of the fetus or newborn after birth. This weight should be measured preferably within the first hour of life before significant postnatal weight loss has occurred.

The definition of LBW is less than 2,500 g (up to, and including 2,499 g), regardless of gestational age. Birth weight under 1,500 g is classified as very LBW.

Table 1.9 also shows the rate of LBW newborns between 1980 and 2007.

The assessment of the true incidence of PB has been compromised by difficulty in differentiating growth-restricted fetuses/newborns from preterm babies. This problem explained that some decades ago newborns who had birth weight under 2,500 g were classified as "premature".

While PB is associated with maternal factors in most pregnant women (Iams and Creasy, 2004), LBW-IUGR in general connected with fetal factors. Recently the term intrauterine growth restriction is recommended for this phenomenon because IUGR was frequently confused with mental retardation (Resnik and Creasy, 2004).

However, the diagnosis of IUGR depends on the accuracy/reliability of the measurement of birth weight and gestational age. The measurement of birth weight if delivery takes place in hospital is an accurate and reliable variable. However, the gestational age calculated from the first day of the last menstrual period is not a reliable and accurate index, if the mother was not seen early in gestation, or had history of irregular menstrual cycles or conception occurred soon after discontinuation of oral contraceptives. However, ultrasonographic scanning is particularly useful in dating pregnancies if it is performed before 22 week of gestation, i.e. before a significant biological variation begins. Thus IUGR is rarely diagnosed before 22–24 weeks of gestation.

The data of both birth weight and gestational age were medically recorded based on the discharge summary of mothers' delivery in the data set of the HCCSCA. Unfortunately the gestational age was rarely measured and/or confirmed by ultrasonographic evaluation in pregnant women during the study period particularly in the 1980s. However, this measurement bias was similar in both study groups of our newborn cohorts (i.e. with or without exposure studied).

1.8 The Data Set of the HCCSCA, 1980–1996

At the evaluation of cases and controls we excluded subjects who had undelivered address when the explanatory letter, questionnaire, etc was mailed to them and later regional nurses were also not able to find them.

The flow (inclusion or exclusion) of cases and controls is summarized in Fig. 1.5.

Of 2,822 case mothers visited at home, 2,640 were evaluated according to their lifystyle on the basis of family consensus. In addition 200 non-respondent control mothers, furthermore 600 other control mothers were visited at home in two validation studies (XIV, XV).

The demographic features, as maternal characteristics of pregnant women, i.e. case, matched control and malformed control mothers are shown in Table 1.10.

Table 1.10 Demographic features of pregnant women

Variables	Cases with CA (*N* = 22,843)		Matched controls without CA (*N*= 38,151)		Malformed controls (*N*= 834)	
	No.	%	No.	%	No.	%
Maternal age (year)						
19 or less	2,220	9.7	3,075	8.1	57	6.8
20–29	15,815	69.2	27,406	71.8	415	49.8
30–39	4,469	19.6	7,180	18.8	265	31.8
40 or more	339	1.5	490	1.3	97	11.6
Mean ± S.D.		25.5±5.4	25.5 ± 5.2		29.1 ± 7.5	
Birth order (parity)						
1	10,708	46.9	18,217	47.8	295	35.4
2–3	10,506	46.0	18,398	48.2	421	50.5
4 or more	1,629	7.1	1,536	4.0	118	14.1
Mean ± S.D.		1.9 ± 1.1	1.7 ± 0.9		2.3 ± 1.5	
Marital status						
Never	642	2.8	694	1.8	14	1.7
Married	19,716	86.3	35,139	92.1	709	85.0
Divorced	2,485	10.9	2,318	6.1	111	13.3
Employment status						
Professional	1,901	8.3	4,356	11.4	79	9.5
Managerial	4,968	21.8	10,142	26.6	200	24.0
Skilled	6,329	27.7	11,693	30.7	200	24.0
Semiskilled	3,869	16.9	5,782	15.1	150	18.0
Unskilled	1,503	6.6	1,857	4.9	54	6.5
Homemaker	2,128	9.3	2,028	5.3	67	8.0
Others (student, premature retired, unemployment)	2,145	9.4	2,293	6.0	84	10.1

The pregnancy outcomes of informative offspring, and mean gestational age and birth weight, in addition the rate of PB and LBW newborns among live-born babies are demonstrated in Table 1.11.

The male excess of males among cases is explained mainly by the high incidence of two CAs, i.e. hypospadias and undescended testis in the male genital organs. The controls were matched to the sex of cases therefore there is a male predominance among control newborns as well.

1.8.1 Maternal Diseases

Finally the numbers of maternal diseases and the so-called pregnancy complications are shown according to the WHO classification in control, case and malformed control mothers (Table 1.12). The possible association of these maternal pathological

Table 1.11 Data of cases (informative offspring), controls (live-born newborn infants without CA) and malformed controls (cases with Down syndrome)

Variables	Cases (*N*= 22,843)		Controls (*N*= 38,151)		Malformed controls (*N*= 834)	
Informative offspring	No.	%	No.	%	No.	%
Electively terminated malformed fetuses	70	0.3	0	0.0	1	0.1
Stillborn fetuses	381	1.7	0	0.0	4	0.5
Live-born infants	22,392	98.0	38,151	100.0	829	99.4
Males	14,913	65.3	24,796	65.0	437	52.4
Twins	421	1.8	410	1.1	13	1.6
Livebirths						
Preterm birth	3,431	15.3	3,536	9.3	140	16.9
Low birthweight newborns	4,385	19.6	2,157	5.7	195	23.5
	Mean	S.D.	Mean	S.D.	Mean	S.D.
Gestational age (week)	38.7	3.2	39.4	2.1	38.1	2.7
Birth weight (g)	2,990	719	3,279	515	2,801	557

conditions with CAs and two adverse birth outcomes: PB and LBW newborns will be presented in the second Part II of the book mainly on the basis of our previous studies.

Our plan was to evaluate the possible association of *all maternal diseases* with higher risk for CA, PB and LBW if the number of cases and controls allowed us an appropriate statistical power.

Finally it is worth showing the numerical distribution of maternal diseases and pregnancy complications in the pregnant women of study groups in the data set of the HCCSCA (Table 1.13). One pregnant woman may have more than one pathological condition.

Thus the mean number of maternal diseases/pregnancy complications was about 2 in pregnant women studied, but this figure was somewhat higher in control mothers.

1.8.2 Statistical Analysis

The statistical analysis of data SAS version 8.02 (SAS Institute Ins., Cary, North Carolina, USA) was used.

1.8.2.1 Case-Control Approach

The objective of these studies was to evaluate the possible association of a given maternal disease with the higher risk of different CAs in their offspring.

Table 1.12 Number of maternal diseases in control, case and malformed control mothers in the HCCSCA, 1980–1996

Disease	Control mothers	Case mothers	Malformed control mothers
I. Certain infectious and parasitic diseases			
Salmonellosis (salmonella gastroenteritis)	23	15	1
Infectious diarrhoea (dysenteric?)	70	82	1
Tuberculosis	26	15	0
Chickenpox (varicella)	56	31	0
Herpes zoster	18	13	0
Genital herpes	228	160	0
Herpes simplex, orofacial	574	435	15
Measles (morbilli, rubeola)	7	8	0
Viral genital warts (condyloma accuminatum)	25	17	2
Cytomegalic inclusion disease	19	16	1
Mumps	50	33	0
Rubella (German measles)	38	32	1
Viral hepatitis	16	9	0
Syphilis	2	3	0
Other or unspecified viral infections	49	80	2
Gonococcal infection	0	1	0
Candidiasis of vulva and vagina	307	215	2
Thrichomoniasis, urogenital	418	190	4
Dermatomycosis	71	48	0
Ascariasis	10	7	0
Toxoplasmosis	27	35	1
Scabies	1	3	1
II. Neoplasms			
Malignant neoplasm of breast (breast cancer)	4	3	1
Malignant neoplasm of cervix uteri	5	6	1
Lymphoid leukemia	0	1	0
Malignant neoplasm of thyroid gland	2	2	0
Benign neoplasm of adrenal gland	0	1	0
Uterine leiomyoma (myoma)	71	34	3
Haemangioma, large	1	0	0
Neurofibromatosis (Recklinghausen's disease)	1	0	0
III. Disease of the blood and blood-forming organs			
Iron deficiency anaemias	6,358	3,242	98
Von Willebrand's disease	3	1	0
Polycythaemia	1	0	0
IV. Endocrine, nutritional and metabolic diseases			
Goitre	3	2	0

Table 1.12 (continued)

Disease	Control mothers	Case mothers	Malformed control mothers
Hypothyroidism	31	14	4
Congenital hypothyroidism	5	2	0
Acquired hypothyroidism	2	0	0
Hyperthyroidism	116	71	5
Diabetes mellitus	458	276	13
Obesity	29	11	0
Hyperparathyroidism	0	1	0
Diabetes insipidus	2	1	0
Cushing's syndrome	3	1	0
Addison's disease	1	0	0
Wilson's disease	0	1	0
V. Mental disorders			
Schizophrenic psychosis	1	0	0
Maniac-depressive disorders	22	21	5
Panic disease	187	210	10
Other anxiety-neurotic disorders	17	7	0
Alcohol dependence syndrome	0	5	0
Drunkenness	1	0	0
Drug dependence	0	1	0
Mental retardation	4	7	1
VI. Diseases of the nervous system			
Multiple sclerosis	6	3	0
Epilepsy	90	95	2
Migraine	713	565	24
Headache, others	1,268	538	19
VII. Diseases of eye and adnexa			
Glaucoma	0	1	0
Myopia	6	3	0
VIII. Diseases of ear and mastoid process			
Otitis media	55	58	3
Deafness	1	1	0
IX. Diseases of the circulatory system			
Mitral stenosis due to rheumatic fever	2	2	0
Essential hypertension	1,579	1,030	36
Gestational hypertension	1,098	580	19
Preeclampsia-eclampsia	1,286	739	19
Myocardial infarction, old	0	3	0
Angina pectoris	12	22	4
Myocarditis, acute	1	1	0
Conduction disorders	7	2	1
Paroxismal supraventricular tachycardia	149	103	5
Extrasystolic arrhythmia	4	8	0
Transient cerebral ischaemia	1	1	0

Table 1.12 (continued)

Disease	Control mothers	Case mothers	Malformed control mothers
Arterial embolism and thrombosis	3	1	0
Phlebitis and thrombophlebitis	970	338	21
Pulmonary embolism	1	3	0
Varicose veins of lower extremities	566	332	29
Haemorrhoids	1,617	795	34
Vulvar varices	0	1	0
Hypotension	1,268	538	19
X. Diseases of the respiratory system			
Common cold (acute nasopharyngitis)	5,475	3,827	144
Epistaxis (haemorrhage from nose)	5	4	0
Sinusitis, acute	250	141	10
Pharyngitis, acute	1,048	641	25
Tonsillitis, acute	1,165	674	30
Laryngitis and tracheitis, acute	804	404	13
Bronchitis and bronchiolitis, acute	398	339	17
Pneumonia	182	116	7
Allergic rhinitis (hay fever)	379	176	7
Asthma	757	511	5
Influenza	1,838	1,328	37
Chronic bronchitis	16	13	0
Emphysema	1	1	0
Pleurisy	12	8	0
Pneumothorax	1	2	0
XI. Diseases of the digestive system			
Diseases of the teeth (mainly severe caries)	12	6	0
Periodontal diseases (pulpitis, gingivitis, etc)	18	21	2
Nausea/vomiting in pregnancy	20,013	10,906	389
Gastric ulcer	45	13	1
Duodenal ulcer	13	7	0
Dyspepsia (incl. gastro-oesophageal reflux)	270	175	5
Gastritis and duodenitis	78	67	1
Appendicitis	25	21	1
Inguinal hernia	17	3	0
Ventral (incisional) hernia	4	4	0
Colitis ulcerosa	95	71	5
Crohn disease	9	3	0
Peritonitis	1	0	0
Constipation	797	465	13
Intrahepatic cholestatis of pregnancy	7	2	0
Cirrhosis of liver	2	1	0

Table 1.12 (continued)

Disease	Control mothers	Case mothers	Malformed control mothers
Cholelithiasis	119	62	4
Cholecystitis	145	109	2
Cholangitis	10	9	0
Pancreatitis	4	4	0
XII. Diseases of the skin and subcutaneous tissue			
Carbuncle and furuncle	2	1	0
Lymphadenitis, acute	3	3	0
Dermatitis, atopic	91	80	1
Erythema nodosum	1	1	0
Psoriasis	40	18	0
Pruritus	25	8	3
Alopecia	1	2	0
Chronic ulcer of skin	1	1	0
Allergic urticaria	187	95	9
XIII. Diseases of the musculoskeletal system and connective tissue			
Systemic lupus erythematosus	2	1	0
Rheumatoid arthritis	68	36	2
Pain in hip join	10	6	0
Ankylosing spondylitis (Bechterew's disease)	1	2	0
Lumbago (intervertebral disc disorders)	80	41	1
Rheumatism, myalgia, neuralgia, etc.	33	28	0
Scoliosis, kyphosis, acquired	4	2	0
XIV. Diseases of the genitourinary system			
Glomerulonephritis	479	309	12
Bacteruria, significant	1,767	1,250	37
Cystitis, acute	178	149	14
Pyelonephritis, acute	243	143	8
Calculus of kidney	147	69	1
Kidney disease, chronic with secondary hypertension	49	34	3
Nephroptosis	1	0	0
Vesicoureteric reflux	0	2	0
Adnexitis	126	65	4
Salpingitis	30	20	0
Endometritis	2	2	0
Vulvovaginitis, bacterial vaginosis	3,326	2,027	40
Abscess of Bartholin's gland	8	5	1
Endometriosis	26	16	0
Ovarian cysts	94	60	3
Polyp of corpus uteri	12	5	0
Erosion of cervix	25	40	1
Incompetence of cervix	2,795	1,170	13

Table 1.12 (continued)

Disease	Control mothers	Case mothers	Malformed control mothers
Others disorders of vagina and vulva	25	11	0
Diseases of breast	4	1	0
XV. Pregnancy, childbirth and the purperium			
Threatened abortion (haemorrhage)	5,534	2,999	112
Threatened abortion (uterine spasm)	976	498	8
Together	6,510	3,497	130
Placenta praevia	471	239	9
Premature separation of placenta (abruption placetae.)	86	37	2
Antepartum haemorrhage	36	20	0
Together	593	296	11
Polyhydramnios	191	211	15
Oligohydramnios	14	33	1
Oedema or excessive weight gain	912	428	17
Threatened preterm delivery	3,191	1,688	70
Isoimmunisation	73	83	4
Trauma, burn poisoning	91	67	1
Together	593	296	11
XVII. Congenital anomalies			
Spina bifida aperta	2	0	0
Cong. cerebral cyst	0	1	0
CAs of eye	4	7	0
Cardiovascular CAs	41	32	1
CAs of uterus	67	58	2
CAs of kidney	4	0	0
Cong. dislocation of hip	30	18	0
Scoliosis	2	1	0

The main characteristics of the mothers of cases and controls were evaluated using Student *t*-test for quantitative and chi square test for categorical variables. The prevalence of pregnancy complications, other maternal diseases, drugs and pregnancy supplements used during pregnancy were compared between the group of cases and controls with the given maternal disease studied and *odds ratios* (OR) with 95% *confidence intervals* (CI) were calculated using unconditional logistic regression model. We examined confounding variables by comparing the OR for the given maternal diseases studied in the models with and without inclusion of the potential confounding variables and in general maternal age (<20, 20–29, and 30 year or more), birth order (first delivery or one or more previous deliveries), employment status, high fever related influenza-common cold (yes/no), drugs used for the treatment for the given maternal disease studied (yes/no), and use of folic

Table 1.13 Number and percentage figures of maternal diseases and pregnancy complications in control, case and malformed control pregnant women

Number of maternal diseases	Control mothers ($N = 38{,}151$)		Case mothers ($N = 22{,}843$)		Malformed control mothers ($N = 834$)	
	No.	%	No.	%	No.	%
0	4,953	13.0	3,620	15.8	125	15.0
1	12,565	32.9	7,604	33.3	290	34.8
2	10,600	27.8	6,072	26.6	217	26.0
3	5,760	15.1	3,158	13.8	108	12.9
4	2,598	6.8	1,434	6.3	57	6.8
5	1,003	2.6	578	2.5	21	2.5
6	446	1.2	218	1.0	9	1.1
7	141	0.4	104	0.5	6	0.7
8	51	0.1	36	0.2	1	0.1
9	25	0.1	12	0.1	0	0.0
10 or more	9	0.0	7	0.0	0	0.0
Mean		1.86		1.77		1.78
S.D.		1.54		1.48		1.55
Number of pregnancy complications						
0	6,103	16.0	4,263	18.7	147	17.6
1	13,635	35.7	8,116	35.5	291	34.9
2	10,059	26.4	5,849	25.6	217	26.0
3	5,003	13.1	2,738	12.0	108	13.0
4	2,097	5.5	1,148	5.0	41	4.9
5	811	2.1	443	1.9	16	1.9
6	295	0.8	190	0.8	11	1.3
7	90	0.2	63	0.3	2	0.2
8	36	0.1	18	0.1	1	0.1
9	18	0.1	13	0.1	0	0.0
10	4	0.0	2	0.0	0	0.0
Mean		1.68		1.61		1.66
S.D.		1.30		1.31		1.32

acid/folic acid containing multivitamin supplement (yes/no) were included in the models. The prevalence of the given maternal disease studied during the study pregnancy in 25 or less (including at least 3 cases) specified CA groups (Table 1.5) was compared with the frequency of the given maternal disease in their all matched controls and adjusted OR were evaluated using conditional logistic regression models to estimate the risk of CAs in the informative offspring of pregnant women affected with the disease studied.

1.8.2.2 Cohort Approach

The objective of this study design is based on the so-called controls (i.e. newborns without any CA and matched to each case according to sex and birth year/week of cases and the residents of their mothers) and these controls without CA born to mothers with or without the given maternal disease studied was compared to estimate the risk of PB and LBW newborns.

First, characteristics of newborn infants born to mothers with and without the given disease studied as reference were compared using chi-square test for categorical variables, while Student *t*-test for quantitative variables. Second, the characteristics of pregnant women with or without the given disease were compared. Third frequencies of other pregnancy complications, acute and chronic maternal diseases, in addition maternal drug uses and vitamin supplementations were compared in mothers with or without the given disease studied in ordinary logistic regression models and OR were evaluated. Finally, the birth outcomes, i.e. mean gestational age at delivery and birth weight, in addition the rate of PB and LBW newborns was evaluated in mothers with the given disease studied and mothers without the given disease studied as reference using adjusted Student *t*-test and OR with 95% CI.

The major drawback of the data in the HCCSCA was that the evaluation of drug exposures based on the usual clinical doses of drugs did not allow to estimate a dose-teratogenic/fetotoxic effect relationship and to determine the threshold level of teratogenicity/fetotoxicity (XXVIII). These difficulties stimulated me to establish a special monitoring system.

1.9 Budapest Monitoring System of Self-Poisoning Pregnant Women

Pregnant women, who survive suicide attempts by taking large doses of drugs, may represent a unique model for the study of human teratogenicity and fetotoxicity of drugs (XVII, LXXXIII). This type of attempted suicide has been termed *self-poisoning* and our monitoring system is based on pregnant women who attempted suicide by drugs and were admitted to the central toxicological hospital in Budapest from the population of about 3 million people of Budapest and the surrounding area. Pregnant women were identified among self-poisoned females by a pregnancy test to determine the teratogenic and fetotoxic effect of large doses of drugs in their *exposed children*. Previously born and subsequent unexposed child(ren) of self-poisoned pregnant women were used as *sib controls*.

The doses and effects of drugs used for suicide attempt are estimated on the basis of (i) information obtained from the pregnant women, (ii) drug levels in their blood and (iii) the clinical pictures of intoxication. The date of suicide attempt is known according to the pregnancy day/hour and sometimes minute. Live-born exposed children and their sibs are examined personally by experts. Further details regarding the study period between 1960 and 1993 were presented previously (XVII), in addition the publications of specific studies of drugs regarding their teratogenic/fetotoxic effect are shown in the Appendix at the end of the book, and mentioned in the Part II of the monograph.

The strength of monitoring system of self-poisoned pregnant women is the personal examination of exposed children and their sib controls by the same methods Thus all CAs can be diagnosed by the well-defined diagnostic criteria, in addition the exposure data (drugs, doses, time according to the day of pregnancy) are based on multiple sources of information and there is chance for dose-effect and teratogenic threshold estimation. The lack of CAs after the use of very large doses of a drug during the critical period of CAs, it is an important argument against its teratogenicity.

However, the limitations of the monitoring system of self-poisoned pregnant women are also obvious. The number of pregnant women who attempt suicide – fortunately – is limited particularly in the critical period of major CAs. In addition several pregnancies are terminated after the suicide attempt. Many drugs get probably never or only very rarely used for self-poisoning.

Nevertheless, the self-poisoning model seems to be an effective human approach for the evaluation of drug teratogenicity/fetotoxicity therefore it would be worth establishing an international monitoring system of self-poisoned pregnant women.

1.10 Final Conclusions

The results of studies presented in Part II of the book were based on the data set of the HCCSCA.

There were three objectives of this long description of data sets and methods. The first aim was to summarize my 50 years' experiencies in human teratology which may help younger experts to use them. The second objective of this Part I of our monograph was to show the methodological weaknesses of previous studies and to recommend the use of up-to-date knowledge in the study design of new studies. Third, and mainly, this description provides the methodological background for the studies presented in the major Part II of the monograph.

References

Botto LD, Olney RS, Erickson JD. Vitamin supplements and the risk for congenital anomalies other than neural tube defects. Am J Med Genet C 2004; 125C: 12–21.

Briggs GG, Freeman RK, Yaffe SJ. Drugs in Pregnancy and Lactation: A Reference Guide to Fetal and Neonatal Risk. 7th ed. Lippincott Williams and Wilkins, Philadelphia, 2005.

Creasy RK, Resnik R, Iams JD (eds.) Maternal-Fetal Medicine. Principles and Practice. 5th ed. Saunders, Philadelphia, 2004.

Friedman JM, Polifka JE. The Effects of Drugs on the Fetus and Nursing Infant. Johns Hopkins Univ Press, Baltimore, 2000.

Goldenberg RL, Culhane JF, Iams JD, Romero R. Epidemiology and causes of preterm birth. Lancet 2008; 371: 75–84.

Hernandez-Diaz S, Werler MM, Walker AM, Mitchel AA. Folic acid antagonists during pregnancy and the risk of birth defects. N Engl J Med 2000; 343: 1608–1914.

Iams JD, Creasy RK. Preterm labor and delivery. In: Creasy RK, Resnik R, Iams JD (eds.) Maternal-Fetal Medicine. Principles and Practice. 5th ed. Saunders, Philadelphia, 2004. pp. 623–661.

Meadow KJ, Baker GA, Browning N et al. Cognitive function at 3 years of age after fetal exposure to antieplileptic drugs. N Engl J Med 2009; 360: 1597–1605.

Nishimura H, Yamamura H. Comparison between man and some other mammals of normal and abnormal developmental processes. In: Nishimura H, Miller JR (eds.) Method of Teratological Studies in Experimental Animals and Man. Igaku Shoin, Tokyo 1969. pp. 223–240.

Opitz JM. The developmental field concept in clinical genetics. J Pediatr 1982; 101: 803–809.

Perneger TV. What's wrong with Bonferroni adjustment. Br Med J 1998; 316: 1236–1238.

Resnik R, Creasy RK. Intrauterine growth restriction. In: Creasy RK, Resnik R, Iams JD (eds.) Maternal-Fetal Medicine. Principles and Practice. 5th ed. Saunders, Philadelphia, 2004. pp. 495–512.

Shaffer JP. Multiple hypothesis testing. Ann Rev Psychol 1995; 46: 561–584.

Shepard TH, Lemire RJ. Catalog of Teratogenic Agents. 11th ed. Johns Hopkins University Press, Baltimore, 2004.

Smith DW. Classification, nomenclature and naming of morphologic defects. J Pediatr 1975; 87: 162–164.

Spranger L, Benirschke K, Hall J et al. Errors of morphogenesis concept and terms. J Pediatr 1982; 100: 160–165.

Yoon PW, Rasmussen SA, Lynberg, MC et al. The national birth defects prevention study. Public Health Rep 2001; 116 (Suppl. 1): 32–40.

Own Publications

I. Czeizel A. First 25 years of the Hungarian Congenital Abnormality Registry. Teratology 1997; 55: 299–305.

II. Czeizel AE, Telegdi L, Tusnady G. Multiple Congenital Abnormalities. Akadémiai Kiadó, Budapest, 1988.

III. Czeizel AE, Kovács M, Kiss P, Méhes K, Szabó L, Oláh É, Kosztolányi G, Szemere G, Kovács H, Fekete G. Nationwide evaluation of multiple congenital abnormalities in Hungary. Genetic Epid 1988; 5: 183–202.

IV. Czeizel A. Schisis association. Am J Med Genet 1981; 10: 25–35.

V. Czeizel AE, Ludányi I. VACTERL association. Acta Morph Hung 1984; 32: 75–79.

VI. Pazonyi I, Bod M, Czeizel A. Postural associations. Acta Paediatr Acad Sci Hung 1983; 23: 431–445.

VII. Czeizel A. Genital anomalies of males: GAM-complex. Eur J Pediatr 1987; 146: 181–183.

VIII. Kis-Varga A, Rudas T, Czeizel A. A new approach to germinal mutation surveillance: pair-wise evaluation of component elements in unidentified multiple congenital abnormalities. Mutat Res 1990; 238: 87–97.

IX. Czeizel AE, The activities of the Hungarian Centre for Congenital Anomaly Control. WHO Stat Quart Rep 1988; 41: 219–227.

X. Czeizel A. The ethical issues of the postmarketing surveillance of drug teratogenicity in Hungary. Pharmacoepid Drug Saf 2001; 10: 635–639.

XI. Czeizel AE, Intõdy Zs, Modell B. What proportion of congenital abnormalities can be prevented? Br Med J 1993; 306: 499–503.

XII. Czeizel AE, Tusnady G. Aetiological Studies of Isolated Common Congenital Abnormalities in Hungary. Akadémiai Kiadó, Budapest, 1984.

XIII. Czeizel A. Epidemiological studies of congenital abnormalities in Hungary. In: Kalter H (ed.) Issues and Reviews in Teratology 1993; 6: 85–124.

XIV. Czeizel AE, Petik D, Vargha P. Validation studies of drug exposures in pregnant women. Pharmacoepid Drug Saf 2003; 12: 409–416.

XV. Czeizel AE, Vargha P. Periconceptional folic acid/multivitamin supplementation and twin pregnancy. Am J Obstet Gynecol 2004; 191: 790–794.
XVI. Czeizel AE, Petik D, Puhó E. Smoking and alcohol drinking during pregnancy: the validity of retrospective maternal self-reported information. Centr Eur J Publ Health 2004; 12: 179–183.
XVII. Czeizel AE, Gidai J, Petik D, Timmermann G, Puho H. Self-poisoning during pregnancy as a model for teratogenic estimation of drugs. Toxic Indust Health 2008; 24: 11–28.
XVIII. Czeizel AE, Tóth M. Birth weight, gestational age and medications during pregnancy. Int J Gynecol Obstet 1998; 60: 245–249.
XIX. Czeizel AE, Pazonyi I. Increase of upper-limb-reduction deformities in Hungary. Lancet 1976; 1: 701.
XX. Czeizel AE, Keller S, Bod M. An aetiological evaluation of increased occurrence of congenital limb reduction abnormalities in Hungary, 1975–1978. Int J Epidemiol 1983; 12: 442–449.
XXI. Czeizel AE, Elerk Cs, Gundy S, Métneki J, Nemes E, Reis K, Sperling K, Timár L, Tusnády G. Virágh Z. Environmental trichlorfon and cluster of congenital abnormalities. Lancet 1993; 34: 539–542.
XXII. Czeizel AE, Rockenbauer M, Siffel Cs, Varga E. Description and mission evaluation of the Hungarian Case-Control Surveillance of Congenital Abnormalities, 1980–1996. Teratology 2001; 63: 176–185.
XXIII. Czeizel A. The role of pharmacoepidemiology in pharmacovigilance: rational drug use in pregnancy. Pharmacoepid Drug Saf 1999; 8: 555–561.
XXIV. Czeizel A. Drug use during pregnancy in Hungary. Acta Med Hung 1989; 46: 53–62.
XXV. Czeizel AE, Rácz J. Evaluation of drug intake during pregnancy in the Hungarian Case-Control Surveillance of Congenital Anomalies. Teratology 1990; 42: 505–512.
XXVI. Czeizel A. Drug exposure in pregnant women. Lupus 2004; 13: 740–745.
XXVII. Bánhidy F, Lowry RB, Czeizel A. Risk and benefit of drug use during pregnancy. Int J Med Sci 2005; 2: 100–106.
XXVIII. Czeizel A. The estimation of human teratogenic/fetotoxic risk of exposures to drugs on the Hunagraian experience: a critical evaluation of clinical and epidemiological models of human teratology. Exp Opin Drug Saf 2009; 8: 283–303.
XXIX. Czeizel AE, Révész C. Major malformations of the central nervous system in Hungary. Br J Prev Soc Med 1970; 24: 205–222.
XXX. Czeizel A. Anencephaly-spina bifida cystica. In: Czeizel AE, Tusnady G. Aetiological Studies of Isolated Common Congenital Abnormalities in Hungary. Akadémiai Kiadó, Budapest, 1984. pp. 49–83.
XXXI. Medveczky E, Puho E, Czeizel A. An evaluation of maternal illnesses in the origin of neural-tube defects. Arch Gynecol Obstet 2004; 270: 244–251.
XXXII. Medveczky E. Puho E. Parental employment and neural-tube defects and folic acid/multivitamin supplementation in Hungary. Eur J Obstet Gynecol Reprod Biol 2004; 115: 178–184.
XXXIII. Medveczky E, Puho E, Czeizel A. The use of drugs in mothers of offspring with neural-tube defects. Pharmacoepid Drug Saf 2004; 13: 443–455.
XXXIV. Czeizel AE, Tusnády G. An epidemiological study of cleft lip with or without cleft palate and posterior cleft palate in Hungary. Hum Hered 1971; 21: 17–38.
XXXV. Czeizel AE, Tusnády G. A family study on cleft lip with or without cleft palate and posterior cleft palate in Hungary. Hum Hered 1972; 22: 405–416.
XXXVI. Sárközi A, Wyszynski DF, Czeizel A. Oral clefts with associated anomalies: findings in the Hungarian Congenital Abnormality Registry. BMC Oral Health 2005; 5: 4–18.
XXXVII. Wyszinsky DE, Sárközy A, Vargha P, Czeizel A. Birth weight and gestational age of newborns with cleft lip with or without cleft palate and with isolated cleft palate. J Clin Pediat Dent 2003; 27: 185–190.

XXXVIII. Czeizel AE, Sárközy A, Wyszinsky D. Protective effect of hyperemesis gravidarum for non-syndromic oral cleft. Obstet Gynecol 2003; 101: 737–744.
XXXIX. Wyszynski DF, Sárközi A, Czeizel A. Oral clefts with associated anomalies: methodological issues. Cleft Palate-Craniofacial J 2006; 43: 1–6.
XL. Métneki J, Puho E, Czeizel A. Maternal disease and isolated orofacial clefts in Hungary. Birth Defects Res A 2005; 73: 617–623.
XLI. Puho HE, Métneki J, Czeizel A. Drug treatment during pregnancy and isolated orofacial clefts in Hungary. Cleft Palate-Craniofacial J 2007; 44: 194–202.
XLII. Puho E, Métneki J, Czeizel A. Maternal employment status and isolated orofacial clefts in Hungary. Cent Eur J Publ Health 2005; 13: 144–148.
XLIII. Szendrey T, Danyi G, Czeizel A. Etiological study on isolated esophageal atresia. Hum Genet 1985; 70: 51–58.
XLIV. Czeizel A. Birthweight distribution in congenital pyloric stenosis. Arch Dis Child 1972; 47: 978–980.
XLV. Czeizel A. Congenital hypertrophic pyloric stenosis. In: Czeizel AE, Tusnady G. Aetiological Studies of Isolated Common Congenital Abnormalities in Hungary. Akadémiai Kiadó, Budapest, 1984. pp. 197–120.
XLVI. Czeizel AE, Toth J, Czvenits E. Increased birth prevalence of isolated hypospadias in Hungary. Acta Paediatr Hung 1986; 27: 329–337.
XLVII. Czeizel AE, Toth J, Erödi E. Aetiological study of hypospadias in Hungary. Hum Hered 1979; 29: 166–171.
XLVIII. Czeizel AE, Toth J. A correlation between the birth prevalence of isolated hypospadias and parental subfertility. Teratology 1990; 41: 167–172.
XLIX. Fritz G, Czeizel A. Abnormal sperm morphology and function in the fathers of hypospadiacs. J Reprod Fertil 1996; 106: 63–66.
L. Czeizel AE, Erődi É, Toth J. An epidemiological study on undescended testis. J Urol 1981; 126: 524–527.
LI. Czeizel AE, Erődi É, Toth J. Genetics of undescended testis. J Urol 1981; 126: 528–529.
LII. Czeizel AE, Vitéz M. Etiological study of omphalocele. Hum Genet 1981; 58: 390–395.
LIII. Abdel-Salam GMH, Vogt G, Halász A, Czeizel A. Microcephaly with normal intelligence and chorioretinopathy. Ophthal Genet 1999; 20: 259–264.
LIV. Czeizel AE, Abdel-Salam GMH. A case-control etiologic study of microcephaly. Epidemiology 2000; 11: 1–5.
LV. Abdel-Salam GMH, Svékus A, Pelle Z. Microcephaly, microphthalmia, congenital cataract, with calcification of the basal ganglia: MCA/MR syndrome. Genet Counsel 2000; 4: 391–397.
LVI. Abdel-Salam GMH, Vogt G, Czeizel A. Microcephaly with chorioretinal dysplasia: characteristic facial features. Am J Med Genet 2000; 95: 513–515.
LVII. Abdel-Salam GMH, Halász AA, Czeizel A. Association of epilepsy with different groups of microcephaly. Develop Med Child Neurol 2000; 42: 760–767.
LVIII. Abdel-Salam GMH, Gyenis G, Czeizel A. Antropometric craniofacial pattern profiles in microcephaly. Anthrop Rev 2002; 65: 65–74.
LIX. Vogt G, Horvath-Puho E, Czeizel A. A population-based case-control study of isolated primary congenital glaucoma. Am J Med Genet 2006; 140A: 1148–1155.
LX. Vogt G, Szunyogh M, Czeizel A. Birth characteristics of different ocular congenital abnormalities in Hungary. Ophthalmic Epidemiology 2006; 13: 159–166.
LXI. Vogt G, Puhó E, Czeizel A. A population-based case-control study of isolated ocular coloboma. Ophthalmic Epidemiol 2005; 12: 191–197.
LXII. Vogt G, Puhó E, Czeizel A. A population-based case-control study of isolated congenital cataract. Birth Defects Res A 2005; 73: 997–1005.
LXIII. Vogt G, Puhó E, Czeizel A. A population-based case-control study of isolated anophthalmia and microphthalmia. Eur J Epidemiol 2005; 20: 939–946.

LXIV. Puhó HE, Vogt G, Czeizel A. Maternal demographic and socioeconomic characteristics of live-born infants with isolated ocular congenital abnormalites. Ophthal Epid 2008; 15: 257–263.

LXV. Czeizel AE, Kamarás J, Balogh Ö, Szentpéteri J. Incidence of congenital heart defects in Budapest. Acta Paediatr Acad Sci Hung 1972; 13: 191–202.

LXVI. Mészáros M, Nagy A, Czeizel A. Incidence of congenital heart disease in Hungary. Hum Hered 1975; 25: 513–519.

LXVII. Mészáros M, Czeizel A. Point prevalence at birth of ventricular septal defect in Hungary. Acta Paediatr Acad Sci Hung 1978; 19: 51–54.

LXVIII. Czeizel AE, Mészáros M. Two family studies of children with ventricular septal defects. Eur J Paediatr 1981; 136: 81–85.

LXIX. Mészáros M, Czeizel A. ECG-conduction disturbance in the first-degree relatives of children with ventricular septal defect. Clin Genet 1981; 19: 298–301.

LXX. Czeizel AE, Pornoi A, Péterffy E, Tarczal E. Study of children of parents operated on for congenital cardiovascular malformation. Br Heart J 1982; 47: 290–293.

LXXI. Bellyei Á, Czeizel A. A higher incidence of congenital structural talipes equinovarus in gypsies. Hum Hered 1983; 33: 58–59.

LXXII. Czeizel AE, Bellyei Á, Kránicz J, Mocsai L, Tasnády G. Confirmation of multifactorial threshold model for congenital structural talipes equinovarus. J Med Genet 1981; 19: 99–100.

LXXIII. Czeizel AE, Evans JA, Kodaj I, Lenz W. Congenital Limb Deficiencies in Hungary. Genetic and Teratologic Epidemiological Studies. Akadémiai Kiadó, Budapest, 1994.

LXXIV. Czeizel AE, Kodaj I, Lenz W. Smoking during pregnancy and congenital limb deficiency. Br Med J 1994; 308: 1473–1476.

LXXV. Czeizel AE, Kovács M. A family study of congenital diaphragmatic defects. Am J Med Genet 1985; 21: 105–115.

LXXVI. Fraser FC, Czeizel AE, Hanson C. Increased frequency of neural tube defects in sibs of children with other malformations. Lancet 1982; 2: 144–145.

LXXVII. Puho HE, Czeizel AE, Ács N, Bánhidy F. Birth outcomes of cases with unclassified multiple congenital abnormalities and pregnancy complicationbs in their mothers depending on the number of component defects. Population-based case-control study. Cong Anom (Kyoto) 2006; 48: 126–136.

LXXVIII. Rockenbauer M, Olsen J, Czeizel AE, Pedersen L, Sorensen HT, EuroMAP group et al. Recall bias in a case-control study on the use of medicine during pregnancy. Epidemiology 2001; 12: 401–406.

LXXIX. Czeizel A. The first trimester concept is outdated. Cong Anom (Kyoto) 2001; 41: 204.

LXXX. Czeizel AE, Puho HE, Ács N, Bánhidy F. The use of specified critical periods of different congenital abnormalities instead of the first trimester concept. Birth Defects Res A 2008; 82: 139–146.

LXXXI. Czeizel A. Specified critical period of different congenital abnormalities: a new approach for human teratology. Cong Anom (Kyoto) 2008; 48: 103–109.

LXXXII. Gönczi L, Czeizel A. Integrating smoking cessation into periconceptional care. Tobacco Control 1996; 5: 160.

LXXXIII. Christian MS, Czeizel A. Introduction and history of the Hungarian project for monitoring suicide attempts in pregnant women. Toxic Indust Health 2008. 24: 5–9.

Part II
Results of Studies and Their Interpretation

Nándor Ács and Ferenc Bánhidy

Chapter 2
Certain Infectious and Parasitic Diseases

When evaluating pregnant women affected with certain infectious or parasitic diseases we followed the ICD classification (WHO) (see Table 1.12), though the experts of handbooks and review papers preferred the etiological classification according to the types of agents (virus, bacterium, parasite) or the route of infections (e.g. sexually transmitted infections/diseases). However, some acute infectious diseases did not occur in the data set of the HCCSCA, though have important role in the origin of adverse pregnancy outcomes, such as spontaneous abortions (e.g. parvovirus), fetal diseases (e.g. listeriosis or again parvovirus) and birth outcomes such as PB (e.g. chlamidial infection). According to the ICD classification we had to present the data of common cold and influenza in Chapter 11, *Diseases of the Respiratory System*. Finally, we inserted bacterial vaginosis, vaginal candidiasis, and trichomoniasis in the Chapter 16, *Diseases of Genital Organs* because microbial agents were not identified in most pregnant women with vulvovaginitis-bacterial vaginosis; therefore, it seemed to be better to evaluate them together.

The aim of this monograph is to evaluate the possible associations between maternal pathological conditions and increased risk of CAs and PB. Therefore, maternal morbidity and mortality are not discussed; in addition, the data set of the HCCSCA was not appropriate for the analysis of miscarriages. As we discussed in Chapter 1, the main focus of the HCCSCA has been CAs, i.e. the developmental error of organogenesis. However, fetopathies, i.e. fetal diseases were also notified frequently to the HCAR; therefore, we can evaluate fetal varicella and cytomegalic diseases, fetal toxoplasmosis, etc. These fetal diseases are the inflammatory reactions against these microbial agents after the maturation of the fetal immune system from IV gestational month.

The number of controls without CA is 38,151 in our data set corresponding to nearly 2% of newborn population. This control population can represent not only the live-born but indirectly the pregnancy population in Hungary. The data of birth outcomes of control newborns without CA born to mothers with different infectious diseases are summarized in Table 2.1. The distribution of CAs in cases will be presented in the subchapters of this chapter.

N. Ács et al., *Congenital Abnormalities and Preterm Birth Related to Maternal Illnesses During Pregnancy*, DOI 10.1007/978-90-481-8620-4_2,

Table 2.1 Birth outcomes of "control" newborns without CA in different infectious diseases

		Quantitative				Categorical			
		Gestational age (week)		Birth weight (g)		PB		LBW newborns	
Study groups	No.	Mean	S.D.	Mean	S.D.	No.	%	No.	%
Control reference	38,151	39.4	2.1	3,279	515	3,536	9.3	2,157	5.7
Salmonellosis	23	39.9	1.4	3,395	442	0	0.0	0	0.0
Infectious diarrhea	70	40.0**	1.4	3,298	446	1	1.4*	3	4.3
Tuberculosis	26	39.8	1.7	3,492*	545	2	7.7	0	0.0
Chickenpox	56	39.7	1.9	3,235	552	3	5.4	3	5.4
Herpes zoster	18	40.1	2.1	3,060	477	2	11.1	1	5.6
Herpes, orofacial[a]	572	39.7***	1.7	3,309	498	20	3.5***	24	4.2
Herpes, genital[b]	86	38.9*	2.0	3,163*	534	12	14.0	9	10.5*
Measles	7	39.3	2.8	3,257	640	1	14.3	1	14.3
Rubella	38	39.7	2.3	3,386	534	3	7.9	2	5.3
Viral hepatitis	16	39.4	1.9	3,412	406	1	6.3	1	6.3
Mumps	49	39.5	2.4	3,260	485	6	12.2	3	6.1
Genital viral warts	25	38.0***	3.0	2,980***	570	7	28.0***	3	12.0
Cytomegalic inclusion disease	19	39.4	1.3	3,144	388	1	5.3	3	15.8*
Viral infections, unspecified	49	39.8	1.6	3,327	518	3	6.1	3	6.1
Syphilis	2	39.5		3,700		0	0.0	0	0.0
Gonococcal infections	0	–	–	–	–	–	–	–	–
Dermatomycosis	71	39.1	2.0	3,271	504	9	12.7	2	2.8
Toxoplasmosis	27	39.1	2.3	3,300	485	3	11.1	1	3.7
Ascaris	10	39.8	1.1	3,192	264	0	0.0	0	0.0
Scabies	1	41.0	–	2,200	–	0	0.0	1	(100.0)

*$p < 0.05$; **$p < 0.01$; ***$p < 0.001$.
[a]Out of 574 pregnant women, 572 with recurrent orofacial herpes were evaluated here.
[b]Out of 228 pregnant women, 86 with medically recorded recurrent genital herpes were evaluated.

2.1 Intestinal Infectious Diseases with the Leading Symptom of Diarrhea

Intestinal infectious diseases with the leading symptom of diarrhea in general are not presented in the well-known handbooks (e.g. Creasy et al., 2004); however, a number of pregnant women with these diseases are in the data set of the HCCSCA.

The meaning of diarrhea is explained by two Greek words: "dia" and "rein" which means "through" and "flow", respectively. Therefore, diarrhea is an increase in the volume and frequency of bowel movement with a change in the consistence of the stools. In the clinical practice diarrhea may be defined as the passage of two or more stools daily that conform to the shape of the container or the passage of liquid stools exceeding 300 g/day (DeHovitz et al., 1986). Diarrhea is usually the results of either secretion of fluid into the intestinal lumen or inflammatory destruction of the ileal or colonic mucosa caused by microbes.

2.1.1 Salmonellosis (Salmonella Gastroenteritis)

Among the causes of infectious diarrhea, *Salmonella gastroenteritis* (SGE) is caused by motile, gram negative bacili. There are 3 species of Salmonella: S. typhi, S. choleraesuis and S. enteritidis having over 1,500 serotypes. Salmonellosis is a major cause of foodborne (mainly poultry and eggs) outbreaks of gastroenteritis. SGE occurs if a sufficient number of Salmonella bacilli survive the acid pH of the host's stomach and reach the small bowel. Salmonella organisms penetrate the mucosa of the ileum and colon and reach the lamina propria where an inflammatory response is elicited. SGE occurs 8–72 h after ingestion of contaminated food or water. The onset is usually abrupt, with nausea and vomiting followed by abdominal cramps and diarrhea sometimes fevers. These symptoms generally subside within 5–7 days.

2.1.1.1 Results of the Study (I)

Out of 22,843 cases with CA, 15 (0.07%) had mothers with the diagnosis of SGE, while out of 38,151 controls, 23 (0.06%) were born to pregnant women affected with SGE. All mothers had prospectively and medically diagnosis of SGE in the prenatal logbook.

There is no characteristic onset of SGE according to gestational months, though the lack of this disease in the first and last gestational month is noteworthy.

Mean maternal age and birth order, in addition to the distribution of their marital and employment status did not show significant difference between case and control mothers with SGE. The use of folic acid during pregnancy was higher in control mothers (65.2%) than in case mothers (46.7%) with SGE.

Other acute and chronic diseases in pregnant women with or without SGE did not show significant difference.

Among pregnancy complications, the incidence of threatened abortion (21.7% vs. 17.1%) was somewhat higher in pregnant women with SGE than in the reference sample.

Antidiarrheal (activated charcoal 7.9% vs. 0.1%, diphenoxylate-atropine mixture 8.7% vs. 0.1%), antimicrobial (ampicillin 23.7% vs. 7.0%, cotrimoxazole 15.8% vs. 1.3%) and antispasmodic (drotaverine 21.1% vs. 9.1%) drugs were used mainly for the treatment of pregnant women with SGE.

The mean gestational age was longer and mean birth weight was larger in 23 control babies born to mothers with SGE therefore PB and LBW did not occur (Table 2.1).

15 cases had 12 CA-groups (Table 2.2). Cardiovascular CAs occurred in 6 cases but different types (ventricular septal defect 2, atrial septal defect type II, stenosis of pulmonary valve, coarctation of the aorta and unspecified defect). The possible overlapping of SGE with the critical period of 6 cardiovascular CAs and 3 hypospadias was not found in most cases.

In conclusion, a higher risk of adverse birth outcomes was not found in the pregnancies of women with SGE during the study pregnancy.

2.1.2 Infectious Diarrhea

There are several microbial agents which can cause infectious diarrhea beyond *Salmonella* species, and these organisms are classified as bacteria (*Vibrio cholera* and *Vibrio parahaemolyticus*, *Escherichia coli*, *Staphylococcus aureus*, *Bacillus cereus*, *Clostridium perfringens*, *Shigella* species, *Yersinia enterocolitica*, *Campylobacter*, *Aeromonas hydrophila*, *Clostridium difficile*), viruses (Rotavirus, Norwalk-like Agents, enteral adenoviruses) and protozoas (*Giardia lamblia*, *Entamoeba histolytica*, *Cryptosporidium*, *Isospora belli*).

In the date set of HCCSCA, 152 women with *infectious diarrhea during pregnancy* (IDP) were recorded. We did not find previous controlled epidemiological studies regarding the possible associations between IDP and adverse pregnancy/birth outcomes particularly CA therefore we decided to evaluate these associations.

2.1.2.1 Results of the Study (I)

Out of 22,843 cases with CA, 82 (0.36%), while out of 38,151 controls, 70 (0.18%) mothers have been affected by IDP. Only mothers with prospectively and medically recorded IDP diagnosis in the prenatal logbook were evaluated.

IDP was assumed to be caused by Shigellae in 20 (24.3%) of the case mothers and 18 (25.6%) of the control mothers during the study pregnancy but documented laboratory findings were missing. Shigellae, i.e. non-motile, gram-negative bacilli, all of the Shigella species, e.g. S. dysenteriae can cause dysentery or shigellosis. Affected persons can infect other subjects, therefore, most dysentery is caused by person-to-person transmission, but waterborne and foodborne outbreaks are also known. There is a 24–72 h incubation period after the ingestion of these bacilli

Table 2.2 Estimation of risk of different CAs in pregnant women with SGE and IDP during the entire period of pregnancy and II and/or III gestational month, based on the comparison of cases to their matched controls

		SGE								IDP							
		Entire pregnancy				II ± III month				Entire pregnancy				II ± III month			
Study groups	Grand total No.	No.	%	OR[a]	95% CI	No.	%	OR[a]	95% CI	No.	%	OR[a]	95% CI	No.	%	OR[a]	95% CI
Controls	38,151	23	0.06	Reference		6	0.02	Reference		70	0.18	Reference		21	0.06	Reference	
Isolated CAs																	
Neural-tube defects	1,202	0	0.00	–	–	0	0.00	–	–	4	0.33	1.9	0.7–5.3	2	0.17	3.1	0.7–13.2
Cleft lip ± palate	1,374	0	0.00	–	–	0	0.00	–	–	11	0.80	**5.0**	**2.6–9.4**	8	0.58	**12.3**	**5.4–28.0**
Cardiovas-cular CAs	4,479	6	0.13	2.4	0.9–5.9	1	0.02	1.9	0.2–15.6	16	0.36	**2.2**	**1.3–3.8**	5	0.11	2.4	1.0–6.3
Hypospadias	3,038	3	0.10	1.7	0.5–5.7	0	0.00	–	–	9	0.30	1.8	0.9– 3.5	1	0.03	0.7	0.1–4.9
Undescended testis	2,051	1	0.05	0.9	0.1–6.7	0	0.00	–	–	4	0.20	1.1	0.4–3.1	2	0.10	1.9	0.4–8.1
Clubfoot	2,424	0	0.00	–	–	0	0.00	–	–	5	0.21	1.2	0.5–3.0	3	0.12	2.4	0.7–8.2
Limb deficiencies	548	0	0.00	–	–	0	0.00	–	–	5	0.91	**5.4**	**2.1–13.3**	4	0.73	**14.1**	**4.8–41.4**
Poly/syndactyly	1,744	2	0.11	2.0	0.5–8.6	1	0.06	4.4	0.5–36.6	8	0.46	**2.8**	**1.3–5.8**	1	0.06	1.1	0.2–8.3

Table 2.2 (continued)

Study groups	Grand total No.	SGE										IDP							
		Entire pregnancy				II ± III month						Entire pregnancy				II ± III month			
		No.	%	OR[a]	95% CI	No.	%	OR[a]	95% CI			No.	%	OR[a]	95% CI	No.	%	OR[a]	95% CI
Other isolated CAs	4,634	3[b]	0.05	1.2	0.4–4.0	0	0.00	–	–			14[c]	0.30	1.8	0.9–3.1	7	0.15	**2.9**	**1.2–6.8**
Multiple CAs	1,349	0	0.00	–	–	0	0.00	–	–			6[d]	0.44	2.8	1.2–6.4	3	0.22	**4.6**	**1.4–15.5**
Total	22,843	15	0.07	1.2	0.6–2.2	2	0.01	0.7	0.1–3.3			82	0.36	**2.1**	**1.5–2.9**	36	0.16	**3.1**	**1.8–5.2**

[a]OR adjusted for maternal age, marital and employment status, birth order, and use of folic acid.

[b]Oesophageal atresia, double urethra, exomphalos.

[c]Cleft palate only 2, cong pyloric stenosis, microcephaly, congenital hydrocephalus, web of larynx, lung hypoplasia, intestinal atresia, doubling of the uterus, agenesis of vagina, renal agenesis, cystic kidney, congenital stricture of the ureter, exstrophy of the urinary bladder.

[d]Congenital hydrocephaly + complex cardiovascular CA (ventricular septal defect + persistent ductus arteriousus), tetralogy of Fallot + cleft lip + limb deficiency with syndactyly, complex cardiovascular CA (atrial septal defect + persistent ductus arteriosus) + renal dysgenesis and cystic kidney with lung hypoplasia, and microcephaly + complex cardiovascular CAs and other 2 multiple CAs.

followed by the so-called "small-bowel phase" consisting of abdominal pain, watery diarrhea, and fever due to the enterotoxin of these microbes. In the next phase, these organisms invade and kill mucosal cells of the terminal ileum and colon due to inflammatory destruction resulting in the classical symptoms of dysentery such as bloody or mucoid stools associated with rectal urgency and tenesmus.

Other 20% of IDP was assumed to be caused by *Escherechia coli*, *Yersinia enterocolitica*, Norwalk-like Agents and enteral Adenoviruses but again without documented laboratory confirmation. Finally, only clinical symptoms (diarrhea with abdominal discomfort or pain, nausea or vomiting, anorexia and fever) were recorded without the specification of microbial agents in the prenatal care logbook in the rest of pregnant women with IDP. These pregnant women were evaluated together.

The onset of IDP occurred in all gestational month with a maximum in III–V months.

Many women with IDP were characterised by fever ("fever or high fever related to infectious diarrhoea") in the prenatal care logbook, in addition, 8 case mothers with IDP were visited at home, and 5 (62.5%) reported high fever (over 38.5°C) due to their IDP.

Maternal age and birth order, in addition to the distribution of their marital and employment status did not show significant difference between case and control mothers with IDP, but control mothers had somewhat better socioeconomic status. The use of folic acid during pregnancy was higher in control mothers (68.6%) than in case mothers (58.6%) with IDP.

Both case (19.5%) and control (20.0%) mothers with IDP had a higher incidence of acute infectious diseases of respiratory system compared to pregnant women without IDP (9.1%). The occurrence of chronic maternal diseases did not show significant difference among the study groups.

IDP did not associate with a higher risk of pregnancy complications, but the occurrence of anaemia was lower in mothers with IDP (8.6% vs. 15.8%) likely to their higher rate of iron supplementation 82.9% vs. 70.2%).

Women with IDP used antidiarrheal (activated charcoal 11.2% vs. 0.1%, diphenoxylate-atropine mixture 19.1% vs. 0.2%, bismuth 9.2% vs. 0.1%, loperamide 4.6% vs. 0.1%), antimicrobial (ampicillin 15.8% vs. 7.0%, cotrimoxazole 5.3% vs. 1.3%, penamecillin 13.2% vs. 6.3%), and antispasmodic (drotaverine 13.2% vs. 9.1%) drugs more frequently. In addition, women with IDP were treated frequently by antipyretic-antiinflammatory drugs such as acetylsalicylic acid, paracetamol, and dipyrone as well (31.6% vs. 9.2%).

The mean gestational age at delivery of babies born to mothers with IDP was longer and PB did occur (Table 2.1). Their mean birth weight was higher only by 19 g, and the rate of LBW newborns reflected it. Therefore, the longer gestational age associated with some intrauterine growth retardation in the fetuses of mothers with IDP

The data of Table 2.2 show a higher risk for some CAs, particularly cleft lip ± palate and limb deficiency based on 11 and 5 cases born to mothers with IDP. In addition 16 cases with cardiovascular CA had mainly conotruncal types (transposition of the great vessels, tetralogy of Fallot and mainly ventricular septal defect) and 8 cases with poly/syndactyly also showed association with maternal IDP. 4 out of 6 multiple CA cases had also complex cardiovascular CA. By the evaluation of IDP only in II and/or III gestational months, the association of IDP with limb deficiencies, cleft lip ± palate, cardiovascular CA was confirmed and two other CA-groups showed also association with IDP during this time window. Previously, the predominance of complex cardiovascular CAs were stressed among multimalformed cases. The significant association of other isolated CA group with IDP has disappeared after the exclusion of 2 cases with cleft palate.

2.1.2.2 Interpretation of Results

As far as we know, this is the first controlled epidemiological study to evaluate the possible association between maternal IDP and CAs of their offspring. This population-based case-control study showed a higher risk of some CAs in the children of women with IDP.

The secondary result of the study is the detection of a longer gestational age in the newborns of women with IDP, which did not associate with a larger mean birth weight. Our hypothesis is that these short infectious diseases during pregnancy were followed a more conscious prenatal care and healthier lifestyle, in addition IDP related antibiotic treatment had beneficial effect for asymptomatic or untreated vulvovaginal infections which may explain the longer gestational age. However, the IDP may have some adverse affect for the intrauterine fetal growth.

When evaluating the possible association between IDP and higher risk of some CAs in their offspring, the effect of IDP itself (including fever), the causes of IDP (i.e. the microbial agents), related drug treatments, other confounders and chance effect should be considered.

The classic presentation of IDP includes fever, and it was frequently recorded in the prenatal care logbook or in the questionnaire. Some previous studies indicated an association between CA and high fever during the critical period of orofacial cleft (II), limb deficiencies (III), cardiovascular CA (Tikkanen and Heinonen, 1991; Botto et al., 2001, IV), and multiple CA (V). Therefore, the common denominator of these findings may be the high fever because the teratogenic effect of high fever/hyperthermia is well-established (VI, VII).

We did not find any data regarding the possible association between the microbial causes of IDP and these CAs (Shepard and Lemire, 2004). Only one experiment showed that the Shigella toxin inhibited the development of mouse blastocysts in vitro (Olsen and Storeng, 1986).

The drugs might have a role in the origin of CAs, particularly cotrimoxazole (Hernandez-Diaz et al., 2000; 19, 20), some types of sulfonamides (17) and oxytetracycline (8). Ampicillin (4), penamecillin (3), acetylsalicylic acid (75, 76), paracetamol (77), drotaverine (83) and dipyrone (81) were used more frequently by case mothers with IDP, but only ampicillin showed a somewhat higher risk of cleft palate in the HCCSCA.

Previous intervention trials showed some protective effect of folic acid containing multivitamins during the periconceptional period for cardiovascular CAs and limb deficiencies (VIII, IX); therefore, these supplementations were evaluated in the study as confounders.

Finally, the effect of chance cannot be excluded at the interpretation of the association between IDP and these specific CAs.

Our hypothesis is that the cause of the possible association between IDP in early pregnancy and a higher risk for high fever sensitive CAs (such as orofacial clefts, cardiovascular CAs, and limb deficiencies) may be the high fever which is characteristic for IDP. Previous studies have shown that this fever related risk is preventable by antipyretic drug therapy (IV, VI); therefore, it is necessary to combine antimicrobial and antipyretic drugs in the treatment of IDP in pregnant women.

In conclusion, a higher risk of PB was not found in the pregnancies of women with IDP, but an association between IDP in early pregnancy and a higher risk for high fever sensitive specific CAs was found and might be explained by high fever.

2.2 Tuberculosis

Tuberculosis caused by Mycobacterium tuberculosis and bovis was very common in the Hungarian population until the 1930s, thus, it was called as "Morbus Hungaricus". After this time, there was a successful public health program to reduce this infection and to treat patients more effectively. As a result, the occurrence of tuberculosis reduced drastically. Unfortunately, recently an increasing trend of "new" tuberculosis patients has been found mostly because of the increasing proportion of people with low socioeconomic status, the negligence of obligatory chest radiography screening, and the emergence of drug-resistant tuberculosis.

Females have a higher progression from infection to disease and a higher case-fatality rate as well (Holmes et al., 1998). The symptoms of active pulmonary tuberculosis in pregnant women are cough (74%), weight loss (41%), fever (30%), malaise, fatigue (30%), and hemoptysis (19%) (Good et al., 1981).

The finding of acid-fast bacilli in early morning sputum specimens (at least one of three necessary specimen examinations) confirms the diagnosis of pulmonary tuberculosis. However, most pregnant women with tuberculosis are asymptomatic, therefore pregnant women at high risk for tuberculosis should be screened with subcutaneous administration of PPD (intermediate-strength purified protein derivative) with 90–99% sensitivity for exposure to tuberculosis. However, this screening cannot be used in a vaccinated population like Hungary. The extrapulmonary tuberculosis is rare in pregnancy (Hamadeh and Glassroth, 1992).

Pregnant women with tuberculosis may have a vertical, i.e. transplacental transmission of mycobacterium through the utero-placental circulation and it may cause the so-called congenital tuberculosis (Cantwell et al., 1994), correctly fetal tuberculosis disease. This can be diagnosed by the lesions of primary hepatic complex or cavitating hepatic granuloma and by the characteristic intrauterine growth retardation. However, these microbial agents and related drug treatments do not induce CA (Snider et al., 1980). Pregnant women with active tuberculosis should be treated with isoniacid, sometimes combined with rifampicin, or if resistance to isoniazid is recognized, ethambutol and other drugs are used.

We checked the possible teratogenic effect of antituberculotic drugs such as isoniazid, rifampicin, pyrazinamide, ethambutol (21), and streptomycin (15) and higher risk of CA was not found. However, the ototoxic effect (i.e. congenital anomaly) of streptomycin is well-known (Shepard and Lemire, 2004).

2.2.1 Interpretation of Data in the HCCSCA

Fifteen out of 22,843 cases (0.07%) and 26 out of 38,151 controls (0.07%) had mothers infected by tuberculosis during the study pregnancy.

Among maternal characteristics, only the lower socioeconomic status of pregnant women with tuberculosis is worth mentioning. Among pregnancy complications, threatened abortion showed a higher incidence (26.9% vs. 17.1%).

Our data did not confirm the fetal growth retardation of fetuses in the pregnancy of women with tuberculosis. The mean birth weight was larger in newborns and LBW newborns did not occur among 26 controls. Therefore, the treatment and lifestyle of these patients may have some benefit for the development of fetuses.

Fifteen cases had 8 different CA-groups, and among them, 5 cases were affected with hypospadias and 3 cases with neural-tube defects (anencephaly 1 and spina bifida 2).

In conclusion, the changing lifestyle and appropriate treatment of pregnant women with tuberculosis might help the development of their fetuses.

2.3 Varicella (Chickenpox) and Herpes Zoster

The *varicella zoster virus* (VZV) belongs to the family of herpes virus, i.e. a DNA virus (Heininger and Seward, 2006). This highly contagious acute disorder occurred about 90% of persons in childhood age; therefore, it was rare during pregnancy in the past. However, recently increasing numbers of pregnant women with varicella disease have been reported in Hungary (X) due to the change of public hygiene and the drastic drop of child number within families.

After the incubation period (mean of 15 days with the range of 10–21 days), the typical skin lesions are manifested which progress from macules and papules to vesicles and pustules. Uncomplicated maternal varicella disease does not appear to pose a severe risk to pregnant women, but previously varicella pneumonia caused high mortality. Recently the high doses of acyclovir seem to be effective.

The primary infection of pregnant women with VZV may associate with a low risk (about 1%) of congenital anomaly in their fetuses (Enders et al., 1994) because of 20 pregnant women with varicella disease, 3 (15%) had evidence of transplacental infection (Trlifajova et al., 1986). Maternal antibodies due to previous infection (or vaccination) usually protect the fetus. The affection of the fetus is not a typical CA-syndrome but a fetopathy, thus, we use the term *fetal varicella disease*. The latter is explained by the critical period of fetal varicella disease, which is between 10th and 21st gestational (i.e. 8th and 19th postconceptional) weeks. The symptoms of fetal varicella disease are the consequences of fetal varicella skin lesions which consist of cuteneous scars and secondary limb hypoplasia (caused by the massive scars of skin in the flexible developing bones), and anomalies of auricles (e.g. microtia) (Enders et al., 1994; Jones et al., 1994). Rarely the inflammatory lesions of eyes and central nervous system (epilepsy, mental retardation) may occur. The ultrasound appears to be appropriate at 21–22 weeks for the confirmation of the possible risk, i.e. abnormal limb development sometimes with polyhydramnios (Pretorius et al., 1992).

Herpes zoster is the recurrent form of VZV infection when the latent VZV is reactivated in older or immunocompromised persons. Herpes zoster is manifested as painful vesicular lesions that occur along segmental dermatomes.

2.3.1 Results of the Study (X)

Out of 22,843 cases, 31 (0.14%) had mothers with medically recorded varicella disease during pregnancy, while out of 38,151 controls, 56 (0.15%) were born to mothers with varicella disease.

Among pregnancy complications, only threatened abortion showed a higher incidence (21.4% vs. 17.1%).

Birth outcomes of 56 control newborns without CA had no adverse pattern; in fact there was a longer gestational age with a lower rate of PB (Table 2.1).

Out of 31 CAs, 28 cases had isolated and 3 had multiple CAs. Out of these 28 isolated CAs, 3 were considered as fetal varicella disease due to maternal infection during the study pregnancy. Two fetuses showed characteristic sequence of secondary complex skeletal CAs (one of them is shown in Fig. 2.1) due to the primary serious skin scars, while the third case had deformed microtia due to skin scars. The mothers of these children were affected with varicella disease in IV, IV and V

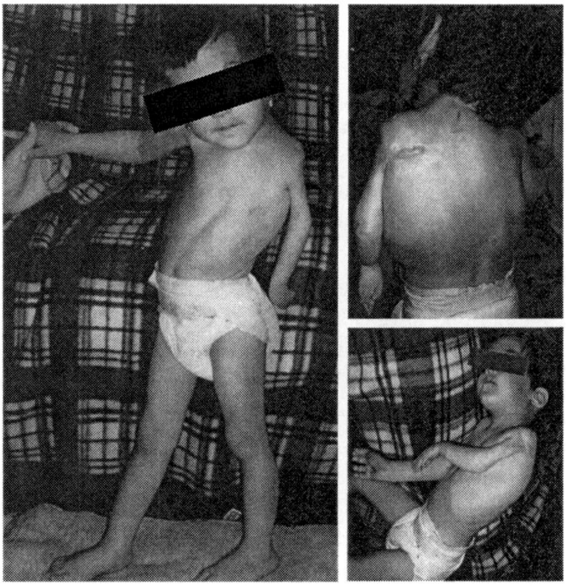

Fig. 2.1 Symptoms of fetal varicella disease: cuteneous scars of fetal varicella disease with secondary bone hypoplasia and disruption of the *left* shoulder and *upper* limb

gestational months, respectively. The other 25 isolated CAs did not seem to be associated with maternal varicella disease, i.e. these CA were considered as coincidental events. Out of 3 multiple CAs, two may be associated with maternal varicella disease (atypical microtia and anal atresia, microphthalmia and atypical microtia after the occurrence of maternal varicella disease in III and V gestational month, respectively). The third multimalformed case was affected with congenital hydrocephaly, complex cardiovascular CA (ventricular and atrial septal defects) and atresia of auditory canal with normal auricle. His mother was affected with varicella disease in III gestational month, but the critical period of this multiple CA was estimated on II gestational month.

In the data set of the HCCSCA 13 cases with different CA (0.06%) and 18 controls without CA (0.05%) had mothers with medically recorded *herpes zoster* during pregnancy.

Among pregnancy complications, again threatened abortion had a higher incidence (22.2% vs. 17.1%).

Control newborns showed an unusual pattern of birth outcomes (Table 2.1). The gestational age was much longer but the mean birth weight was lower and it indicates intrauterine fetal growth retardation. However, the rate of PB was higher, while the rate of LBW newborns did not differ from the figure of reference sample.

The risk of CAs was not higher in the group of cases and characteristic pattern of CAs could not be recognized; only hypospadias occurred in two cases.

2.3.2 Interpretation of Results

The risk of characteristic pattern of fetal varicella disease is low; however, this low fetal risk causes serious anxiety in pregnant women. Therefore, it is very important to stress that fetal varicella disease is preventable by vaccination which is available as attenuated virus vaccine (Varivax, Varilrix, Okavax) (Kuter et al., 2004; Shinefeld et al., 2005). These vaccines contain a live attenuated virus, therefore, pregnant women should not be vaccinated or women who are planning their conception should avoid pregnancy for 1 month after injection. However, out of 371 pregnant women with inadvertent vaccination before or during pregnancy, no case had fetal varicella disease (CDC, 1996).

If pregnant women are affected with varicella disease, administration of VZIG (varicella-zoster immune globulin) within 96 h of exposure is recommended. In addition, ultrasound may demonstrate severe limb defects around the 20th gestational week of pregnancy (Pretorius et al., 1992).

Varicella in newborns is out of our topic; nevertheless, this very severe pathological condition cannot be neglected here. If an infant is born after the maternal viraemia but before a maternal antibody response, there is a high risk for life-threatening (about 30%) neonatal varicella infection. Neonates are at risk if the mother has contracted VZV between 5 days before and 2 days after delivery.

If pregnant women are affected with herpes zoster, the risk of CA in the fetus is most unlikely.

In conclusion, an important task is to clarify previous varicella disease in the history of every woman in the preconceptional period. In case of negative or unsure history of varicella, it is necessary to recommend the administration of varicella vaccine in prospective pregnant women.

2.4 Herpes Simplex

Herpes simplex virus 1 (HSV-1) and *Herpes simplex virus 2* (HSV-2) are known as human pathogens. HSV-1 is normally associated with orofacial infections, whereas HSV-2 usually causes genital infections (Riley et al., 1998; Whitley and Roizman, 2001). However, both viruses are capable of causing either genital or orofacial infections. Furthermore, both viruses can cause neonatal herpes which is a perinatally acquired infection (Florman et al., 1973; Hutto et al., 1985; Baldwin and Whitley, 1989; Jacobs, 1998; Guitierrez et al., 1999; Rudnick et al., 2002). In the majority of cases, neonatal HSV is acquired via the birth canal, but rare cases of intrauterine infections have been described (South et al., 1969; Brown et al., 1987; Whitley, 2001); hence transplacental transmission of the infection is possible. In developed countries seroconversion has been reported in about 20% of children younger than 5 years with a second seroconversion peak (40–60%) at the age of 20–40 years (Nahmias et al., 1990).

There were three aims of our study based on the data set of the HCCSCA. First, we wanted to evaluate the incidence of pregnancy complications and to compare these variables in pregnant women with orofacial and genital herpes. The second aim was to estimate the association between maternal orofacial and genital herpes during pregnancy and birth outcomes, particularly gestational age at birth and birth weight of control newborns without CA. Thirdly, the possible association between orofacial and genital herpes during pregnancy with CAs in a case-control study was evaluated.

2.4.1 Orofacial Herpes

Orofacial herpes (OFH) commonly affects women of childbearing age including pregnant women. Previous studies showed associations between genital herpes, i.e. mainly HSV-2 and CA, however, Florman et al. (1973) reported an infant infected with HSV-1 who had microcephaly, intracranial calcification and owl eye inclusion body in the urine. Baldwin and Whitley (1989) reviewed and evaluated 71 cases with intrauterine acquired herpes infection. HSV-2 accounted for 61% of these cases, while HSV-1 was found in 7%. (The origin and/or type of HSV were not reported in 32% of cases.) Chorioretinitis, hydranencephaly, and cutaneous lesions as main findings were diagnosed in the newborns within the first 48 h of delivery.

First, the data of pregnant women with OFC in the HCCSCA are summarized.

2.4.1.1 Results of the Study (XI, XII)

Out of 22,843 cases with CA, 435 (1.9%) were born to mothers with OFH. Out of 38,151 controls, 574 (1.5%) had mothers who had OFH during pregnancy.

The OFH was differentiated into two types: Primary infection and recurrent OFH on the basis of maternal information only, medical records only, or both. Out of 435 case mothers, 429 (98.6%) and of 574 control mothers, 572 (99.7%) reported recurrent OFH, therefore only 6 case and 2 control mothers had primary OFH. These primary OFH cases were medically recorded in the prenatal logbook, but their limited numbers avoided their evaluation. Recurrent OFH was recorded rarely in the prenatal care logbooks or the discharge summaries; therefore, it was mostly reported by mothers (81.0% of cases and 72% of controls). Finally, 429 case and 572 control mothers with *recurrent OFH* were evaluated in the study (crude OR: 1.3, 1.1–1.4).

The maximum of recurrent OFH was found in III gestational month (21.1% in case and 17.2% in control mothers), followed by II, IV and I gestational month. The occurrence of recurrent OFH was rare after V gestational month, it occurred only in 6 case and 8 control mothers during the last 2 months of gestation.

Mothers with recurrent OFH were somewhat older (26.1 vs. 25.4 year) than mothers without OFH; while their mean birth order was lower (1.4 vs. 1.6) due to the larger proportion of primiparae (72.3% vs. 59.4%). There was no difference in the proportion of unmarried pregnant women among the study groups. Recurrent OFH was more frequent among professional (26.5% vs. 11.2%), while less frequent in semi- and unskilled workers and housewives (10.1% vs. 25.6%).

Among pregnancy supplements, the use of folic acid was more frequent by mothers with recurrent OFH than by mothers without OFC (case mothers: 57.1% vs. 49.2%, control mothers: 65.9% vs. 54.3%). A similar trend was seen in the use of multivitamins (case mothers: 11.7% vs. 5.7%, control mothers: 15.5% vs. 6.5%). However, control mothers used folic acid and multivitamins more frequently than case mothers.

The occurrences of acute infectious maternal diseases showed significant difference in influenza-common cold with secondary complications (case mothers with or without OFC: 39.4% vs. 21.4%, control mothers with or without OFC: 36.2% vs. 18.2%) and acute diseases of respiratory system, mainly tonsillitis (in case groups: 18.9% vs. 9.1% and in control groups: 22.0% vs. 8.9%). Therefore, influenza-common cold was 1.9, while respiratory diseases were 2.6 fold frequent in mothers with recurrent OFH than in mothers without OFH, respectively. Chronic maternal diseases, such as diabetes mellitus and epilepsy did not show difference among the study groups.

Among frequently used drugs, antipyretic (acetylsalicylic acid, aminophenazone, dipyrone, paracetamol), antimicrobial (ampicillin, clotrimazole, metronidazole, penamecillin), and prednisolone had a more frequent use in mothers with recurrent OFH than in pregnant women without OFH probably due to the higher prevalence of the previously mentioned acute maternal diseases. In the data set of the HCCSCA, only 15 mothers with recurrent OFH were treated with acyclovir introduced in Hungary during the 1990s.

The incidence of pregnancy complications showed that preterm delivery (11.5% vs. 8.3%, 1.4, 1.1–1.8) occurred more frequently in mothers with recurrent OFH than in mothers without recurrent OFH, while the incidence of preeclampsia-eclampsia was lower among them (5.9% vs. 9.2%, 0.6, 0.5–0.9).

The second objective of the study was the evaluation of birth outcomes of children without CA born to mother with recurrent OFC and without OFC as reference. Mean gestational age was 0.4 week longer in mothers with OFH compared with mothers without OFH and the rate of PB was 2.7 fold lower in mothers with recurrent OFH. The difference was only 30 g in the mean birth weight between live-born babies born to mothers with or without OFH, therefore the rate of LBW did also not show significant difference between the two study groups.

The third objective of the study was to evaluate the possible association between recurrent OFH during pregnancy and particularly in II and/or III gestational month and different CAs (Table 2.3).

There was a higher risk for five CA-groups: isolated limb deficiencies, cleft lip ± palate, cardiovascular CAs, neural-tube defects and multiple CAs if maternal recurrent OFC occurred in II and/or III gestational months.

In the next step, we differentiated pregnant women with recurrent OFH according to the use or without the use of antipyretic drugs in II and/or III gestational month. The above associations were lost in all but one previous CA-groups, the exception was the groups of cardiovascular CAs.

Finally, we evaluated the possible association between recurrent OFH in II and/or III gestational month and different CAs according to the supplementation of folic acid in II and/or III gestational months. The supplementation of folic acid was able to prevent the risk for neural-tube defects, cleft lip ± palate and cardiovascular CAs, but not for limb deficiencies and multiple CAs associated with recurrent OFH. In fact, the risk was higher in the group of multiple CAs.

2.4.1.2 Interpretation of Results

Our study resulted in some unexpected findings. First, there was a higher incidence of threatened preterm delivery and a lower incidence of preeclampsia-eclampsia in pregnant women with recurrent OFH, while the occurrence of PB was less frequent.

Second, maternal recurrent OFH associated with a somewhat longer gestational age of newborn infants and a lower proportion of PB, but there was no change in mean birth weight and the rate of LBW newborns. Our findings do not agree with the results of previous studies in which intrauterine HSV infection was associated with more frequent PB (Hutto et al., 1985; Brown et al., 1987) and intrauterine growth retardation (Brown et al., 1987, 1997). The explanation for these discrepancies may be that adverse effects were found after primary HSV infection during pregnancy in previous studies while our pregnant women had recurrent OFH.

In the study, higher maternal age, larger proportion of professionals and folic acid/multivitamin usage in pregnant women with recurrent OFH may be associated with longer gestational age and smaller proportion of PB. On the other hand, the larger proportion of primiparae and semi- or unskilled workers, housewives may

Table 2.3 The estimation of risk for different CAs in the offspring of pregnant women with OFH in II ± III gestational months, in addition, their stratification by the use of antipyretic drugs or folic acid

	Total			Antipyretic drug[a]		Folic acid	
Study groups	No.	%	OR (95% CI)	No OR (95% CI)[b]	Yes OR (95% CI)[b]	No OR (95% CI)[b]	Yes OR (95% CI)[b]
Controls	191	0.5	Reference	Reference	Reference	Reference	Reference
Isolated CAs							
Neural-tube defects	11	0.9	**2.0 (1.1–3.6)**	**2.1 (1.1–4.0)**	1.0 (0.1–7.3)	**2.3 (1.2–4.6)**	1.2 (0.3–4.9)
Cleft lip ± palate	19	1.4	**3.1 (1.9–5.0)**	**2.9 (1.7–5.0)**	3.0 (0.9–9.1)	**3.4 (2.0–5.9)**	2.5 (0.9–6.3)
Cleft palate only	4	0.7	1.4 (0.5–3.8)	0.8 (0.2–3.4)	2.8 (0.6–12.6)	1.5 (0.5–4.8)	1.2 (0.2–8.7)
Oesophageal atresia/stenosis	3	1.4	2.8 (0.9–9.0)	3.3 (0.9–10.3)	–	2.7 (0.7–11.1)	3.2 (0.4–23.8)
Obstructive CA of urinary tract	3	0.6	1.2 (0.4–3.7)	1.0 (0.2–3.8)	1.9 (0.2–14.8)	1.2 (0.3–4.8)	1.3 (0.2–9.1)
Hypospadias	12	0.4	0.9 (0.5–1.5)	0.8 (0.4–1.5)	1.0 (0.2–4.1)	0.7 (0.3–1.5)	1.2 (0.5–2.9)
Undescended testis	6	0.3	0.6 (0.3–1.4)	0.5 (0.2–1.3)	2.0 (0.5–8.7)	0.5 (0.2–1.5)	1.0 (0.3–3.1)
Cardiovascular CA	44	1.0	**2.2 (1.6–3.0)**	**1.9 (1.3–2.8)**	**2.8 (1.4–5.8)**	**2.3 (1.6–3.4)**	1.9 (0.9–3.4)
Clubfoot	5	0.2	0.4 (0.2–1.1)	0.5 (0.2–1.2)	–	0.4 (0.1–1.2)	0.5 (0.1–2.2)
Limb deficiencies	8	1.5	**3.2 (1.6–6.5)**	**3.3 (1.5–7.1)**	1.8 (0.2–13.6)	**2.9 (1.2–7.1)**	**4.0 (1.2–12.8)**
Poly/syndactyly	11	.6	1.4 (0.7–2.5)	1.6 (0.9–2.9)	–	1.7 (0.9–3.3)	0.7 (0.2–3.0)
Other isolated CAs	22	0.7	1.5 (0.9–2.3)	1.6 (0.9–2.6)	0.5 (0.1–3.5)	1.5 (0.9–2.6)	1.3 (0.6–2.9)
Multiple CAs	15	1.1	**2.5 (1.5–4.3)**	**2.2 (1.2–4.1)**	3.0 (0.9–8.9)	1.9 (0.9–3.9)	**4.1 (1.8–8.9)**
Total	163	0.7	**1.6 (1.3–1.9)**	**1.5 (1.2–1.9)**	1.6 (0.9–2.8)	**1.6 (1.2–2.0)**	**1.6 (1.1–2.2)**

[a]Use of antipyretic drugs (acetylsalycylic acid, aminophenazone, dipyrone, paracetamol) in II and/or III months of pregnancy.
[b]ORs adjusted for maternal age, birth order, maternal employment status.

be associated with a shorter gestational age and larger proportion of PB. However, these variables were considered at the calculation of adjusted risk values.

An obvious discrepancy was observed between the higher rate of threatened preterm birth as pregnancy complications and the lower rate of PB in the group of pregnant women with recurrent OFH. One explanation might be that the treatment to prevent premature delivery was effective. In addition, the significantly longer gestational age and smaller proportion of PB did not associate with a significantly larger mean birth weight and lower proportion of LBW. These findings agreed with the results of some previous studies indicating relative intrauterine fetal growth retardation in women with OFH (Brown et al., 1987, 1997).

It is a well-known fact that immune suppression plays a fundamental role in maintaining pregnancy. Recurrent OFH usually develops in a suppressed state of the immune system (Whitley and Roizman, 2001). Therefore, we may hypothesize that this immune suppression may explain at least partly the longer pregnancy duration and lower proportion of PB.

The third and major unexpected finding of the study was a possible association between maternal recurrent OFH in II and/or III gestational months and five CA-groups, namely according to the magnitude of risks: limb deficiencies, cleft lip ± palate, multiple CAs, cardiovascular CAs, and neural-tube defects. These associations may be connected with the higher rate of influenza–common cold and acute infectious diseases of the respiratory system in these pregnant women, because there is a well-known association between fever and recurrent OFH. In addition, the parallel use of antipyretic drugs was able to prevent this risk in all but one CA-group. In addition, the high dose of parallel folic acid supplementation reduced the risk for neural-tube defects, cardiovascular CAs, and cleft lip ± palate due to recurrent OFH.

These CAs did not show similarity with CAs associated with HSV-infection found in previous studies (Florman et al., 1973; Karesh et al., 1983; Brown et al., 1987, 1997; Eskild et al., 2000; Vasileiadis et al., 2003). Our hypothesis may solve this discrepancy: the possible association between recurrent OFH and neural-tube defects, cleft lip ± palate, limb deficiencies, cardiovascular CAs, and multiple CAs can be explained by the high fever related acute infectious diseases in the pregnant women which preceded and triggered recurrent OFH. Therefore, the order of events may be (i) pregnancy with suppressed state of immune system, (ii) followed by high fever related maternal diseases (iii) which trigger the recurrence of OFH and (iv) in parallel induce some hyperthermia-related CAs (Smith et al., 1978; Edwards et al., 1995).

The teratogenic effect of hyperthermia is well-known (Edwards, 1967; Jones, 1988, VI). Another study showed a higher prevalence of maternal influenza during II and III months of pregnancy in women who later had offspring with cleft lip ± palate, cleft palate only, neural-tube defects, and cardiovascular CAs (IV). In addition, another important argument for the teratogenic effect of high fever is that antipyretic drugs were able to reduce or prevent the risk for these CAs.

Antipyretic and antimicrobial drugs were not used more frequently by case mothers than control mothers, in addition, previous studies did not indicate the teratogenic effect of acetylsalicylic acid (75, 76), dipyrone (81), paracetamol (77), clotrimazole (28), metronidazole (41–44), penamecillin (3) and prednisolone (70). Ampicillin associated with a low risk for cleft palate (4). Acyclovir and other antiviral drugs did not show human teratogenic effect (Whitley et al., 1991).

Finally, it is worth mentioning that folic acid or folic acid containing multivitamin supplementations can reduce the first occurrence of neural-tube defects (XII) and some others CAs (VIII, IX, Botto et al., 2004). However, this study showed that the high dose of folic acid can also reduce the hyperthermia related risk for some candidate CAs associated with recurrent OFH.

In conclusion, recurrent OFH may be associated with a higher risk of some CAs and it may be the indirect effect of high fever related maternal diseases which triggered the recurrence of OFH. However, the major message of the study is that the possible association between recurrent OFH and some CAs probable is caused by the high fever and this risk can be reduced by antipyretic drugs in the above CA-groups except cardiovascular CAs. In addition, the risk of neural-tube defects, cleft lip $\pm$ cleft palate, and cardiovascular CAs was reduced by the high dose of folic acid supplementation. Therefore, it is necessary to use antipyretic therapy and folic acid supplementation in pregnant women with fever related diseases in order to prevent CAs.

2.4.2 Genital Herpes

HSV infection of the genital tract is one of the most common viral sexually transmitted infections/diseases (Wald et al., 1995; Fleming et al., 1997; Xu et al., 2002; Pebody et al., 2004), mostly caused by HSV-2 but can be caused by HSV-1 as well.

Women are more likely to become infected than men. The chance of infection has a positive correlation with the number of sexual partners. About 5% of reproductive-aged women reported a history of genital herpes in our periconceptional clinic (XIV) and it corresponded to the figure found in other countries (Monif et al., 1985). However, between 4.2% (in England and Wales) and 27.1% (in the USA) of the female populations have antibodies against HSV-2 (Nahmias et al., 1990; Arvin et al., 2007).

Intrauterine infection of HSV-2 during pregnancy may occur in women who have not completed seroconversion by the onset of labor; however, transplacental HSV infection is extremely rare. It may occur in less than 5% of primary infections (Monif et al., 1985). Primary HSV infection in the absence of cross-protecting antibodies may result in hematogenous dissemination of HSV to the fetus, particularly between 6th and 14th weeks of gestation and may induce a typical triad of CAs such as (i) skin manifestations such like vesicles and/or scarring, (ii) eye CAs: microphthalmia and cataract, in addition, chorioretinitis, (iii) neurological involvement with the secondary consequence of microcephaly and intracranial calcification (South et al., 1969; Chalhub et al., 1977; Hutto et al., 1983; Monif et al., 1985). In addition, some case reports showed a possible association between CAs and clinical recurrence of previously described genital herpes infections (Avgil and Ornoy, 2006).

The aims of the study (similar to the OFC) were described in the previous subchapter, here the data of genital herpes are summarized.

2.4.2.1 Results of the Study (XV)

The symptoms of clinically recognized genital herpes show grouped vesicles localized to a small area of the external genitalia with or without progression to ulceration and crusting. Maternal genital herpes was differentiated into two types: first occurrence, i.e. primary and recurrent, based on maternal information only, medical records only, or both. The definition of recurrent genital herpes was the reactivation of genital herpes from the previous lesions of genital organs in the study.

Out of 22,843 cases with CA, 160 (0.70%) were born to mothers with reported and/or recorded genital herpes during the study pregnancy. Out of 38,151 controls, 228 (0.60%) had mothers with reported and/or recorded genital herpes during the study pregnancy.

Out of 160 case mothers, 60 (37.5%) and out of 228 control mothers, 88 (38.6%) had prospectively and medically recorded genital herpes in the prenatal logbook. Case and control mothers with genital herpes based on only maternal retrospective self-reported information were excluded from the study because in general the type (first occurrence and recurrent) and the time (according to gestational months) of genital herpes were not mentioned, in addition, the validity of these diagnoses were low. Out of 60 case mothers, one, while out of 88 control mothers, two had medically recorded primary genital herpes in the prenatal logbook. These cases were also excluded from this analysis due to the low number of pregnant women; in addition, we wanted to evaluate a group of recurrent genital herpes as homogeneous as possible. Finally, only 59 (0.26%) cases and 86 (0.23%) controls born to mothers with prospectively and medically recorded *recurrent genital herpes* (RGH) were evaluated in the study (1.2, 0.8–1.6).

The evaluation of onset of RGH according to gestational months showed that the maximum of incidence was found in IV gestational month in case mothers followed by III and VII gestational month. In control mothers the maximum of incidence was found in V gestational month, followed by IV and II–III gestational months. The occurrence of RGH was rare in the last month of gestation.

Mothers with RGH were somewhat younger (24.7% vs. 25.5 year) than mothers without RGH as reference therefore the mean birth order (1.5 vs. 1.7) was lower due to the larger proportion of younger age group (less than 24 years: 58.1% vs. 47.1%) and primiparae (65.1% vs. 47.7%). The proportion of unmarried pregnant women was larger in pregnant women with RGH (7.0% vs. 3.9%), and RGH was less frequent among skilled workers (22.1% vs. 30.7%).

Folic acid was used more frequently by case mothers (64.4% vs. 49.5%) and controls mothers (58.1% vs. 46.2%) with RGH than by mothers without this disease. There was no difference in the use of multivitamins among the study groups.

The evaluation of acute infectious maternal diseases showed that influenza-common cold with secondary complications (25.4% vs. 21.7% in case and 22.1% vs. 18.5%) was more frequent in mothers with RGH than in mothers without RGH.

However, these differences were not significant. The acute diseases of respiratory (15.3% vs. 9.3%) and digestive system (10.2% vs. 3.2%) showed a higher incidence only in case mothers with RGH but not in control mothers with RGH. The prevalence of chronic maternal diseases did not have differences among the study groups.

Among drugs, some antimicrobial drugs such as ampicillin (11.0%), penamecillin (10.3% vs. 6.3%), sulfamethoxazole+trimethoprim (4.8% vs. 1.3%) had more frequent use in mothers with RGH due to the higher prevalence of the previously mentioned acute maternal diseases. Acyclovir was not used by pregnant women with RGH during the study period.

There was no significant difference in the incidence of pregnancy complications between control mothers with or without RGH.

The data of birth outcome in pregnant women with RGH are shown in Table 2.1. Mean gestational age at delivery was 0.5 week shorter and the rate of PB was higher compared to the newborns of pregnant women without RGH. The shorter gestational age was reflected in mean birth weight which was 113 g smaller with a higher rate of LBW newborns.

We evaluated birth outcomes according to the RGH in different trimesters of the study pregnancies. There was an obvious time trend (mean gestational age: 39.5, 39.2, and 38.7 week, mean birth weight: 3,348, 3,147, and 3,112 g, rate of PB: 6.7, 15.4, and 23.5%, rate of LBW: 3.3, 12.8 and 17.7%) in the first, second, and third trimesters of pregnancy. The third trimester infections associated with the shortest gestational age and the highest rate of PB (2.6, 1.5–4.5).

The main objective of the study was to evaluate the possible association between RGH anytime during pregnancy and particularly in the critical period of different CAs. Originally, we wanted to evaluate II and/or III gestational months, however, the analysis of pregnant women with RGH showed that RGH in I gestational month frequently extended to II gestational month. Therefore, finally we evaluated the first trimester, as the time window of critical period of CAs. Adjusted OR did not show a higher risk for any CA group either during the entire pregnancy or in the first trimester exposure of RGH.

2.4.2.2 Interpretation of Results

Overall 0.5–2% of women acquires HSV during pregnancy (Kulhanjian et al., 1992; Brown et al., 1997). The prevalence of symptomatic RGH was 0.6–0.7% in our study, but we evaluated only prospectively recorded RGH diseases. About 70% of newly acquired HSV infections among pregnant women are asymptomatic or unrecognized, and the reactivations of genital herpes are also most commonly unrecognized (Brown et al., 1991, 2005).

In our study the lower maternal age with a larger proportion of primiparae and unmarried women were found in pregnant women with RGH. These variables may be connected to the higher number of sexual partners. Finally, pregnant women with RGH had a higher rate of folic acid supplementation during pregnancy.

Our study showed a statistically significant association between maternal RGH and the rate of PB (14.0% vs. 9.3%) demonstrating the higher rate of PB in pregnant women with RGH during the third trimester compared to healthy controls. The gestational age specific birth weight groups did not show a significant retardation; therefore, the lower birth weight and higher rate of LBW were mainly connected with the shorter gestational age at delivery. Therefore, we did not find an association between RGH and intrauterine growth retardation.

The primary maternal genital infection with HSV in early pregnancy associated with a 3 fold increase in the rate of spontaneous abortion (Monif et al., 1985), although this finding was not confirmed later. Both symptomatic (clinical) and asymptomatic (subclinical) primary HSV infection in the second and third trimesters of pregnancy increased the risk for PB and LBW, i.e. small-for-gestational-age newborns in other studies (Whitley et al., 1988; Brown et al., 1987, 1996). However, some studies did not find association between genital herpes and PB and/or LBW (Boehm et al., 1981; Vontver et al., 1982; Harger et al., 1983; Catalano et al., 1991; Proper et al., 1992). Our study confirmed an association between RGH in the second part of pregnancy and higher risk of PB birth but did not show association with a higher risk of LBW.

Infections caused by HSV are defined clinically as *symptomatic or asymptomatic*. In our study only symptomatic RGH in pregnant women were evaluated, based on the clinical symptoms. However, as ACOG (2007) recommended: "All suspected herpes virus infections should be confirmed by viral or serological testing" due to the poor sensitivity (about 40%) and high false positive rate (about 20%) of clinical diagnosis (CDC, 2006). Our study was based on medically recorded symptomatic RGH in pregnant women without mentioning the proportion and/or method of viral and serological testing.

Infections caused by HSV are defined serologically as *primary and secondary infections*. The cellular targets of HSV are epithelial cells of the skin and mucosa, in addition to neurons. During the primary infections in the skin and/or mucosa caused by sexual contact with infected partners, HSV enters into sensory and autonomic neurons through the axons that extend to the location of the lesions. Once HSV is in the neuron nucleus, it can be latent for the entire life of the host (Whitley, 2001; Arvin et al., 2007). However, physical or emotional stress can reactivate HSV which transport back through the axon to the original point of entry, and shed in the genital area inducing clinical symptoms, i.e. disease, although it may be also asymptomatic. The reactivation of HSV may occur despite of the presence of the immune response followed the primary infections. Almost 100% of women with HSV-2 infection have symptomatic or asymptomatic RGH throughout their lives (Wald et al., 1995; Eskild et al., 2000).

RGH was likely caused by HSV-2 in the study because the frequency of genital reactivation is much less with HSV-1 which rarely recurs symptomatically or asymptomatically after the first year of infection (Reeves et al., 1981; Bendetti et al., 1994).

In conclusion, our study showed a higher risk of PB in pregnant women with RGH during the second part of pregnancy but no association between clinically recognized, i.e. symptomatic RGH and higher risk for any CA.

Finally, as the first aim of our studies, we attempted to compare recurrent OFH and RGH. Both birth outcomes and risk of CAs showed different patterns. Our study showed that mothers with recurrent OFH during pregnancy had a somewhat longer (0.4 week) gestational age and an obviously lower rate of PB while RGH mainly in the third trimester associated with a shorter gestational age and a higher rate of PB. On the other hand, there was an association between recurrent OFH and higher risk for high fever sensitive CAs but we were unable to find similar association between CAs and RGH. Therefore, the direct teratogenic effect of HSV is probably very limited and it is necessary to consider the indirect (confounder) teratogenic effect of high fever which precedes and triggers recurrent HSV-manifestation. Our studies first showed these unexpected differences in the two manifestations of recurrent HSV in the same data set of the HCSCA and these findings need further studies and explanation.

2.5 Measles (Rubeola, Morbilli)

Measles is caused by a single-stranded RNA measles virus which belongs to the family of paramyxovirus family. This virus is highly contagious through respiratory droplets; therefore, essentially all children developed measles in the past. After 10–14 days incubation period of measles infection, there are 5 important symptoms of measles: (i) characteristic rash, i.e. a generalized nonpruritic maculopapular rash that begins on the face and neck and then spreads to the trunk and extremities lasting longer than 3 days, (ii) fever of 38.3°C or higher, (iii) cough, (iv) coryza, (v) conjunctivitis. The duration of measles is 7–10 days, and it results in a lifelong immunity.

Measles occurred rarely during pregnancy because of the acquired immunity in the childhood age. However, if measles infection occurs during pregnancy, this disease associated with a higher risk of complications and mortality (Gibbs et al., 2004). Some studies reported a higher rate of spontaneous abortion and PB, but not a higher risk of CAs in pregnancies after measles infection (Creasy et al., 2004).

The first measles vaccine was licensed in 1963; the first hope was that this primary preventive method, i.e. a single injection of life measles vaccine when a child was approximately 15 months of age could eradicate the occurrence of this disease, i.e. provided lifelong immunity. Later measles outbreaks occurred in the United States (Gibbs et al., 2004) where the public health authorities now recommend that all individuals who have not been infected with the live virus should receive a second dose of vaccine at 4–6 years of age. In addition, if this second vaccination was not given, it is worth administrating it before a woman plans her first pregnancy.

2.5.1 Interpretation of Data in the HCCSCA

Out of 22,843 cases, 8 (0.04%), while out of 38,151 controls, 7 (0.02%) had mothers with measles during pregnancy. Pregnancy complications were not more frequent in 15 women with measles during the study pregnancy than in the reference sample. Birth outcomes of 7 control newborns did also not show difference from the figures of reference sample (Table 2.1). Out of 8 cases with CA, only hypospadias occurred twice.

2.6 Rubella

CAs caused by rubella-virus are important from historical and medical aspect in the human teratology. On one hand, this virus was the first infectious teratogen proved by Gregg in Australia, 1941. On the other hand the introduction of rubella vaccination was the first and good example for the primary prevention of a specific CA-entity, i.e. fetal rubella syndrome.

Rubella is caused by a RNA (ribonucleic acid) virus, spread by respiratory droplet. After the infection of upper respiratory system, the virus runs first to the cervical lymph nodes and later disseminates hematogenously throughout the organism. The characteristic symptoms of rubella are manifested after the incubation period of 2–3 weeks. The principal clinical presentations of rubella are nonpruritic, erythematous, maculopapular rash with postauricular adenopathy and mild general symptoms such as malaise, headache, myalgia, and arthralgia within the 3–5 days of this disease. The symptoms of rubella may be mild or sometimes lacking, therefore, the serological diagnosis, i.e. the characteristic increase of IgG titer (persisting throughout the lifetime of patients) and the identification of IgM antibody (with a peak 7–10 days after the onset of rubella and then decline over a period of 4 weeks) is crucial. In Hungary only 10.6% of females were seronegative before the first pregnancy (XIV); however, about 40% of women with negative rubella history were seropositive.

Rubella-virus crosses the placenta during the time of hematogenous dissemination and causes a typical CA-syndrome when rash occurred in II and III (about 80% of fetuses) gestational months. If rash was diagnosed in IV gestational month, 54% of newborns had some symptoms of typical rubella CA syndrome; mainly deafness (Miller et al., 1982). The typical triad of fetal rubella CA-syndrome covers (i) CA of the eyes, mainly cataract (sometimes corneal opacity, microphthalmia) (52%), (ii) cardiovascular CA, mainly persistent ductus arteriosus and supravalvular pulmonic stenosis (sometimes septal defects) (22%), and (iii) deafness (96%). This triad can be completed by microcephaly, in addition to mental (10%) and growth (50%) retardation (Menser et al., 1967). Since the identification of the virus (Alford et al., 1964), the rubella CA-syndrome was expanded to characteristic symptoms of rubella fetopathy, i.e. disease after the infection of III and/or IV gestational months including hepatosplenomegaly, hemolytic anemia and thrombocytopenia, pneumonia, encephalitis (Plotkin et al., 1965).

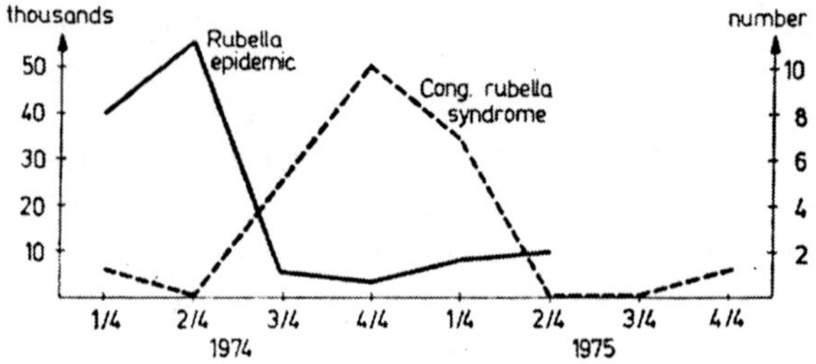

Fig. 2.2 The cluster of cases with fetal rubella CA-syndrome based on the registry diagnosis after the rubella epidemic in Hungary, 1974

The triad of fetal rubella CA-syndrome is characteristic, however frequently unrecognized by medical doctors. Therefore, we introduced the registry diagnosis of fetal rubella CA-syndrome in the HCAR based on the combination of congenital cataract and persistent ductus arteriosus with or without microcephaly. Our validation study confirmed the correctness of this registry diagnosis in about 90% of cases, and it helped us to identify the consequences of rubella epidemics in Hungary, e.g. in 1974 (Fig. 2.2) (XVI).

The rubella vaccination was introduced in 1989 and all children have been vaccinated. About 95% of people show seroconversion after vaccination and adverse effects of vaccination are minimal. Women who have received the vaccine cannot transit infection to susceptible persons. Pregnancy is not recommended at least 1 month after vaccination, even though fetal rubella CA-syndrome was not found in the offspring of approximately 400 pregnant women who received the rubella vaccine within 3 months of conception (CDC, 1994).

2.6.1 Interpretation of Data in the HCCSCA

Out of 22,843 cases, 32 (0.14%), while out of 38,151 controls, 38 (0.10%) had mothers with rubella during the study pregnancy.

The evaluation of pregnancy complications showed a higher incidence of severe nausea and vomiting in pregnancy (15.8% vs. 10.1%), threatened preterm delivery (18.4% vs. 14.3%) and anemia (28.9% vs. 16.7%).

Out of 38 newborn infants born to mothers with rubella infection during pregnancy, only 3 were preterm baby, this 7.9% rate of PB is lower than the reference figure because gestational age was 0.3 week longer (Table 2.1). The mean birth weight was also larger, but there was no difference in the rate of LBW newborns.

The evaluation of CAs in 32 cases showed two groups. The first group may associate with rubella infection because its components corresponded to the expected CAs. However, it is necessary to consider that deafness could not be diagnosed immediately after birth in Hungary during the study period. There were 4 multiple CAs and three had typical fetal rubella CA syndrome in newborns of pregnant women with rubella infection in II and/or III gestational month: (i) microcephaly + microphthalmia-congenital cataract + ventricular septal defect-persistent ductus arteriosus, (ii) microcephaly + congenital cataract + ventricular septal defect,

(iii) microphthalmia-congenital cataract + persistent ductus arteriosus. Out of 28 isolated CAs, microcephaly in 4 cases (with the rubella infection between III and V gestational month), ductus arteriosus in 4 cases, ventricular septal defect in 3 cases, and complex cardiovascular CAs (ventricular + atrial septal defects and ventricular septal defect + persistent ductus arteriosus) in 2 cases may be associated with rubella infection due to the type of CAs and the time of exposure. The group of other CAs may have only with coincidental association with maternal rubella infection/diseases. Out of the rest 15 CAs, 3 cases with cleft lip+cleft palate and 3 cases with syndactyly are worth mentioning.

In conclusion, rubella virus is a good example of teratogens inducing specific CAs and a particular CA syndrome. It is important to know that this severe CA-entity is preventable.

2.7 Viral Hepatitis

The most common cause of jaundice during pregnancy is hepatitis caused by viruses and other agents. Here only hepatitis viruses are discussed, while other viruses such as herpes viruses (herpes simplex virus and cytomegalovirus) and Epstein-Barr virus (mononucleosis) are neglected because these types of hepatitis did not occur in the data set of the HCCSCA.

Six primary subtypes (A, B, C, D, E, G) of hepatitis virus are known but only hepatitis A, hepatitis B and C occurred in pregnant women in the HCCSCA.

The main characteristics of these 3 viruses are summarized in Table 2.4. Their diagnosis is based on serological markers because unspecific clinical symptoms cannot help to diagnose these diseases.

Table 2.4 Comparative data of hepatitis A, B, C viruses

Viral hepatitis	A	B	C
Viral type	RNA	DNA	RNA
Transmission	Oral	Parenteral	Parenteral intravenous drug use
Source	Feces	Blood, seminal fluid, vaginal	Blood transfusion
Incubation (d)	14–50	30–180	30–160
Symptoms	Jaundice, malaise	Nausea/vomiting, headache, fatigue	Diarrhea, anorexia
Diagnosis	Serology (IgM, 1–6 months after infection)	Serology (HBsAg, anti-HBs HBeAg, anti-HBc HBV-DNA)	Serology (C-antibody)
Risk for carrier status (%)	0	10–15	50–85
Chronic state	None	Yes (persistent)	Yes (persistent)
Consequences	–	Cirrhosis	Cirrhosis
Fetal transmission	No	Yes	Yes

Pregnant women with hepatitis A cannot infect their fetuses.

Hepatitis in adult persons is frequently caused by hepatitis B virus due to mainly sexual contacts (i.e. hepatitis B is sexually transmitted disease) and after the acute phase the so-called chronic carrier condition is common (Dienstag, 2008). After the acute disease, there is a complete recovery due to the developing immunity in 85–90% of patients. Recently, more effective and less resistance-prone antiviral agents have become available to treat hepatitis B infection. However, the virus is remaining in the organism of 10–15% of the infected patients, and 15–30% of these chronically infected patients will have chronic acute hepatitis or cirrhosis or primary liver cancer. In Hungary, the rate of hepatitis B surface antigen (HbsAg) carriers is 0.9%.

The prevalence of acute hepatitis B infection is 1–2 per 1,000 pregnant women (Dinsmoor, 1997). However, the prevalence of chronic hepatitis B infections is 5–15 per 1,000 (Syndman, 1985) and there is a vertical transmission of HbsAg from carrier pregnant women to their offspring. Schweitzer et al. (1973) evaluated 31 infants born to mothers with hepatitis B during or shortly after pregnancy. Out of 10 pregnant women infected in the first and second trimesters, 1, while out of 21 pregnant women infected in the third trimester, 16 had infants with neonatal infection. Out of these 17 infected infants, 6 (35.3%) had LBW. Similar findings were reported by Heiber et al. (1977), while Drew et al. (1978) reported a male predominance among newborns (60 males and 24 females) of mothers with HbsAg positivity.

This high risk explains that screening of hepatitis B serological status was introduced in the Hungarian periconception service or prenatal care clinics and the neonates of seropositive pregnant women should be vaccinated within 12 h of birth. As Beasley et al. (1981) showed there was a significant reduction in the carrier rate in the newborn infants of HbsAg carrier mothers after immunization with hepatitis B immune globulin (HBIG) after birth.

A higher rate of CA was not found in any of the study done by Siegel and Fuerst (1966) in pregnant women with hepatitis without subtype specification, in the study of Zhaomeng et al. (1988) in pregnant women with positive HbsAg titers, or in the study of Ayoola and Johnson (1987) in pregnant women with hepatitis B vaccination in the third trimester. There was no higher rate of fetal death in 34 pregnant women in the study of Adams and Combes (1965).

Hepatitis C is a leading cause of chronic hepatitis, cirrhosis and hepatocellular carcinoma in Europe and the United States (Maheshwari et al., 2008). In general, acute hepatitis C is a mild disease, frequently undiagnosed. After the acute disease, chronic hepatitis is common and nearly 20% of these patients eventually develop cirrhosis and in 1–6% will be affected with hepatocellular cancer (Seeff et al., 1992). Unfortunately, vaccine is not yet available for hepatitis C.

The prevalence of hepatitis C infections was estimated from 1 to 5% in pregnant women (Berger, 1998). Pregnant women affected with hepatitis C less frequently (about 5%) infect their fetuses through transplacental passage than hepatitis B (Granovsky et al., 1998; Conte et al., 2000). When evaluating birth outcomes in pregnant women with viral hepatitis C, a slightly higher rate of PB and perinatal mortality was found but the occurrence of miscarriages, intrauterine growth retardation, and CA did not exceed the population-based figures (Landon, 2004; Jabeen et al., 2000).

2.7.1 Interpretation of Data in the HCCSCA

Out of 22,843 cases, 9 (0.04%), while out of 38,151 controls, 16 (0.04%) had mothers with viral hepatitis during the study pregnancy. Jaundice was characteristic in these pregnant women which was associated with nausea and vomiting in 62.5% of control pregnant women with viral hepatitis. (This figure was 10.1% in the reference sample.) Other pregnancy complications did not show deviation from the usual figures.

The evaluation of birth outcomes of 16 control newborns showed that the mean gestational age was the same than in the reference sample but mean birth weight was 133 g larger; therefore, there was a seemingly fetal growth promoting effect of viral hepatitis (Table 2.1).

Out of 9 cases, 6 different CAs were recorded. Three cases were affected with different manifestations of clubfoot and two boys had undescended testis.

In conclusion, the data of 25 children born to mothers with viral hepatitis did not indicate a higher risk for adverse birth outcomes.

2.8 Mumps

Mumps is caused by a RNS virus that belongs to the family of paramyxovirus. This virus is transmitted by saliva and droplet contamination of patients. The usual incubation period of this virus infection is between 14 and 18 days followed by the prodrome of 1 day with symptoms such a fever, malaise, myalgia, and anorexia.

Mumps itself is an acute non-exanthematous infectious disease of the parotid and salivary glands. In general, parotitis is obvious due to the swollen and tender parotid glands, generally both sides. The parotitis sometimes is followed by involvement of submaxillary glands and rarely of sublinqual glands. However, the generalized manifestation of mumps might involve gonads, brain, and pancreas.

Monif (1974) reported a two-fold increase in the rate of spontaneous abortion in pregnant women affected by mumps during the first trimester (27.3% vs. 13.0%) but a higher rate of PB and LBW newborns were not found. Siegel (1973) and Garcia et al. (1980) did not find higher rate of CAs in infants born to mumps-virus infected pregnant women compared to the infants of uninfected mothers. On the other hand, there was a higher rate of positive skin reactivity to mumps virus antigen in children born with endocardial fibroelastosis (Noren et al., 1963; Shone et al., 1966). This finding was not confirmed (Gersony et al., 1966). Nevertheless, St. Geme et al. (1966) reported a higher risk of endocardial fibroelastosis in newborn infants of pregnant women with mumps. However, the role of mumps-virus remains controversial in the origin of CAs.

The treatment of mumps is symptomatic in general and in pregnant women as well. The live attenuated mumps vaccine is available for the prevention of mumps but is not recommended during the time of planning of pregnancy because mumps is generally benign during pregnancy. There is no evidence that this vaccine virus is teratogenic in humans. Nevertheless, women vaccinated with monovalent mumps vaccine should not become pregnant for at least 1 month. Even if it happens, similarly to the mumps disease during pregnancy, pregnancy termination should not be considered.

2.8.1 Interpretation of Data in the HCCSCA

Out of 22,843 cases, 33 (0.14%), while out of 38,151 controls, 49 (0.13%) had mothers with mumps during the study pregnancy; therefore, mumps was relatively frequent. Among pregnancy complications, the incidence of threatened abortion (24.5% vs. 17.1%), severe nausea and vomiting in pregnancy (14.3% vs. 10.1%), and anemia (24.5% vs. 16.7%) was higher.

Birth outcomes did not show significant deviation from the usual pattern (Table 2.1).

Out of 33 cases, 8 were affected with ventricular septal defect. Other cardiovascular CAs did not show similar cluster (only 1 case was affected with teralogy of Fallot) and it was not characteristic for other CAs as well.

In conclusion, mumps does not seem to have any risk for fetal development, the cluster of ventricular septal defect found in the study likely is chance effect, but it needs to be studied in other databases.

2.9 Viral Genital Warts (Condylomata Acuminata)

Viral genital warts (VGW) (previously called as condylomata acuminate) in females are pedunculated masses in the vulva with very wide range of size from the pinhead to the entire vulva. Sometimes VGW is expanded to the warm and moist environment of anorectal region. Therefore, the diagnosis of this visible VGW is easy on the basis of physical examination. However, as it appeared after the recognition of their causes, most part of this maternal disease are asymptomatic or atypical (Beutner et al., 1998).

The causes of VGW are certain types of *human papillomavirus* (HPV). More than 100 types of HPV have been identified, and about 35 associated with the affection of the epithelium of genital organs. Within these genital organ associated HPVs, two categories were differentiated. The first group includes the high oncogenic risk HPV types such as 16, 18, 20, 31, 45, 54, 55, 56, 64, and 68. The second group involves low oncogenic risk HPV types, i.e. 6, 11, 42, 43, and 44, sometimes with low-grade squamous intraepithelial lesions. VGW are caused by low risk HPV types 6 and 11, rarely types 42, 43, 44, and 54; only the latter belongs to the high oncogenic risk category (Beutner et al., 1998; Gibbs et al., 2004).

VGW belongs to the *sexually transmitted infections/diseases* (STD) category and about 40% of sexually active women are affected with HPV in their genital organs. About 65% of women are infected after the sexual contact of infected partner followed by a long incubation period with a mean of 2.8 months (its range is between 3 weeks and 8 months). The prevalence of VGW is the highest between

16 and 25 years, because the younger age is a predisposition for VGW. Therefore, VGW occurs frequently in pregnant women also with a more rapid growth due to the decrease of cell-mediated immunity.

VGW needs treatment during pregnancy as well. The previously used podophyllin is not recommended in pregnant women. Cryotherapy and surgical excision are preferred; however, tri- and dichloroacetic acids can also be used.

The transplacental transmission of HPV is known but its adverse consequences like CAs in the fetus have not been recognized. The vertical transmission of HPV at delivery may infect the neonate and causes layngeal (respiratory) papillomatosis. However, this complication is very rare (Watts et al., 1998; Tenti et al., 1999).

2.9.1 Results of the Study (XVII)

Out of 22,843 cases, 17 (0.07%), while out of 38,151 controls, 25 (0.07%) had mothers affected with VGW during the study pregnancy.

The mean age of pregnant women with VGW (21.7 vs. 25.5 year) was lower with a higher proportion of primiparae (85.7% vs. 47.4%) than in pregnant women without VGW. Out of 17 case mothers, 3, while out of 25 control mothers 6 were treated locally by podophyllum. Pregnancy complications of pregnant women with VGW did not deviate from the figures of the reference sample.

However, birth outcomes of control newborns are noteworthy (Table 2.1). An obvious female excess among newborns (there was 17% male deficit). This phenomenon associated with the obvious reduction of gestational age ($p = 0.002$) and a much higher rate of PB (28.0%; 3.6, 1.5–8.6). The mean birth weight was also somewhat smaller ($p = 0.33$) and associated with a 2.1 fold increase in the rate of LBW (0.9, 0.2–4.7); however, these differences were not significant at the calculation of gestational age corrected figures. Therefore, VGW drastically shortened the fetal period and a higher rate of fetal death also cannot be excluded due to the change of sex ratio of live-born babies.

The distribution of CAs in 17 cases did not indicate any cluster of CAs, 4 cases with cardiovascular CA including 2 cases with rare transposition of the great vessels, 2 cases with neural tube defects (anencephaly and spina bifida), 2 cases with hypospadias, 2 cases with syndactyly, while other 7 CAs occurred only once.

In conclusion, the birth outcomes of pregnant women with VGW showed very high rate of PB therefore this viral infection needs further studies.

2.10 Cytomegalovirus

Cytomegalovirus (CMV) is a very large (molecular weight is 60 million) double-stranded DNA-virus which belongs to the family of herpesvirus. Infections occur in close personal contact, mainly in sexual partnership by contaminated seminal fluid, urine, saliva or blood. The incubation period is long; the mean is 40 days with the range between 28 and 60 days.

The diagnosis is a difficult task because most acquired CMV infections are asymptomatic or even if symptomatic, the clinical presentation of CMV disease is unspecific similar to mononucleosis. Symptoms, such as malaise, fever, lymphadenopathy and hepatosplenomegaly may occur. Therefore, the diagnosis is based on serologic method. After CMV infection CMV-specific IgM antibody is present in serum with a decline after 30–60 days to a low level detectable for many months. The four-fold or greater increase in the IgG titer also indicates a CMV infection. The most exact diagnosis of CMV infection is the isolation of virus in tissue culture (Brown, 1998).

In general, CMV remains latent in host cells after the primary infection, like herpes virus. CMV disease may also be caused by the reactivation of latent virus.

The so-called *fetal cytomegalovirus disease* (FCD) may be the consequence of the primary CMV infection of pregnant women after hematogeneous dissemination of the virus across the placenta. The reactivation of the latent CMV infection in general does not cause FCD (Fowler et al., 1992). The occurrence of primary CMV infection was found to be 1–5% in pregnant women by serological methods (Sever et al., 1962; Yow et al., 1988) followed by the infection of every fourth (about 25%) fetuses (Melish and Hanshaw, 1973), and 0.6–0.7% of all infants are born with intrauterine CMV infection (Dollard et al., 2007). Symptoms of FCID can be diagnosed at birth in about 11% of newborn infants after intrauterine infection (Stagno and Ewhitley, 1985; Yow et al., 1988; Gibbs et al., 2004; Kebbeson et al., 2007).

However, the time of the primary infection in pregnant women is also important. CMV is large virus; therefore, its transplacental transmission in general does not occur before the 12th gestational week (Alexander, 1967). Therefore, CMV has not been shown to cause spontaneous abortion. Fetuses could be infected during the last two trimesters, but the highest risk is expected after the primary infection of CMV between IV and VI gestational months (Krech et al., 1971).

If we calculate with 2.2% rate of primary infection in pregnant women (Yow et al., 1988), we can expect intrauterine infection in 0.55% of fetuses and FCD somewhat less than in 0.1% of births.

The most obvious symptoms of FCD are microcephaly and intrauterine growth retardation at birth, completed by chorioretinitis and optic atrophy (blindness). After birth, hepatosplenomegaly with hyperbilirubinemia, i.e. jaundice and elevated serum transaminase level, intracranial calcification, and seizures may occur. The long-term consequences of FCID are mental retardation, sensorineural hearing loss, and vision problems, although sometimes these anomalies can be diagnosed only after several months after birth, usually until the 2 years of life (Pass et al., 1980).

Unfortunately, there is no real prevention of CMV infections because effective vaccine and MV hyperimmune globulin have the potential to decrease incident cases of maternal and congenital CMV infection (Pass et al., 2009; Nyholm and Schless, 2010). After the diagnosis of CMV infection during pregnancy, sonographic findings may be suggestive in the detection of serious fetal anomalies such as microcephaly, ventriculomegaly, intracerebral calcification with intrauterine growth retardation and sometimes with oligohydramnios (Donner et al., 1993).

2.10.1 Interpretation of Data in the HCCSCA

There were 16 (0.07%) cases and 19 (0.05%) controls in the data set of the HCCSCA. The maternal characteristics did not show any special pattern. The occurrence of maternal diseases and pregnancy complications did not show difference from the values of reference sample.

The mean gestational age was the same in 19 control babies born to mothers with CMV infection and in the reference sample (Table 2.1), however, the mean birth weight was 135 g smaller and it indicated some intrauterine fetal growth retardation confirmed by the higher rate of LBW newborns.

Out of 16 cases, 6 were affected by cardiovascular CA: 2 cases with transposition of the great vessels, 2 ventricular septal defects, 1 persistent ductus arteriosus, and 1 case with unspecified CA. Transposition of the great vessels is a rare CA. Its doubling is an interesting finding but this CA is not considered as part of FCD. All other non-cardiovascular CAs occurred only once. Among them one case with microcephaly and one case with multiple CA including microcephaly and unspecified eye CA are worth mentioning because they may fit FCD.

In conclusion, some intrauterine growth retardation was found in the fetuses of pregnant women with CMV infection. The defects/diseases of FCID are difficult to detect on the basis of usual CAs, therefore, its diagnosis occurred rarely in the HCCSCA.

2.11 Other or Unspecified Viral Infections

This category of the ICD is very heterogeneous including the suspected virus infections caused by Coxsackie virus, ECHO virus, Adenovirus, Rhinovirus or others that could not be proven by laboratory methods or virus infection which had unspecified nature or site.

Coxsackie viruses are RNA viruses and belong to the groups of enteroviruses. Their transplacental transmission was demonstrated but adverse effect on the development of the fetus was not found (XVIII, Gibbs et al., 2004).

Echoviruses also belong to the group of enteroviruses and their infection may cause severe diseases in neonates, however, a higher risk of fetal death or CA was not found (Philip and Larsen, 1973).

Adenoviruses and parvoviruses have a role in the origin of non-immune hydrops but their contribution to the origin of other CAs is debated (Wilkins, 2004). Myco- and ureaplasmas are also blamed to have a role in the origin of fetal death, intra-amniotic infection, PB, LBW, and neonatal infection but their role in the origin of CA has not been proven (Gibbs et al., 2004).

2.11.1 Interpretation of Data in the HCCSCA

The data set of the HCCCA is comprised of 129 subjects with this diagnosis. Out of 22,843 cases, 80 (0.35%), while out of 38,151 controls, 49 (0.13%) were born to pregnant women with *other or unspecified viral infections* (OUVI). The nearly 3 fold higher rate of OUVI in the case group is noteworthy, though of the 77 cases, only 3 and of the 49 controls, 0 was medically recorded in the prenatal care logbook.

The onset of OUVI was rare in the third trimester in both case and control mothers, and about one-third of the infections occurred in the first trimester (38.8% in case and 32.7% in control mothers) with the duration of 1–4 weeks. However, all OUVI with the onset in I gestational month continued in II month.

Pregnant women with OUVI were about 1 year older but mean birth order did not show difference compared to the reference sample. The proportion of professional and skilled worker women (53.5% vs. 40.7%) was higher in pregnant women with OUVI than in pregnant women without OUVI. The use of folic acid showed obvious difference between case (48.8% and 49.4%) and control (57.1% and 54.5%) women but not with or without OUVI within these study groups.

The evaluation of maternal diseases revealed an unusual finding. The incidence of influenza-common cold with secondary complications was less frequent in pregnant women with OUVI both in the case (7.5% vs. 21.4%) and control (8.2% vs. 18.4%) mother groups. Therefore, it is not possible to exclude that some pregnant women in this group had influenza or common cold with secondary complications. Other acute and chronic diseases did not show difference among the study groups.

There was another unusual finding among pregnancy complications. Case mothers with or without OUVI did not show difference in the incidence of pregnancy complications. However, control mothers with OUVI had a much higher rate of threatened abortion (34.7% vs. 17.0%) and preterm delivery (20.4% vs. 14.3%) than control mothers without OUVI. This threatened abortion rate was the highest among all infectious diseases.

Pregnant women with OUVI were frequently treated by ampicillin (26.4% vs. 7.0%), penamecillin (24.0% vs. 6.3%), cotrimoxazole: sulfamethoxazole+trimethoprim (7.8% vs. 1.3%), doxycycline (5.4% vs. 0.2%), cefalexin (5.4% vs. 1.0%) and parenteral penicillin (3.9% vs. 0.3%), in addition to clotrimazole (14.0% vs. 7.7%) compared to pregnant women without OUVI. The use of antipyretic drugs such as acetylsalicylic acid, paracetamol, aminophenazone, dipyrone (46.2% vs. 9.3%) was also common.

Birth outcomes showed some "benefit" of OUVI in the children without CA of control mothers (Table 2.1). Mean gestational age at delivery was longer and mean birth weight was somewhat larger, therefore there was a lower rate of PB.

However, the risk of some CAs was unusual high in the offspring of pregnant women with OUVI (Table 2.5).

The higher risk for congenital hydrocephalus and renal a/dysgenesis was based only on 2 cases, while the very high risk of intestinal atresia/stenosis and CA of diaphragm occurred in 3–3 cases. The high risk of neural-tube defects was more obvious if these cases were evaluated after maternal OUVI in II gestational month, i.e. when neural-tube defects have their critical period. Isolated cleft lip $\pm$ cleft palate and cleft palate have different etiology; nevertheless, similar environmental agents have a role in their origin. UVIP is an exception because cleft lip $\pm$ cleft palate occurred in 11 cases resulting in a high risk for this anomaly, while cleft palate

Table 2.5 Estimation of risk of different CAs in cases born to pregnant women with OUVI

Study groups	Grand total No.	Entire pregnancy No.	%	OR	95% CI	II–III gestational months No.	%	OR	95% CI
Controls	38,151	4,923	0.1	Reference		16	0.04	Reference	
Isolated CAs									
Neural-tube defects	1,202	6	0.5	**3.9**	**1.7–9.1**	6	0.50	**14.7**	**5.6–38.8**
Cong. hydrocephalus	314	2	0.6	**5.0**	**1.2–20.6**	0	0.0	**6.6**	**1.2–34.8**
Cleft lip ± palate	1,375	11	0.8	**6.3**	**3.3–12.1**	6	0.44	2.3	0.6–8.3
Cardiovascular CAs	4,480	19	0.4	**3.3**	**1.9–5.6**	6	0.07	–	–
Intestinal atresia/stenosis	158	3	1.9	**15.1**	**4.6–48.8**	1	0.63	–	–
Renal a/dysgenesis	126	2	1.6	**12.5**	**3.0–52.1**	0	0.0	–	–
Hypospadias	3,036	4	0.1	1.0	0.4–2.8	1	0.03	–	–
Undescended testis	2,052	3	0.1	1.1	0.4–3.7	1	0.05	–	–
Clubfoot	2,425	10	0.4	**3.2**	**1.6–6.4**	2	0.08	1.8	0.4–12.2
Poly/syndactyly	1,744	6	0.3	**2.7**	**1.1–6.3**	1	0.06	–	–
CAs of the diaphragm	244	3	1.2	**9.7**	**3.0–31.3**	1	0.41	–	–
Other isolated CAs	3,203	5[a]	0.2	1.2	0.5–3.1	1	0.03	–	–
Multiple CAs	1,349	2	0.1	1.2	0.3–4.8	2	0.15	**4.4**	**1.0–19.3**
Total	22,843	80	0.4	**2.7**	**1.9–3.9**	31	0.14	**3.7**	**2.0–7.0**

[a]Microtia, cleft palate only, oesophageal atresia, anorectal atresia, exomphalos.

was recorded only once. The distribution of 19 cases with cardiovascular CAs was the following: 1 tetralogy of Fallot, 1 common ventricle, 8 ventricular septal defect, 1 atrial septal defect type II, 1 congenital insufficiency of the aortic valve, 2 coarctation of the aorta, 1 stenosis of the pulmonary artery, 1 CA of the cerebral vessels, 3 unspecified. The groups of clubfoot (talipes equinovarus and calcaneovarus, talipes calcaneovalgus, metatarsus varus, mild deformations) and poly/syndactyly include subgroups with heterogeneous origin.

The secondary results of the study showed a longer gestational age at delivery and somewhat larger mean birth weight in newborns of pregnant women with OUVI. These short infectious diseases likely stimulated pregnant women to practice more conscious prenatal care and to live a healthier lifestyle, in addition OUVI related antibiotic treatment may have a beneficial effect for asymptomatic or untreated vulvovaginal infections.

When evaluating the possible association between OUVI and higher risk of some CAs in their offsprings, the effect of OUVI itself (including fever), the causes of OUVI (i.e. the microbial agents), and related drug treatments, other confounders and chance effect should be considered.

Most OUVI usually presents with fever which was frequently but not always mentioned in the questionnaires. Some previous studies indicated an association between neural-tube defects (XIX) or cleft lip ± cleft palate (II) and high fever.

Of course, the direct teratogenic effect of viruses cannot be excluded. The possible association of OUVI with intestinal atresia/stenosis is also worth mentioning because this CA may have a critical period after the first trimester and viruses were blamed to have some role in their origin.

Drugs have a role in the origin of CAs and cotrimoxazole (Hernandez-Diaz et al., 2000; 19, 20) and oxytetracycline (8) are well known human teratogens. Ampicillin also was used more frequently by the mothers with OUVI but ampicillin was evaluated in the HCCSCA without showing any effect on neural-tube development (4). However, parenteral penicillin (1), penamecillin (3), cotrimoxazole (28), doxycycline (9), cefalexin (11), and antipyretic drugs such as acetylsalicylic acid (75. 76), paracetamol (77), and dipyrone (81) had no human teratogenic effect.

Previous intervention trials showed an obvious protective effect of folic acid or folic acid-containing multivitamins during the periconceptional period for neural-tube defects (XIII) and some others CAs such as cardiovascular CAs (VII, VIII), therefore, these supplementations were evaluated as confounders in our study.

This evaluation was based on retrospective maternal information, therefore, strong recall bias need to be considered. Recall bias can double the observed risk of CA (XX) but even higher risks were found in this study in some CAs.

In conclusion, an unexpectedly high risk of some CAs was found in the pregnancies of women with OUVI; therefore, it is necessary to further study viral infections during pregnancy to understand the specific role of these viruses in inducing CAs.

2.12 Syphilis

Syphilis is caused by the spirochete *Treponema pallidum* and in general it is spread by sexual contact and results in chronic systemic infectious process including 4 stages: primary, secondary, latent, and tertiary syphilis (Sanchez and Wendel, 1997).

After exposure, there is an average 21 days incubation period (with a range of 10–90 days) followed by the primary stage. The primary stage is manifested in the form of chancre, i.e. a painless ulcerated lesion with a raised border and indurated base in addition to painless inguinal lymphadenopathy. This primary chancre spontaneously disappears after 2–6 weeks without treatment. Primary chancre is followed by the secondary stage of syphilis. The secondary stage means spirochetemia with the clinical manifestation of generalized lymphadenopathy, condylomata, and generalized maculopapular rash mainly on the palms, soles, and mucous patches. These symptoms again spontaneously disappear within 2–6 weeks, although at this point of the infection spirochetes are disseminated into any organ including central nervous system. The next stage of syphilis as its name suggests is latent without apparent clinical disease. After 1–2 years of infection, patients do not infect their partners by sexual transmission. About one third of the untreated patients get affected by the tertiary stage of syphilis with the involvement of central nervous, cardiovascular, and musculocutaneous systems.

In pregnant women affected with first, second, and rarely latent stage of syphilis, *Treponema* can be transferred across the placenta and can infect the fetus as early as the 6th gestational weeks. However, the typical manifestation of the so-called congenital syphilis is the consequence of cutaneous and mucous inflammatory lesions, i.e. fetal disease developed after the 16th week of pregnancy when fetal immunocompetence starts. The risk of fetal syphilis disease is about 50% in pregnant women with primary and secondary syphilis. They have a higher rate of adverse pregnancy outcomes such as stillbirths, PB, and LBW newborns (i.e. intrauterine growth retardation). The classic late manifestation of "fetal syphilis disease" includes saddle nose, Hutchinson teeth, mulberry molars, interstitial keratitis, eight nerve deafness, rhagades, saber shins, and the symptoms of central nervous system's infections: hydrocephalus, general paresis, optic nerve atrophy, mental retardation, while the early manifestation represents the symptoms of active syphilis at birth (maculopapular rash that may progress to desquamation or formation of vesicles and bullae, snuffles, mucous patches in the oropharyngeal cavity, hepatosplenomegaly, jaundice, lymphadenopathy, chorioretinits, etc.). However, most infected newborns are asymptomatic at birth therefore the diagnosis needs laboratory tests (Gibbs et al., 2004).

After the introduction of penicillin in the 1940s, syphilis has become treatable and fetal syphilis disease is preventable in the offspring of infected pregnant women. In Hungary all pregnant women are screened for syphilis at the first visit in the prenatal care clinics, and positive cases are treated.

2.12.1 Interpretation of Data in the HCCSCA

Out of 22,843 cases, 3 (0.01%), while out of 38,151 controls, 2 (0.01%) had mothers with syphilis during the study pregnancy. These unexpectedly low numbers of cases and controls can be explained by the very effective public health action against the syphilis in Hungary from the 1960s; in addition, most pregnancies with syphilis infections are terminated.

Two control newborns without CA had 4,150 and 3,250 g birth weight with 39 and 40 gestational weeks at delivery, respectively. Three cases had isolated microcephaly, ventricular septal defect, and renal dysgenesis, respectively.

In conclusion, fetal syphilis disease is rare in Hungary.

2.13 Gonococcal Infection

Gonorrhea caused by *Neisseria gonorrhoeae* was the most common classical sexually transmitted disease in Hungary. The risk of transmission of gonorrhea from an infected man to an exposed woman is about 70%. After a 3–5 days incubation period, the characteristic symptoms are vaginal discharge and dysuria. However, gonococcal infections are most commonly asymptomatic and/or undiagnosed in pregnant women (Gibbs et al., 2004). Among the adverse effects of infection with gonorrhea in pregnant women, first the so-called "gonococcal ophthalmia neonatorum" was recognized. Pregnant women with gonoccocal infection, particularly during the second and third trimesters, have an increased risk for disseminated infection which may induce the "amniotic infection syndrome" due to gonorrheal chorioamnionitis (Handsfield et al., 1973; Engebretsen, 1974). The consequence of this syndrome is intrauterine growth retardation, premature rupture of the membranes, therefore PB and neonatal sepsis is common. However, the possible role of gonococcal infection in the origin of CAs was not reported.

The diagnosis of gonococcal infection is based on the clinical symptoms and history of pregnant women but it needs confirmation by laboratory methods. Both symptomatic and asymptomatic infections should be treated in pregnant women. The first recommended treatment was penicillin, but now it has to be considered that about 10% of N. gonorrhea had become resistant to penicillin and a major part of pregnant women with gonococcal infection also have chlamidial infection. At present the first recommended treatment protocol includes cephalosporins and amoxicillin.

2.13.1 Interpretation of Data in the HCCSCA

Only one case with ventricular septal defect was recorded in the HCCCA.

2.14 Dermatomycosis

There are two main groups of these superficial fungal infections. On one hand, dermatophytons such as *Trichophyton, Epidermophyton, and Microsprorums* cause diseases in the stratum corneum, nails, and hair. On the other hand, *Candida albicans* causes candidiasis-moniliasis in the moist intertriginosus regions of skin and mucous membranes, in addition, in nailbed after intrauterine infection (Holmes et al., 1983; Ambrus-Rudolph et al., 2006).

2.14.1 Interpretation of Data in the HCCSCA

Out of 22,843 cases, 48 (0.24%), while out of 38,151 controls, 71 (0.19%) had mothers with dermatomycosis in the study pregnancy.

Among pregnancy complications, nearly all showed lower incidence in women with recorded dermatomycosis: threatened abortion (11.3% vs. 17.1%) and preterm delivery (11.3% vs. 14.3%), severe nausea and vomiting in pregnancy (5.6% vs. 10.1%), preeclampsia-eclampsia (1.4% vs. 3.0%), and anemia (9.9% vs. 16.7%). Only edema/excessive weight gain without hypertension was more frequent in pregnant women with dermatomycosis (7.0% vs. 2.4%).

Birth outcomes of newborns without CA did not show difference from the figures of the reference sample (Table 2.1).

However, 48 cases with CA showed some clusters of CA: 6 cases with cardiovascular CA (common ventricle 1, ventricular septal defect 2, endocardial cushion defect 1, unspecified CA 2), 6 cases were affected with the different manifestations of clubfoot, other 6 cases with hypospadias, and further 6 cases with orofacial cleft (1 cleft palate only, 3 cleft lip, 3 cleft lip with cleft palate), 5 cases with undescended testis, 3 cases with neural-tube defects (1 anencephaly, 2 spina bifida), and 3 cases with multiple CA (with different component CAs).

In conclusion, dermatomycosis were reported with low incidence of pregnancy complications and showed some association with certain CA-groups. It would be necessary to clarify whether these associations are explained by the maternal disease (investigating all agents separately), drug treatments, confounders, or chance.

2.15 Toxoplasmosis

Toxoplasmosis is caused by a parasite: *Toxoplasma gondii* that belongs to the family of coccidia. The natural host of this parasite is the cat because the sexual cycle of *T. gondii* happens only in the intestinal tract of cats; therefore, the main source of infection is coccidian oocysts from cat feces. This facultative parasite causes disease, i.e. toxoplasmosis only in immunosuppressed adult patients (e.g. AIDS) or immunological unprotected fetuses.

The serological screening of *T. gondii* infection in 8,289 Austrian pregnant women detected 20 primary infections. This 0.24% rate may reflect the incidence of "new" infections (Fuith et al., 1988). In Hungary 42.9% of reproductive aged women were seropositive, i.e. had previous asymptomatic infection (XXI) and our estimation regarding to the new infection of pregnant women was 0.20% in Hungary (XXII). Congenital toxoplasmosis or correctly fetal/connatal toxoplasmosis (i.e. a fetal disease) may occur after the primary infection of pregnant women after the first trimester. Partly because, these large parasites cannot cross the placenta before the 14th gestational week (Paul, 1962), and also because fetal immunocompetence develops after this period when the fetus can react to this infection with inflammatory disease as the result of maturing fetal immune system. The risk of fetal toxoplasmosis in previously infected seropositive pregnant women is minimal because chronic or latent infection can be manifested only in immunosuppressed pregnant women.

After the primary infection of pregnant women, about 40% of fetuses are infected. However, the proportion of fetuses with toxoplasmosis, i.e. disease that had symptoms at birth was estimated between 28% (Romana et al., 2001) and 5% (Daffos et al., 1988), i.e. a very wide range and the rate also depends on the treatment. For example, all infected pregnant women were treated with pyrimethamine and sulfadiazine and none of the infants had clinical signs of fetal toxoplasmosis in the previously mentioned Austrian study (Fuith et al., 1988). The symptoms of fetal toxoplasmosis are the consequences of fetal meningoencephalitis classified by Sabin (1942) as a tetrad: (i) chorioretinitis (99%), and the secondary symptoms of inflammatory disease of the central nervous system such as (ii) brain, mainly periventricular calcification (63%), (iii) secondary microcephaly or hydrocephaly (ventriculomegaly) (50%), i.e. they are not true CAs, (iv) and seizures, paresis, and mental retardation (59%). The occurrence of these symptoms was estimated by Feldman (1968) and in their study toxoplasmosis also showed a higher risk for PB (31%). Later in neonatal life, these symptoms are completed by hepatosplenomegaly, ascites, and rash (Daffos et al., 1988), i.e. the symptoms of generalized fetal toxoplasmosis.

The seroconversion proves the primary infection in pregnant women, but not the infection and/or disease of the fetus. There are two important tasks after the diagnosis of primary infection of *T. gondii* during pregnancy. The first is the treatment of pregnant women by pyremethamine, sulfonamides and spiramycin, but their combination was found more effective than single-agent therapy. The second is the ultrasound diagnosis of expected symptoms of fetal disease, i.e. ventriculomegaly, microcephaly, intracranial calcification, hepatosplenomegaly with fetal growth retardation because it helps to concretize the risk for fetal infection.

A *T. gondii* specific gene was identified by Hohlfield et al. (1994), therefore, now it is possible to diagnose this parasitic infection from the amniotic fluid utilizing a PCR test. Out of 339 pregnant women with seroconversion, 34 (10.0%) had fetal toxoplasmosis. The overall sensitivity of this PCR test in amniotic fluid specimens was 64% (Romana et al., 2001) with the greatest sensitivity between 17 and 21 gestational weeks, while the specificity and positive predictive value of the test were 100%. In the study of Daffos et al. (1988), out of 746 pregnant women with serologically confirmed primary infection with spiramycin treatment, 39 (5.2%) had infected fetuses based on the examination of umbilical blood sample. The pregnant women in their study were treated with pyrimethamine plus either sulfadoxine or sulfadiazine. Out of these 39 infected fetuses, 24 were not born because those pregnancies were terminated. Out of the rest 15 fetuses, 13 (86.7%) newborn infants were found healthy during a 3-month observation period, while chorioretinitis was diagnosed in 2 infants.

Unfortunately, vaccine is not available for the prevention of fetal toxoplasmosis at present time. Preconceptional serological examination helps to differentiate seropositive (i.e. protected) and seronegative women before conception. Seronegative pregnant women should be advised to avoid contact with stray cats or cat litter, to wash their hand after preparing row meat for cooking and never to eat raw or "bloody" meat, in addition to wash fruits and vegetables carefully to remove all possible contamination by oocysts (Egerman and Beazley, 1998; Gibbs et al., 2004). In some countries seronegative women are suggested to have another serological examination during the second part of pregnancy to identify seroconversion and seroconvert pregnant women are treated.

2.15.1 Interpretation of Data in the HCCSCA

Out of 22,843 cases, 35 (0.15%), while out of 38,151 controls, 27 (0.07%) had mothers with toxoplasma infection during the study pregnancy.

In general, the incidence of pregnancy complications was lower in pregnant women with suspected toxoplasma infection: threatened abortion (14.8% vs. 17.1%)

and preterm delivery (11.1% vs. 14.3%), severe nausea and vomiting in pregnancy (0.0% vs. 10.1%) and anemia (7.4% vs. 16.7%).

Birth outcomes of 27 newborns with CA showed unusual pattern: gestational age was somewhat (0.3 week) shorter with a higher rate of PB; the mean birth weight was somewhat larger with lower rate of LBW newborns.

The rate of reported toxoplasmosis in case pregnant women (0.15%) who had child with CAs exceeded the rate of suspected toxoplasmosis (0.07%) in control pregnant women by 2.1 fold. The distribution of CAs, however, did not show characteristic pattern, only 2 cases with hydrocephalus and of the 3 cases with multiple CA, two (one preterm boy had congenital hydrocephalus + persistent ductus arteriosus + stenosis of small intestine + undescended testis and microcephaly + buphthalmos + ear CA) may have some association of fetal toxoplasmosis. Other most frequent CAs were cardiovascular CAs (4 ventricular septal defect, 1 hypoplastic left heart, 2 unspecified), orofacial clefts (1 cleft lip, 3 cleft lip with cleft palate), 3 undescended testis and 3 hypospadias.

In conclusion, suspected toxoplasmosis in pregnant women associated with a lower incidence of pregnancy complications and showed a higher risk for some CA-groups. It is necessary to further investigate whether these associations are explained by the maternal disease, drug treatments, confounders, or chance.

2.16 Ascaris

There are five important intestinal worms or nematodes: Ascaris lumbricoides, hookworm, Strongyloides stercoralis, Trichuris trichuria, and Enterobius vermicularis (pinworm). Ascariasis associates with mild abdominal discomfort and eosinophilia, but intestinal and common bile duct obstruction may develop in severe illness (Jones and DeHovitz, 1986).

2.16.1 Interpretation of Data in the HCCSCA

Out of 22,843 cases, 7 (0.03%), while out of 38,151 controls, 10 (0.03%) had mothers with reported ascariasis.

Pregnancy complications did not differ from the distribution of pregnancy complications of the reference sample.

Birth outcomes of 10 newborns without CA showed contradictory pattern (Table 2.1): while mean gestational age at delivery was longer by 0.4 week and PB did not occur; the mean birth weight was 87 g smaller.

Seven cases had CA, only one CA (syndactyly) occurred twice. Atrial septal defect type II, anal atresia, hypospadias, torticollis and multiple CA were detected in 1–1 case.

In conclusion, ascaris infection during pregnancy does not seem to have a risk for adverse birth outcomes.

2.17 Scabies

The cause of this high contagious ectodermal disease is Sarcoptes scabei which insert themselves into the stratum corneum of the skin and lay their eggs into the stratum corneum. The incubation period of 30–40 days is followed by pruritic papules.

2.17.1 Interpretation of Data in the HCCSCA

Out of 22,843 cases, 3 (0.01%), while out of 38,151 controls, 1 (0.002%) had mothers with scabies during the study pregnancy.

One newborn without CA was born on the 41st gestation week with very low birth weight (2200 g). Two cases were affected with polydactyly, while one with obstructive CA of urinary tract (stricture of ureteropelvic junction).

The available data do not allow drawing any conclusion.

2.18 Final Conclusions

The evaluation of population based data set of the HCCSCA regarding to infectious diseases/infections during pregnancy showed the following basic observations:

(1) Some virus infections during pregnancy do not associate with a higher risk of CA.
(2) Rubella-virus in II and III gestational months induces a characteristic pattern of CA-syndrome, while varicella-virus, cytomegalovirus, and rubella-virus after the first trimester are associated with characteristic patterns of fetal diseases.
(3) The indirect teratogenic effect of high fever may occur in viral diseases associated with high fever.
(4) An unexpectedly high risk of some CAs was found in the pregnancies of women with unspecified virus infection; therefore, it is necessary to identify these agents to better understand which viruses and how can induce these CAs.
(5) The population-based surveillances of CA is useful to evaluate the virus associated CAs, but is not appropriate for the detection of long-term consequences and functional symptoms of fetal diseases.
(6) The proportion of CAs caused by infection is about 1% while on the basis of HCCSCA data infectious origin of other fetal diseases is estimated higher. In addition, the proportion of PB due to microbial agents is very large but these data will be presented in detail when evaluating infectious diseases of the female genital organs.
(7) Fetal rubella CA-syndrome and fetal disease, in addition to fetal varicella disease are preventable with vaccination, also, the indirect teratogenic effect of high fever related maternal diseases due to infections can be reduced by antipyretic drugs.

References

ACOG Practice Bulletin. Management of herpes in pregnancy. Obstet Gynecol 2007; 109: 1489–1498.

Adams RH, Combes B. Viral hepatitis during pregnancy. J Am Med Ass (JAMA) 1965; 192: 195–198.

Alexander ER. Maternal and neonatal infection with cytomegalovirus in Taiwan. Pediat Res 1967; 1: 210 only.

Alford CA, Neva FA, Weller TH. Virologic and serologic studies on human products of conception after maternal rubella. N Engl J Med 1964; 271: 1275–1281.

Ambros-Rudolph CM, Müllegger RR, Vaughan-Jones SA et al. The specific dermatoses of pregnancy revisited and reclassified: results of a retrospective two-center study on 505 pregnant patients. J Am Acad Dermatol 2006; 54: 395–404.

Arvin A, Campadielli-Fiume G, Mocarski E et al. (eds.) Human Herpesviruses. Biology, Therapy and Immunoprophylaxis. Cambridge University Press, Cambridge, 2007-04-17.

Avgil M, Ornoy A. Herpes simplex virus and Epstein-Barr virus infections in pregnancy: consequences of neonatal or intrauterine infection. Reprod Toxicol 2006; 21: 436–445.

Ayoola EA, Johnson AOK. Hepatitis B vaccine in pregnancy: immunogenicity and transfer of antobodies to infants. Int J Gynaecol Obstet 1987; 25: 297–301.

Baldwin S, Whitley RJ. Intrauterine herpes simplex virus infection. Teratology 1989; 39: 1–10.

Beasley RP, Lin C-C, Wang K-Y et al. Hepatitis B immune globulin (HBIG) efficiency in the interruption of perinatal transmission of Hepatitis B virus carrier state. Lancet 1981; 2: 388–393.

Benedetti J, Corey L, Ashley RL. Recurrence rate in genital herpes after symptomatic first-episode infection. Ann Intern Med 1994; 121: 847–885.

Berger A. Mother to child transmission of hepatitis C virus: prospective study of risk factors and timing of infection in children born to women seronegative for HIV-1. Science commentary: behaviour of hepatitis C virus. Br Med J (BMJ) 1998; 317: 440.

Beutner KR, Reitano MV, Richwald GA et al. External genital warts: report of the American medical association conference. Clin Infect Dis 1998; 27: 796–806.

Boehm FH, Estes W, Wright PF, Growdon JF. Management of genital herpes simplex virus infection occurring during pregnancy. Am J Obstet Gynecol 1981; 141: 735–740.

Botto LD, Lynberg MC, Erickson JD. Congenital heart defects, maternal febrile diseases and multivitamin use: a population-based study. Epidemiology 2001; 12: 485–490.

Botto LD, Olney RS, Erickson JD. Vitamin supplements and the risk for congenital anomalies other than neural-tube defects. Am J Med Genet C 2004; 125C: 12–21.

Brown HL, Abernathy MP. Cytomegalovirus infection. Semin Perinatol 1998. 45: 260–266.

Brown ZA, Vontver LA, Benedetti J et al. Effects on infants of a first episode of genital herpes during pregnancy. N Engl J Med 1987; 317: 1246–1250.

Brown ZA, Benedetti J, Ashley R et al. Neonatal herpes simplex virus infection in relation to asymptomatic maternal infection at the time of labor. N Engl J Med 1991; 324: 1247–1352.

Brown ZA, Benedetti J, Selke S et al. Asymptomatic maternal shedding of herpes simplex virus at the onset of labor: relationship to preterm labor. Obstet Gynecol 1996; 87: 483–488.

Brown ZA, Zelke S, Zeh J et al. The acquisition of herpes simplex virus during pregnancy. N Engl J Med 1997; 337: 509–515.

Brown ZA, Gardella C, Wald A, Morrow RA, Corey L. Genital herpes complicating pregnancy. Obstet Gynecol 2005; 106: 845–856.

Cantwell MF, Shehab AM, Costello AM. Congenital tuberculosis. N Engl J Med 1994; 330: 1051.

Catalano PM, Meritt AO, Mead PB. Incidence of genital herpes simplex virus at the time of delivery in women with known risk factors. Am J Obstet Gynecol 1991; 164: 1303–1306.

CDC: Centers for Disease Control and Prevention. Rubella and congenital rubella syndrome – United States, January 1, 1991–May 7, 1994. MMWR (Morb Mortal Wkly Rep) 1994; 43: 391–401.

CDC: Centers for Disease Control and Prevention. Prevention of varicella. Recommendation of the Advisory Committee on Immunization Practices (ACIP). MMWR (Morb Mortal Wkly Rep) 1996; 45: (RR-11).

CDC: Centers for Disease Control and Prevention. Sexually Transmitted Diseases Treatment Guidelines. MMWR (Morb Mortal Wkly Rep) 2006. 55. (RR-7).

Chalhub EG, Baenziger J, Feigen RD, Middlekamp JN, Shackelford GD. Congenital herpes simplex type II infection with extensive hepatic calcification bone lesions and cataracts, complete post-mortem examination. Dev Med Child Neurol 1977; 19: 527–534.

Conte D, Fraquelli M, Prati D et al. Prevalence of clinical course of chronic hepatitis C virus (HCV) infection and rate of HCV vertical transmission in a cohort of 15,250 pregnant women. Hepatology 2000, 31: 751–755.

Creasy RK, Resnik R, Lams DJ. (eds.) Maternal-Fetal Medicint. 5th ed. Saunders, Philadelphia, 2004.

Daffos F, Forestier F, Capella-Pavlovsky M et al. Prenatal management of 746 pregnancies at risk for congenital toxoplasmosis. N Engl J Med 1988; 318: 271–275.

DeHovitz JA, Johnson WD Jr, Pape JW. Gastrointestinal infections. In: Roberts BR (ed.) Infectious Diseases: Pathogenesis, Diagnosis, and Therapy. Year Book Medical Publ., Chicago, 1986. pp. 116–131.

Dienstag JL. Hepatitis B virus infection. N Engl J Med 2008; 359: 1486–1500.

Dinsmoor MJ. Hepatitis in the obstetric patient. Infect Dis North Am 1997; 11: 77–91.

Dollard SC, Grosse SD, Ross DS. New estimates of the prevalence of neurological and sensory sequelae and mortality associated with congenital cytomegalovirus infection. Rev Med Virol 2007; 17: 355–363.

Donner C, Liesnard C, Content J et al. Prenatal diagnosis of 52 pregnancies at risk for congenital cytomegalovirus infection. Obstet Gynecol 1993; 82: 481–486.

Drew JS, London WT, Lustbader ED et al. Hepatitis B virus and sex ratio of offspring. Science 1978; 201: 687–692.

Edwards MJ. Congenital defects in guinea pigs following induced hyperthermia during gestation. Arch Pathol 1967; 84: 42–49.

Edwards MJ, Shiota K, Walsh DA, Smith MS. Hyperthermia and birth defects. Reprod Toxicol 1995; 9: 411–425.

Egerman RS, Beazley D. Toxoplasmosis. Semin Perinatol 1998; 22: 332–338.

Enders G, Miller E, Cradock-Watson J et al. Consequences of varicella and herpes zoster in pregnancy: prospective study of 1739 cases. Lancet 1994; 343: 1548–1551.

Engerbretsen T. Gonorrheal chorioamninitis. Tids Nor Laegeforen 1974; 94: 1903.

Eskild A, Jeansson S, Hagen JA et al. Herpes simplex virus type 2 antibodies in pregnant women: the impact of the stage of pregnancy. Epidemiol Infect 2000; 125: 685–692.

Feldman HA. Toxoplasmosis. N Engl J Med 1966; 279: 1370 or 1431.

Fleming DT, McGuillan GM, Johnson RE et al. Herpes simplex virus type 2 in the United States, 1976 to 1994. N Engl J Med 1997; 337: 1105–1111.

Florman AL, Gershon AA, Blackett PR, Nahmias AJ. Intrauterine infection with herpes simplex virus. Resultant congenital anomalies. J Am Med Ass 1973; 225: 129–132.

Fowler KB, Stagno S, Pass RF et al. The outcome of congenital cytomegalovirus infection in relation to maternal antibody status. N Engl J Med 1992; 326: 663–667.

Fuith LC, Reibnegger G, Honlinger M, Wachter H. Screening for toxoplasmosis in pregnancy. Lancet 1988; 2: 1196.

Garcia AGP, Pereira LMS, Vidigal N et al. Intrauterine infection with mumps virus. Obstet Gynecol 1980; 56: 756–759.

Gersony WM, Katz SL, Nadas AS. Endocardial fibroelastosis and mumps virus. Pediatrics 1966; 37: 430–434.

Gibbs RS, Sweet RL, Duff WP. Maternal and fetal infectious disorders. In: Creasy RK, Resnik R, Iams JD (eds.) Maternal-Fetal Medicine. 5th ed. Saunders, Philadelphia, 2004. pp. 741–801.

Good JT, Iseman MD, Davidson PT et al. Tuberculosis in association with pregnancy. Am J Obstet Gynecol 1981; 140: 492–498.

Granovsky MO, Minkoff HL, Tess BH et al. Hepatitis C virus infection in the mothers and infants cohort study. Pediatrics 1998; 102: 355–359.

Gregg NM. Congenital cataract following German measles in the mothers. Trans Ophthalmol Soc Aust 1941; 3: 35–46.

Gutierrez KM, Halpern MSF, Maldonado Y, Arvin AM. The epidemiology of neonatal herpes simplex infection in California from 1985 to 1995. J Infect Dis 1999; 180: 199–202.

Hamadeh MA, Glassroth J. Tuberculosis in pregnant women. Chest 1992; 101: 1114.

Hansfield HH, Hodson A, Holmes KK. Neonatal gonoccal infection: I. Orogastric contamination of Neissaria gonorrhoeae. J Am Med Ass (JAMA) 1973; 225: 697–701.

Harger JH, Pazin GJ, Armstrong JA et al. Characteristics and management of pregnancy in women with genital herpes simplex virus infection. Am J Obstet Gynecol 1983; 145: 784–791.

Heiber JO, Dalton D, Shorey J, Combes B. Hepatitis in pregnancy. J Pediatr 1977; 91: 545–549.

Heininger U, Seward JE. Varicella. Lancet 2006; 368: 1365–1376.

Hernandez-Diaz S, Werler MM, Walker AM, Mitchell AA. Folic acid antagonists during pregnancy and the risk of birth defects. N Engl J Med 2000; 343: 1608–1614.

Hohlfeld P, Daffos E, Costa JM et al. Prenatal diagnosis of congenital toxoplasmosis with a polymerase-chain reaction test on amniotic fluid. N Engl J Med 1994; 331: 695–699.

Holmes CB, Hausler H, Numm P. A review of sex difference in the epidemiology of tuberculosis. Int F Tuberc Lung Dis 1998; 2: 96–104.

Holmes RC, Black MM. The specific dermatoses of pregnancy J Am Acad Dermatol 1983; 8: 405–412.

Hutto C, Arvin A, Jacobs R, Steele R, Stagno S, Lyrene R et al. Herpes virus simplex virus and congenital malformations. South Med J 1983; 76: 1561–1563.

Hutto C, Willett L, Yeager A, Whitely R. Congenital herpes simplex virus (HSV) infection. Early vs. late gestational acquisition. Pediatr Res 1985; 19: 296A.

Jabeen T, Cannōn B, Hogan M et al. Pregnancy and pregnancy outcome in hepatitis C type 1b. Q J Med 2000; 93: 597–601.

Jacobs RF. Neonatal herpes simplex virus infections. Semin Perinatol 1998; 22: 64–71.

Jones KL. Smith's Recognizable Patterns of Human Malformation. 4th ed. W.B. Saunders Co., Philadelphia, 1988. pp. 516–519.

Jones KL, Johnson KA, Chambers CD. Offspring of women infected with varicella during pregnancy: a prospective study. Teratology 1994; 49: 29–32.

Jones TC, DeHovitz JA. Infectious diseases common to the tropics and subtropics. In: Roberts BR (ed.) Infectious Diseases: Pathogenesis, Diagnosis, and Therapy. Year Book Medical Publ., Chicago, 1986. pp. 132–157.

Karesh JW, Kapur S, MacDonald M. Herpes simplex virus and congenital malformations. South Med J 1983; 76: 1561–1563.

Kebbeson A, Cannon MJ. Review and meta-analysis of the epidemiology of congenital cytomegalovirus (CMV) infection. Rev Med Virol 2007; 17: 253–276.

Krech UH, Jung M, Jung F. Cytomegalovirus Infections of Man. Karger, Basel, 1971.

Kulhanjian J, Soroush V, Au D et al. Identification of women at unsuspected risk of primary infection with herpes simplex virus type 2 during pregnancy. N Engl J Med 1992; 326: 916–920.

Kuter B, Matthews H, Shinefeld H et al. Ten year follow-up of healthy children who received one or two injections of varicella strategy. Pediatr Infect Dis J 2004; 23: 132–137.

Landon MB. Viral hepatitis. In: Creasy RK, Resnik R, Iams JD (eds.) Maternal-Fetal Medicine. 5th ed. Saunders, Philadelphia, 2004. pp. 1132–1137.

Maheswari A, Ray S, Thuluvath PJ. Acute hepatitis C. Lancet 2008; 372: 321–332.

Melish ME, Hanshaw JB. Congenital cytomegalovirus infection: developmental progress of infants detected by routine screening. Am J Dis Child 1973; 126: 190–194.

Menser MA, Dods L, Harley JD. A twenty-five year follow-up of congenital rubella. Lancet 1967; 2: 1347–1350.

Miller W, Cradock-Watson JE, Pollack TM. Consequences of confirmed maternal rubella at successive stages of pregnancy. Lancet 1982; 2: 781–784.

Monif GRG. Maternal mumps infection during gestation. Observations in the progeny. Am J Obstet Gynecol 1974; 119: 549–551.

Monif GRG, Kellner KR, Donnnelly WH Jr. Congenital herpes simplex type II infection. Am J Obstet Gynecol 1985; 152: 1000–1002.

Nahmias AJ, Lee FK, Bechman-Nahmias S. Sero-epidemiological and sociological patterns of herpes simplex virus infection in the world. Scand J Infect Dis 1990; 69: 19–36.

Noren GR, Adams P, Anderson RC. Positive skin reactivity to mumps virus antigen in endocardial fibroelastosis. J Pediat 1963; 62: 604–606.

Nyholm JL, Schleiss MR. Prevention of maternal cytomegalovirus infection: current status and future prospects. Int J Women's Health 2010; 2: 225–230.

Olsen WM, Storeng R. Effect of shigella toxin on preimplantation of mouse embyros in vitro. Teratology 1986; 33: 234–246.

Pass RF, Stagno S, Myers GJ, Alford CA. Outcome of symptomatic congenital cytomegalovirus infection: results of long-term longitudinal follow-up. Pediatrics, 1980; 66: 758–762.

Pass RF, Zhang C, Evans A et al. Vaccine prevention of maternal cytomegalovirus infection. N Engl J Med 2009; 360: 1191–1199.

Paul J. Frühgeburt und Toxoplasmose. Urban und Schwarzenberg, München-Berlin, 1962.

Pebody RG, Andrews N, Brown D, Gopal R, De Melker H, Francois G et al. The seroepidemiology of herpes simplex virus types 1 and 2 in Europe. Sex Transm Infect 2004; 80: 185–191.

Philip AGC, Larsen EJ. Overwhelming neonatal infection with echo 19 virus. J Pediatr 1973; 82: 391–397.

Plotkin SA, Oski F, Hartnett EM et al. Some recently recognized manifestations of the rubella syndrome. J Pediatr 1965; 67: 182–191.

Pretorius DH, Hayward I, Jones KL et al. Sonographic evaluation of pregnancies with maternal varicella infection. J Ultrasound Med 1992; 11: 459–463.

Pridjian G, Puschett JB. Preeclampsia. Part 2: experimental and genetic consideration. Obstet Gynecol Surv 2002; 57: 619–640.

Proper C, Corey L, Brown ZA et al. The management of pregnancies complicated by genital infections with herpes simplex virus. Clin Infect Dis 1992; 15: 1031–1038.

Reeves WC, Corey L, Adams HG. Risk of recurrence after the first episode of genital herpes. Relation to HSV type and antibody response. N Engl J Med 1981; 305: 315–319.

Riley LE. Herpes simplex virus. Sem Perinatol 1998; 22: 284–292.

Romana S, Wallon M, Franck J et al. Prenatal diagnosis using polymerase chain reaction on amnitoc fluid for congenital toxoplasmosis. Obstet Gynecol 2001; 97: 296–300.

Rudnick CM, Hoekzema GS. Neonatal herpes simplex virus infections. Am Famil Physician 2002; 65: 1138–1143.

Sabin AB. Connatal toxoplasmosis. Advanc Pediat 1942; 1: 1.

Sanchez PJ, Wendel GD. Syphilis in pregnancy. Clin Perinatol 1997; 24: 71–90.

Schweitzer IL, Dunn AEG, Peters RL, Spears RL. Viral hepatitis B in neonates and infants. Am J Med 1973; 55: 762–771.

Seeff LB, Buskell-Bales Z, Wright EC et al. Long-term mortality after transfusion-associated non-A, non-B hepatitis. The National Heart, Lung, and Blood Institute Study Group. N Engl J Med 1992; 327: 1906–1911.

Sever JL, Huebner RJ, Castellano GA, Bell JA. Serological diagnosis "en masse" with multiple antigens. Am Rev Resp Dis Supl 1962; 88: 342–359.

Shepard TH, Lemire RJ. Catalog of Teratogenic Agents. 11th ed. Johns Hopkins Univ Press, Baltimore, 2004.

Shinefeld H, Black S, Digillo L et al. Evaluation of a quadrivalent measles, mumps, rubella, and varicella vaccine in healthy children. Pediatr Infect Dis J 2005; 24: 665–669.

Shone J, Armas SM, Manning JA, Keith JD. The mumps antigen skin test in endocardial fibroelastosis. Pediatrics 1966; 37: 423–429.

Siegel M. Congenital malformations following chickenpox, measles, mumps, and hepatitis. Results of a chart study. J Am Med Ass (JAMA) 1973; 226: 1521–1524.
Siegel M, Fuerst HT. Low birth weight and maternal virus diseases. A prospective study of rubella, measles, mumps, chicken pox and hepatitis. J Am Med Ass (JAMA) 1966; 197: 680–684.
Smith DW, Clarren SK, Harvey MA. Hyperthermia as a possible teratogenic agent. J Pediatr 1978; 92: 878–883.
Snider DE, Layde PM, Johnson MW, Lyle MA. Treatment of tuberculosis during pregnancy. Am Rev Resp Dis 1980; 122: 65–79.
South MA, Thompkins WAF, Morris CR, Rawls WE. Congenital malformations of the central nervous system associated with genital type (type 2) herpes virus. J Pediatr 1969; 75: 13–15.
Stagno S, Whitley RJ. Herpes virus infections of pregancy. Part I: cytomegalovirus and Epstein-Barr virus infections. N Engl J Med 1985; 313: 1270–1274.
St. Geme JW Jr, Noren GR, Adams P. Proposed embyopathic relationship between mumps virus and primary endocardial fibroelastosis. N Engl J Med 1966; 275: 339–347.
Syndman DR. Hepatitis in pregnancy. N Engl J Med 1985; 313: 1398–1401.
Tenti P, Zappatore R, Migliora P et al. Perinatal transmission of human papillomavirus from gravidas with latent infections. Obstet Gynecol 1999; 3: 475–479.
Tikkanen J. Heinonen OP. Maternal hyperthermia during pregnancy and cardiovascular malformation in the offspring. Eur J Epidemiol 1991; 7: 628–635.
Trlifajova J, Benda R, Benes C. Effect of maternal varicella-zoster virus infection on the outcome of pregnancy and analysis of transplacental virus transmission. Acta Virol 1986; 30: 249–255.
Vasileiadis GT, Ronkema HW, Romano W et al. Intrauterine herpes simplex infection. Am J Perinatol 2003; 20: 55–58.
Vontver LA, Hickok DE, Brown ZA et al. Recurrent genital herpes simplex virus infection in pregnancy: infant outcomes and frequency of asymptomatic recurrences. Am J Obstet Gynecol 1982; 143: 75–84.
Wald A, Zeh J, Selke S, Ashley RL, Corey L. Virologic characteristics of subclinical and symptomatic genital herpes infections. N Engl J Med 1995; 333: 770–775.
Watts DH, Koutsky LA, Holmes KK et al. Low risk of perinatal transmission of human papilomavirus: results of a prospective cohort study. Am J Obstet Gynecol 1998; 178: 365–373.
Weigel MM, Weigel R. Nausea and vomiting of early pregnancy and pregnancy outcome. An epidemiological study. Br J Obstet Gynecol 1989; 96: 1304–1311.
Whitley RJ, Corey L, Arvin A et al. Changing presentation of herpes simplex virus infection in neonates. J Infect Dis 1988; 158: 109–116.
Whitley R, Arvin A, Prober C et al. A controlled trial comparing vidarabine with acyclovir in neonatal herpes simplex virus infection. N Engl J Med 1991; 324: 444–449.
Whitley RJ. Herpes simplex virus. In: Howley RM, Knipe DM (eds.) Fields Virology. 4th ed. Lipincott Press, New York, 2001.
Whitley RJ, Roizman B. Herpes simplex virus infection. Lancet, 2001; 357: 1513–1518.
Wilkins I. Nonimmune hydrops. In: Creasy RK, Resnik R, Iams JD (eds.) Maternal-Fetal Medicine. 5th ed. Saunders, Philadelphia, 2004. pp. 503–576.
Xu F, Schillinger JA, Sternberg MR et al. Seroprevalence and coinfection with herpes simplex virus type 1 and type 2 in the United States, 1988–1994. J Infect Dis 2002; 185: 1019–1924.
Yow MD, Williamson DW, Leeds LJ et al. Epidemiologic characteristics of cytomegalovirus infection in mothers and infants. Am J Obstet Gynecol 1988; 158: 1189–1195.
Zhaomeng H. The relationship between congenital malformation of newborn and hepatitis B virus infection in pregnant women. Chin J Epidemiol 1988; 9: 360–363.

Own Publications

I. Ács N, Bánhidy F, Puhó E, Czeizel AE. Possible association of maternal infectious diarrheas in pregnant women and congenital abnormalities in their offspring. Scand J Infect Dis. 2010 (in press).

II. Métneki J, Puhó E, Czeizel AE. Maternal diseases and isolated orofacial clefts in Hungary. Birth Defects Res A 2005; 73: 617–622.
III. Czeizel AE, Evans JA, Kodaj I, Lenz W. Congenital Limb Deficiencies in Hungary. Akadémiai Kiadó, Budapest, 1994.
IV. Ács N, Bánhidy F, Puhó E, Czeizel AE. Maternal influenza during pregnancy and risk of congenital abnormalities in offspring. Birth Defects Res A 2005; 73: 989–996.
V. Czeizel AE, Puho HE, Ács N, Bánhidy F. High fever-related maternal diseases as a possible cause of multiple congenital abnormalities. A population-based case-control study. Birth Defects Res A 2007; 79: 544–551.
VI. Czeizel AE, Ács N, Bánidy F et al. Primary prevention of congenital abnormalities due to high fever related maternal diseases by antifever therapy and folic acid supplementation. Curr Woman Health Rev 2007; 3: 1–12.
VII. Czeizel AE, Ács N, Bánhidy F, Vogt G. Possible association between maternal disease during pregnancy and congenital abnormalities. In: Engel JV (ed.) Birth Defects: New Research. Nova Science Publ., New York, 2006. pp. 55–70.
VIII. Czeizel AE. Reduction of urinary tract and cardiovascular defects by periconceptional multivitamin supplementation. Am J Med Genet 1996; 62: 179–183.
IX. Czeizel AE, Dobó M, Vargha P. Hungarian two-cohort study of periconceptional multivitamin supplementation to prevent congenital abnormalities. Birth Defects Res Part A 2004; 70: 853–861.
X. Gidai J, Bács É, Czeizel AE. Magzati varicellabetegség (Fetal varicella disease). Orvosi Hetilap (Hungarian with English abstract) 2007; 148: 1373–1379.
XI. Bánhidy F, Puhó HE, Ács N, Czeizel AE. Possible association between maternal recurrent orofacial herpes in pregnancy and lower rate of preterm birth. J Mat-Fet Neonat Med 2006; 19: 537–542.
XII. Bánhidy F, Puho E, Ács N, Czeizel AE. Possible indirect association between maternal recurrent orofacial herpes on pregnancy and higher risk for congenital abnormalities. J Turkish-German Gynec Ass 2007. 8: 1–11.
XIII. Czeizel AE, Dudás I. Prevention of the first occurrence of neural-tube defects by periconceptional vitamin supplementation. N Engl J Med 1992; 327: 1832–1835.
XIV. Czeizel AE. Ten years of experience in periconceptional care. Eur J Obstet Gynec Reprod Biol 1999; 84: 43–49.
XV. Ács N, Bánhidy F, Puho E, Czeizel AE. No association between maternal recurrent genital herpes in pregnancy and higher risk for congenital abnormalities. Acta Obstet Gynecol Scand 2008; 87: 292–299.
XVI. Czeizel AE, Kiss P, Osztovics M, Pazonyi I. Nationwide investigation of multiple malformations. Acta Paediat Acad Sci Hung 1978; 19: 275–280.
XVII. Bánhidy F, Ács N, Puhó HE, Czeizel AE. Birth outcomes among pregnant women with genital warts. Int J Gynecol Obstet 2010; 108: 153–154.
XVIII. Czeizel AE. Coxsackievirus and congenital malformations. J Am Med Ass (JAMA) 1967; 201: 153.
XIX. Medveczky E, Puhó E, Czeizel AE. The evaluation of maternal illnesses in the origin of neural-tube defects. Arch Gynec Obstet 2004; 270: 244–251.
XX. Rockenbauer M, Olsen J, Czeizel AE et al. Recall bias in a case-control surveillance system on the use of medicine during pregnancy. Epidemiology 2001; 12: 461–466.
XXI. Janko M, Czeizel AE. Epidemiology of toxoplasmosis in Hungary. Parasit Hung 1970; 3: 119–132.
XXII. Czeizel AE, Janko M. An estimation on the incidence of toxoplasmosis infection during pregnancy. Am J Obstet Gynecol 1970; 106: 776–779.

Chapter 3
Neoplasms

Neoplasms are differentiated into benign and malignant ("cancer") tumors. The incidence of cancer in pregnant women is approximately 0.1% (Berman et al., 2004), though it depends on the maternal age due to the increasing occurrence of malignant tumors with advanced age.

The most common cancers in 700 pregnant women were, in order of frequency, breast cancer, leukemias, lymphomas, melanoma, gynecologic cancers, and bone tumors (Barber and Brunschwig, 1968). The hormonal (particularly in tissues and organs under hormonal control), hemodynamic (due to increased vascularity in the breasts and genital organs), and immunological (explained by increased immunotolerance) changes during pregnancy resulted in the hypothesis of faster growing and earlier dissemination of the malignant process during pregnancy. However, as Berman et al. (2004) stated: "the validity of such conclusions lacks solid supporting clinical data."

Gestational trophoblastic neoplasias following hydatidiform moles did not occur in the HCCSCA because in general this disease is diagnosed after the end of pregnancy.

3.1 Breast Cancer

Pregnancy associated breast cancer is uncommon because breast cancer is rare under age 35. However, because of the increasing number of women with delayed pregnancy and women who are carriers of BRCA1 or BRCA2 mutations, pregnant women may have breast cancer by age 40. The incidence of breast cancer is 1 in 3,000 pregnancies (National Cancer Institute, 2002).

3.1.1 Interpretation of Data in the HCCSCA

Three case mothers and 4 control mothers with breast cancer were recorded in the HCCSCA. The children of 3 case mothers were affected with intestinal atresia, clubfoot (talipes equinovarus), and amputation type upper limb deficiency.

N. Ács et al., *Congenital Abnormalities and Preterm Birth Related to Maternal Illnesses During Pregnancy*, DOI 10.1007/978-90-481-8620-4_3,

The mean gestational age of 4 control newborns was much shorter (37.3 vs. 39.4 week) with lower mean birth weight (2,900 vs. 3,276 g) compared to the reference sample.

In conclusion, pregnant women with breast cancer had a higher risk for adverse birth outcomes.

3.2 Cervical Cancer

Cervical cancer is the most frequently diagnosed malignant tumor in pregnant women; its incidence is 1 in 2,000–2,500 pregnancies (Shivvers and Miller, 1997). About 3% of all cervical cancers are diagnosed during pregnancy due to necessary medical examinations at the beginning of the pregnancy (Hacker et al., 1982). Cervical cancer of pregnant women is most often diagnosed at an early phase, CIN (cervical intraepithelial neoplasia) I–III which is followed by cone biopsy. After biopsy, the histological diagnosis defines the management. If invasive cancer is identified the necessary management is radical hysterectomy, radiotherapy. Recently if pregnancy is desired and the disease has an early stage, trachelectomy can be attempted.

3.2.1 Interpretation of Data in the HCCSCA

Out of 22,843 cases, 6 (0.03%), while out of 38,151 controls, 5 (0.01%) had mothers with cervical cancer diagnosis. This 3 fold difference seems to indicate a higher risk of CAs even with limited number of pregnant women. However, each case was affected by different CA: ventricular septal defect, cleft palate, dilatation of oesophagus, atresia of the bile duct, undescended testis, and multiple CA including occipital encephalocele and ventricular septal defect. Of the 834 patient controls affected with Down syndrome, one had mother with cervical cancer.

The mean gestational age was somewhat longer (39.6 vs. 39.4 week), while the mean birth weight (3,230 vs. 3,276 g) of control newborns was somewhat lower compared to the value of the reference sample.

3.3 Thyroid Cancer

Although, the majority of thyroid cancers are diagnosed over age 50, about 15% of thyroid carcinomas are detected below age 30 and about 65% of all patients are women. Therefore, thyroid carcinoma may occur in pregnant women. Thyroid cancer is not an absolute indication to terminate the pregnancy and thyroidectomy can be performed even during pregnancy (Tan et al., 1996).

3.3.1 Interpretation of Data in the HCCSCA

There were 2 case mothers and 2 control mothers with thyroid cancer in the study pregnancy.

Two cases were affected with hypospadias and cystic kidney, while the mean gestational age (39.6 week) and mean birth weight (3,230 g) of 2 control newborns was in the normal range.

3.4 Uterine Leiomyoma

Leiomyoma is a benign tumor of the uterus involving submucosal fibroids. Compressive effect of leiomyoma may distort the intrauterine cavity and alter the endometrium; therefore, after conception it may interfere with implantation, placental development, and the growth of the conceptus mechanically (Ouyang and Hill, 2002). In addition, there is an increased uterine irritability and contractility secondary to rapid fibroid growth. Therefore, the direct mechanical effect and indirect alteration in oxytocinase activity may disrupt the normal progression of uterus and the development of the fetus, therefore, leiomyoma might be a cause of pregnancy loss (Rice et al., 1989; Probst and Hill, 2000).

The onset of leiomyoma is increasing with advanced maternal age but this pathological condition occurs in pregnant women as well. The objective of our study was to evaluate possible associations between maternal uterine *leiomyoma in pregnancy* (LP) and pregnancy complications, in addition to adverse birth outcomes, particularly CAs in our data set.

3.4.1 Results of the Study (I)

The diagnosis of LP was based on the personal manual and ultrasound examination of pregnant women by obstetrician and was recorded in the prenatal care logbook.

The case group consisted of 22,843 malformed newborns or fetuses ("informative offspring") of whom 34 (0.15%) had mothers with LP. Of the 38,151 controls, 71 (0.19%) were born to mothers with LP (0.8, 0.5–1.2). Most case (88.2%) and control mothers (84.5%) had diagnosed LP in the first visit of prenatal care clinic; therefore, the onset of this pathological condition was prior to conception.

The mothers with LP were older (32.0 vs. 25.4 year) due to the larger proportion of women within the age group of 30 or more years (64.8% vs. 19.0%). They were more frequently unmarried (8.6% vs. 4.5%) with professional/managerial employment status (56.3% vs. 38.5%), but case mothers used folic acid less frequently than control pregnant women (47.1% vs. 54.9%). The mean birth order was higher in control mother with LP (1.9 vs. 1.7), while it was somewhat lower in case pregnant women with LP (1.8 vs. 1.9)

The incidence of acute maternal diseases was similar in the study groups but essential hypertension (19.5% vs. 7.0%), hemorrhoids (18.1% vs. 4.0%), and constipation (7.4% vs. 2.1%) were more frequent in women with LP.

Threatened abortion (22.5% vs. 17.1%) occurred more frequently in women with LP but it was not characteristic for threatened preterm delivery (14.1% vs. 14.3%).

The use of vitamin E (13.3% vs. 6.1%), human chorionic gonadotropin (2.9% vs. 0.3%), and hydroxyprogesterone (5.7% vs. 1.2%) was more frequent in pregnant women with LP than in pregnant women without LP.

Birth outcomes are shown in only control newborns without CA (Table 3.1). The mean gestational age was somewhat (0.2 week) longer and mean birth weight was 95 g larger in the newborns of mothers with LP. However, these differences were not reflected in the rate of PB and LBW newborns. The rate of PB was higher in newborns of mother with LP while there was no significant difference in the rate of LBW. However, there was a somewhat higher proportion of postterm births and large birthweight newborns, although the latter difference was more obvious in babies weighting more than 3,500 g (46.5% vs. 34.4%).

There was no higher risk for the total group of CA (0.7, 0.5–1.1). The distribution of CAs was the following: hypospadias 9 (1.3, 0.5–3.3), cardiovascular CAs 6 (0.9, 0.3–2.4), cleft lip ± cleft palate 3, undescended testis 3, cong. limb deficiencies 3, neural-tube defects 2, cleft palate only 2, branchial cyst 1, torticollis 1.

3.4.2 Interpretation of Results

A higher risk of threatened abortion and of preterm birth was found in women with LP. The rate of postterm births was also somewhat more frequent indicating U-shaped curve of gestational age, i.e. predominance in the preterm and postterm period. Unfortunately, the expected higher occurrence of miscarriages could not be evaluated in the HCCSCA. Babies of mothers with LP had no higher risk for the developing CAs.

The study confirmed the well-known fact that LP is more frequent in elder pregnant women and it explains their higher prevalence of essential hypertension, hemorrhoids, and constipation.

In conclusion, a higher occurrence of threatened abortion, but not threatened preterm delivery was found at the evaluation of pregnancy complications of mothers with LP. There was a higher risk of preterm and postterm birth of babies born to mothers with LP, but higher risk of CAs was not found among them.

3.5 Others

One case mother was affected by *lymphoid leukemia*. She delivered a baby with lethal multiple CA including high number of component CA: buphthalmos, bilateral microtia, cleft lip + cleft palate, cor biloculare, renal dysgenesis, undescended testis with hypoplasia of penis, and agenesis of spleen.

Another case mother had *benign adrenal tumor*. Her son was affected with hypospadias.

Table 3.1 Birth outcomes of control newborn infants without congenital abnormalities born to mothers with or without leiomyoma in pregnancy (LP)

Gestational time (week)	31 or less		32–36		Preterm		37–41		42 or more		Total											
Birth weight (g)	with LP	without	with LP	without	with LP	without	with LP	without	with LP	without	with LP No.	%	Birth weight Mean	S.D.	Gest. time Mean	S.D.	without LP No.	%	Birth weight Mean	S.D.	Gest. time Mean	S.D.
1,499 or less	0	90	0	39	0	129	0	18	0	0	0	0.0	0		0.0		147	0.4	1240	152	31.3	3.4
1,500–1,999	0	75	1	243	1	318	0	99	0	9	1	1.4	1700	0	35.0	0.0	426	1.1	1775	136	34.4	3.1
2,000–2,499	0	19	2	814	2	833	1	715	0	42	3	4.2	2150	132	36.3	3.5	1590	4.2	2275	136	36.3	2.8
Total LBW	0	184	3	1096	3	1280	1	832	0	51	4	5.6	2037	221	36	2.6	2163	5.7	2106	335	35.6	3.2
2,500–2,999	0	1	5	2035	5	2036	7	4821	0	309	12	16.9	2748	121	38.0	2.6	7166	18.8	2767	135	38.1	2.1
3,000–3,499	0	2	1	140	1	142	18	14340	3	1158	22	**31.0**	3227	140	39.5	1.7	15640	**41.1**	3236	143	39.5	1.4
4,000 or more	0	0	0	1	0	1	3	1729	4	1135	7	9.9	4281	215	41.7	2.0	2865	7.5	4198	200	41.0	1.1
Total No.	0	187	9	3300	9	3487	54	30739	8	3854	71	100.0	3370	575			38080	100.0	3275	511		
%	0.0	0.5	12.7	8.7	12.7	9.2	76.1	80.7	11.3	10.1												
Gest. Mean	0.0	29.8	35.0	35.0	35.0	34.8	39.9	39.5	42.6	42.2	39.6							39.4				
time S.D.		1.1	1.0	1.1	0.9	1.6	1.0	0.2	1.1	0.5	2.2							2.0				
Birth Mean	0	1540	2580	2536	2580	2483	3433	3323	3833	3615												
Weight S.D.		401	439	373	417	436	472	429	560	485												

Finally, one control mother was reported with *large hemangioma*, she delivered a boy with 2,850 g on the 42nd gestational week, while another control mother with *neurofibromatosis* delivered a newborn with 3,500 g born on the 40th week (the skin symptoms of this genetic anomaly was not seen at birth).

3.6 Conclusions

There were only a very low number of pregnant women with cancer in the data set of HCCSCA. Fortunately, cancer in pregnant women is not frequent in Hungary; in addition, if cancer occurs in pregnant women, most medical doctors recommend therapeutic abortion due to the teratogenic effect of necessary radio- and/or chemotherapy, and for the better protection of the pregnant women's life.

The sex ratio of cases and controls born to mothers with different neoplasms was not mentioned due to the limited number of pregnant women. However, is seems to be interesting that of the 13 cases, 11 (84.6%) and of the 13 controls, 10 (76.9%) were boys.

References

Barber HRK, Brunschwig A. Carcinoma of the bowel: radiation and surgical management and pregnancy. Am J Obstet Gynecol 1968; 100: 926–933.

Berman ML, Di Saia PhJ, Tewari KS. Pelvic malignancies, gestational trophoblastic neoplasia, and nonpelvic malignancies. In: Creasy RK, Resnik R, Iams JD (eds.) Maternal-Fetal Medicine. 5th ed. Saunders, Philadelphia 2004. pp. 1213–1242.

Hacker NF, Berek JS, Lagasse LD et al. Carcinoma of the cervix associated with pregnancy. Obstet Gynecol 1982; 59: 735–746.

National Cancer Institute. Breast cancer in pregnancy. Cancer-Net. Available at www.cancernet.nci.nih.gov/cgi-bin/srchcgi.exe. Accessed April 24, 2002.

Ouyang D, Hill JA. Leiomyoma, pregnancy and pregnancy loss. Infert Reprod Med Clin N Am 2002; 13: 325–339.

Probst AM, Hill JA. Anatomic factors associated with recurrent pregnancy loss. Semin Reprod Med 2000; 18: 341–350.

Rice JP, Kay HH, Mahony BS. The clinical significance of uterine leiomyoma in pregnancy, Am J Obstet Gynecol 1989; 160: 1212–1216.

Shivvers SA, Miller DS. Preinvasive and invasive breast and cervical cancer prior to or during pregnancy. Clin Perinatol 1997; 24: 369–389.

Tan GH, Gharib H, Goellner JR et al. Management of thyroid nodules in pregnancy. Arch Intern Med 1996; 156: 2317–2320.

Own Publications

I. Bánhidy F, Ács N, Puhó EH, Czeizel AE. Birth outcomes and pregnancy complications of women with uterine leiomyoma – a population-based case-control study. Health 2010 (in press).

Chapter 4
Diseases of the Blood and Blood-Forming Organs

There is normally a 36% increase in the blood volume during pregnancy with a maximum at the 34th gestational week (Peck and Arias, 1979). This dramatic change is caused by the 47% plasma volume increase and 17% red blood cell mass increase. The latter reaches its maximum at term. This difference results in a relative hemodilution throughout pregnancy with a maximum between 18th and 34th gestational weeks.

4.1 Anemia

Anemia is defined as a hemoglobin value below the lower limits of its normal range. However, anemia is not a disease but a sign similar to fever and is very common in pregnant women. The symptoms of anemia are caused by tissue hypoxia such as fatigue, lightheadedness, weakness, and exertional dyspnoe. In general, a mild anemia caused by iron deficiency is hardly harmful to either the pregnant women or the fetus (Kilpatrick and Laros, 2004).

The aim of the study was to check the possible interaction between anemia and other diseases, pregnancy complications, and birth outcomes in pregnant women.

4.1.1 Results of the Study (I)

The normal hemoglobin level for adult female is 14.0 ± 2.0 g/dL (Laros, 1986). However, if the previously mentioned definition of anemia, i.e. "hemoglobin value below the lower limits of normal range not explained by the state of dehydration" (Kilpatrick and Laros, 2004) is accepted, 20–60% of pregnant women will be found to be anemic at some time during the pregnancy (Alper et al., 2000). Therefore, CDC defined anemia in pregnancy as a hemoglobin level below 11 g/dL in the first and third trimesters and below 10.5 g/dL in the second trimester (CDC, 1998). Unfortunately, we were not able to clarify the diagnostic criteria of anemia in Hungarian pregnant women evaluated in the study; therefore, we accepted this diagnosis if it was prospectively and medically recorded in the prenatal care

N. Ács et al., *Congenital Abnormalities and Preterm Birth Related to Maternal Illnesses During Pregnancy*, DOI 10.1007/978-90-481-8620-4_4,

logbook by obstetricians. We trusted in the clinicians' diagnosis, because laboratory examinations including hemoglobin level, red blood cell count, and hematocrit measurement in pregnant women is the obligatory part of the prenatal care in Hungary.

Out of 22,843 cases with CA, 3,242 (14.2%), while out of the 38,151 controls without CA, 6,358 (16.7%) had mothers with medically recorded anemia in the prenatal care logbooks.

The onset of anemia was recorded in I gestational month, i.e., before the conception in 332 (10.2%) case mothers and in 688 (10.8%) control mothers. Their anemia remained present during the study pregnancy; therefore, their anemia was considered as chronic anemia. In about 90% of pregnant women, the anemia was diagnosed during the study pregnancy. The peak of new onset anemia was in III gestational month (16.4% in case mothers and 17.9% in control mothers) explained by the laboratory examination of their blood at the first visit in the prenatal case clinics. These figures were 9.3% in case mothers and 9.2% in control mothers with an earlier visit/examination in the prenatal care clinic. After III gestational month there was a decreasing trend in the diagnosis of anemia: 15.2% and 15.5% in IV, 13.9% and 12.1% in V, 9.3% and 9.0% in VI, and 7.4% and 7.6% in VII gestational months in case and control pregnant women, respectively. Later, the diagnosis of anemia was less frequent. The question is whether these pregnant women had a true new onset anemia or their anemia was only diagnosed in these gestational months.

The origin of anemia was specified as iron deficiency in the prenatal care logbook in 1,999 (56.4%) case mothers and in 4,444 (69.9%) control mothers. Hereditary spherocytosis was recorded only in 2 pregnant women (II); megaloblastic anemia was diagnosed in nobody. Thus, iron deficiency anemia was presumed in the rest of the pregnant women with unspecified anemia in agreement with nearly 95% use of iron derivatives. However, about 60% of pregnant women without anemia had similar iron supplementation. The use of folic acid was also much more frequent in control mothers (71.8% vs. 51.0%) and case mothers (69.7% vs. 46.0%) with anemia than in women without anemia. There was no difference in the use of folic acid-containing multivitamins among the study groups.

The mean age of anemic pregnant women was somewhat lower (25.3 vs. 25.5 year) due to the higher proportion of young age group (19 year or less). The distribution of maternal employment status as indicator of socioeconomic status did not show characteristic pattern.

The data of lifestyle were evaluated based on the so-called family consensus in pregnant women visited at home. The rate of smokers during the study pregnancy was 13.6 and 23.4% of case mothers with or without anemia, while these figures were 12.9 and 19.7% in control mothers with or without anemia, respectively. The drinking habit was also evaluated and the rate of regular drinkers was about 1% in all subsamples.

The evaluation of maternal diseases showed only two associations. Anemic pregnant women had a higher rate of constipation related hemorrhoids (6.3% vs. 3.8%) and hypotension (5.8% vs. 2.8%).

There was no significant difference in the distribution and frequency of other drug usage between women with and without anemia.

The evaluation of birth outcomes resulted in three important findings (Table 4.1). On one hand, the rate of twins was two-fold higher (2.0% vs. 1.0%). On the other hand, the birth outcomes of pregnant women with anemia supplemented with iron did not show any adverse effect for birth outcomes of pregnant women without anemia. The mean gestational age was the same, therefore, the rate of PB was similar as well. There was no real difference in the mean birth weight, but the rate of LBW newborns was somewhat but significantly lower in newborns of anemic pregnant women.

There was no difference in the rate of postterm births, i.e. 42 week of more gestational weeks (10.3% vs. 10.1%) and large newborns, i.e. 4,000 g or more birth weight (7.2% vs. 7.6%) in control mothers with and without anemia (The latter data are not shown in Table 4.1.)

Finally, it is worth making a comparison of anemic control pregnant women without iron supplementation matched to anemic pregnant women without iron supplementation. The matching was based on age and socioeconomic status (Table 4.2). There was 0.4 week shorter mean gestational age at delivery and 33 g smaller mean birth weight in the newborns of 214 anemic pregnant women without iron supplementation compared to the newborns of 1,576 anemic pregnant women with iron treatment. The rate of PB was lower in the iron treated subgroup than in untreated subgroup but somewhat higher than in the group of pregnant women with anemia (Table 4.1). The rate of LBW newborns was higher but not significantly in untreated anemic pregnant women compared to iron treated anemic pregnant women.

In addition the birth outcomes of newborn infants born to anemic pregnant woman treated with iron + folic acid or folic acid alone can also be evaluated (Table 4.2). The longest mean gestational age and lowest rate of PB were found after iron + folic acid supplementation in anemic pregnant women, but the mean birth

Table 4.1 Birth outcomes of newborns without CA (controls) born to pregnant women with anemia or without anemia as reference

Birth outcomes	Pregnant women: Without anemia ($N = 31{,}793$)		Pregnant women: With anemia ($N = 6{,}358$)		Comparison: Crude		Comparison: Adjusted	
Quantitative	Mean	S.D.	Mean	S.D.	$t =$	$p =$	$t =$	$p =$
Gestational age (week)	39.4	2.0	39.4	2.2	1.5	0.13	1.6[a]	0.10
Birth weight (g)	3,275	513	3,278	500	0.3	0.74	0.2[b]	0.81
Categorical	No.	%	No.	%	OR (95% CI)		OR (95% CI)	
PB	2,919	9.2	577	9.1	0.99 (0.90–1.08)		0.97 (0.88–1.07)[a]	
LBW	1,850	5.8	317	5.0	*0.85 (0.75–0.96)*		*0.85 (0.74–0.99)*[b]	

[a]Adjusted for maternal age, birth order and maternal socio-economic status.
[b]Adjusted for maternal age, birth order, maternal socio-economic status and gestational age.

Table 4.2 Birth outcomes of newborns without CA (i.e. controls) born to anemic pregnant women without iron treatment and with iron treatment, in addition with folic acid (FA) and with iron + folic acid and treatment

Birth outcomes	Treatment									
	Without iron ($N = 214$)		With iron ($N = 1,576$)		Comparison		With FA ($N = 1,567$)		With iron+FA ($N = 4,419$)	
Quantitative	Mean	S.D.	Mean	S.D.	$t =$	$p =$	Mean	S.D.	Mean	S.D.
Gestational age (week)	38.9	2.3	39.3	2.1	*2.2*[a]	*0.03*	39.4	2.0	39.5	2.0
Birth weight (g)	3,234	545	3,267	482	0.1[b]	0.91	3,348	470	3,282	505
Categorical	No.	%	No.	%	OR (95% CI)		No.	%	No.	%
PB	32	15.0	168	10.7	*0.67 (0.44–0.99)*[a]		14	9.4	363	8.2
LBW	16	7.5	70	4.4	0.73 (0.35–1.55)[b]		5	3.4	226	5.1

[a]Adjusted for maternal age, birth order and maternal socio-economic status.
[b]Adjusted for maternal age, birth order, maternal socio-economic status and gestational age.

weight was lower and the rate of LBW newborns was higher than in the group of anemic pregnant women with folic acid alone treatment. After folic acid alone supplementation the largest mean birth weigh and the lowest rate of LBW was found but mean gestational age and rate of PB corresponded to the population figures. Thus folic acid may have a more obvious effect for birth weight and the rate of LBW newborns than iron.

There was no higher risk in the group of total CAs or in any specific CA groups. We attempted to evaluate these associations only in women with recorded anemia in II and/or III gestational months, i.e. critical period of most major congenital abnormalities, again without any association.

4.1.2 Interpretation of Results

When evaluating possible interactions between anemia during pregnancy and other maternal disease, only the association of constipation related hemorrhoids and hypotension was found to be associated to anemia during pregnancy. In addition, pregnant women with anemia showed a healthier lifestyle and a more conscious prenatal and medical care.

The main message of the study is that the newborns of pregnant women with early diagnosis of anemia but without iron treatment had a significantly shorter gestational age at delivery and somewhat higher rate of PB. However, this higher rate of PB was not found in newborn infants of anemic pregnant women with iron supplementation from the first trimester of pregnancy.

A higher rate of CAs was not found in the offspring of pregnant women with iron deficiency but supplemented with iron, the prevalence of anemia during pregnancy was 15.7% in our study with a higher figure in case mothers (16.7%) than control mothers (14.2%). The etiology of anemia during pregnancy was mostly iron deficiency. These facts are explained by the increasing demand of iron during pregnancy and by the "dilution" model of pregnancy, i.e. expansion of the plasma volume.

As the classical study of Scott and Pritchard (1967) showed, the iron stores in healthy women are marginal at best due to the menstrual blood loss (25–30 ml containing 12–15 mg of element iron) in every female cycle. However, pregnancy presents substantial demands on iron balance above and beyond what is saved by 9 months of amenorrhea. Thus the usual diet in general cannot supply this large demand of iron, therefore, supplementation of iron is necessary during pregnancy (Pritchard et al., 1969).

Previous studies showed a higher risk of PB and LBW newborns (Klebanoff et al., 1991; Lu et al., 1991; Scholl et al., 1992; Goldenberg et al., 1996), in addition to stillbirth (Sagen et al., 1984; Stephansson et al., 2000). However, recent studies including a meta-analysis of available data reported significant association only between anemia in early pregnancy and higher risk of PB (Scanlon et al., 2000; Xiong et al., 2000; Bondevik et al., 2001).

The main message of our study is that anemia in most pregnant women is due to iron deficiency. However, it does not pose any risk for the mothers or their fetuses, not even the risk of PB. Our explanation for this beneficial finding is based on three suppositions/facts: (i) most pregnant women may have mild anemia, (ii) nearly all were treated with iron and folic acid, (iii) anemic women are considered as a high risk group of pregnant women with higher standard of preconceptional and prenatal care and they also live healthier lifestyle.

There were three findings in the study that needs attention. First, the rate of twin pregnancies was higher in pregnant women with anemia. The explanation is that two fetuses needs more iron thus pregnant women with multiple fetuses need a higher level of iron supplementation. Second, there is an association of anemia with constipation related hemorrhoids. This observation can be explained by the well-known relation between constipation and hemorrhoids and frequent anal bleeding in our pregnant mothers. The cause of the so-called new-onset "pregnancy constipation" mainly in III and IV gestational months is connected with the common oral iron therapy pregnancy which also may exacerbate constipation (Williamson, 2001; Welsh, 2005).

The third finding is the association of anemia and hypotension, the question is whether they have common or independent origin.

In conclusion, anemia in 9,600 pregnant women treated with iron and folic acid does not pose a real risk for pregnant women or their fetuses. Thus there are significant benefits to birth outcomes of newborn infants born tor pregnant women who were anemic and took iron supplement.

4.2 Von Willebrand's Disease

Von Willebrand's disease (VWD) is characterized by abnormal bleeding with varying severity due the inheritance of a mutant dominant autosomal gene. VWD has three subtypes. All of them are related to reduced production or abnormal structure (or both) of the von Willebrand factor (v WF) which is a necessary element of the normal platelet adhesion and aggregation.

The first choice of treatment is DDAVP (l-deamino-8-D-argenine-vasopressin). Burlingame et al. (2001) reported 6 pregnancies in 2 women with VWD treated appropriately and these pregnancies ended with normal birth outcomes.

4.2.1 Interpretation of Data in the HCCSCA

There were 3 controls and one case born to pregnant women affected by VWD. The case was also affected with undescended testis, while 3 controls were born on the 39th gestational week with 2,700, 3,400, and 3,450 g.

In conclusion, pregnancies in women with VWD should be treated according to the international recommendation and after appropriate care normal birth outcomes can be expected.

4.3 Others

The so-called "other group" included only one control mother with *polycythemia* who delivered a son with 3,300 g on the 40th gestational week. In Hungary, thalassemia syndromes, sickle cell anemia did not occur or were extremely rare; therefore, there was no pregnant woman with these diseases in the data set of HCCSCA.

4.4 Conclusion

The evaluation of blood disorders showed that only iron deficient anemia occurs frequently among Hungarian pregnant women and their appropriate medical management seems to be successful.

References

Alper BS, Kimber R, Reddy AK. Using ferritin levels to determine irondeficiency anemia in pregnancy. J Fam Oract 2000; 49: 829–832.

Bondevik GT, Lie RT, Ulstein M et al. Maternal hematological status and risk of low birth weight and preterm delivery in Nepal. Acta Obstet Gynaecol Scand 2001; 80: 402–408.

Burlingame J, McGaraghan A, Kilpatrick S et al. Maternal and fetal outcomes in pregnancies affected by von Willebrand disease type 2. Am J Obstet Gynecol 2001; 184: 229–230.
CDC: Centers for Disease Control and Prevention. Recommendation to prevent and control iron deficiency anemia in the Unites States MMWR (Morb Mortal Wkly Rep) 1988; 47: 1–29.
Goldenberg RJ, Tamura T, DuBard M et al. Plasma ferritin and pregnancy outcome. Am J Obstet Gynecol 1996; 175: 1356–1359.
Kilpatrick SJ, Laros RK. Maternal hematologic disorders. In: Creasy RK, Resnik R, Iams JD (eds.) Maternal-Fetal Medicine. 5th ed. Saunders, Philadelphia, 2004. pp. 975–1004.
Klebanoff MA, Shiono PH, Shelby JV et al. Anemia and spontaneous preterm birth. Am J Obstet Gynecol 1991; 164: 59–63.
Laros RK Jr (ed.) Blood Disorders in Pregnancy. Lea and Febiger, Philadelphia, 1986.
Lu ZM, Goldenberg RL, Cliver SP et al. The relationship between maternal hematocrit and pregnancy outcomes. Obstet Gynecol 1991; 77: 190–194.
Peck TM, Arias F. Hematologic changes associated with pregnancy. Clin Obstet 1979; 22: 785–798.
Pritchard JA, Whalley PJ, Scott DE. The influence of maternal folate and iron deficiency on intrauterine life. Am J Obstet Gynecol 1969; 104: 388–396.
Sagen N, Nilsen ST, Kim HC et al. Maternal hemoglobin concentration is closely related to birth weight in normal pregnancy. Acta Obstet Gynaecol Scand 1984; 63: 245–248.
Scanlon KS, Yip R, Schieve LA, Cogswell ME. High and low hemoglobin levels during pregnancy. Differential risks for preterm birth and small for gestational age. Obstet Gynecol 2000; 96: 741–748.
Scholl TO, Hediger ML, Fischer RL et al. Anemia vs. iron deficiency: Increased risk of preterm delivery in a prospective study. Am J Clin Nutr 1992; 55: 985–988.
Scott DE, Pritchard JA. Iron deficiency in healthy young college women.JAMA (J Am Med Ass) 1967; 199: 147–150.
Stephansson O, Dickman PW, Johansson A et al. Maternal hemoglobin concentration during pregnancy and risk of stillbirth.JAMA (J Am Med Ass) 2000; 284: 2611–2617.
Welsh A. Hyperemesis, gastrointestinal and liver disorders in pregnancy. Curr Obstet Gynaecol 2005; 15: 123–131.
Williamson C. Gastrointestinal disease. Best Pract Res Clin Obstet Gynaecol 2001; 15(5): 937–952.
Xiong X, Buekens P, Alexander S et al. Anemia during pregnancy and birth outcomes: a meta-analysis. Am J Perinatol 2000; 17: 137–146.

Own Publications

I. Bánhidy F, Ács N, Puho HE, Czeizel AE. Iron deficiency anemia: Pregnancy outcomes with or without iron supplement. Nutrition 2010 (in press).
II. Czeizel AE, István L. Spherocytosis with autosomal dominant inheritance (Hungarian with English abstract) Medicus Universalis 1998; 31: 17–21.

Chapter 5
Endocrine, Nutritional and Metabolic Diseases

Pregnancy is accompanied by a series of metabolic changes such as hyperinsulinemia, insulin resistance, relative fasting hypoglycemia, increased circulating plasma lipids, and hypoaminoacidemia due to the function of maternal-placental-fetal unit/complex (Liu, 2004). These metabolic changes can provide an uninterrupted supply of metabolic fuels to the growing fetus and these changes are directed by hormones and elaborated mainly by the placenta. Thus placenta is an endocrine organ and can synthesize virtually every hormone, in addition to growth factors and cytokines.

There are many endocrine, nutritional and metabolic diseases and some of them are modified during pregnancy due to the interaction with fetoplacental unit. However, only thyroid diseases, diabetes mellitus, and obesity occurred frequently in pregnant women in the data set of the HCCSCA

5.1 Thyroid Diseases in Pregnancy

Thyroid gland consisting of two lobes and connected by the isthmus is located in the central region of the anterior neck. The average weight of thyroid gland is 20–25 g. Each lobe of thyroid gland consists of lobules and each lobule is built of 20–40 follicles containing a glycoprotein material called colloid.

Thyroid gland produces two hormones: thyroxine (T4) and triiodothyronine (T3) from the uptake of dietary iodine and regulated by thyrotropin (TSH, previous name was thyroid stimulating hormone). The production of TSH is increased by thyrotropin releasing hormone (TRH) produced in the paraventricular nucleus of the hypothalamus while suppressed via a negative feedback by circulating thyroid hormones.

Iodine is an essential dietary element for humans being required for the synthesis of the thyroid hormones. The natural sources of iodine for humans are found in food and water. The latter was the major source of iodine intake (8–30 mcg/day assuming a consumption of 1.5–2 water L/day) (WHO, 1988). The recommended mean population intake for iodine is 100–150 mcg/day, but for pregnant women this dose is 200 mcg/day (WHO, 1996).

N. Ács et al., *Congenital Abnormalities and Preterm Birth Related to Maternal Illnesses During Pregnancy*, DOI 10.1007/978-90-481-8620-4_5,

Major part of dietary iodine (80–100 mcg daily) is concentrated in the thyroid gland, and the excess is being excreted by the kidneys into the urine. Thus, the average adult thyroid gland contains about 8–15 mg iodine which is 70–80% of the total body iodine amount (about 10–20 mg). The intake of iodine can be measured by its urinary excretion; the values below 50 mcg/L indicate moderate iodine deficiency (Hollowell et al., 1998). The recent NHANES survey (2003–2004) reported that 37.2% of women of childbearing age had urinary iodine values below 100 mcg/L in the USA which suggest mild iodine deficiency (Caldwell et al., 2008).

Dietary iodine is transformed to iodide and iodide is actively used by the thyroid gland for hormone synthesis. First iodide is converted back to iodine; in the second step iodine is organified by binding to tyrosyl residues by the help of thyroid peroxidase producing a glycoprotein called thyroglobulin. The third step results in T4 and T3. These thyroid hormones are stored in the previously mentioned colloid follicles of the thyroid gland, and partly they are transferred into capillaries. The daily secretion rate is about 90 mcg of T4 with one week half-life and 30 mcg of T3 with one day half-life. Only a minor part of circulating hormones is free (0.03% of T4 and 0.3% of T3). The rest is bound to a protein called thyroxin-binding globulin (TBG). Free thyroid hormones enter the cell and bind to nuclear receptors resulting in their diverse effect on cellular growth, development, and metabolism.

There are profound alterations in the mechanism of thyroid function during pregnancy explained mainly by six factors: (i) the high production of human chorionic gonadotropin (hCG) in the placenta during the first trimester of pregnancy decreases the production of TSH. (ii) There is a 2–3 fold increase in the level of TBG due to effect of higher production of estrogens, thus, the proportion of free T4 and T3 is lower by 10–15% and it stimulates the hypothalamic-pituitary-thyroid gland axis. (iii) The placenta provides the selective transfer for major components of thyroid related hormones. TSH does not cross the placenta while T4 does. (iv) There is an alteration in peripheral metabolism of thyroid hormones due to the effect of the placenta (Nader, 2004). (v) The clearance of thyroidal iodine is increased about 3 fold in the kidney. (vi) In the second part of pregnancy a significant amount of iodine is used by fetus for the function of its own thyroid gland mainly from 18 to 20 gestation weeks (Glinoer and Delange, 2000) and it can also interact with the maternal thyroid function. The above factors explain that pregnancy is a strong environmental effect for the thyroid function and it may associate frequently with thyroid disorders during pregnancy.

The association between severe iodine deficiency and the high risk of cretinism has been known but recent studies showed that even mild iodine deficiency may have adverse effects on the cognitive function of children (De Escobar et al., 2004). Thus, the iodine supplementation is an important public health task (Leung et al., 2009). In addition, it would be worth to follow the recommendation of the American Association of Clinical Endocrinologists (Gharib et al., 1999) to introduce routine TSH measurements before or in early pregnancy and thyroxine should be administered promptly even if the TSH elevation is mild.

5.2 Simple Goiter

Goiter is the enlargement of the thyroid gland. Iodine deficiency is associated with goiter, low serum T4, and suboptimal brain functions such as apathy and low capacity for initiative and decision making. Goiter is initially diffuse but later becomes nodular with the appearance of autonomous nodules. The appearance of large goiter may cause obstruction of the trachea and the oesophagus and it also increases the risk of thyroid dysfunction and thyroid cancer. Hypothyroidism is the usual consequence of iodine deficiency, although the latter may also cause hyperthyroidism by the production of uncontrollable TSH.

Pregnancy is goiterogenic, therefore, an increased amount of iodine intake is required to prevent the development of goiter and to keep the serum levels of free T4 and T3 stable.

5.2.1 Interpretation of Data in the HCCSCA

Out of 22,843 cases with CA, 2 (0.01%), while out of 38,151 controls without CA, 3 (0.01%) had mothers with simple goiter without the diagnosis of hypo- or hyperthyroidism. The above mentioned 2 cases were affected with undescended testis and clubfoot. The mean gestational age at delivery was 39.7 week and the mean birth weight was 3,260 g of the 3 control newborns.

5.3 Hypothyroidism

The prevalence of hypothyroidism was estimated 1 in 1,600–2,000 pregnancies (Montoro, 1997); however, it depends on the definition of the disease. For example there is a population-based neonatal screening of peroxidase deficiency, an inborn error of metabolism, in Hungary and the prevalence of positive cases was 0.23 per 1,000 (I). However, the most common form of hypothyroidism in adult persons including pregnant women is related to iodine deficiency. The WHO (1996) recommends 150 mcg iodine per day for adults and 200 mcg for pregnant women. This higher dose is needed for pregnant women because of the increased renal iodine clearance and the significant transplacental iodine transfer to the fetal thyroid to produce its own hormones.

Another common cause of hypothyroidism is Hashimoto's thyroiditis (chronic lymphocytic thyroiditis due to antithyroid antibodies) because hypothyroidism subsequently develops in many patients.

The characteristic symptoms of hypothyroidism, beyond goiter, are modest weight gain, decrease in exercise capacity, mental sluggishness-lethargy, intolerance of cold, dry skin, edema, puffy face, hair loss, hoarse voice etc. due to reduced metabolic rate.

Hypothyroidism is treatable with 0.1–0.15 mg/day dose of T4 and later the dose should be adjusted to the level of blood TSH concentration measured every 4 week.

The major complications of untreated or not appropriately treated pregnant women are higher risk of fetal death (both miscarriages and stillbirths), PB, LBW newborns, placental abruption, and preeclampsia. However, the major risk of iodine related hypothyroidism is mental retardation and other neurological defects such as deafness of the fetus.

There are three major developmental phases of central nervous system. The first phase is related to the structural development of the neural-tube, i.e. brain and spinal cord. The second phase includes neuron cell division and the organization of neuron cells during the second trimester. The third phase covers the time frame from the third trimester to 2–3 years after birth comprising the maximum fetal brain growth and the development of synaptic network among neurons. In the second phase, the fetus gets the necessary supply of thyroid hormones almost exclusively from the mother and if she is affected by iodine related hypothyroidism, irreversible neurological developmental defects are expected. However, even moderate iodine deficiency can reduce the potential mental capacity of the fetus measured by IQ tests later in life.

5.3.1 Interpretation of Data in the HCCSCA

Out of 22,843 cases with CA, 14 (0.06%), while out of 38,151 controls without CA, 31 (0.08%) had mothers with hypothyroidism recorded in the prenatal maternity logbook. The onset of this maternal disease was before the conception in all pregnant women and hypothyroidism was treated by thyroxin. Obviously this prevalence is under-ascertained due to the inclusion of only severe patients. Of the 14 case mothers, 6 were treated orally by liothyronine, 1 was treated by triiodothyronine + levothyroxine (Thyreotom) and 7 mothers were given thyreoidea pulvis (Thyranon), while out of 31 control mothers, 13 mothers were treated by liothyronine, 6 patients were given triiodothyronine + levothyroxine and 12 mothers took thyreoidea pulvis during the entire pregnancy.

Mean maternal age was older in pregnant women with hypothyroidism (28.2 vs. 25.5 year) but there was no difference in the mean birth order (1.7 $\pm$ 1.0). The proportion of skilled workers (41.9% vs. 31.2%) was higher among pregnant women with hypothyroidism compared to pregnant women without this disease. The use of folic acid was lower in control mothers (45.2% vs. 54.5%) and particularly in case mothers (14.3% vs. 49.2%) affected with hypothyroidism than in control and case mothers without this disease.

The occurrence of acute and other chronic diseases was similar in pregnant women with or without hypothyroidism.

The evaluation of pregnancy complications showed a lower incidence of threatened abortion (9.7% vs. 17.1%). The mean gestational age was somewhat longer in newborns of mothers with hypothyroidism (39.6 vs. 39.4 week) but it did not associate with a larger mean birth weight (3,264 vs. 3,276 g) indicating some intrauterine growth delay of fetuses. This phenomenon was confirmed by the higher proportion of postterm babies (16.1% vs. 10.1%) without an excess among large babies (4,000 or more g) (6.5% vs. 7.5%).

The evaluation of different CAs and the rate of total CAs in informative offspring (0.8, 0.4–1.4) did not result in any association with maternal hypothyroidism. Of the 14 cases with CA, 3–3 had common cardiovascular CA (0.8, 0.3–2.7) and hypospadias (1.2, 0.4–4.0), all other CA occurred in only one case.

In conclusion, our data showed longer gestational age with intrauterine growth retardation of fetuses in severe hypothyroidism. Unfortunately, our study was unable to measure possible mental retardation of children. Finally, pregnant women with subclinical or unrecognized hypothyroidism would require more medical attention and help.

In addition there were 2 cases and 5 controls born to mothers with *congenital hypothyroidism* in the HCCSCA. One case boy was affected with undescended testis while one case female with clubfoot (talipes equinovarus). The mean gestational age at delivery was 39.8 wk with 3,314 g mean birth weight in 5 controls.

Two controls were born to mothers with *acquired hypothyroidism* due to surgical intervention of goiter. The gestational age at delivery of these newborns was 42 and 41 wk with birth weight of 3,550 and 3,800 g, respectively.

5.4 Hyperthyroidism

The prevalence of hyperthyroidism in pregnant women was found between 0.05% and 0.2% in different studies (Fernandez-Soto et al., 1998). The typical symptoms of hyperthyroidism are weight loss, tachycardia (more than 100 beats/min), diffuse goiter, and ophthalmopathy (Bahn, 2010).

Most (90–95%) of hyperthyroid pregnant women have Graves disease which is an autoimmune disease caused by antibodies that activate the TSH receptor and stimulate the thyroid follicular cells. The optimal onset of treatment is before pregnancy and frequently treatment is continued during pregnancy as well. As autoimmune responses are usually weakening in pregnancy due to gestational immunotolerance, the symptoms of Graves disease are frequently ameliorated during pregnancy. Some drugs (namely methimazole) used for the treatment of hyperthyroidism were shown to have teratogenic potential. Nevertheless, it is necessary to stress that the risk of antithyroid medication is less than the risk of untreated hyperthyroidism regarding to birth outcomes (Millar et al., 1994; Phooojaroenchanachai et al., 2001). The aim of our study was to evaluate the pregnancy complications of hyperthyroid women and birth outcomes, particularly CAs in their children.

5.4.1 Results of the Study

Out of 22,843 cases with CA, 71 (0.31%), while out of 38,151 controls without CA, 116 (0.30%) had mothers with hyperthyroidism in our data set. This maternal pathological condition was medically recorded in the prenatal maternity logbooks.

The onset of hyperthyroidism was before the conception in 56 (78.9%) case and 89 (76.7%) control mothers. The peak of new onset hyperthyroidism was in the second trimester. The question is whether these pregnant women had a true new onset disease or their disease was only diagnosed in these gestational months.

The mean maternal age was somewhat elder (27.1 vs. 25.5 year) with a higher mean birth order (1.8 vs. 1.7) in mothers with hyperthyroidism compared to mothers without this disease. The proportion of skilled workers was larger among them (38.8% vs. 26.9%). The use of folic acid was higher in control (58.6% vs. 54.4%) and case (60.6% vs. 49.3%) mothers with hyperthyroidism than in pregnant women without hyperthyroidism.

The incidence of acute maternal diseases did not show obvious difference between pregnant women with or without hyperthyroidism However, hyperthyroidism in pregnant women showed important associations with some chronic diseases: the prevalence of essential hypertension (21.9% vs. 5.4%), hemorrhoids (13.9% vs. 3.9%), migraine (5.9% vs. 2.1%), constipation (5.4% vs. 2.1%), and diabetes mellitus (2.7% vs. 0.6%) was higher in pregnant women with hyperthyroidism.

The incidence of several pregnancy complications was higher in control mothers with hyperthyroidism as well compared to control pregnant women without this disease: threatened abortion (22.4% vs. 17.0%), preeclampsia-eclampsia (5.2% vs. 3.0%, but 8.5% vs. 2.9% in case mothers), threatened preterm delivery (19.8% vs. 14.3%).

There was some difference in the frequency of drug uses between pregnant women without and with hyperthyroidism explained by the higher prevalence of chronic diseases (e.g. essential hypertension with antihypertensive drugs) in the latter group. Of the 71 case mothers with hyperthyroidism, only 4 (methimazole 3, propylthiouracyl 1), while out of 116 control mothers with this disease, only 8 (methimazole 7, propylthiouracyl 1) used pharmacologic products appropriate for the treatment of hyperthyroidism, however, prior to pregnancy most of them were treated by these drugs. Medical doctors suggested stopping these drugs because of their teratogenic potential.

The mean gestational age was somewhat shorter (39.3 vs. 39.4 week) with a somewhat smaller mean birth weight (3,210 vs. 3,276 g) and these birth outcomes associated with a higher rate of preterm births (10.3% vs. 9.2%) and low birthweight newborns (6.9% vs. 5.7%).

Table 5.1 shows the risk of different CA (including at least 3 cases) in the informative offspring of pregnant women with hyperthyroidism compared to their matched controls without CA born to mothers with hyperthyroidism.

There was no higher risk in the group of total CAs but a higher risk was found in the groups of obstructive CA of the urinary tract, oesophageal atresia/stenosis, and congenital pyloric stenosis in the children of mothers with hyperthyroidism. We attempted to evaluate these associations only in pregnant women with hyperthyroidism in II and/or III gestational months, i.e. critical period of most major CAs. However, this approach is debatable because the critical period of congenital pyloric stenosis is after this time frame; in addition, the onset of hyperthyroidism during pregnancy is questionable because this date may show only the delay of diagnosis.

Table 5.1 Estimation of risk of different CAs in the offspring of mothers affected with hyperthyroidism comparing to matched controls newborns without CA born to mothers with hyperthyroidism

Study groups	Grand total No.	Entire pregnancy No.	%	OR	95% CI*
Controls	38,151	116	0.3	Reference	
Isolated CAs					
Neural-tube defects	1,202	5	0.4	1.4	0.6–3.4
Ear CA	354	3	0.8	2.8	0.9–8.9
Cleft lip ± palate	1,375	3	0.2	0.7	0.2–2.3
Cleft palate only	601	4	0.7	2.2	0.8–6.0
Cardiovascular CAs	4,480	10	0.2	0.7	0.4–1.4
Oesophageal atresia/stenosis	217	3	1.4	**4.7**	**1.5–15.0**
Cong. pyloric stenosis	241	3	1.2	**4.1**	**1.3–13.2**
Obstructive CAs of urinary tract	343	5	1.5	**4.9**	**2.0–12.9**
Hypospadias	3,038	7	0.2	0.8	0.4–1.6
Clubfoot	2,425	3	0.1	0.4	0.1–1.3
Poly/syndactyly	1,744	5	0.3	0.9	0.4–2.3
CAs of musculo- skeletal system	585	3	0.5	1.9	0.5–5.3
Other isolated CAs	4,889	13**	0.3	0.8	0.4–1.5
Multiple CAs	1,349	4	0.3	0.9	0.4–2.6
Total	22,843	71	0.3	1.0	0.8–1.4

*adjusted for maternal age and employment status, birth order, hyperthyroidism related drugs and related chronic disease, folic acid use.
** cong. hydrocephalus 2, primary microcephaly 2, undescended testis 2, cong. limb deficiencies 2, buphthalmos, anal atresia, vaginal atresia, CA of diaphragm, gastroschisis 1-1.

5.4.2 Interpretation of Results

In conclusion hyperthyroidism induces a high risk for pregnant women. On the one hand, hyperthyroidism is associated with some other maternal diseases such as essential hypertension, migraine, and diabetes mellitus. On the other hand, chronic maternal hyperthyroidism induces a higher incidence of pregnancy complications, e.g. preeclampsia-eclampsia. Finally, a higher risk of some specific CA was found in the study and this association cannot be explained by the drugs used for the treatment of hyperthyroidism. In fact the lack of appropriate treatment of these pregnant women seems to be the major problem because the risk of antithyroid medication in pregnant women affected with hyperthyroidism is much lower than the risk of untreated hyperthyroidism regarding to pregnancy complications and adverse birth outcomes such as CAs.

5.5 Carbohydrate Metabolism

The glucose homeostasis is changed in the direction of diabetes mellitus in normal pregnancy. Thus glucose tolerance gradually deteriorates for which reason pregnancy is often called "diabetogenic".

The placenta is a highly potent endocrine organ producing steroid and protein hormones, this strongly influences maternal metabolism. Glucose freely passes through the placenta, but maternal insulin does not. The fetus begins to produce insulin from the 11th gestational week. Permanent glucose oversupply to the fetus stimulates the fetal pancreatic islet cells to increase insulin production and it gradually induces their hypertrophy and hyperplasia.

The mean blood glucose in normal pregnancy is 5.0–5.6 mmol/L (90–100 mg/dL). The fasting blood glucose level sinks to 3.3–3.9 mmol/L (60–70 mg/dL) during the course of normal pregnancy. The postprandial blood glucose level in pregnancy elevated to 7.2–7.8 mmol/L (130–140 mg/dL) due to the result of placental anti-insulin hormones.

Glucose tolerance improves in normal early pregnancy due to the effect of human chorionic gonadotropin; however, there is a progressive decrease in glucose tolerance after the 20th gestational week associated with placental anti-insulin hormones.

Insulin secretion is increased during normal pregnancy with gestational age. However, the effect of insulin is enhanced by insulinotropic hormones before the 20th gestational week, but is decreased thereafter by the effect of anti-insulin hormones.

5.6 Diabetes Mellitus

Diabetes mellitus (DM) is a common disease, recently with an increasing prevalence in childbearing age, therefore, in pregnant women as well. The major part of the previously found high fetal morbidity including CAs in pregnant women affected by DM is preventable by the high standard of preconceptional and prenatal care.

The first level classification of DM differentiates 3 types:

Type 1 (DM-I) is a chronic autoimmune disease due to inadequate insulin production by the islet beta cells due to the interaction of genetic and environmental factors causing progressive islet cell destruction in the pancreas. These patients with low to absent insulin level and acute or subacute appearance of DM symptoms need insulin treatment for life. The onset of DM-I is predominantly under 30 years with a peak of 9 years (explaining its previous term: juvenile-onset DM or insulin dependent DM: IDDM); in general, in non-obese persons who are prone to ketosis.

Type 2 (DM-II) is a chronic disease arising from progressive tissue insulin resistance caused again by the interaction of genetic and environmental factors. These patients with variable insulin level and in general slow appearance of symptoms need diet control and/or oral hypoglycemic drugs. The onset of DM-II is predominantly over 30 years (explaining its previous term: adult-onset DM or non-insulin dependent DM: NIDDM, although the past 12–20 years have seen a dramatic increase in the prevalence of DM-II in children and adolescents), commonly in obese (often central or masculine obesity type), however, ketosis is less likely. Insulin treatment may also be required later in these patients to control hyperglycemia.

Gestational DM (GDM) is defined as glucose intolerance of any degree that begins or is first recognized during pregnancy. This pregnancy complication occurs about 4% of pregnancies (Ben-Haroush et al., 2004). The explanation of GDM is the maternal tissue insulin resistance due to the drastic hormonal changes in pregnant women. GDM is similar to DM-II, thus most of them are a preclinical state of DM-II with a later onset. Pregnant women with GDM need medical nutritional therapy and insulin when necessary. Insulin treatment in GDM is primarily important for the fetus, thus insulin treatment is indicated when, despite diet, fasting blood glucose value repeatedly exceed 6.1 mmol/L (110 mg/dL) and in pregnant women with a mean blood glucose exceeding 7.2 mmol/L (130 mg/dL) even when the fasting blood glucose is below 6.1 mmol/L (110 mg/dL). Women with GDM have a considerably increased risk of perinatal morbidity/mortality and of developing manifest DM-II later on (Weiss and Coustan, 1988). Shortly after delivery, glucose homeostasis is restored to non-pregnancy levels, but affected women remain at high risk of developing DM-II, obesity and metabolic syndrome in the future (Reece et al., 2009).

DM and pregnancy "do not like" each other. On one hand pregnancy can modify the maternal DM because interprandial hypoglycemia becomes more severe parallel with the progress of pregnancy therefore the status of DM has become worse with the necessary change of treatment. On the other hand DM can cause pregnancy complications and adverse pregnancy/birth outcomes including CAs. This dangerous interaction can be explained by the growing fetal glucose demand and the function of placenta with increasing level of diabetogen steroids and peptide hormones (estrogens, progesterone, and chorionic somatomammotropin). The increase of these hormonal levels results in a progressively rising tissue resistance to maternal insulin action. Thus the hypoglycemia is more severe between meals and at night in pregnant women therefore insulin production in the pancreas increases more than two-fold compared with non-pregnant level during feeding. However, the failure in the increase of pancreatic insulin output induces maternal and fetal hyperglycemia; therefore it is necessary to increase exogenous insulin treatment. Fetal hyperglycemia is followed by fetal hyperinsulinemia which is dangerous for fetal well-being and consequently fetal growth because promotes storage of excess nutrients and consequently macrosomia.

The maternal complications of diabetic pregnant women (retinopathy, nephropathy, cardiovascular complication, diabetic ketoacidosis) are not discussed here (Moore, 2004), the focus of this chapter is fetal morbidity, although the mortality, i.e. miscarriages was also more frequent in diabetic pregnant women with poor glucose control (Greene, 1999).

Intrauterine growth retardation and CAs are highlighted within fetal morbidity.

The weight of fetus/newborns of pregnant women with DM-II generally is skewed in both sides of their distribution, thus, there is a higher risk of low and high birth weight newborns. This U-shaped higher risk is explained by the characteristics of diabetic pregnant women.

Macrosomia, i.e. high birth weight (above 4,500 g or above the 90th percentile for gestational age) is caused mainly by fetal obesity due to fetal hyperinsulinemia particularly in the third trimester. Skeletal growth is largely unaffected. Fetal obesity is concentrated mainly in the truncal region thus the measurement of abdominal circumference by ultrasound after the 24th gestational week but mostly from the 32nd weeks can detect it (Combs et al., 2000). High birth weight was found 3-fold higher in the newborn infants of diabetic pregnant women compared to normoglycemic control pregnant women (Combs et al., 1992), especially in females with underlying vascular diseases. Of course, macrosomia associates with a higher risk of birth injury, mainly shoulder dystocia and branchial plexus trauma.

LBW newborns, i.e. intrauterine growth retardation were also found in a significantly higher rate in diabetic pregnant women, particularly with vasculopathy (retinal, renal and heart complications), preeclampsia, and hypertension after the exclusion of offspring with CA. Thus uteroplacental vasculopathy may be the common denominator in the origin of intrauterine growth retardation of fetuses in the pregnancy of diabetic women.

The risk of CAs in the offspring of pregnant women with overt DM prior to conception was 4–8-fold higher (Reece et al., 1998). This high risk is explained by the maternal teratogenic effect of DM because there is no higher risk of CA in the children of diabetic fathers, normoglycemic pregnant women and women with GDM if its onset was after the first trimester. Another important argument for the maternal teratogenic effect of DM is that this maternal disease associated with specific CAs (Becerra et al., 1990) and a CA-syndrome with specific component CAs ("diabetic embryopathy") as it was shown in our previous study of pregnant women with DM-I as well (III).

The spectrum of maternal DM associated CAs encompasses neural-tube defects (Milunsky et al., 1982), cardiovascular CAs particularly transposition of the great vessels, double outlet right ventricle, and common truncus (Ferencz et al., 1990; Loffredo et al., 2001), kidney CA (renal a/dysgenesis), CAs of the urinary tract, congenital limb deficiency (mainly the lack of femoral head), and CAs of the skeletal system, mainly CAs of spine (Rusnak and Driscoll, 1965). There is also a CA-syndrome in the offspring of pregnant women with DM and it is the caudal dysplasia sequence (its previous name was caudal regression syndrome/complex) (Kucera et al., 1965; Passarge and Lenz, 1966). The primary CA of the caudal region is incomplete development of the sacrum associated with the CA of the lumbar vertebrae (sometimes with typical spina bifida aperta) and femoral head, renal a/dysgenesis, imperforate anus, and sometimes orofacial clefts. While the secondary consequences of the primary CAs are clubfoot, flexion and abduction deformity of hips, popliteal webs, in addition to urine and feces incontinence due to neurologic impairment of the distal spinal cord.

The primary cause of maternal DM associated CAs is hyperglycemia which may promote excessive formation of oxygen radicals in susceptible fetal organs and tissues which are inhibitors of prostacyclins (Moore, 2004). The secondary consequence is the predominance of thromboxanes causing a disruption of the vascularization of embryonic organs.

There is a higher risk of neonatal morbidity (polycythemia, hyperviscosity, hypoglycemia, cardiomyopathy, respiratory distress syndrome, etc) and associated mortality of the infants of diabetic pregnant women but this important topic is again out of our experiences (Moore, 2004).

5.6.1 Results of the Study (IV, V)

In the case group including 22,843 offspring with CA, there were 79 (0.35%) pregnant women with DM treated with insulin (they were considered to have DM-I), 77 (0.34%) pregnant women with DM without treatment of insulin (they were presumed to have DM-II). All together we had 156 (0.68%) diabetic case pregnant women and 120 (0.53%) pregnant women with GDM.

The control group comprises 38,151 newborns without CA, 88 (0.23%) and 141 (0.37%), together 229 (0.60%) had mother with DM-I and DM-II. In addition, 229 (0.60%) control pregnant women were affected with GDM. Thus, there was a higher rate of pregnant women with DM-I in the case group as a preliminary indication of its maternal teratogenic effect.

The onset of GDM happened after III gestational month in 92.8% of pregnant women, while DM-I and DM-II were considered as chronic disease with an effect during the entire pregnancy.

The mean maternal age was the highest in control mothers with DM-I (28.7 year), and the lowest in pregnant women with DM-II (26.0 year) with an intermediate value in control mothers with GDM (27.7 year). All these numbers exceeded the mean age of reference sample without diabetic pregnant women (25.4 year). There was no obvious difference in the mean birth order and the distribution of marital or socioeconomic status among the study groups.

The evaluation of maternal diseases showed only one obvious difference among the study groups and it was essential hypertension. Here the data of control mothers are shown: DM-I: 18.2%, DM-II: 22.0%, GDM: 14.0% vs. 6.9% in non-diabetic mothers. Case mothers showed a similar tendency.

The incidence of pregnancy complications are shown in Table 5.2.

Here only the data of control mothers are commented. The rate of threatened abortion was higher in pregnant women with GDM and lower in mothers with DM-I and DM-II. There was a much lower rate of severe nausea and vomiting in pregnant women with DM-I and DM-II. The incidence of threatened preterm delivery was somewhat higher in pregnant women with DM-I and GDM. Mothers with DM-I were affected more frequently with pregnancy related renal diseases and preeclampsia-eclampsia. However, the occurrence of anemia was lower in all diabetic groups compared to the values of non-diabetic pregnant women as reference.

Table 5.2 Pregnancy complications in case and control mothers with DM-I and DM-II, in addition to mothers with GDM and without DM ("none") as reference

Pregnancy complications	None ($N = 22{,}567$)		DM-I ($N = 79$)		DM-II ($N = 77$)		Together ($N = 156$)		GDM ($N = 120$)		None ($N = 37{,}693$)		DM-I ($N = 88$)		DM-II ($N = 141$)		Together ($N = 229$)		GDM ($N = 229$)	
	No.	%	No.	%	No.	%	No.	%	No.	%	No.	%	No.	%	No.	%	No.	%	No.	%
Threatened abortion	3,451	15.3	7	8.9	12	15.6	19	12.2	27	22.5	6,427	17.1	11	12.5	16	11.3	27	11.8	56	24.5
Nausea/vomiting, severe	1,724	7.6	3	3.8	4	5.2	7	4.5	11	9.2	3,826	10.2	4	4.5	5	3.5	9	3.9	20	8.7
Preeclampsia-eclampsia	652	2.9	6	7.6	2	2.6	8	5.1	10	8.3	1,142	3.0	4	4.5	4	2.8	8	3.5	8	3.5
Pregnancy related renal disease	330	1.5	1	1.3	3	3.9	4	2.6	4	3.3	481	1.3	5	5.7	3	2.1	8	3.5	3	1.3
Edema (excessive weight gain)	426	1.9	0	0.0	1	1.3	1	0.6	1	0.8	905	2.4	0	0.0	2	1.4	2	0.9	5	2.2
Placental disorders[a]	286	1.3	1	1.3	0	0.0	1	0.6	9	7.5	588	1.6	0	0.0	3	2.1	3	1.3	2	0.9
Polyhydramnios	205	0.9	1	1.3	0	0.0	1	0.6	5	4.2	183	0.5	1	1.1	1	0.7	2	0.9	6	2.6
Threatened preterm delivery[b]	2,568	11.4	8	10.1	19	24.7	27	17.3	11	9.2	5,370	14.2	16	18.5	20	14.2	36	15.7	41	17.9
Anemia	3,202	14.2	10	12.7	8	10.4	18	11.5	22	18.3	6,304	16.7	11	12.5	13	9.2	24	10.5	30	13.1
Others[c]	286	1.3	1	1.3	0	0.0	1	0.6	2	1.7	669	1.8	0	0.0	0	0.0	0	0.0	6	2.6

[a] Incl. placenta previa, premature separation of placenta, antepartum hemorrhage.
[b] Incl. cervical incompetence as well.
[c] For example, trauma, poisoning, blood immunization, etc.

Table 5.3 Birth outcomes of newborn infants without CA born to mothers with DM-I and DM-II, in addition to mothers with GDM and without DM ("none") as reference

Birth outcomes	None ($N = 141$)		DM-I. ($N = 88$)		DM-II. ($N = 141$)		Together ($N = 229$)		GDM ($N = 229$)	
Quantitative	Mean	S.D.	Mean	S.D.	Mean	S.D.	Mean	S.D.	Mean	S.D.
Gestational age, wk	39.4	2.1	38.9	2.0	39.7	1.7	39.4	1.8	39.4	1.8
Birth weight, g	3,275	510	3,324	672	3,273	438	3,292	539	3,390	551
Categorical	No.	%	No.	%	No.	%	No.	%	No.	%
PB	3,463	9.2	11	12.5	6	4.3	17	7.4	16	7.0
LBW	2,139	5.7	11	12.5	4	2.8	15	6.6	13	5.7

The use of drugs showed difference only in antidiabetic (insulin and oral antidiabetics) and antihypertensive drugs between diabetic and non-diabetic pregnant women.

The supplementation of folic acid was less frequent in case mother with DM-II and GDM than in control mothers with DM-II and GDM, however, there was no real difference in case and control mothers with DM-I.

Table 5.3 shows the birth outcomes of control newborns without CA of pregnant women with DM-I, DM-II, and GMD.

There was no difference in the sex ratio and the rate of twins among the study groups. The mean gestational age at delivery was the same in the group of GDM and the reference sample, while DM-I had significantly shorter, and DM-II had longer gestational age. These differences were reflected in the rate of PB, although it was somewhat lower in the group of GDM than in the reference sample. The mean birth weight did not follow this pattern; it was largest in the newborns of pregnant women with GDM followed by DM-I, while the mean birth weight in the group of DM-II did not differ from the reference value. On the contrary of babies with largest mean birth weight born to mothers with GDM, their rate of LBW was not lower than in the reference sample, in addition, the larger mean birth weight in the groups of DM-I associated with the higher (the highest) rate of LBW newborns in the study. The rate of postterm birth was somewhat lower in the groups of GDM but the rate of large birthweight newborns was the highest. Thus, these data indicate a higher risk of both small and large birthweight newborns in DM-I and a higher risk of large birthweight newborns in the groups of GDM.

Finally, the total (birth + fetal) prevalences of different CAs are shown in Table 5.4. The major finding of this analysis is that the total rate of cases with CA was higher only in the group of DM-I and within them specific types/groups of CAs had a higher risk in the offspring of mothers with DM-I. Three CA groups: isolated renal a/dysgenesis and obstructive CA of the urinary tract (including 2 cases with cystic dysplasia), isolated cardiovascular CA (including 12 cases with ventricular septal defect, but the second most common CA was transposition of the great vessels in 5 cases) and multiple CA.

Table 5.4 Estimation of risk for different CAs in the offspring of pregnant women with DM-1, DM-2 and GDM compared to their all matched controls

Study groups	Grand total No.	DM-1			DM-2			GDM		
		No.	Percent	OR 95% CI[a]	No.	Percent	OR 95% CI[a]	No.	Percent	OR 95% CI[a]
Controls	38,151	88	0.2	Reference	141	0.4	Reference	229	0.6	Reference
Isolated CAs										
Neural-tube defects	1,202	3	0.2	1.1 0.3–3.4	5	0.4	1.1 0.5–2.8	7	0.6	1.0 0.5–2.1
Cleft lip ± palate	1,375	5	0.4	1.6 0.6–3.9	8	0.6	1.6 0.8–3.2	8	0.6	1.0 0.5–2.0
Cleft palate	601	3	0.5	2.2 0.7–6.8	1	0.2	0.4 0.1–3.2	1	0.2	0.3 0.0–2.0
Oesophageal atresia/stenosis	217	1	0.5	2.0 0.3–14.4	0	0.0	0.0 0.0–0.0	1	0.5	0.8 0.1–5.5
Intestinal atresia/stenosis	158	0	0.0	0.0 0.0–0.0	0	0.0	0.0 0.0–0.0	2	1.3	2.1 0.5–8.6
Rectal/anal atresia/stenosis	231	1	0.4	1.9 0.3–13.6	0	0.0	0.0 0.0–0.0	3	1.3	2.2 0.7–6.8
Renal a/dysgenesis	126	3	2.4	*10.4 3.3–33.5*	0	0.0	0.0 0.0–0.0	0	0.0	0.0 0.0–0.0
Obstructive urinary CAs	343	4	1.2	*5.2 1.9–14.3*	3	0.9	2.4 0.8–7.7	8	2.3	*4.0 2.0–8.2*
Hypospadias	3,038	7	0.2	1.0 0.5–2.2	9	0.3	0.8 0.4–1.6	14	0.5	0.8 0.4–1.3
Undescended testis	2,052	3	0.1	0.6 0.2–2.0	2	0.1	0.3 0.1–0.0	7	0.3	0.6 0.3–1.2
Exomphalos/gastroschisis	255	0	0.0	0.0 0.0–0.0	1	0.4	1.1 0.1–7.6	1	0.4	0.7 0.1–4.7
Hydrocephaly, congenital	314	0	0.0	0.0 0.0–0.0	1	0.3	0.9 0.1–6.2	3	1.0	1.6 0.5–5.0
Ear CAs	354	2	0.6	2.4 0.6–10.0	1	0.3	0.8 0.1–5.5	1	0.3	0.5 0.1–3.4
Cardiovascular CAs	4,480	26	0.6	*2.5 1.6–3.9*	16	0.4	1.0 0.6–1.6	28	0.6	1.0 0.7–1.5
Clubfoot	2,425	5	0.2	0.9 0.4–2.2	7	0.3	0.8 0.4–1.7	12	0.5	0.8 0.5–1.5
Limb deficiencies	548	1	0.2	0.8 0.1–5.7	1	0.2	0.5 0.1–3.5	3	0.5	0.9 0.3–2.8
Poly/syndactyly	1,744	3	0.2	0.7 0.2–2.4	10	0.6	1.5 0.8–2.9	5	0.3	0.5 0.2–1.2
CAs of musculo-skeletal system	585	1	0.2	0.7 0.1–5.3	2	0.3	0.9 0.2–3.7	2	0.3	06 0.1–2.3
Diaphragmatic CAs	244	0	0.0	0.0 0.0–0.0	3	1.2	*3.4 1.1–10.6*	2	0.8	1.4 0.3–5.6
Other isolated CAs	1,202	2[b]	0.2	0.7 0.2–2.9	3[c]	0.2	0.7 0.2–2.1	6[d]	0.5	0.8 0.4–1.9
Multiple CAs	1,349	9	0.7	*2.9 1.5–5.8*	4	0.3	0.8 0.3–2.2	6	0.4	0.7 0.3–1.7
Total	22,843	79	0.3	*1.5 1.1–2.0*	77	0.3	0.9 0.7–1.2	120	0.5	0.9 0.7–1.1

[a] Adjusted for maternal age and employment status, birth order and maternal hypertension.
[b] Congenital stenosis of trachea, congenital hiatus hernia.
[c] Cleft nose, double urethra, absent of breast.
[d] Ankyloglossia, Hirschsprung's disease, transposition of intestine, atresia of bile duct, exstrophia of urinary bladder, congenital angulation of tibia.

Out of 9 multiple CAs, 4 (44.4%) were diagnosed as caudal dysplasia sequence: (i) CA of the sacral spine with clubfoot + renal agenesis + transposition of the great vessels; (ii) sacral agenesis with lumbar spina bifida + renal dysgenesis + transposition of the great vessels and persistent ductus arteriosus, + abdominal situs inversus + CA of the ear; (iii) femur aplasia with unspecified CAs of the spine + ectopic anus + cleft palate + CA of the ear; (iv) renal dysgenesis + anal atresia + sacral agenesis. In addition, one-one multimalformed case had transposition of the great vessels (with cleft lip and palate + clubfoot) and occipital encephalocele (with deformity of the ear which is likely to be a secondary CA, thus it would have been better to classify this case as isolated neural-tube defect).

If we consider the annual distribution of cases with DM-I related CAs, out of 42 cases, 30 (71.4%) were born in the 1980s.

In the group of pregnant women with GDM only CAs of the urinary tract showed a higher occurrence. In general, the onset of GDM occur after III gestational months (i.e. the critical period of most major CAs), however, the critical period of some obstructive CAs of the urinary tract is in the later gestational months. Thus, this finding needs further studies to confirm or exclude this possible association. The marginal risk of diaphragmatic CAs in the offsprings of mothers with DM-II may have happened by chance as we only had 3 cases. Four and 6 multimalformed offsprings of mothers with DM-II and GDM, respectively, did not fit the pattern of caudal dysplasia sequence.

Finally, offsprings of pregnant women with DM-I were evaluated according to folic acid supplementation (Table 5.5).

The estimated daily dose of folic acid was 5.6 mg. There was no offspring with neural-tube defect and renal a/dysgenesis in the folic acid supplemented subgroup, in addition, there was an obvious reduction in the rate of cleft lip ± palate, cleft palate, and obstructive CAs of the urinary tract, some reduction in the rate of cardiovascular CAs and no reduction in the occurrence of multiple CAs. Obviously, this preventive effect is expected only at the folic acid supplementation in the critical period of the given CA.

5.6.2 Interpretation of Results

Our data confirmed the well-known association of DM-I with hypertension and preeclampsia (Moore, 2004). The lower rate of severe nausea and vomiting is interesting because severe nausea and vomiting showed some protective effect not only for early fetal death (Weigel and Weigel, 1989) but for some CAs as well (VI). The lower rate of anemia may be related to the higher standard of prenatal care of diabetic pregnant women.

The birth outcomes are determined very much by the type of DM. The U-shaped increased risk of LBW and large birthweight newborns was seen in the newborns of pregnant women with DM-I. DM-II is associated with intrauterine fetal growth delay (longer gestational age was not associated with expected larger birth weight) while GDM was associated with larger birth weight.

Table 5.5 Estimation of risk for different CAs in the offspring of pregnant women with DM-1 with or without folic acid supplementation

					Folic acid supplementation					No folic acid supplementation				
	Grand total	DM-1			No DM-1		DM-1			No DM-1		DM-1		
Study groups	No.	No.	Percent	OR 95% CI[a]	No.	Percent	No.	Percent	OR (95% CI)	No.	Percent	No.	Percent	OR (95% CI)
Controls	38,151	88	0.23	Reference	20,518	54.4	54	0.14	Reference	17,175	45.5	34	0.09	Reference
Isolated CAs														
Neural-tube defects	1,202	3	0.25	1.1 0.3–3.4	528	43.9	0	0.00	– (–)	671	56.1	3	0.25	2.3 (0.7–7.4)
Cleft lip ± palate	1,375	5	0.36	1.6 0.6–3.9	678	49.4	1	0.07	0.5 (0.1–3.3)	692	50.6	4	0.29	*2.9 (1.0–8.3)*
Cleft palate	601	3	0.50	2.2 0.7–6.8	285	47.6	1	0.17	1.0 (0.1–7.4)	313	52.4	2	0.33	3.3 (0.8–13.6)
Renal a/dysgenesis	126	3	2.38	*10.4 3.3–33.5*	61	48.4	0	0.00	– (–)	62	51.6	3	2.38	*24.7 (7.4–82.5)*
Obstructive CAs of urinary tract	343	4	1.17	*5.2 1.9–14.3*	160	46.9	1	0.29	1.8 (0.2–13.0)	179	53.1	3	0.87	*8.5 (2.6–28.1)*
Hypospadias	3,038	7	0.23	1.0 0.5–2.2	1,469	48.5	5	0.16	1.0 (0.4–2.6)	1,562	51.5	2	0.07	0.7 (0.2–2.7)
Undescended testis	2,052	3	0.15	0.6 0.2–2.0	1,060	51.8	2	0.10	0.6 (0.2–2.7)	989	48.2	1	0.05	0.5 (0.1–3.8)
Cardiovascular CAs	4,480	26	0.58	*2.5 1.6–3.9*	2,161	48.6	14	0.31	*2.1 (1.1–3.5)*	2,293	51.4	12	0.27	*2.7 (1.4–5.2)*
Clubfoot	2,425	5	0.21	0.9 0.4–2.2	1,213	50.1	3	0.12	0.8 (0.2–2.5)	1,207	49.9	2	0.08	0.8 (0.2–3.5)
Poly/syndactyly	1,744	3	0.17	0.7 0.2–2.4	908	52.1	1	0.06	0.4 (0.1–2.8)	833	47.9	2	0.11	1.2 (0.3–5.1)
Other isolated CAs	4,109	8[b]	0.19	0.8 0.3–2.9	2,109	50.8	5	0.12	0.8 (0.2–1.7)	1,992	49.2	3	0.07	0.8 (0.3–2.7)
Multiple CAs	1,349	9	0.67	*2.9 1.5–5.8*	624	46.8	7	0.52	*3.1 (1.4–6.9)*	716	53.2	2	0.15	1.4 (0.3–5.9)
Total	22,843	79	0.35	*1.5 1.1–2.0*	11,256	49.3	40	0.18	1.1 (0.7–1.7)	11,508	50.4	39	0.17	*1.7 (1.1–2.7)*

Atresia of external auditory canal, microtia.

[a]Adjusted for maternal age and employment status, birth order and hypertension.

[b]Congenital stenosis of trachea, oesophageal atresia, rectal stenosis, limb deficiency, congenital hiatus hernia, torticollis.

The teratogenic effect of maternal DM was also shown but only in the offsprings of mothers with DM-I without the appropriate treatment, thus, our data suggests that the teratogenic risk of maternal DM depends on the type and severity of the DM (White, 1937; Molsted-Pedersen et al., 1964), and also on the duration and efficacy of the treatment. The status of the pathological condition in pregnant women with DM can be measured by laboratory methods, like the measurement of glucose threshold (Langer, 2002) or glycosylated hemoglobin (Nielsen et al., 1997).

Our data confirmed the association between maternal DM-1 and caudal dysplasia sequence. Out of 79 pregnant women with DM-1, 4 (5.1%) had children with caudal dysplasia sequence. Beyond this characteristic type of diabetic embryopathy, a higher rate of renal a/dysgenesis-obstructive CAs of the urinary tract and cardiovascular CAs, particularly, transposition of the great vessels have been shown to have an association with maternal DM-I.

The unchanged risk of neural-tube defects, congenital limb deficiencies, and CAs of the spine in the offsprings of our diabetic mothers necessitates some discussion. On one hand, the decreased rate of isolated neural-tube defects can be explained by the periconceptional high dosage (4 mg) of folic acid (MRC Vitamin Study, 1991) or folic acid-containing multivitamin supplementation (VII). In addition, as our previous trials demonstrated, periconceptional folic acid-containing multivitamin supplementation was able to reduce the occurrence of cardiovascular (particularly conotruncal) and urinary tract (mainly obstructive) CAs both in our randomized control and cohort trials (VIII, IX). The evaluation of cases in the HCCSCA showed that the high dosage of folic acid was able to reduce the occurrence of isolated orofacial clefts (X). However, none of the two trials (XI) or the data of HCCSCA (XII) indicated any reduction in the rate of multiple CAs. On the other hand, two previous case-control studies have found association between maternal DM and congenital limb deficiencies and CA of the spine in their offspring based on 4 and 9 cases (Becerra et al., 1990; Martinez-Frias et al., 1998). Sheffield et al. (2002) found only one case with CA of the skeleton in 410 children born to mothers with DM. Thus, the explanation for this discrepancy may be the low birth prevalence of these CAs, because the specific diabetic associated limb deficiency, i.e. femur or femoral head aplasia, is represented only in some percent in the total group of congenital limb deficiencies (0.5/1,000) (XIII). In addition, the rare CAs of the spine are underrepresented in the HCAR because the lack of radiological documents in several cases.

We hope that the lower risk figures of specific CAs (1.5-fold instead of the previous 4- to 8-fold) reflects the recent progress in the specific medical care of diabetic pregnant women.

An important message of this study is that insulin and other antidiabetic drugs can reduce the teratogenic risk of hyperglycemia during the critical period of CAs in diabetic pregnant women. Thus, it is worth introducing the term of "antiteratogenic drugs" for drugs, such as insulin.

Unfortunately, the special periconceptional and prenatal care was not provided in all diabetic pregnant women in Hungary during the study period, particularly in the 1980s, thus the preventable maternal DM associated CAs were not prevented in several newborns. The use of folic acid was much lower in case mothers with DM-I than in control mothers with DM-I. One of the most important purposes of the Hungarian periconceptional service introduced in 1984 was to provide a special care for diabetic pregnant women. The evaluation of about 15,000 pregnant women showed that this service was able to prevent the maternal teratogenic effect of DM (XIV). In addition, the diagnosis of GDM sometimes happened too late or it was not diagnosed at all, subsequently, these pregnant women were often undertreated.

In conclusion, the maternal teratogenic effect of DM is preventable with appropriate periconceptional and prenatal care.

5.7 Obesity

Obesity is defined as a body mass index greater than or equal to 30. This pathological condition has a growing importance among poor reproductive outcomes. First, there is an increasing trend in the rate of obesity among women; second, studies have indicated the role of obesity in the origin of infertility, fetal death, fetal macrosomia, preeclampsia, DM-II, and GDM (Creasy et al., 2004)

5.7.1 Interpretation of Data in the HCCSCA

Out of 22,842 cases with CA, 11 (0.05%), while out of 38,151 controls without CA, 29 (0.08%) had mothers with obesity. This pathological condition was reported by the mothers in the questionnaire. The onset of obesity happened before conception in all women.

There was no significant difference in the mean age of mothers and mean birth order among the study groups. However, the proportion of professional and managerial women was lower in pregnant women with obesity compared to pregnant women without obesity (27.6% vs. 38.5%) and the usage of folic acid was also lower among them (44.8% vs. 54.5%).

The incidence of acute disease groups did not show differences between pregnant women with or without obesity. However, the prevalence of DM (3.4% vs. 0.6%), migraine (17.2% vs. 1.8%), and essential hypertension (13.8% vs. 7.0%) was higher.

Among pregnancy complications, severe and treated nausea and vomiting in pregnancy (24.1% vs. 10.1%) and preeclampsia-eclampsia (10.3% vs. 3.0%) showed a higher incidence in pregnant women with obesity.

The mean gestational age was much longer in the newborns of pregnant women with obesity (39.9 vs. 39.4 week) and it was associated with a larger mean birth weight (3,566 vs. 3,275 g). PB and LBW newborns did not occur among these babies.

Of the 11 cases with CA, 3 were affected with hypospadias, 2 were affected by cardiovascular CA and 2 were affected by obstructive CA of the urinary tract. Other 4 CAs occurred only once. The adjusted OR did not show significant association between maternal obesity and any CA in their offspring.

In conclusion this sample is not appropriate for valid analysis due to the limited number of pregnant women with obesity and because the diagnosis of obesity was based on maternal information. Nevertheless, the higher risk of some pregnancy complications and a concomitant occurrence of some diseases are obvious, in addition, there is an association between maternal obesity and longer gestational age with larger babies.

5.8 Others

5.8.1 Hyperparathyroidism

Serum calcium level is regulated and maintained within normal limits by parathyroid hormones and vitamin D. The production of parathyroid hormone in the parathyroid glands are stimulated by hypocalcaemia and suppressed by high concentrations of calcium, magnesium and active form of vitamin D.

Hyperparathyroidism is very rare during pregnancy (Mestman, 1998). In the data set of HCCSCA, only one case was affected by syndactyly on the feet.

5.8.2 Diabetes Insipidus

The location of pituitary gland is in the sella turcica of the sphenoidal bone lined by the dura mater. The pituitary gland consists of two lobes: anterior (adenohypophysis) and posterior (neurohypophysis). The pituitary stalk comprises a direct neural connection between the hypothalamic nuclei and the posterior lobe of pituitary gland. Vasopressin and oxytocin are produced in the supraoptic and paraventricular nuclei of the hypothalamus and are released into the posterior lobe of the pituitary gland and into the circulation. The lack of vasopressin results in diabetes insipidus with the symptoms of polyuria, polydipsia, and low urinary specific gravity. There are several different types of diabetes insipidus during pregnancy (Durr and Lindheimer, 1996).

One case with hypospadias was born to pregnant women with diabetes insipidus, while two controls with 2,850 and 4,150 g birth weight were born on the 37th and 39th gestational week, respectively.

5.8.3 Cushing's Syndrome

Cushing's syndrome is the disease of the anterior lobe of the pituitary gland of the hypophysis. The cause of this disease is the excess ACTH production (e.g. by a tumor) and the hypercortisolism with the symptoms of striae, pigmentation, weight gain, hypertension, and edema. Pregnancy is uncommon in patients with Cushing's syndrome because of its association with anovulation and menstrual disturbances (Buescher, 1996).

One case with clubfoot (talipes equinovarus) and three controls with birth weight of 3,050, 3,360 and 3,500 g were born on the 40th, 38th and 40th gestational weeks, respectively, reported to HCCSCA.

5.8.4 Addison Disease

Addison disease is a primary adrenocortical insufficiency caused by the atrophy or damage of the adrenal gland mainly due to autoimmune activity, hemorrhage, infections, tumors, etc. The symptoms of increased pigmentation, abdominal pain, nausea and vomiting with anorexia, decreased systolic blood pressure help to diagnose this disease. Replacement hormone therapy is effective (Albert et al., 1989).

One control without CA was born to mother with Addison disease with 3,350 g on the 40th gestational week in the HCCSCA.

5.8.5 Wilson Disease

Wilson disease is a rare disorder of copper metabolism characterized by liver failure and neurologic dysfunction (intellectual disturbance, abnormal movements, etc) and caused by the autosomal recessive mutant gene-pair on the long arm of chromosome 13. Previously a higher rate of miscarriages was found but recently successful pregnancies have been reported in treated pregnant women with Wilson disease (Toaff et al., 1997, XV)

One case with malposition of the heart and congenital heart block was registered in the HCCSCA.

5.9 Final Conclusion

Placenta is an endocrine organ thus during pregnancy can modify the function of the previous non-pregnant endocrine orchestra. In general the interaction of placenta and other endocrine organs associate with conflicts resulting in a higher risk of pregnancy complications in the mothers and adverse birth outcomes of the offspring. However, the recent progress in the treatment of diabetes mellitus promises a lower risk, however, similar beneficial progress was not seen in the care and treatment of pregnant women with hyperthyroidism and obesity in Hungary. Thus an urgent task is to improve the quality of treatment of pregnant women with these endocrine and/metabolic diseases.

References

Albert E, Dalaker K, Jorde R et al. Addison's disease and pregnancy. Acta Obstet Gynaecol Scand 1989; 68: 185–187.

Bahn RS. Graves' ophthalmopathy. N Engl J Med 2010; 362: 726–738.

Becerra JE, Khoury MJ, Cordero JF et al. Diabetes mellitus during pregnancy and the risk for specific birth defects: a population-based case-control study. Pediatrics 1990; 85: 1–9.

Ben-Haroush A, Yogev Y, Hod M. Epidemiology of gestational diabetes mellitus and its association with type 2 diabetes. Diabet Med 2004; 21: 103–113.

Buescher MA. Cushing's syndrome in pregnancy. Endocrinologist 1996; 6: 357–361.

Caldwell KL, Miller GA, Wang RY et al. Iodine status of the US population. National Health and Nutrition Examination Survey 2003–2004. Thyroid 2008; 18: 1207–1214.

Combs CA, Gunderson E, Kitzmiller J et al. Relationship of fetal macrosomia to maternal postprandial glucose control during pregnancy. Diabetes Care 1992; 15: 1251–1257.

Combs CA, Rosenn B, Miodovnik M et al. Sonographic EFW and macrosomia: is there an optimum formula to predict diabetic fetal macrosomia? J Matern Fetal Med 2000; 9: 55–61.

Creasy RK, Resnik R, Iams JS (eds.) Maternal-Fetal Medicine. 5th ed. Saunders, Philadelphia, 2004.

De Escobar DM, Obregon MJ, del Rey FE. Maternal thyroid hormones early in pregnancy and fetal brain development. Best Pract Res Endocrinol Metab 2004; 18: 225–248.

Durr JA, Lindheimer MD. Diagnosis and management of diabetes insipidus during pregnancy. Endocr Pract 1996; 2: 353–361.

Ferencz C, Rubin JN, NcCarter RJ, Clark EB. Maternal diabetes and cardiovascular Malformations: predominance of double outlet right ventricle and truncus arteriosus. Teratology 1990; 41: 319–326.

Fernandez-Soto ML, Jovanovic LG, Gomzalez-Jimenez A et al. Thyroid function during pregnancy and the postpartum period iodine metabolism and disease status. Pract 1998; 4: 97–105.

Gharib H, Cobin RH, Dickey RA. Subclinical hypothyroidism during pregnancy: position statement from the American Association of Clinical Endocrinologist. Endocrine Pract 1999; 5: 367–368.

Glinoer D, Delange F. The potential repercussions of maternal, fetal and neonatal hypothyroxinemia on the progeny. Thyroid 2000; 10: 871–887.

Greene MF. Spontaneous abortions and major malformations in women with diabetes mellitus. Semin Reprod Endocrinol 1999; 17: 127–136.

Hollowell JG, Staehling NW, Segal MN et al. Iodine nutrition in the United States. Trend from public health implications: iodine excretion data from National Health and Nutrition Examination Survey I and III (1971–1974 and 1988–1994). J Clin Endocrinol Metab 1998; 83: 3401–3408.

Kucera J, Lenz W, Maier W. Missbildungen der Beine und der kaudalen Wirbelsaule bei Kindern diabetischer Mütter. Dtsch Med Wochenschr 1965; 90: 901–905.

Langer O. A spectrum of glucose thresholds may effectively prevent complications in the pregnant diabetic patient. Semin Perinatol 2000; 26: 196–205.

Leung AM, Pearce EN, Braverman LE. Iodine content of prenatal multivitamins in the United States. N Engl J Med 2009; 360: 939–940.

Liu JH. Endocrinology of pregnancy. In: Creasy RK, Resnik R, Iams JS (eds.) Maternal-Fetal Medicine. 5th ed. Saunders, Philadelphia, 2004. pp. 121–134.

Loffredo CA, Wilson PD, Ferencz C. Maternal diabetes: an independent risk factors for major cardiovascular malformations with increased mortality of affected infants. Teratology 2001; 64: 98–106.

Martinez-Frias NL, Bemejo E, Rodriguez-Pinilla E et al. Epidemiological analysis of outcomes of pregnancy in gestational diabetic mothers. Am J Med Genet 1998; 78: 140–145.

Mestman JH. Parathyroid disorders of pregnancy. Semin Perinatol 1998; 22: 485–496.

Millar LK, Wing DA, Leung AS et al. Low birth weight and preeclampsia in pregnancies complicated by hyperthyroidism. Obstet Gynecol 1994; 84: 946–949.

Milunsky A, Alpert E, Kitzmiller JL et al. Prenatal diagnosis of neural tube defects. The importance of serum alfa-fetoprotein in diabetic pregnant women. Am J Obstet Gynecol 1982; 142: 1030–1032.

Molsted-Pedersen L, Tygstrup I, Pedersen J. Congenital malformations in newborn infants of diabetic women. Correlation with maternal diabetes and vascular complications. Lancet 1964; 1: 1124–1126.

Montoro MN. Management of hypothyroidism during pregnancy. Clin Obstet Gynecol 1997; 40: 65–80.

Moore TR. Diabetes in pregnancy. In: Creasy RK, Resnik R, Iams JS (eds.) Maternal-Fetal Medicine. 5th ed. Saunders, Philadelphia, 2004. pp. 1023–1061.

MRC Vitamin Study Research Group. Prevention of neural-tube defects: results of the Medical Research Council Vitamin Study. Lancet 1991; 338: 131–137.

Nader S. Thyroid disease and pregnancy. In: Creasy RK, Resnik R, Iams JS (eds.) Maternal-Fetal Medicine. 5th ed. Saunders, Philadelphia, 2004. pp. 1063–1081.

Nielsen GL, Sorensen HT, Nielsen PH et al. Glycosylated haemoglobin as predictor of adverse fetal outcome in type 1 diabetic pregnancies. Acta Diabetol 1997; 34: 217–222.

Passarge E, Lenz W. Syndrome of caudal regression in infants of diabetic mothers: observations of further cases. Pediatrics 1966; 37: 672–675.

Phooojaroenchanachai M, Sriussadapom S, Peerpatdir T et al. Effect of maternal hyperthyroidism during late pregnancy on the risk of neonatal low birth weight. Clin Endocrinol 2001; 54: 365–370.

Reece EA, Sivan E, Francis G et al. Pregnancy outcomes among women with and without diabetic microvascular disease (White's classes B to FR) versus non-diabetic controls. Am J Perinatol 1998; 15: 549–555.

Reece EA, Leguizamón G, Wiznitzer A: Gestational diabetes: the need for a common ground. Lancet 2009; 373: 1789–1797.

Rusnak SL, Driscoll SG. Congenital spinal anomalies in infants of diabetic mothers. Pediatrics 1965; 35: 989–995.

Sheffield JS, Butler-Koster EL, Casey BM et al. Maternal diabetes mellitus and Infant's malformations. Obstet Gynecol 202; 100: 925–930.

Toaff R, Toaff M, Peyser M et al. Hepatolenticular degeneration (Wilson's disease) and pregnancy. Obstet Gynecol Surv 1977; 32: 497–507.

Weigel MM, Weigel R. Nausea and vomiting of early pregnancy and pregnancy outcome. An epidemiological study. Br J Obstet Gynaecol 1989; 96: 1304–1311.

Weiss PAM, Coustan DR (eds.) Gestational Diabetes. Springer Verlag, Wien-New York, 1988.

White P. Diabetes complicating pregnancy. Am J Obstet Gynecol 1937; 33: 380–385.

WHO (World Health Organization). Toxicological evaluation of certain food additives and contaminants. FAS 1988; 24: 267–294.

WHO (World Health Organization). Trace elements in human nutrition and health. WHO Geneva, 1996.

Own Publications

I. Czeizel AE, Intõdy Zs, Modell B. What proportion of congenital abnormalities can be prevented? Br Med J 1993; 306: 499–503.

II. Czeizel AE. Ten years experience in periconceptional care. Eur J Obstet Gynecol Reprod Biol 1999; 84: 43–49.

III. Nielsen GL, Norgard B, Puhó E, Rothman KJ, Sorensen HT, Olsen J. Risk of specific congenital abnormalities in offspring of women with diabetes. Diabet Med 2005; 22: 693–696.

IV. Czeizel AE, Ács N, Bánhidy F. Diabetes mellitus in pregnant women and adverse birth outcomes. In: Swahn E (ed.): Diabetes in Women. NOVA Science Publ. New York, 2010. pp. 1–25.

V. Bánhidy F, Ács N, Czeizel AE. Congenital abnormalities in the offspring of pregnant women with type 1, type 2, gestational diabetes mellitus and prevention with high dose of folic acid – a population-based case-control study, 2010 (in press).

VI. Czeizel AE, Puhó E, Ács N, Bánhidy F. Inverse association between severe nausea and vomiting in pregnancy and some congenital abnormalities. Am J Med Genet 2006; 140A: 453–462.

VII. Czeizel AE., Dudás I. Prevention of the first occurrence of neural-tube defects by periconceptional vitamin supplementation. N Engl J Med 1992; 327: 1832–1835.

VIII. Czeizel AE. Reduction of urinary tract and cardiovascular defects by periconceptional multivitamin supplementation. Am J Med Genet 1996; 62: 179–183.

IX. Czeizel AE, Dobó M, Vargha P. Hungarian two-cohort study of periconceptional multivitamin supplementation to prevent congenital abnormalities. Birth Defects Res A 2004; 70: 853–861.

X. Czeizel AE, Timár L, Sárközi A. Dose-dependent effect of folic acid on the prevention of orofacial clefts. Pediatrics 1999; 104: e66.

XI. Czeizel AE, Medveczi E. No difference in the occurrence of multimalformed offspring after periconceptional multivitamin supplementation. Obstet Gynecol 2003; 102: 1255–1261.

XII Czeizel AE, Puhó E, Bánhidy F. No association between periconceptional multivitamin supplementation and risk of multiple congenital abnormalities. A population-based case-control study. Am J Med Genet A 2006; 140A: 2469–2477.

XIII. Czeizel AE, Evans JA, Kodaj I, Lenz W. Congenital Limb Deficiencies in Hungary. Genetic and Teratologic Epidemiological Studies. Akadémiai Kiadó, Budapest, 1994.

XIV. Czeizel AE. Periconceptional care: An experiment in community genetics. Community Genetics 2000; 3: 119–123.

XV. Pilsihegyi J, Lacza T, Kazy, Czeizel AE. Genetic counseling and successful pregnancy in a patient with Wilson disease. (Hungarian with English abstract). Orvosi Hetilap 1993; 134: 1813–1816.

Chapter 6
Mental and Behavioural Disorders

Pregnancy may occur during the course of established psychiatric diseases, or, conversely, psychiatric illnesses may start first during pregnancy or more frequently shortly after delivery in the postpartum period. Specific psychiatric disorder related to pregnancy is not known, but all psychiatric diseases occurring in the reproductive period may affect pregnant women. However, pregnant women are different from non-pregnant women; therefore, the treatment of their psychiatric diseases needs special attention. On one hand, it is necessary to consider the possible teratogenic/fetotoxic effect of treatment. On the other hand, pregnant women are different from the psychopathologic aspect partly depending on their attitude regarding pregnancy (planned, not planned but accepted, don't want).

Nevertheless, psychiatric diseases and psychoses in pregnant women are frequently underestimated and/or undertreated; therefore, their recognition and management have critical importance both for the mothers and their fetuses. The symptoms of psychiatric disorders are similar in pregnant and non-pregnant women except the postpartum period. However, maternity blues and postpartum depression/psychoses are not topic of this monograph because the study period in our study is ending with the delivery.

6.1 Schizophrenia

Schizophrenia is a common disorder with a life-time prevalence of 0.8–1.0%. Diagnosis of schizophrenia is not an easy task because there is no universally accepted definition for schizophrenia with a central feature such as mood change in manic-depression disorders. Nevertheless, a constellation of symptoms such as hallucination and psychotic delusions, disordered thinking and concentration, erratic behavior, severely inappropriate emotional responses, social and occupational deterioration help the experts to get to the correct diagnosis. In general, the onset of schizophrenia occurs in young adults; therefore, pregnant women can be affected.

In the study of Rieder et al. (1975) the rate of fetal and neonatal deaths was 7.5% in 186 pregnant women who, or their husbands, had been hospitalized due to schizophrenia compared to 4.3% in the control group. However, an association of

N. Ács et al., *Congenital Abnormalities and Preterm Birth Related to Maternal Illnesses During Pregnancy*, DOI 10.1007/978-90-481-8620-4_6,

schizophrenia and related drug treatments with a higher risk of CA was not found. Bennedsen et al. (2001) studied 2,230 pregnancies of women with schizophrenia and higher rate of stillbirths and neonatal deaths of their offsprings have not been experienced. However, there was a marginally increased rate of CAs (RR: 1.70 with 95% CI: 1.04–2.77) and sudden infant death of their infants.

6.1.1 Interpretation of Data in the HCCSCA

Only one control was born to mother with schizophrenia. This very low number of subjects may indicate the limited chance of these patients to find partners and to become pregnant, in addition, patients frequently do not inform medical doctors about their schizophrenia in the prenatal care clinic. Additionally, there is a strong medical recommendation to terminate the pregnancies due to the higher genetic recurrence risk, the teratogenic potential of drugs used for maternal treatment, and mainly because of the serious difficulties to take care of the babies.

6.2 Manic-Depression Disorders

Two categories of the so-called affective disorders are differentiated: unipolar and bipolar diseases. Unipolar diseases include the rare manic diseases (about 0.1% in population) and the very frequent depression (about 2–6% with an obvious dominance in females). The bipolar manic-depression is diagnosed in about 1% of the population.

The criteria of major depressive episodes are well-defined (APA, 1994):

> Five (or more) of the following symptoms have been present during the same 2-week period and represent a change from previous functioning; at least one of the symptoms is either (i) depressed mood or (ii) loss of interest in pleasure. (iii) Depressed mood most of the day, nearly every day, as indicated by either subjective report (e.g. feels sad or empty) or observation made by others (e.g. appears tearful). (iv) Markedly diminished interest or pleasure in all or almost all activities most of the day, nearly every day (as indicated by either subjective account or observation by others). (v) Significant weight loss or weight gain when not dieting (e.g. a change of more than 5% of body weight in a month), or decrease or increase in appetite nearly every day

1. Insomnia or hypersomnia nearly every day
2. Psychomotor agitation or retardation nearly every day (observable by others, not merely subjective feelings of restlessness or being slowed down)
3. Fatigue or loss of energy nearly every day
4. Feelings of worthlessness or excessive or inappropriate guilt (which may be delusional) nearly every day (not merely self-reproach or guilt about being sick)
5. Diminished ability to think or concentrate, or indecisiveness, nearly every day (either by subjective account or as observed by others)
6. Recurrent thoughts of death (not just fear of dying), recurrent suicidal ideation without a specific plan, or a suicide attempt or a specific plan for committing suicide (Parry, 2004)

We cited word by word this criterion system because it was followed at the diagnosis of Hungarian pregnant women with affective disorders. It is necessary to recognize these symptoms as early as possible because early treatment dramatically improves the prognosis of this disorder group. The onset of these diseases in general prior to pregnancy. The symptoms usually do not increase during pregnancy but the severity of the symptoms often gets more serious in postpartum period. The results of several studies showed that untreated depression in pregnant women can impair neurocognitive development of the child (Dawson et al., 1992; Murray, 1992). Therefore, the risk of major depression and other psychiatric illnesses are much worse for the brain and other organs of fetuses than the potential adverse effects of psychotropic medication (Parry, 2004).

Kallen and Tandberg (1983) evaluated the pregnancy outcomes of 350 women with manic-depressive disorders. They found that the rate of fetal death before the 26th week was 16.6% while the perinatal death rate was 4.3%. Out of these 350 pregnant women, 59 were treated by lithium. Kinney et al. (1993) found significantly higher rate of pregnancy complications in 16 women with bipolar disease compared to the data of their unaffected siblings.

6.2.1 Interpretation of Data in the HCCSCA

Out of 22,843 cases, 21 (0.09%) had mothers with medically recorded manic-depressive disorders, while out of 38,151 controls, 22 (0.06%) were born to pregnant women with these diseases. The distribution of CAs in 21 cases was the following: congenital hydrocephalus 1, cleft lip 1, cleft lip + cleft palate 2, cardiovascular CA 3 (ventricular septal defect, left heart hypoplasia, dextrocardia), cystic kidney 1, obstructive CA of the urinary tract 1, undescended testis 5, hypospadias 3, polydactyly 1, clubfoot 2, multiple CA 2. The higher number of 2 CAs of the male genital organs is noteworthy, but their separate adjusted OR did not indicate significant association. However, it is important to stress that only 6 case mothers were treated with antidepressive drugs because medical doctors did not recommend the use of these drugs during pregnancy due to the hypothetical teratogenic risk

The mean gestational age of 22 control newborns was 38.0 week with the mean birth weight of 2,896 g. The rate of PB was 31.8%, while the rate of LBW was 22.7%. These high figures of adverse birth outcomes showed the hazard of this maternal disease group for the fetal development. Out of 22 control mothers, 6 were treated with antidepressive drugs, the gestational age of their newborns was 39.3 week with mean birth weight of 3,268 g, i.e. much better than the values of babies born to untreated mothers.

In conclusion, the prevalence of manic-depression disorders is strongly under-ascertained in the data set of the HCCSCA.

6.3 Panic Disorders

Anxiety disorders ("i.e. various combination of physical and mental manifestations of anxiety, not attributable to real danger and occurring either in attacks or as a persisting state") cover a wide spectrum including panic disorder ("the anxiety is usually diffuse and may extend to panic") (WHO, 2007).

Most pregnant women with anxiety disorders were diagnosed as *panic disorder* (PD) in Hungary; therefore, we focused our study on these patients. PD occurs in females during childbearing years, thus in pregnant women as well. A number of clinical challenges then arise due to prenatal exposure to psychotropic drugs for the fetuses of women with PD (Cohen and Rosenbaum, 1998; Ericson et al., 1999) and for the pregnant women (George et al., 1987; Cowley et al., 1989; Villeponteaux et al., 1992; Klein et al., 1994; Roy-Byrne et al., 1999). On the other hand, some studies also suggest adverse effects of untreated maternal PD or other anxiety disorders on neonatal outcome (Istran, 1986; Steer et al., 1992; Orr and Miller, 1995).

PD was the most frequent anxiety disorder reported for pregnant women in the HCCSCA. The objectives of the study were to investigate the occurrence of pregnancy complications, in addition to possible associations between maternal PD and drug treatments during pregnancy and adverse birth outcomes, particularly CAs.

6.3.1 Results of the Study (I, II)

The case group consisted of 22,865 malformed newborns or fetuses ("informative offspring"), of whom 210 (0.9%) had mothers with PD. Of the 38,151 controls, 187 (0.5%) were born to mothers suffering from PD (crude OR: 1.9, 1.5–2.3).

Nearly all maternal PD were medically recorded in the prenatal maternity logbooks (93.8% in case and 96.8% in control mothers). Pregnant women with other anxiety disorders, like depression, etc. were excluded from the study.

The mean maternal age (26.1 vs. 25.4 year) and birth order (1.7 vs. 1.6) was somewhat higher in pregnant women with PD compared to pregnant women without PD as reference. There was a larger proportion of unmarried status (7.0% vs. 3.2%) and their employment status showed a smaller proportion of professional and managerial women (26.8% vs. 38.0%) and larger proportion of unskilled workers and housewives (20.4% vs. 10.2%) in pregnant women with PD.

The proportion of smokers was 20% and 18% in case and control pregnant women, however, this figure was 2-times higher in case mothers with PD (42.1%). Hard drinking was rarely found in both case and control mothers during the study pregnancy. The reported use of illegal recreational drugs was very limited among pregnant women during the study period.

The evaluation of different pregnancy supplements showed a drastic difference in the use of folic acid in case mothers with or without PD (35.2% vs. 49.5%) compared to control mothers with or without PD (51.3% vs. 54.5%). The use of multivitamins did not show obvious differences in case (7.1% vs. 5.8%) and control (6.4% vs. 6.6%) mothers with or without PD. Finally, it is worth mentioning the use of iron in case (53.8% vs. 64.6%) and control (66.3% vs. 70.2%) mothers with or without PD.

Out of 187 control and 210 case mothers with PD, 51 (27.3%) and 46 (21.9%) had no other diseases during the study pregnancy, respectively. The prevalence of all but one acute maternal disease did not show obvious difference between the study groups. The exception was influenza and/or common cold generally with secondary complications which was more frequent in case mothers with PD than in case mothers without PD (31.4% vs. 21.7%). Similar difference was not seen in the two subgroups of control mothers (19.3% vs. 18.5%), thus this disease group occurred more frequently in case than in control mothers with PD (1.9, 1.2–3.1).

Among chronic diseases, hemorrhoid (7.5% vs. 3.3%) was more frequent in pregnant women with PD than in pregnant women without PD.

The first objective of the study was to evaluate pregnancy complications (Table 6.1).

Table 6.1 Incidence of pregnancy complications in control pregnant women with or without PD

	With PD (*N* = 187)		Without PD (*N* = 37,964)		Difference
Pregnancy complications	No.	%	No.	%	OR (95% CI)
Threatened abortion	35	18.7	6,477	17.1	1.1 (0.8–1.6)
Nausea-vomiting, severe	21	11.2	3,848	10.1	1.1 (0.7–1.8)
Preeclampsia-eclampsia	22	11.8	3,199	8.4	1.4 (0.9–2.3)
Threatened preterm delivery[a]	19	10.2	5,983	15.8	**0.6 (0.4–1.0)**
Placental disorders[b]	1	0.5	591	1.6	0.3 (0.0–2.4)
Gestational diabetes	2	1.1	268	0.7	1.5 (0.4–6.2)
Polyhydramnios	3	1.6	188	0.5	**3.3 (1.0–10.3)**
Anemia	46	24.6	6,310	16.6	**1.6 (1.2–2.3)**

[a]Including cervical incompetence.
[b]Including placenta previa, premature separation of placenta, antepartum hemorrhage.

The proportion of polyhydramnios (however, this possible association was based on only 3 mothers and its power is very wide with a lower figure of 1) and anemia was higher in control mothers with PD than in the control mothers without PD. However, the incidence of threatened preterm delivery was marginally lower in mothers with PD.

Drugs were evaluated in two categories. (i) Of course, all drugs for PD such as diazepam (34.2% vs. 10.7%), chlordiazepoxide (20.9% vs. 0.6%), phenobarbitals (9.1% vs. 1.0%), meprobamate (5.9% vs. 0.3%), tofisopam (5.4% vs. 0.1%), nitrazepam (2.7% vs. 0.0%), medazepam (1.6% vs. 0.0%), and alprazolam (1.1% vs. 0.0%) were much more commonly used by women with PD. Together 73.1% of case and 73.9% of control mothers with PD were treated with these drugs (ii) Among most frequently used other drugs, four: promethazine (32.6% vs. 15.7%), allylestrenol (19.3% vs. 14.0%), dipyrone (12.3% vs. 5.0%), and dimenhydrate (8.6% vs. 4.5%) also showed a higher prevalence in mothers with PD.

The second aim of the study was the evaluation of birth outcomes of control newborns without CA born to mothers with or without PD (Table 6.2)

Table 6.2 Distribution of birth weight and gestational age groups in newborn infants born to mothers with or without PD

Gestational age (week)		37 or less		38–41		42 or more		Total				Gestational age[b]			
		With PD	Without PD	With PD	Without PD	With PD	Without PD	With PD		Without PD		With PD		Without PD	
Birth weight (g)		No.	No.	No.	No.	No.	No.	No.	%	No.	%	Mean	S.D.	Mean	S.D.
2,499 or less		12	1,271	3	830	1	50	16	8.6	2,151	5.7	35.5	3.5	35.6	3.2
2,500–3,499		20	2,164	78	19,108	8	1,462	106	56.7	22,734	59.9	38.6	2.1	39.1	1.8
3,500 or more		0	29	55	10,719	10	2,331	65	34.8	13,079	34.5	40.4	1.0	40.5	1.1
Total	No.	32	3,464	136	30,657	19	3,843	187	100.0	37,964	100.0	39.0	2.4	39.4	2.1
	%	17.1	9.1	72.7	80.8	10.2	10.1	100.0	–	–	–	–	–	–	–
Birth weight[a]	Mean	2,510	2,483	3,320	3,323	3,588	3,616	3,209	–	3,276	–	–	–	–	–
	S.D.	409	437	441	430	620	485	560	–	511	–	–	–	–	–

[a]Adjusted t-test for birth weight for maternal employment status, use of pregnancy supplements: $t = 1.4$, $p = 0.16$.
Adjusted OR for LBW for employment status, use of pregnancy supplements, maternal age: 1.4 (0.8–2.3).
[b]Adjusted t-test for gestational age for maternal employment status, use of pregnancy supplements: $t = 2.3$, $p =$ **0.02**.
Adjusted OR for PB for employment status, use of pregnancy supplements, maternal age: **1.9 (1.3–2.8)**.

Sex ratio, i.e. the proportion of males was larger in newborn infants born to mothers with PD with about 5% compared to newborns of mothers without PD ($p < 0.001$). Mean gestational age was 0.4 week shorter in the mothers with PD and the shorter gestational age was seen in all birthweight groups, but particularly in the group of 2,500–3,499 g. The proportion of PB was 1.9 times larger in the newborn infants of mothers with PD. The shorter gestational age resulted in a somewhat lower (67 g) birth weight as well. The proportion of LBW newborns was also larger – but not significantly – in the group of mothers with PD. These associations remained unchanged when male and female newborns were evaluated separately.

We attempted to differentiate the effect of PD and their related drug treatments for gestational age and preterm birth (Table 6.3).

Table 6.3 Differentiation of the effect of PD and related drug treatments for gestational age and preterm birth (PB)

		Antipanic disorder drugs[a]	
Panic disorders		Yes	No
Yes	No.	151	59
	Gestational age (mean, S.D.)	38.9 ± 2.4	39.0 ± 2.3
	t-test	$p = \mathbf{0.03}$	$p = 0.14$
	PB (%)	14.8	22.0
	χ^2test	$p = \mathbf{0.009}$	$p = \mathbf{0.0002}$
No	No.	4,686	33,278
	Gestational age (mean, S.D.)	38.9 ± 2.2	39.4 ± 2.0
	t-test	$p < \mathbf{0.0001}$	Reference[b]
	PB (%)	14.3	8.4
	χ^2test	$p < \mathbf{0.0001}$	Reference[b]

[a]Diazepam, Chlordiazepoxide, Phenobarbitals, Meprobamate, Tofisopam, Nitrazepam, Medazepam, Alprazolum.
[b]Without PD and antipanic drug treatment.

The largest proportion of PB was seen in the group of PD without treatment. However, mean gestational age was shorter, but similar in the groups of PD with antipanic drugs and pregnant women without PD but treated with these drugs than in pregnant women without PD and without treatment of antipanic drugs as referent.

Finally – as the third objective of the study – 15 CA-groups (including at least 3 cases) were evaluated by two statistical approaches (Table 6.4).

The evaluation of cases with different CAs showed a higher prevalence of maternal PD for two CA-groups: cleft lip ± palate and multiple CAs. Nineteen cases with multiple CAs had 69 component CAs and the more frequent component CAs were the following: cardiovascular CA 9, particularly ventricular septal defect 4, cleft lip ± palate 5, hypospadias 4, congenital hydrocephalus 3, neural-tube defect 3, polydactyly 3, and the rare CAs of the spine 3. Most multiple CAs might be caused by monogenic conditions or new mutations but clinicians were unable to identify these CA-syndromes.

Table 6.4 Comparison of PD's prevalence in the mothers of cases with different CAs and their all matched controls or matched case-control pairs

Study groups	Grand total no.	Panic disorder No.	%	One case – all controls Adjusted OR[a] (95% CI)		One case – one control pair Adjusted OR[a] (95% CI)	
Isolated CAs							
Neural-tube defects	1,202	13	1.1	1.1	(0.5–2.4)	1.2	(0.5–2.9)
Cleft lip± palate	1,374	15	1.1	**3.4**	**(1.3–9.0)**	**5.4**	**(1.5–19.4)**
Cleft palate only	582	6	1.0	2.2	(0.5–8.5)	1.4	(0.4–5.4)
Oesophageal atresia/stenosis	217	4	1.8	–		–	
Hypospadias	3,038	26	0.9	1.6	(0.9–2.9)	1.2	(0.6–2.3)
Undescended testis	2,051	19	0.9	1.6	(0.8–3.3)	1.4	(0.7–3.1)
Exomphalos/gastroschisis	238	3	1.3	3.4	(0.5–23.8)	5.4	(0.5–61.1)
Congenital hydrocephaly	314	3	1.0	0.8	(0.2–4.0)	0.9	(0.1–5.1)
Cardiovascular CAs	4,479	46	1.0	1.4	(0.9–2.2)	1.2	(0.7–2.0)
CAs of the genital organs	123	3	2.4	3.1	(0.3–33.1)	–	
Clubfoot	2,424	19	0.8	1.5	(0.8–2.9)	1.6	(0.7–3.5)
Limb deficiencies	548	4	0.7	1.2	(0.3–5.4)	2.0	(0.2–18.8)
Poly/syndactyly	1,744	13	0.8	1.4	(0.7–3.1)	1.1	(0.5–2.6)
Other isolated CAs	3,160	17*	0.5	1.4	(0.7–3.4)	1.5	(0.7–3.3)
Multiple CAs	1,349	19	1.4	**3.0**	**(1.2–7.2)**	**3.7**	**(1.2–11.4)**
Total cases	22,843	210	0.9	**1.6**	**(1.3–2.0)**	**1.5**	**(1.2–1.9)**
Total controls	38,151	187	0.5	Reference[b]		Reference[b]	

[a]OR with 95% CI adjusted for maternal age, birth order, maternal employment status, influenza-common cold, antipanic disorder drugs, use of folic acid and compared to controls as reference using a conditional regression model.
[b]The data of controls were considered as an etalon.
[c]CA of diaphragm 2, torticollis 2, hydronephrosis, cong. stricture of ureteropelvic junction, primary microcephaly, porencephaly, microtia, branchial cyst, cleft nose, intestinal atresia, anal atresia, Hirschsprung's disease, atresia of bile duct, pectus excavatum, CA of spine.

Finally, we attempted to differentiate the effect of PD or their related drug treatments on cleft lip ± palate or multiple CAs (Table 6.5).

PD in mothers without antipanic drugs had a higher adjusted OR than mothers with antipanic drug treatments in both of these two CA groups. In fact, drugs used for the treatment of this disease seemed to be protective for cleft lip ± palate and multiple CAs.

6.3.2 Interpretation of the Results

The major finding of our study is that the offsprings of pregnant women with PD had a higher risk for cleft lip ± palate and multiple CAs if they were untreated with antidepressant drugs. However, the offsprings of pregnant women with PD treated with drugs, mainly benzodiazepines, had no higher risk in any of the CA groups. Therefore, we can conclude that PD itself is teratogenic.

Table 6.5 Estimation of the associations between maternal PD with or without related drugs and cleft lip ± palate and multiple CAs

	All		With antipanic disorder drugs[a]		Without antipanic disorder drugs	
Study groups	No.	Adjusted OR[b]	No.	Adjusted OR[b] (95% CI)	No.	Adjusted OR[b] (95% CI)
Controls	187	Reference[c]	128	Reference[c]	59	Reference[c]
Cleft lip ± palate	15	**2.1 (1.2–3.5)**	8	1.5 (0.7–3.2)	7	**3.1 (1.4–6.9)**
Multiple CAs	19	**2.6 (1.6–4.2)**	13	1.7 (0.9–3.1)	6	**2.9 (1.2–6.7)**

[a]Including Alprazolam, Chlordiazepoxide, Diazepam, Medazepam, Meprobamate, Nitrazepam, Phenobarbital, and Tofisopam.
[b]OR with 95% CI adjusted for maternal age, birth order, maternal employment status, influenza-common cold, use of folic acid.
[c]The data of controls were considered as an etalon.

The secondary results of the study showed a higher prevalence of anemia in pregnant women with PD. It may be associated with the lower socioeconomic status of pregnant women with PD without appropriate treatment (we refer the low rate of iron supplementation). The higher rate of PB is probably explained by the lower socioeconomic status and lifestyle of pregnant women with PD (Orr and Miller, 1995; Abelson et al., 1997; Ericson et al., 1999; Hoffmann and Hatch, 2000; Orr et al., 2002; Dole et al., 2003).

The prevalence of PD was 0.5% in our study and this rate is lower than it was expected based on other studies (Halbreich, 2004). However, we only evaluated medically recorded PDs, which were probably more severe cases than subjects in prior studies.

In the study, a significant male excess was found among cases with PD. Further studies are needed to explain this phenomenon because it is hard to believe that maternal PD can modify the sex ratio of zygotes at the time of conception. A higher proportion of fetal death particularly including more females has not been reported in pregnant women with depression and panic disorders (Klein et al., 1994).

Cleft lip ± palate and multiple CAs were more prevalent in informative offspring of case mothers with PD. The question is whether these possible associations are causal or explained by biases, confounders or happened by chance. The role of possible biases might be limited. The effect of confounders particularly related drug treatment was restricted by the calculation of adjusted OR for the analysis of matched case-control pairs. In addition, the potential teratogenic effect of benzodiazepines such as diazepam (54), chlordiazepoxide (55), nitrazepam, medazepam, tofisopam, alprazolam (56) in the data set of the HCCSCA without any association with cleft lip±palate and multiple CAs. Phenobarbital (58), promethazine (74), allylestrenol (66), dipyrone (81), and dimenhydrate (71) treatment during pregnancy also did not show any association with these two groups of CAs. Finally, no higher risks of CAs have been reported in mothers who attempted suicide with extremely large doses of diazepam (106), chlorodiazepoxide (107), alprazolum (109), medazepam (110), phenobarbital (115) meprobamate (117), or promethazine (111) during pregnancy.

Our recent findings suggest that CAs in the offspring of pregnant women with psychiatric disorders are mainly caused by the psychiatric disorders and the related lifestyle, and not by the drugs used for their treatment.

Among direct effects of PD, different quantity and/or pathogenic effect of neurotransmitters or other brain chemicals of the disease itself can be considered. Among PD related lifestyle factors a higher occurrence of substance use/abuse behaviors, alcohol drinking was not found in the study, in addition cleft lip ± palate and the pattern of component CAs in our multiple CA cases did not fit the characteristics of fetal alcohol syndrome (Jones et al., 1973; Abel, 1983). However, the proportion of smokers was larger in pregnant women with PD in the study. Ericson et al. (1979) found a significant increase in smokers among 66 women who gave birth to infants with isolated oral clefts. In another Swedish study, the data of two registries were evaluated and an association was found between maternal smoking and isolated cleft palate (OR: 1.35; 1.12–1.63) (Källen, 1997). In addition, a gene-environmental interaction has been proposed behind the occurrence of oral clefts in children with the rare C2 allele of the transforming growth factor alpha (TGF-alpha) gene born to women who smoked during pregnancy (Hwang et al., 1995).

Finally, the use of folic acid was less frequent in mothers with PD. A low dose (0.8 mg) of a folic acid-containing multivitamin in the early part of pregnancy may have some preventive effect for neural-tube defects, cardiovascular CAs, CAs of the urinary tract and limb deficiencies, but not for oral clefts (III–V). However, periconceptional use of a multivitamin and a very high dose of folic acid (10 mg) together were able to reduce the recurrence risk of cleft lip ± palate (Tolarova, 1982). In general, also a high dose of folic acid (about 6 mg) was used for the prevention of neural-tube defects in Hungary (thus in this data set as well) and it reduced the occurrence of oral clefts by about 30% (VI). In addition, Shaw et al. (1998) found evidence for an interaction between the TGF-alpha marker and folic acid-containing multivitamin use. Thus, the interaction of maternal disorder itself, the lifestyle of patients and the lower rate of periconceptional folic acid supplementation may be the multicausal factor in the origin of cleft lip ± palate and multiple CAs found in the offspring of mothers with PD.

PD typically has a chronic and recurrent course (Pollack et al., 1990; Cohen, 1996). Pregnancy may ameliorate symptoms of PD in some patients (George et al., 1987; Cowley et al., 1989; Villeponteaux et al., 1992; Klein et al., 1994); of course, there is no need for treatment if symptoms of PD are ameliorated during pregnancy. However, other pregnant women with PD appear to experience persistence or exacerbation of symptoms (Cohen, 1996; Roy-Byrne et al., 1999). Untreated anxiety may have an adverse effect for neonatal outcome (Istran et al., 1986; Steer et al., 1992; Perkin et al., 1993; Orr and Miller, 1995; Abelson et al., 1997). However, a recent study did not reveal differences in neonatal outcome between women with antenatal depressive disorders and/or anxiety disorders and healthy subjects (Field et al., 2003). However, only those pregnant women were included into the study who had mental disorders in the second trimester of pregnancy. Abrupt discontinuation of antipanic medication is not recommended (Ballanger et al., 1998). Drugs used for the treatment of PD are not proved human teratogenic drugs; in fact this study suggested some protective effect of CAs after adequate drug treatment. Therefore, antipanic treatment, a strong control of lifestyle (e.g. without alcohol consumption and smoking) together with adjunctive cognitive-behavioral therapy may be pursued to minimize risk for CAs and adverse birth outcomes during pregnancy of women with PD. This strategy may help to avoid the withdrawal symptoms of benzodiazepine treatment in newborn infants.

In conclusion, our study showed a somewhat shorter gestational age in pregnant women with PD and related lifestyle and it explains the significantly higher rate of PB. In addition, a higher occurrence of cleft lip ± palate and multiple CAs was found in the offspring of mothers with PD without antipanic drugs, but no higher risk of these CAs was found in the treated group. Higher risk of CAs in untreated group may be the results of an interaction between maternal PD and lifestyle factors.

6.4 Other Anxiety Disorders

6.4.1 Interpretation of Data in the HCCSCA

Out of 22,843 cases, 7 (0.03%), while out of 38,151 controls, 17 (0.04%) had mothers with the other types of anxiety disorders (mainly different phobic states). Of the 7 cases, each had different CAs, while birth outcomes of controls did not deviate significantly from the Hungarian average birth weight and gestational age at delivery.

There was only one case born to mother with drug dependence during the study pregnancy and he was affected with hypospadias.

6.5 Alcohol Dependence Syndrome and Drunkenness

6.5.1 Interpretation of Data in the HCCSCA

Out of 22,813 cases, 5 had mothers with alcohol dependence syndrome, while out of 38,151 controls, 1 was recorded with drunkenness in the prenatal care logbook. The latter was born on 37th gestational week with 1,240 g without visible CA. Five cases (4 boys and 1 girl) were affected by CAs: lethal left heart hypoplasia, cystic kidney, multiple CA (complex cardiovascular CA: atrial septal + ductus, ductus persistent arteriosus, and lung hypoplasia) and undescended testis in 2 boys (VII).

There was only one case born to mother with *drug dependence* during the study pregnancy and he was affected with hypospadias.

6.6 Mental Retardation

The diagnosis of mental retardation is based on psychometric (IQ of less than 70), social (educational incompetence) and biological (developmental anomaly) criteria and is classified as severe, medium, or mild. From medical aspect, pathological and familial-cultural categories are differentiated. The Hungarian data and results of researches were summarized previously (VIII).

6.6.1 Interpretation of Data in the HCCSCA

Out of 22,843 cases, 7 (0.03) had mothers with mental retardation (recorded in the prenatal logbook) while similar diagnosis occurred in 4 (0.01%) mothers in the control group. The latter 2 boys were born on the 30th and 35th gestational weeks with 1,200 and 2,600 g birth weights and 2 girls were born on 34th and 35th gestational weeks with birth weight of 1,700 and 2,600 g and showed the above adverse birth outcomes. Of the 7 cases, 2 died of lethal left heart hypoplasia and multiple CA including lethal complex heart CA during neonatal period. The other 5 cases were affected by congenital hydrocephalus, ventricular septal defects, undescended testis, syndactyly, and clubfoot in 2 cases.

6.7 Final Conclusions

There are two main results of the evaluation of mental disorders. The first is that the number of pregnant women with these disorders is obviously underdiagnosed and/or underreported, although, mental disorders have an increasing number and public health importance. The second observation is that necessary drug treatments are frequently neglected because of the hypothetic teratogenic effect of drugs. The main message of this chapter is that the withdrawing or withholding the necessary drug treatment is far more dangerous than the drugs themselves.

References

Abel EL. Fetal Alcohol Syndrome and Fetal Alcohol Effects. Plenum Press, New York, 1983.

Abelson JL, Curtis GC, Cameron OG. Hypothalamic-pituitary-adrenal axis activity in panic disorder: effects of alprazolum on secretion of adrenocorticotropin and cortisol. J Psychiatr Res 1997; 30: 79–93.

APA: American Psychiatric Association. Diagnostic and Statistical Manuel for Mental Disorders, 4th ed. American Psychiatric Association, Washington, DC, 1994.

Ballanger JC, Davidson JR, Lecrubier Y et al. Consensus statement on panic disorder from the International Consensus Group on Depression and Anxiety. J Clin Psychiatr 1998; 59(Suppl.8): 47–54.

Bennedsen BE, Mortensen PB, Plesen AV, Henriksen TB. Congenital malformations, stillbirths, and infant deaths among children of women with schizophrenia. Arch Gen Psychitr 2001; 58: 674–679.

Cohen L. Prospective study of panic disorder during pregnancy and the postpartum period. In: Syllabons and Proceedings. Summary of the 1996 Annual Meeting of the American Psychiatric Association. New York, NY, 1996. May 4–9, No.25: 11.

Cohen LS, Rosenbaum JF. Psychotropic drug use during pregnancy: weighing the risk. J Clin Psychiatr 1998; 59(Suppl.2): 18–28.

Cowley LS, Sichel DA, Faraone SV et al. Panic disorder during pregnancy. J Psychosom Obstet Gynecol 1989; 10: 193–210.

Dawson G, Klinger LG, Panagiorides H et al. Frontal lobe activity and affective behavior of infants of mothers with depressive symptoms. Child Develop 1992; 63: 725–737.

Dole N, Savitz DA, Hertz-Picciotto I et al. Maternal stress and preterm birth. Am J Epidemiol 2003; 157: 14–24.

Ericson A, Källen B, Westerholm P. Cigarette smoking as an etiologic factor in cleft lip and palate. Am J Obstet Gynecol 1979; 135: 348–351.

Ericson A, Källen B, Wilholm B-E. Delivery outcome after the use of antidepressants in early pregnancy. Eur J Clin Pharmacol 1999; 55: 503–508.

Field T, Diego M, Hernandez-Reif J et al. Pregnancy anxiety and comorbid depression and anger: effects on the fetus and neonate. Depress Anxiety 2003; 17: 140–151.

George DT, Ladenhlim JA, Nutt DJ. Effect of pregnancy on panic attacks. Am J Psychiatry 1987; 144: 1078–1079.

Halbreich U. Prevalence of mood symptoms and depressions during pregnancy: implications for clinical practice and research. CNS Spectr 2004; 9: 177–184.

Hoffmann S, Hatch MC. Depressive symptomatology during pregnancy: evidence for an association with decreased fetal growth in pregnancies of lower social class women. Health Psychiol 2000; 19: 535–543.

Hwang SJ, Beaty TH, Panny SR et al. Association study of transforming growth factor alpha (TGFA) Taq1 polymorphism and oral clefts: indication of gene-environment interaction in a population-based sample of infants with birth defects. Am J Epidemiol 1995; 141: 629–636.

Istran J. Stress, anxiety, and birth outcome: a critical review of the evidence. Psychol Bull 1986; 100: 331–348.

Jones KL, Smith DW, Ulleland CL et al. Pattern of malformation in offspring of chronic alcoholic mothers. Lancet 1973; 1: 1267–1271.

Källen K. Maternal smoking and orofacial clefts. Cleft Palate Craniofac J 1997; 34: 11–16.

Kallen B, Tandberg A. Lithium and pregnancy. Acta Psychiatr Scand 1983; 68: 134–139.

Klein DF, Skrobala AM, Garfinkel DS. Preliminary look at the effects of pregnancy on the course of panic disorders (technical note). Anxiety 1994; 1: 227–232.

Kinney DK, Yurgelan-Tadd DA, Levy DL et al. Obstetrical complications in patients with bipolar disorders and their siblings. Psychiatr Res 1993; 48: 47–56.

Murray L. The impact of postnatal depression on infant development. J Child Psychol Psychiatr 1992; 33: 543–561.

Orr S, Miller C. Maternal depressive symptoms and risk of poor pregnancy outcome: review of the literature and preliminary findings. Epidemiol Rev 1995; 17: 165–171.

Orr ST, James SA, Prince BC. Maternal prenatal depressive symptoms and spontaneous preterm births among African-American women in Baltimore, Maryland. Am J Epidemiol 2002; 156: 797–802.

Parry BL. Management of depression and psychoses during pregnancy and the puerperium. In: Creasy RK, Resnik R, Iams JD (eds.) Maternal-Fetal Medicine. 5th ed. Saunders, Philadelphia, 2004. pp. 1193–1200.

Perkin MR, Bland JM, Peacock JL et al. The effect of Anxiety and depression during pregnancy on obstetric complications. Br J Obstet Gynaecol 1993; 100: 629–634.

Pollack MH, Otto MW, Rosenbaum JF et al. Longitudinal course of panic disorder: findings from the Massachusetts General Hospital Naturalistic Study. J Clin Psychiatr 1990; 51(Suppl.A): 12–16.

Rieder RO, Rosenthal D, Wender P, Blumenthal H. The offspring of schizophrenics. Arc Gen Psychiatr 1975; 32: 200–211.

Roy-Byrne PP, Dager SR, Cowley DS et al. Relapse and rebound following discontinuation of benzodiazepine treatment of panic attacks: alprazolum versus diazepam. Am J Psychiatry 1999; 146: 860–865.

Shaw GM, Wasserman CR, Murray J, Lammer EJ. Infant TGF-alpha genotype, orofacial clefts, and maternal periconceptional multivitamin use. Cleft Palate Craniofac J 1998; 35: 366–370.

Steer RA, School TO, Hediger ML et al. Self-reported depression and negative pregnancy outcomes. J Clin Epidemiol 1992; 45: 1093–1099.

Tolarova M. Periconceptional supplementation with vitamins and folic acid to prevent recurrence of cleft lip. Lancet 1982; I: 217.

Villeponteaux VA, Lydiard RB, Lavaia MT et al. The effect of pregnancy on preexisting panic disorder. J Clin Psychiatr 1992; 53: 201–203.

WHO (World Health Organization). International Classification of Diseases (ICD), 10th ed. WHO, Geneva, 2007.

Own Publications

I. Ács N, Bánhidy F, Horváth-Puho E, Czeizel AE. Maternal panic disorders and congenital abnormalities: a population-based case-control study. Birth Defects Res A 2006; 76: 253–261.

II. Bánhidy F, Ács N, Puho E, Czeizel AE. Association between maternal panic disorders and pregnancy complications and delivery outcomes. Eur J Obstet Gynecol Reprod Biol 2006; 124: 47–52.

III. Czeizel AE, Dudás I. Prevention of the first occurrence of neural-tube defects by periconceptional multivitamin supplementation. N Engl J Med 1992; 327: 1832–1835.

IV. Czeizel AE. Reduction of urinary tract and cardiovascular defects by periconceptional multivitamin supplementation. Am J Med Genet 1996; 62: 179–183.

V. Czeizel AE, Dobó M, Vargha P. Hungarian cohort-controlled trial of periconceptional multivitamin supplementation shows a reduction in certain congenital abnormalities. Birth Defects Res A 2004; 70: 853–861.

VI. Czeizel AE, Tímár L, Sárközy A. Dose-dependent effect of folic acid on the prevention of orofacial clefts. Pediatrics 1999; 104: e66 (pp. 1–6) .

VII. Agarwall DP, Buda B, Czeizel AE, Goedde HW (eds.) Alcohol Consumption and Alcoholism in Hungary. Akadémiai Kiadó, Budapest, 1997.

VIII. Czeizel AE, Sankararanayeanana K, Szondy M. The load of genetic and partially genetic diseases in man. III. Mental retardation. Mutat Res 1990; 232: 291–303.

Chapter 7
Diseases of the Nervous System

The diseases of the central nervous system may occur during pregnancy as well, although, pregnancy specific disorders of pregnant women are not known. However, certain neurologic diseases may be aggravated or influenced by pregnancy.

7.1 Multiple Sclerosis

Multiple sclerosis is a neurological disorder of the central nervous system due to the demyelination process at different sites which develop at different times. Multiple sclerosis is typically associated with unpredictable exacerbations with increasingly severe neurological symptoms which are followed by remissions during which symptoms may partially or completely resolve.

In general, there is a remission during pregnancy because of gestational immunosuppressive state (Sadovnick et al., 1994) and multiple sclerosis does not modify the natural course of pregnancy or birth outcomes (Poser and Poser, 1983). However, there is an increased frequency of exacerbation of symptoms in women after childbirth within the first 3–6 months (Abramsky, 1994). Nevertheless, there is no association between the number of pregnancies and subsequent neurologic disability; in addition, the higher number of pregnancies did not shorten the life of patients with multiple sclerosis.

7.1.1 Interpretation of Data in the HCCSCA

Out of 22,843 cases, 3 (0.01%), while out of 38,151 controls, 6 (0.02%) had mothers affected with multiple sclerosis. Out of 3 cases 2 has undescended testis and one was affected with hypospadias. The mean gestational age of 6 control newborns was 39.8 week with 3,342 g mean birth weight without PB and LBW.

In conclusion multiple sclerosis does not pose a risk for pregnant women and their offspring.

N. Ács et al., *Congenital Abnormalities and Preterm Birth Related to Maternal Illnesses During Pregnancy*, DOI 10.1007/978-90-481-8620-4_7,

7.2 Epilepsy

Epilepsy is defined as a disorder of the brain function characterized by the periodic and unpredictable occurrence of seizures. Epilepsy is classified as primary generalized, or focal/partial with or without secondary generalization, in addition primary general seizures can be divided into absence, myoclonic, atonic, or tonic-clonic (Tomson et al., 1997; Wyllie, 2001; Aminoff, 2004).

Epilepsy is one of the most frequently studied maternal diseases during pregnancy. Most epilepsy had an early onset; therefore, it occurs in 0.3–0.6% of pregnant women. The higher rate of CA in the children of epileptic women was recognized in the 1960s (Janz and Fuchs, 1964) and later confirmed by several studies (Shepard and Lemire, 2004). However, there was a long debate whether this higher risk is associated with epilepsy itself (genetic predisposition or adverse effect of seizures), antiepileptic drugs, other (e.g. lifestyle) factors, or their interaction.

The relation between epilepsy and pregnancy is variable. About 45% of pregnant women have a higher seizure frequency while about 5% is associated with reduced seizure frequency, and epilepsy remains unchanged in about 50% of pregnant women (Knight and Rhind, 1975). The higher risk for seizure in about 45% of pregnant women may explain that epilepsy may appear first time during pregnancy (the term gestational epilepsy is used for these patients). Therefore, epileptic pregnant women need treatment during pregnancy as well. In addition, serum levels of antiepileptic drugs generally decline in pregnancy (and it may be an explanation for the higher seizure frequency), therefore an increase in dosage is frequently required during pregnancy to maintain the effective plasma level of antiepileptic drugs. According to experiences there is a higher risk for the deterioration of epileptic status in women with frequent seizures (more than one a month) during pregnancy, while if a woman had a seizure free 9 months period before she became pregnant, it is likely that she will not have any seizures during pregnancy.

At the selection of antiepileptic drugs the type of epilepsy is the most important, but other factors (e.g. the duration previous seizure-free interval, pregnancy, others diseases) should also be considered. The first choice is valproate and lamotrigine for the treatment of several seizure types, while carbamazepine and phenytoin are used for the management of partial seizures.

There are five basic observations in epileptic pregnant women. First, the risk of CA is about 3 fold higher in the offspring of epileptic pregnant women, but this rate depends on the spectrum of birth defects, whether only major CAs, all CAs or all CAs and minor anomalies together are evaluated. Second, Holmes et al. (2001) showed that pregnant women with a history of epilepsy and no treatment during pregnancy had no higher risk for CA. However, untreated women are expected to be affected with less severe epilepsy. Third, the risk of CA in the children of pregnant women with monotherapy is lower: 2.8 (1.1–9.7) than after polytherapy: 4.2 (1.1–5.1) (e.g. Kallen, 1986). These findings were confirmed by a meta-analysis of 10 cohort and case control studies regarding to the occurrence of CA in children of pregnant women with or without exposure to antiepileptic drugs compared to the outcome of children of healthy women (Fried et al., 2004). Fourth, certain specific CAs such as cleft lip ± plate, cleft palate only, and cardiovascular CA have a higher risk. Also, the combination of these and other CAs led to the delineation of antiepileptic drug related MCA-syndrome, although some differences in the teratogenic risk of different antiepileptic drugs were found (Meadow et al., 2008). Fifth, the higher dose of antiepileptic drugs is associated with a higher risk of specific CA but the cluster of seizures during pregnancy is associated with an even higher risk of CA.

Previously trimethadione and phenytoin was found to induce a specific multiple CA. The "fetal trimethadione syndrome" comprises characteristic face sometimes with orofacial cleft, cardiovascular CA, and hypospadias (German et al., 1970; Zackai et al., 1975). The characteristic of "fetal hydantoin syndrome" are dysmorphic face frequently with orofacial cleft and distal phalanges/nails hypoplasia of fingers (Meadow et al., 1968; Hanson and Smith, 1975, 57, 58, 60). In addition, both MCA-syndromes are associated with intrauterine growth retardation and a mild mental retardation. Trimethadione was withdrawn from the market.

Later the association of valproic acid/valproate with a higher risk of spina bifida was described (Roberts and Guiband, 1982; Bjerkedahl et al., 1982) and it appeared that this anticonvulsant drug can also induce a broader pattern of CAs, i.e. "fetal valproate syndrome" (DiLiberty et al., 1984) with a high incidence of these CA (10.7%) (Meadow et al., 2008). In addition, valproate is associated with the most severe mental retardation among the recently used antiepileptic drugs (Meadow et al., 2009).

Carbamazepine may be associated with a low risk for spina bifida (Rosa, 1991) and the children of treated pregnant women have a somewhat smaller head circumference (Hiilesmaa et al., 1981) but it does not associate with a higher risk for mental retardation (Meadow et al., 2009). Thus carbamazepine belongs to the group of antiepileptic drugs with low teratogenic risk: 2.2 (1.1–4.6) (Diav-Citrin et al., 2001) and 1.8 (0.8–3.7) (Kaaja et al., 2003).

The teratogenic risk of phenobarbital and diazepam is debated. A higher risk of CA after phenobarbital treatment was found in epileptic pregnant women (Jones et al., 1992) but it was not confirmed in other studies (e.g. Shapiro et al., 1976; Kaaja et al., 2003, 60). There was no higher risk of CA in the children of 88 pregnant women who attempted suicide with very large doses of phenobarbital during pregnancy (15). A higher tertatogenic risk of diazepam was reported in pregnant women with psychiatric diseases (Saxen and Saxen, 1975; Safra and Oakley, 1975; Laegreid et al., 1987, 1992) but not in not-psychiatric pregnant women (51, Rosenberg et al., 1984, 54). No association was found between the usage of very large doses of diazepam by 112 pregnant women who attempted suicide and the CAs in their offspring (100).

A previous Hungarian study showed 17-fold higher risk of CA after the use of sultiame, a carbonic anhydrase inhibitor antiepileptic drug (58). The teratogenic risk of primidone was also shown (Nakane et al., 1988, 58).

The biological mechanisms behind the teratogenic effect of antiepileptic drugs are less-known. The use of some antiepileptic drugs such as carbamazepine, phenobarbital, phenytoin, and primidone reduces the folate level in plasma with increasing levels of these drugs and the folate deficiency is a well-known cause of neural tube defects and some other CAs. Therefore, the possible protective effect of folic acid should be investigated thoroughly. It has been shown by several studies that periconceptional folic acid and folic acid containing multivitamin supplementation can reduce the recurrence and occurrence of neural-tube defect (Smithells et al., 1982; MRC Vitamin Study, 1991, II III; Berry et al., 1999) and some others CA (IV, V, III, Botto el al., 2004). First, the evaluation of the dataset of HCCSCA showed that high dose of folic acid can reduce the teratogenic potential of some antiepileptic drugs (VI) and later the total material of epileptic pregnant women has been evaluated.

7.2.1 Results of the Study (I, VI)

Out of 22,843 cases, 95 (0.42%), while out of 38,151 controls without CA, 90 (0.24%) had mothers with medically recorded epilepsy in the prenatal maternity logbook (1.8, 1.3–2.4). Of the 95 cases and 90 control mothers, 6 (6.3%) and 5 (5.6%) had the onset of epilepsy during the study pregnancy. The onset of this "gestational epilepsy" was in III gestational month in 5 case and 3 control mothers. The epilepsy started in II gestational month in one control mother while it occurred after the first trimester in 1 case and 1 control mother.

The epileptic mothers of the control group was somewhat younger (24.9 vs. 25.5 year) with the same birth order (1.7) compared to non-epileptic mothers. The proportion of unmarried epileptic women (11.1% vs. 3.8%) was larger with a lower proportion of professional-managerial-skilled worker employment status (53.4% vs. 69.7%). The use of folic acid was lower in epileptic control mothers (48.9% vs. 54.5%) than in non-epileptic control mothers, however, case epileptic and non-epileptic mothers had even lower figures (35.8% vs. 49.4%).

Only one acute (in digestive system: 7.8% vs. 0.7%) and one chronic (migraine: 3.3% vs. 1.9%) disease was higher in epileptic mothers compared with non-epileptic mothers. It is worth mentioning that out of the 15 pregnant women with acute diseases of the digestive system, 13 (86.7%) had acute cholecystitis.

The evaluation of pregnancy complications is shown in Table 7.1.

The incidence of threatened abortion was lower in both case and control epileptic mothers, while threatened preterm delivery and anemia occurred less frequently only in epileptic control mothers. The rate of preeclampsia-eclampsia was higher in epileptic case mothers.

Table 7.2 summarizes the distribution of antiepileptic drugs used in Hungary during the study period, 1980–1996.

Antiepileptic drugs (except diazepam, phenobarbitals, and carbamazepine) were used exclusively by epileptic women. The above 3 exceptions can be explained by the other indications of these drugs. In Hungary the most frequently used antiepileptic drugs were phenytoin, diazepam, carbamazepine and primidone. A higher risk for CAs was found after the use of sultiame, valproate, primidone and carbamazepine during pregnancy.

Table 7.1 Incidence of pregnancy complications in case and control mothers with or without epilepsy

Pregnancy complications	Case mothers				Control mothers			
	without epilepsy		with epilepsy		without epilepsy		with epilepsy	
	(*N* = 22,748)		(*N* = 95)		(*N* = 38,051)		(*N* = 90)	
	No.	%	No.	%	No.	%	No.	%
Threatened abortion	3,488	15.3	9	9.5	6,499	17.1	11	12.2
Nausea, vomiting, severe	1,737	7.6	5	5.3	3,846	10.1	9	10.0
Preeclampsia, eclampsia	665	2.9	5	5.3	1,155	3.0	3	3.3
Pregnancy related renal disease	337	1.5	1	1.1	491	1.3	1	1.1
Oedema/excessive weight gain without hypertension	425	1.9	3	3.2	911	2.4	1	1.1
Placental disorders[a]	294	1.3	2	2.1	592	1.6	1	1.1
Polyhydramnios	210	0.9	1	1.1	190	0.5	1	1.1
Oligohydramnios	32	0.1	1	1.1	14	0.0	0	0.0
Threatened preterm delivery[b]	2,595	11.4	11	11.6	5,441	14.3	6	6.7
Anaemia	3,226	14.2	16	16.8	6,352	16.7	6	6.7
Others[c]	287	1.3	2	2.1	674	1.8	1	1.1

[a]Incl. placenta previa, premature separation.
[b]Incl. cervical incompetence.
[c]For example, trauma, poisoning, blood isoimmunisation.

Table 7.3 summarizes birth outcomes of control newborns. Gestational age at delivery was somewhat longer in the newborns of epileptic mothers but it did not associate with a significantly lower rate of PB. The mean birth weight of newborn infants born to epileptic mothers was 21 g smaller with a somewhat higher rate of LBW, thus these data indicate some intrauterine growth retardation in the fetuses of epileptic pregnant women.

Table 7.4 shows the data of CA in cases of epileptic mothers.

Our data confirmed the higher risk of cleft lip ± palate, cleft palate only, and cardiovascular CA but a higher risk for oesophageal atresia/stenosis was also found although this association was based only on 3 cases.

We attempted to characterize the CA pattern of cases born to pregnant women without treatment and treated with mono- or polytherapy according to different antiepileptic drugs (Table 7.5).

The number of epileptic pregnant women was so limited that avoided the evaluation the possible association between maternal epilepsy without antiepileptic drug treatment and different CAs. After monotherapy, a higher risk for neural-tube

Table 7.2 The occurrence of antiepileptic drugs and their association with CA

	Control mothers ($N = 90$)		Case mothers ($N = 95$)												
	No.	%	No.	%	OR	95% CI		NTD	CLP	CPO	OAS	CCM	HGP	MCA	Others
Antiepileptic drugs															
Carbamazepine	17	18.9	27	28.4	**2.7**	**1.4**	**4.9**	3	3	3	1	8	1	0	8
Clomethiazol	0	0.0	2	2.1	–			0	0	0	1	1	0	0	0
Clonazepam	2	2.2.	2	2.1.	1.7	0.2	11.8	0	0	0	0	0	1	1	0
Diazepam	22	24.4	24	25.3	1.8	0.9	3.2	1	5	2	0	6	4	2	4
Ethosuximide	3	3.3	4	4.2	2.2	0.5	9.9	0	1	0	1	2	0	0	0
Mephenytoin	4	4.4	6	6.3	2.5	0.7	8.9	0	1	0	0	2	0	1	2
Morsuximide	4	4.4	4	4.2	1.7	0.4	6.7	0	1	0	0	1	0	1	1
Phenacemid	1	1.1	3	3.2	5.0	0.5	48.2	0	0	1	0	1	0	1	0
Phenobarbital	3	3.3	4	4.2	2.2	0.5	9.9	0	0	1	0	1	1	1	0
Phenytoin	39	43.3	31	32.6	1.3	0.8	2.1	1	7	1	0	8	3	2	9
Primidone	12	13.3	23	24.2	**3.2**	**1.6**	**6.4**	1	4	0	0	7	0	4	7
Sultiame	2	2.2	12	12.6	**10.0**	**2.2**	**44.8**	**0**	3	0	1	4	0	1	3
Trimethadione	1	1.1	4	4.2	6.7	0.7	59.8	0	1	1	0	0	0	1	1
Valproate	7	7.8	14	14.7	**3.3**	**1.3**	**8.3**	2	0	0	1	1	4	1	5

NTD = neural-tube defect, CLP = cleft lip ± palate, CPO = cleft palate only, OAS = oesophageal atresia/stenosis, CCM = congenital cardiovascular malformation, HGP = hypospadias, glandular-penile/perineal, MCA = multiple CA.

Table 7.3 Birth outcomes of newborns without CA born to epileptic and non-epileptic mothers

Birth outcomes	Control newborns born to Non-epileptic (N = 38,061)		Epileptic mothers (N = 90)		Comparison Unadjusted		Adjusted	
Categorical	No.	%	No.	%	OR (95%CI)		OR (95%CI)	
PB	3,488	9.2	8	8.9	1.0 (0.5–2.0)		0.9 (0.4–1.8)[a]	
LBW	2,159	5.7	8	8.9	1.6 (0.8–3.3)		2.1 (0.8–5.3)[b]	
Quantitative	Mean	S.D.	Mean	S.D.	t =	p =	t =	p =
Gestational age (week)	39.4	2.0	39.7	2.2	1.5	0.13	1.8	0.08[a]
Birth weight (g)	3,276	511	3,255	571	0.4	0.70	0.4	0.72[b]

[a]adjusted for maternal age, birth order and maternal socio-economic status.
[b]adjusted for maternal age, birth order, maternal socio-economic status and gestation age.

defects and oesophageal atresia/stenois was found without a higher risk for total CAs. However, after polytherapy, a higher risk for total CAs was observed explained by the higher risk of four CA-groups. Forty-two epileptic mothers had polytherapy, thus it is not possible to estimate the own effect of different antiepileptic drugs separately. These data (not shown here) indicated the teratogenic effect of trimethadione, primidone, sultiame, valproate, and phenytoin, but did not confirm phenobarbital and diazepam as teratogenic drugs (58, VI).

Table 7.4 Estimation of risks of different CAs in cases and all matched controls born to pregnant women with epilepsy

Study groups	Grand total no.	Epilepsy No.	%	OR	95% CI[a]
Controls	38,151	90	0.2	Reference	
Isolated CAs					
Neural-tube defects	1,202	6	0.5	1.9	0.8–4.4
Cleft lip ± palate	1,375	11	0.8	**3.1**	**1.7–5.9**
Cleft palate only	601	5	0.8	**3.4**	**1.4–8.4**
Oesophageal atresia/stenosis	217	3	1.4	**5.4**	**1.7–17.3**
Hypospadias	3,038	13	0.4	1.7	0.9–3.0
Undescended testis	2,052	7	0.3	1.3	0.6–2.8
Cardiovascular CAs	4,480	25	0.6	**2.2**	**1.4–3.4**
Clubfoot	2,425	5	0.2	0.8	0.3–1.9
Poly/syndactyly	1,744	5	0.3	1.1	0.5–2.8
Other isolated CAs	4,360	10	0.2	0.9	0.5–1.7
Multiple CAs	1,349	5	0.4	1.4	0.6–3.4
Total	22,843	95	0.4	**1.6**	**1.2–2.2**

[a]OR adjusted for maternal age, birth order, employment status, folic acid use.

Table 7.5 Estimation of risks of different CA in the offsprings of case pregnant women and matched newborns of control pregnant women affected with epilepsy according to the type of treatment

		Epileptic pregnant women (all)				Without treatment		Monotherapy				Polytherapy			
Study groups	Grand total No.	No.	%	OR[a]	95% CI	No.	%	No.	%	OR[a]	95% CI	No	%	OR[a]	95% CI
Controls	38,151	90	0.2	Reference		13	0.0	48	0.1	Reference		29	0.1	Reference	
Isolated CAs															
Neural-tube defects	1,202	6	0.5	1.9	0.8–4.4	1	0.1	4	0.3	**2.7**	**1.0–7.4**	1	0.1	1.1	0.1–8.1
Cleft lip ± palate	1,375	11	0.8	**3.1**	**1.7–5.9**	0	0.0	2	0.1	1.2	0.3–4.8	9	0.7	**8.7**	**4.1–18.3**
Cleft palate only	601	5	0.8	**3.4**	**1.4–8.4**	0	0.0	2	0.3	2.7	0.6–11.0	3	0.5	**6.6**	**2.1–21.7**
Cardiovascular CAs	4,480	25	0.6	**2.2**	**1.4–3.4**	5	0.1	8	0.2	1.4	0.7–3.0	12	0.3	**3.5**	**1.8–6.9**
Oesophageal atresia/stenosis	217	3	1.4	**5.4**	**1.7–17.3**	0	0.0	2	0.9	**7.4**	**1.8–30.7**	1	0.5	6.1	0.8–45.2
Hypospadias	3,038	13	0.4	1.7	0.9–3.0	3	0.1	7	0.2	1.8	0.8–4.1	3	0.1	1.3	0.4–4.3
Undescended testis	2,051	7	0.3	1.3	0.6–2.8	0	0.0	6	0.3	1.3	1.0–5.4	1	0.0	0.6	0.1–4.7
Clubfoot	2,424	5	0.2	0.8	0.3–1.9	0	0.0	4	0.2	1.3	0.5–3.6	1	0.0	0.5	0.1–4.0
Poly/syndactyly	1,744	5	0.3	1.1	0.5–2.8	2	0.1	1	0.1	0.5	0.1–3.3	2	0.1	1.5	0.4–6.3
Other isolated CAs	4,363	10	0.2	0.9	0.5–1.7	1	0.0	4	0.1	0.8	0.3–2.1	5	0.1		
Multiple CAs	1,349	5	0.4	1.4	0.6–3.4	0	0.0	1	0.1	0.6	0.1–4.3	4	0.3	**3.9**	**1.4–11.1**
Total	22,843	95	0.4	**1.6**	**1.2–2.2**	12	0.1	41	0.2	1.4	0.9–2.2	42	0.2	**2.4**	**1.5–3.9**

[a]OR adjusted for maternal age, birth order, employment status, use of folic acid during pregnancy.

The effect of the high dose folic acid (3–9 mg, the estimated mean about 5.6 mg) supplementation during the time of organogenesis, i.e. the critical period of most major CAs, was also evaluated whether this primary preventive method can reduce the prevalence of total and specific CA among children exposed to these antiepileptic drugs (Table 7.6).

The association between antiepileptic drugs and CAs tended to be lower among offsprings of pregnant women who took folic acid supplement in early pregnancy compared with offspring of mothers who did not. The risk of cleft lip ± palate, neural-tube defect, and hypospadias in the offspring of mothers treated with antiepileptic drugs without folic acid was higher than in the offspring of pregnant women treated with antiepileptics and folic acid together. Thus the risk of 1.5 (1.1–1.5) in the total CA group was reduced to 1.3 (0.8–1.9). In addition, it is worth mentioning that this risk reduction after monotherapy ranged from 1.4 (1.1–1.8) to 1.2 (0.8–1.8) and after polytherapy it ranged from 5.2 (1.4–19.3) to 2.4 (0.5–10.8). However, there is one unexpected finding: the risk of multiple CA increased after the concomitant use of antiepileptic drugs and high dose of folic acid.

Finally, the folic acid CA-reducing effect was evaluated in different antiepileptic drugs (VI). The risk of all CA after carbamazepine treatment without folic acid was 3.3 (1.5–7.5) but with concomitant folic acid supplementation it was only 1.3 (0.4–4.0). A similar risk reduction was found in pregnant women with primidone treatment and folic acid use together from 5.2 (1.7–16.3) to 2.5 (0.8–7.5). There was a risk reduction after the parallel use of phenytoin and folic acid as well, but this reduction did not reach the level of significance. The teratogenicity reducing effect of valproate was not found with the parallel use of folic acid.

7.2.2 The Interpretation of Results

In general, the pregnancy complications of epileptic women were not documented in the studies focused on CA. No difference was found in the incidence of preecalmpsia between epileptic and non-epileptic pregnant women (Watson and Spellacy, 1971), while in another study the rate of preeclampsia was almost twice in the pregnancy of epileptic women than in the unmatched control group (Bjerkedahl and Bahna, 1973). Our data showed a higher risk of preeclampsia only in the epileptic mothers of malformed fetuses, thus an interaction of fetal defect and maternal epilepsy cannot be excluded in the origin of preeclampsia. A higher rate of vaginal bleeding was found in epileptic pregnant women (29.8% vs. 26.0%) particularly with treatment of phenytoin (33.7%) in the study of Monson et al. (1973) and Bjerkedahl and Bahna (1973). Nevertheless, a lower rate of vaginal bleeding (i.e. threatened abortion) was found in our population-based and medically recorded data set. However, the lower occurrence of threatened abortion associated with 5% lower proportion of males among newborns, therefore, it may indicate a higher rate of spontaneous abortion (not recorded in the HCCSCA), i.e. more intensive early selection. Previously a higher rate of stillbirths was found in epileptic pregnant women (Aminoff, 2004).

Table 7.6 Risk (odds ratios) of CAs according to antiepileptic drug exposure and folic acid supplementation between 5–12 gestational weeks

	No epileptic drugs					Epileptic drugs[a]						
	without folic acid		with folic acid			without folic acid			with folic acid			
Study groups	No.		No.	OR[b] (with 95% CI)		No.	OR[b] (with 95% CI)		No.	OR[b] (with 95% CI)		
Controls	27,098		10,869			126			58			
All cases with CA	15,449	1.0	5,195	**0.8**	**(0.8–0.9)**	106	**1.5**	**(1.1–1.9)**	42	1.3	(0.8–1.9)	
Neural-tube defect	918	1.0	272	**0.7**	**(0.6–0.9)**	9	**2.1**	**(1.1–4.2)**	3	1.5	(0.5–4.9)	
Cleft lip ± palate	1,008	1.0	347	**0.9**	**(0.8–1.0)**	14	**3.0**	**(1.7–5.2)**	5	2.4	(0.5–5.9)	
Cleft palate only	430	1.0	146	**0.9**	**(0.7–1.0)**	5	**2.6**	**(1.0–6.3)**	1	1.1	(0.2–8.2)	
Hypospadias	2,283	1.0	731	**0.8**	**(0.7–0.9)**	19	**1.8**	**(1.1–2.9)**	5	1.0	(0.4–2.5)	
Cardiovascular CA	3,374	1.0	1,078	**0.8**	**(0.7–0.9)**	17	1.1	(0.7–1.8)	10	1.4	(0.7–2.7)	
Poly/syndactyly	1,274	1.0	456	**0.9**	**(0.8–1.0)**	11	**1.8**	**(1.0–3.4)**	3	1.1	(0.4–3.5)	
Other isolated CA	3,346	1.0	1,228	**0.9**	**(0.9–1.0)**	19	1.2	(0.7–2.0)	7	1.0	(0.4–2.2)	
Multiple CA	1,027	1.0	311	**0.8**	**(0.7–0.9)**	5	1.0	(0.4–2.5)	6	**2.8**	**(1.2–6.5)**	

[a]Carbamazepine, phenobarbital, phenytoin, primidone.
[b]Adjusted for maternal age and birth order.

The lower rate of threatened preterm delivery and anemia could be explained by the higher standard of prenatal care in epileptic pregnant. These findings are in agreement with a somewhat longer gestational age at delivery and no higher risk for PB. Unfortunately most Hungarian obstetricians believe that folic acid is contraindicated in epileptic pregnant women and this misunderstanding reflects the very low rate of folic acid supplementation.

Among maternal diseases the possible association of higher prevalence of migraine and cholecystitis with epilepsy is noteworthy.

Our data confirmed the teratogenic affect of trimethadione, phenytoin, valproate, primidone, and carbamazepine and completed this list with the teratogenic effect of sultiame and mephenytoin which are not mentioned in the Catalog of Teratogenic Agents (Shepard and Lemire, 2004). However, our material did not confirm the teratogenic effect of diazepam and phenobarbitals in agreement with the results of the recent Cochrane review (Adab et al., 2004). In fact, we were not able to find a higher risk of CA in the children of 112 and 88 pregnant women who attempted suicide with very large doses of diazepam (106) and phenobarbital (115) during pregnancy.

The evaluation of concomitant use of antiepileptics and high dose of folic acid showed some beneficial effect on teratogenic side effect of antiepileptic drugs in general, and particularly in some specific drugs such as carbamazepine and primidone (VI).

In conclusion, pregnancy in epileptic women does not need to be discouraged if they wish to have babies. However, their support with a specific and high standard care is necessary. The first task is to educate epileptic women about the importance of planning their pregnancies. The second task is in the periconceptional care to check their antiepileptic drugs and to attempt changing the teratogenic drugs (e.g. valproate) to a less (e.g. carbamazepine) or non-teratogenic (lamotrigine) drugs under the control of a specialist. In general, drug selection is determined by the type of seizures and the clinical status. If a teratogenic drug is necessary (because the loss of seizure control during pregnancy is more dangerous than the teratogenic epileptic drugs), monotherapy is preferable. In addition, it is recommended to use the lowest effective dose of the given drug because the teratogenic effect of antiepileptic drugs such as valproate is dose dependent. Also, regular blood test is necessary to check the levels of seizure medications because frequently there is a decreased blood concentration during pregnancy. The third task is to strongly recommend periconceptional folic acid supplementation for epileptic women. Unfortunately the optimal dose is still unknown at present time. The fourth task is strictly monitoring the fetal development with a high resolution ultrasound in early pregnancy because principal defects are detectable from the 20th gestational week. Fortunately these defects are diagnosed rarely but when they happen, the pregnant women have the right to decide to keep or terminate their pregnancies. The final fifth task is related to the preparation for delivery. Sometimes clinical or subclinical coagulopathy may occur in newborn infants born to epileptic mothers with some antiepileptic treatment causing vitamin K deficiency. Maternal ingestion of vitamin K1 (10 mg/day) during the last month of pregnancy may prevent this complication (Aminoff, 2004).

7.3 Migraine

Headache is one of the most common disorders of the central nervous system and may have many causes. The duration and course of a headache provide a guide for the detection of underlying causes. The headaches were classified by the Headache Classification Subcommittee of the International Headache Society (HCSIHS, 2004) into five categories:

A. Migraine Headache
B. Tension Headache
C. Hormone Withdrawal Headache
D. Cluster Headache
E. Medication Overuse Headache

First, migraine headache during pregnancy is reviewed here based on the recent international literature and Hungarian studies.

Migraine is a clinically heterogeneous class of craniofacial pain disorders with the alteration of sensory and autonomic functions, dysregulation of mood, and neurological disturbances (Mathew, 2001).

Migraine disorders are broadly classified as migraine with aura or without aura. Migraine without aura is a clinical syndrome characterised by recurrent headache disorder manifesting in attacks lasting 4–72 h with unilateral location, pulsating quality, moderate or severe intensity, aggravated by routine physical activity, and association with nausea/vomiting, photophobia and phonophobia. Migraine with aura is primarily characterised by the focal neurological symptoms that usually precede or sometimes accompany the headache. This recurrent disorder manifesting in attacks of reversible focal neurological symptoms that usually develop gradually over 5–20 min and last for less than 60 min (HCSIHS, 2004; Goadsby, 2003).

First migraines were believed to be vascular headaches due to cerebral vasoconstriction that caused decreased oxygenation followed by vasodilatation which further induced the characteristic headache pain. Later it appeared that the primary event is the release of neuroinflammatory peptides such as serotonin 5-hydroxytriptamine in response to stressors both in peripheral and central portions of the trigeminal nerve. The release of these peptides causes vasoconstriction and later – after the drop of their level – vasodilatation which induces pain around the temples and eyes. In addition, neuroinflammatory peptides result in sensitization of the trigeminal system which usually progresses from peripheral sensitization to central sensitization (Goadsby, 2003).

Emotional stress, fatigue, sleep disturbances, alcohol use especially red wine, ingestion of certain foods such as chocolate and cheese particularly containing additives, e.g. monosodium glutamate, nitrites, aspartame, and last but not least hormonal changes in women may precipitate a migraine attack (Marcus, 2004).

The clinical heterogeneity of migraines probably can be explained by the genetic complexity of migraine (Esterez and Gardner, 2004). The major part of migraines has multifactorial etiology including a genetic predisposition due to a polygenic system triggered by the previously mentioned environmental factors (Russel et al., 1995). This polygenic system explains the tendency to occur in families (Russel et al., 1993) and the higher concordance in monozygotic than in dizygotic twins (Lucas, 1977). Thus, the pattern of familial clusters corresponds to the Mendelian rules only in some exceptional types of migraine, e.g. the rare familial hemiplegic migraine shows autosomal dominant inheritance (Ophoff et al., 1996).

Migraine is among the most frequent chronic diseases and it is more common among females than males. Previously the prevalence of migraine was estimated in women affecting 5% to 12% of the population (Mathew, 2001; MacGregor et al., 2006). However, descriptive epidemiological studies indicated prevalence of 20.4% and 17.5% of women, in addition to 8.6% and 5.7% of men in two U.S European-Caucasian populations, respectively (Stewart et al., 1992; Lipton et al., 2002). Therefore, migraine affects almost 3 times more women than men. The increased susceptibility of females to pain, including migraine is explained at least in part by the influence of cycling estradiol – recently has been reclassified as a neurosteroid – with an important action in neural transmission (Marcus, 2004). The symptoms of 60% of women with migraine show a periodicity linked to the menstrual cycle. These headaches occur just before or during menstruation generally without aura (Aminoff, 2004)

The typical onset of migraine is between 10 and 30 years of age (Reik, 1988; Stewart et al., 1991) and, therefore, it occurs during pregnancy as well.

Migraine typically improves during the first trimester of pregnancy in more than 50% of women with additional improvement in 30% of patients during the later part of the pregnancy (Marcus et al., 1999). The alleviation of migraine during pregnancy may be connected with 50–100 fold increase in the blood level of estradiol. However, in 4–8% of women, migraines worsen during pregnancy. In addition, migraine typically recurs soon after delivery within one week for 34% and within 1 month for 55% of women (Sances et al., 2003). Migraine even can begin for the first time just after delivery. Breastfeeding decreases the risk of recurrence of migraine (Wall, 1992).

Therefore, many women with migraine who needed drug treatment can avoid medication during pregnancy. However, we have to treat pregnant women with severe migraine, because it may result in dehydration and poor nutrition. These pathological conditions may pose a greater risk to the fetus than the potential – and generally exaggerated – risk of the medications (Diamond, 1990; Silberstein and Lipton, 1998).

The possible teratogenic/fetotoxic effects of antimigraine drugs during pregnancy have been evaluated frequently but the possible hazard of underlying maternal diseases, e.g. migraine was studied only in one clinical study. Out of 777 women with migraine, 450 (57.9%), while out of 182 women without migraine, 136 (74.7%) had been pregnant in the migraine clinic of Wainscott et al. (1978). The prevalence of fetal death (miscarriages and stillbirths) was similar in the study groups (27% vs. 29%). There were 924 and 277 livebirths born to mothers with or without migraine, and the rate of CAs was 2.16% and 2.52%, respectively.

There were three objectives of our study: (i) to check the occurrence of pregnancy complications and other maternal diseases in pregnant women with migraine (VII), (ii) to evaluate the birth outcomes of their children (VII), (iii) and particularly the risk for different CAs (VIII).

7.3.1 Results of the Study (VII, VIII)

When evaluating migraine headaches we followed the International Classification of Headache Disorders (HCSIHS, 2004) and the secondary headaches due to other diseases such as trauma, vascular disorders including essential hypertension, infections, neoplasm, etc. were excluded.

The case group comprised 22,843 fetuses or newborns with CAs, of whom 565 (2.5%) had mothers with migraine during the study pregnancy. Of the 38,151 controls without CAs, 713 (1.9%) had migraine during pregnancy (1.3, 1.2–1.5). Out of 834 malformed controls, 24 (2.9%) were born to mothers with migraine anytime during the study pregnancy (0.9, 0.6–1.3).

It is worth mentioning that the prevalence of migraine in pregnant women was lower than in non-pregnant reproductive aged women. This discrepancy can be explained partly by the improving migraine status during pregnancy, and partly by the doctors who recorded only severe migraines into the prenatal maternity logbooks.

Out of 565 cases and 713 controls, 316 (55.9%) and 485 (68.0%) ($p < 0.001$) had mothers with one or more medically recorded migraine attacks during the study pregnancy in the prenatal maternity logbooks, respectively. The number of reported migraine attacks was between 1 and 21 during the study pregnancy. The occurrence of migraine attacks was evaluated according to gestational month (Table 7.7).

Both migraine and other headaches occurred most frequently in III gestational month. Thus, 415 (73.5%) case, 533 (74.8%) control and 20 (83.3%) malformed control mothers had migraine during II and/or III month of pregnancy. Our premise was that CAs caused by migraine could only be due to active attacks during the organogenesis, i.e. the critical period of most CAs.

Mothers with migraine were somewhat older (25.9 vs. 25.4 year) with higher mean birth order (1.8 vs. 1.7) than mothers without migraine as reference. Maternal marital status did not show obvious differences between the study groups but migraine was somewhat more frequent among professionals (14.9% vs. 11.3%). There was a lower use of folic acid (50.8% vs. 54.5%) and multivitamins (4.9% vs. 6.6%) by the mothers with migraine compared with pregnant women without migraine. There was a similar pattern in II and/or III gestational months which reflected the early, in general periconceptional supplementation.

Out of 565 case and 713 control mothers, 192 (34.0%) and 219 (30.7%) had only migraine without any other diseases during the study pregnancy. The incidence of acute maternal diseases did not show any difference among the study groups. However, among chronic disorders, cardiac dysrhythmias (2.5% vs. 0.3%), mainly paroxysmal ventricular-supraventricular tachycardia, and panic disorders (2.2% vs.

Table 7.7 The occurrence of the first migraine attacks according to gestational month during pregnancy

	Migraine				Other headaches			
	Case mothers		Control mothers		Case mothers		Control mothers	
Gestational month	No.	%	No.	%	No.	%	No.	%
I	4[a]	0.7	34[a]	4.8	7	1.3	8	0.6
II	164	29.0	196	27.5	122	22.7	320	25.2
III	247	43.7	303	42.5	244	45.4	543	42.8
IV	43	7.6	54	7.6	54	10.0	133	10.5
V	44	7.8	39	5.5	38	7.1	92	7.3
VI	25	4.4	33	4.6	40	7.4	66	5.2
VII	20	3.5	26	3.6	19	3.5	62	4.9
VIII	15	2.7	21	2.9	9	1.7	30	2.4
IX	3	0.5	7	1.0	5	0.9	14	1.1
Total	565	100.0	713	100.0	538	100.0	1,268	100.0
Difference (χ^2_9)	$p = 0.16$				$p = 0.35$			

[a]Each pregnant woman had recurrent migraine attacks in II and/or III gestational month.

0.4%) occurred more frequently in pregnant women with migraine than in pregnant women without migraine. In addition, the occurrence of thyroid disorders (mainly hyperthyroidism) (1.0% vs. 0.3%) and hemorrhoids (5.8% vs. 3.3%) was somewhat higher in pregnant women with migraine

Three kinds of drug treatments were differentiated in pregnant women with migraine: (i) The so-called antimigraine drugs during migraine attacks prescribed by medical doctors. Ergotamine alone (7.7% vs. 0.0%) or ergotamine in combination with aminophenazone + caffeine + belladonna leaf (3.1% vs. 0.0%) was frequently used in Hungary during the study period. Painkiller drugs such as NSAID (acetylsalicylic acid 10.2% vs. 3.8%, naproxen 1.5% vs. 0.0%), aminophenazone (20.4% vs. 0.8%), dipyrone (61.0% vs. 4.5%) and naproxen (1.5% vs. 0.0%) were also used as supplementary treatment of migraine. The spectrum of these drugs was different from the recently used modern antimigraine drugs (e.g. sumatriptan) in developed countries. (ii) Drugs used during interictal periods for prevention of migraine include beta blockers (propranolol 4.9% vs. 0.1%), antidepressants (amitriptyline 1.0% vs. 0.0%, pizotifene 1.4% vs. 0.0%) and other medications were also used more frequently in the groups of pregnant women with migraine. (iii) All other frequently used drugs did not show difference in II and/or III gestational month between case and control mothers.

The first objective of the study was to evaluate pregnancy complications of mothers with migraine (Table 7.8).

The rate of threatened abortions and threatened preterm delivery was lower while severe nausea/vomiting and preeclampsia-eclampsia was higher in mothers with migraine than in mothers without migraine. Case mothers had no lower rate of

Table 7.8 Incidence of pregnancy complications

	With migraine (*N* = 713)		Without migraine (*N* = 37,438)		
Pregnancy complications	No.	%	No.	%	OR (95% CI)
Threatened abortion	91	12.8	6,421	17.2	**0.7 (0.6–0.9)**
Nausea and vomiting, severe	100	14.0	2,769	10.1	**1.5 (1.2–1.8)**
Preeclampsia-eclampsia	81	11.4	3,140	8.4	**1.4 (1.1–1.8)**
Threatened preterm delivery[a]	82	11.5	5,378	14.4	**0.8 (0.6–0.9)**
Prolonged pregnancy	12	1.7	496	1.3	1.3 (0.7–2.3)
Placental disorders[b]	11	1.5	581	1.6	1.0 (0.5–1.8)
Gestational diabetes	4	0.6	266	0.7	0.8 (0.3–2.1)
Polyhydramnios	3	0.4	188	0.5	0.8 (0.3–2.6)
Oligohydramnios	0	0.0	14	0.0	–
Anemia	118	16.6	6,238	16.7	1.0 (0.8–1.2)

[a]Including cervical incompetence.
[b]Including placenta previa, premature separation of placenta, antepartum haemorrhage.

threatened abortion and preterm delivery, but a higher incidence of preeclampsia-eclampsia (not shown in Table 7.8).

The second objective of our study was to evaluate the birth outcomes of newborns of pregnant women with migraine (Table 7.9). There was no significant difference in the mean gestational age at delivery and mean birth weight of newborn infants born to mothers with or without migraine.

The evaluation of selected CAs (including at least 3 cases) in mothers with migraine during pregnancy was the third main objective of the study (Table 7.10).

The risk of limb deficiencies, neural-tube defects and poly/syndactyly was higher after maternal migraine anytime during the study pregnancy at the comparison of cases and controls. However, the evaluation of migraine attacks during II and/or III

Table 7.9 Birth outcomes of newborn infants without CA born to mothers with and without migraine

Variables	With migraine (*N* = 713)		Without migraine (*N* = 37,438)		Comparison adjusted[a]	
Quantitative	Mean	S.D.	Mean	S.D.	*t*	*p*
Gestational age, week	39.3	2.0	39.4	2.0	0.6	0.54
Birth weight, g	3,266	514	3,276	511	0.6	0.53
Categorical	No.	%	No.	%	OR	95%CI
PB	70	9.8	3,426	9.2	1.1	0.8–1.4
Postterm birth	63	8.8	3,799	10.2	0.9	0.7–1.1
LBW	47	6.6	2,120	5.7	1.2	0.9–1.6
Large birthweight	6	0.8	309	0.8	1.0	0.5–2.3

[a]Adjusted for maternal age and employment status and folic acid use during pregnancy.

Table 7.10 Estimation of risks of different CAs in cases and all matched controls born to pregnant women affected by migraine and other headaches and the data of total malformed controls

		Migraine								Other headaches							
		Anytime during pregnancy				Second and/or third month				Anytime during pregnancy				Second and/or third month			
Study groups	Grand total no.	No.	%	OR[a]	95% CI	No.	%	OR[a]	95% CI	No.	%	OR[a]	95% CI	No.	%	POR[a]	95% CI
Isolated CAs																	
Neural-tube defects	1,202	37	3.1	**2.0**	**1.1–3.5**	29	2.4	1.7	0.9–3.2	37	3.1	1.1	0.7–1.7	27	2.3	1.5	0.8–2.5
Cleft lip± palate	1,375	37	2.7	0.8	0.5–1.4	25	1.8	0.8	0.4–1.4	43	3.1	0.9	0.6–1.3	26	1.9	0.7	0.4–1.1
Cleft palate only	601	9	1.5	0.6	0.2–1.5	8	1.3	0.7	0.3–2.0	8	1.3	0.4	0.2–1.0	8	1.3	0.7	0.3–1.7
Congenital pyloric stenosis	241	7	2.9	0.6	0.2–1.7	4	1.7	0.4	0.1–1.6	2	0.8	0.3	0.1–1.5	1	0.4	0.2	0.0–1.7
Rectal/anal atresia/stenosis	231	7	3.	0.6	0.2–1.8	5	2.2	0.6	0.2–2.0	4	1.8	0.8	0.2–2.9	2	0.9	0.6	0.1–3.5
Renal a/dysgenesis	126	3	2.4	0.9	0.2–5.2	2	1.6	1.0	0.1–7.5	7	6.7	1.9	0.5–6.5	6	5.8	3.0	0.7–12.3
Obstructive urinary CAs	343	3	0.9	1.3	0.3–6.6	2	0.6	2.4	0.3–19.0	9	3.3	0.5	0.2–1.1	9	3.3	0.6	0.3–1.5
Hypospadias	3,038	64	2.1	0.8	0.6–1.2	45	1.5	0.8	0.5–1.2	61	2.0	0.5	0.4–0.7	33	1.1	**0.4**	**0.2–0.5**
Undescended testis	2,052	30	1.5	0.8	0.5–1.3	22	1.1	0.7	0.4–1.1	45	2.2	**0.6**	**0.4–0.9**	31	1.5	**0.6**	**0.4–0.9**
Exomphalos/ gastroschisis	255	6	2.4	1.5	0.4–4.9	5	2.0	1.5	0.4–5.5	7	2.9	1.3	0.5–3.7	3	1.3	0.7	0.2–2.8
Microcephaly, primary	111	4	3.7	2.5	0.5–13.5	4	3.7	4.5	0.7–29.2	3	2.8	1.3	0.3–6.5	2	1.8	1.1	0.2–6.3
Congenital hydrocephaly	314	5	1.6	0.6	0.2–1.8	4	1.3	0.9	0.2–3.7	6	1.9	0.5	0.2–1.4	5	1.6	0.8	0.3–2.4
Ear CAs	354	6	1.7	1.4	0.4–4.9	6	1.7	1.6	0.4–6.0	13	3.7	1.1	0.5–2.5	8	2.3	0.8	0.3–1.9
Cardiovascular CAs	4,480	114	2.6	1.3	0.9–1.7	90	2.0	**1.4**	**1.0–2.0**	106	2.4	**0.7**	**0.6–0.9**	84	1.9	0.8	0.6–1.1
Clubfoot	2,425	56	2.3	1.0	0.7–1.5	38	1.6	1.1	0.7–1.7	66	2.7	**0.7**	**0.5 –0.9**	47	1.9	**0.7**	**0.5–0.9**
Limb deficiencies	548	26	4.7	**2.6**	**1.3–5.5**	19	3.5	**2.5**	**1.1–5.8**	13	2.4	0.6	0.3–1.2	10	1.8	0.6	0.3–1.3

Table 7.10 (continued)

Study groups	Grand total no.	Migraine								Other headaches							
		Anytime during pregnancy				Second and/or third month				Anytime during pregnancy				Second and/or third month			
		No.	%	OR[a]	95% CI	No.	%	OR[a]	95% CI	No.	%	OR[a]	95% CI	No.	%	POR[a]	95% CI
Poly/syndactyly	1,744	46	2.6	**1.9**	**1.2–3.1**	32	1.8	1.6	0.9–2.8	40	2.3	**0.6**	**0.4–0.9**	26	1.5	**0.5**	**0.3–0.9**
CAs of the skeletal system	585	5	0.9	1.4	0.4–5.4	2	0.3	0.7	0.1–4.8	2	0.3	0.4	0.1–1.7	2	0.3	0.4	0.1–2.1
Diaphragmatic CAs	244	10	4.1	3.2	0.9–10.5	7	2.9	3.5	0.8–14.9	4	1.7	0.7	0.2–2.5	2	0.8	0.5	0.1–3.5
Other isolated CAs	1,225	43	35	0.9	0.6–1.5	37	3.0	1.1	0.6–1.8	39	3.2	**0.6**	**0.4–0.9**	29	2.4	**0.6**	**0.4–0.9**
Multiple CAs	1,349	47	3.5	1.0	0.6–1.6	29	2.2	0.7	0.4–1.2	23	1.7	**0.4**	**0.3–0.7**	12	0.9	**0.4**	**0.2–0.7**
Total cases	22,843	565	2.5	1.1	0.9–1.2	415	1.8	1.1	0.9–1.2	538	2.4	**0.6**	**0.5–0.7**	373	1.6	**0.6**	**0.5–0.7**
Total controls	38,151	713	1.9	1.0	–	533	1.4	1.0	–	1,268	3.3	1.0	–	871	2.3	1.0	–
Total malformed controls	834	24	2.9	1.3	0.8–2.0	20	2.4	1.1	0.7–1.8	19	2.3	1.0	0.6–1.6	7	0.8	1.9	0.9–4.0

[a]ORs adjusted for maternal age and employment status, birth order, use of folic acid and antimigraine/antiheadache drugs.

gestational month showed a statistically significant association only with limb deficiency. In addition, there was a borderline association between migraine and cardiovascular CAs including the largest number of cases.

When evaluating only medically recorded maternal migraine during II and/or III month of pregnancy, only limb deficiencies showed association (2.7, 1.1–6.5). Adjusted OR were 1.2, 0.6–2.3 for neural-tube defects, 1.0, 0.7–1.7 for poly/syndactyly and 0.6, 0.4–1.0 for cardiovascular CAs in mothers with migraine attacks during II and/or III month of pregnancy.

At the comparison of cases and malformed controls (these data are not shown here), again only limb deficiencies showed an association with maternal migraine during II and/or III month of pregnancy (1.7, 1.3–3.0). Neural-tube defects (1.1, 0.6–1.8), poly/syndactyly (0.9, 0.6–1.5) and cardiovascular CAs (0.9; 0.7–1.2) did not show association with maternal migraine during II and/or III month.

We also attempted to differentiate the effect of maternal migraine attacks and antimigraine drugs. There was no obvious difference in the prevalence of cases with limb deficiencies born to mothers with migraine attacks during the II and/or III month of pregnancy with or without antimigraine drug treatments.

7.3.2 Interpretation of Results

The prevalence of migraine in our study was lower than expected based on previous studies (Mathew, 2001; MacGregor et al., 2003). This might be explained by two factors. On one hand, the frequency of migraine attacks decreases during pregnancy (Massey, 1977; Villalon et al., 2003). On the other hand, mostly severe migraines were only evaluated in our study. Nearly all pregnant women with migraine were treated by drugs during pregnancy.

Our study was appropriate to evaluate all aspects of pregnant women with migraine (IX). In pregnant women with migraine, a higher incidence of severe nausea/vomiting and preeclampsia-eclampsia and a lower incidence of threatened abortion and preterm delivery were detected.

The higher rate of preeclampsia-eclampsia in pregnant women with migraine is worth discussing because maternal migraine was not mentioned among risk factors for preeclampsia (Dekker and Sibai, 2001). The association between maternal headache and a higher rate of preeclampsia was found previously in other study (Facchinetty et al., 2005) explained by pregnancy-related hypertension. In addition, there may be a common vascular factor in the pathogenesis of these two pathological conditions (Villalon et al., 2003). Several epidemiological studies have suggested that the frequency of preeclampsia is inversely proportional to nutritional calcium intake (Marcoux et al., 1991). A migraine-specific gene at chromosome 19p13 is known to be associated with missense mutations in the brain-expressed voltage-gated alfa1ACa^{2+}-channel subunit gene: CACNA1A (Ophoff et al., 1996). Recently a model of the potential integration of migraine-susceptibility factors into-CACNA1A-dependent pathways has been presented (Esterez and Gardner, 2004).Very rarely migraine with aura has also been linked to a higher risk for ischemic stroke (Kurt, 2007).

The incidence of severe nausea and vomiting during pregnancy was also higher in women with migraine, the latter may associate with a lower rate of early fetal death (Medalie, 1957; Weigel and Weigel, 1989) and this finding was in agreement with the lower occurrence of threatened abortion and preterm delivery in our study. The higher incidence of nausea and vomiting may be related to an interaction between migraine and pregnancy. In addition, a possible association was found between migraine and cardiac dysrhythmias, panic disorder and perhaps hyperthyroidism.

There was no difference in mean gestational age and birth weight in newborn infants born to women with or without migraine. A Swedish study found also a somewhat higher but not significant risk for PB and LBW newborns of pregnant women with migraine treated by sumatriptan (Kallen and Lygner, 2001).

The major finding of our study was the detection of possible teratogenic effect of maternal migraine. An association was found between maternal migraine during early pregnancy and a higher risk for limb deficiencies.

In general, triggering factors, such as meteorological and/or temperature changes, fluorescent lights, dietary factors, serious stress, lack of sleep, etc, cannot be evaluated in the study. We were able to evaluate only the occurrence of migraine during the study pregnancy and it was similar in the case and control groups.

The next point is the evaluation of potential teratogenic effect of related drug treatment (Lance, 1986). Only ergotamine alone and combination with other drugs were considered as specific antimigraine drugs in Hungary during the study period, however, our data did not show any association between limb deficiencies and ergotamine.

Here the use of antimigraine drugs is discussed in more detailed.

(a) *Specific antimigraine drugs*, such as old ergotamine drops and recent triptans, e.g., sumatriptan.

Ergot alkaloids: Ergotamine is a naturally occurring ergot alkaloid that was used first for the treatment of migraine in 1926, and the efficacy of this drug was proved in double-blind trials (Tfelt-Hansen and Saxena, 2000). The ergot alkaloids exhibit wide and various receptor affinity to alfa-adrenoreceptors (alfa-1 and alfa-2), 5-hydroxytriptamine (5-HT), and dopamine D2 receptors. Previously the beneficial effect of ergot alkaloids was explained by its vasoconstrictor properties but later it was completed by the neuronal action of these drugs (Markowitz et al., 1988). Ergotamine was considered as human teratogen; therefore, these drugs were rarely used (84). Our study showed a higher risk for neural-tube defects after the treatment of high dose (1.5 mg or more) ergotamine in II month (6.9, 2.0–24.2) (85); however, previously the high dose of ergotamine was not mentioned as possible cause of neural-tube defects (Mitchell et al., 2004).

Triptans: The first agent of this drug class, sumatriptan was introduced in the treatment of acute migraine attack in 1991. Later other triptans were marketed such as zomitriptan, rizatriptan, eletriptan, almotriptan, naratriptan. Several randomized double-blind, placebo-controlled trial showed good efficacy of triptans mainly sumatriptan in the treatment of migraine attacks. However, the review of Lipton et al. (2004), based on the results of all comparative trials, did not indicate significant differences between triptans and non-steroidal anti-inflammatory drugs (NSAIDs). Clinicians working in the headache field still prefer the use of triptans based on their positive experiences. In addition, most triptans are effective in migraine by oral administration and have good patient's satisfaction results due to pain-free response. Triptans have selective agonist activity on the 5-HT1 receptors and they act in migraine by three mechanisms: intracranial extracerebral vasoconstriction, inhibition of neuropeptic release at the trigemino-vascular afferents, and inhibition of central pain transmission at trigeminal nucleus caudalis. The discovery of the 5-HT1 (particularly 1B/1D) agonist sumatriptan constitutes a substantial advance in the treatment of migraine. Later the second generation triptans (focused agents) exhibit an even higher intrinsic activity on this receptor with appropriate safety and long-lasting action (Giffin et al., 2003). Human studies did not show any teratogenic effect of triptans particularly sumatriptan (Shunaiber et al., 1998; O'Quin et al., 1999; Olesen et al., 2000; Eldridge, 2000; Kallen and Lygner, 2001) and zomitriptan (MacGregor et al., 2003).

In conclusion, ergot alkaloids are not recommended during pregnancy and triptans are preferred for the treatment of acute migraine attacks as specific antimigraine drugs due to their selective activity on the 5-HT1 receptors

(b) Among the so-called *supplementary analgesics*, dipyrone was most frequently used for this indication in Hungary, followed by aspirin and acetaminophen.

Dipyrone:In Hungary, this pyrazolone NSAID was used frequently for the treatment of migraine attacks in pregnant women as well. The critical evaluation of our population-based case-control study did not indicate any teratogenic effect of dipyrone (81).

Aspirin and other NSAIDs: The use of aspirin (i.e. acetylsalicylic acid) was based on empirical experiences in acute migraine treatment for many years and its efficacy was confirmed in controlled clinical trials as well (Tfelt-Hansen and McEwen, 2000). Our study did not find any teratogenic effect of aspirin in early pregnancy (75, 76). Later the beneficial effect of ibuprofen, diclofenac, and naproxen was also shown in migraine attack treatment.

A common primary action of NSAIDs is the inhibition of the synthesis of prostaglandins from arachidonic acid by blocking cyclooxygenase. The effect of NSAIDs in migraine was explained by both peripheral and central action, i.e. in brain neurons with a direct effect on serotonergic and/or opiatergic system. Thus NSADs are not contraindicated in early pregnant women because these drugs are not human teratogenic agents. However, their use should be limited during later pregnancy because some NSAIDs may constrict or close the fetal ductus arteriosus as early as 27th gestational week (Koren et al., 1998).

Acetamoniphen: Acetamoniphen is the less effective drug for the treatment of migraine, but safe and has no effect on the ductus arteriosus (77).

(c) Among *preventive drugs*, beta-blockers such as propranolol, in addition antidepressants and antiemetic metoclopramide, proxibarbal, promethazine were used in pregnant women.

Increased frequency and severity of migraine associated with nausea and vomiting, in addition to dehydration may justify the use of daily preventive treatment as the last resort option (Narbone et al., 2004). Preventive treatments should be considered when patients have at least 3 or 4 prolonged and severe migraine attacks a month. First beta-adrenergic blockers, mainly propranolol have been used. Selective serotonin-reuptake inhibitors such as amitriptyline, pizotifene, fluoxetine, paroxitene, bupropion may be useful for the treatment of migraine with co-morbid depression. However, recently paroxitene and bupropion was labeled as FDA risk category D, because one study identified a higher risk for cardiovascular defects (Hemels et al., 2005). Gabapentin is effective in migraine preventive therapy without any teratogenic risk in early pregnancy (Montouris, 2003). Metoclopramide and promethazine are appropriate – in general with vitamin B6 – for the treatment of severe nausea and vomiting. Our case-control and suicide attempt studies did not show the teratogenic effect of promethazine (74,111).

Therefore, antimigraine drugs cannot be blamed to have any role in the origin of congenital limb deficiencies, and its higher occurrence should be explained by the more severe migraine of their mothers. Non-syndromic limb deficiencies include heterogeneous CAs from both phenotypic manifestations (terminal transverse and amniogenic; longitudinal: radial/tibial, ulnar/fibular, axial: split hand and/or foot; intercalary: phocomelia and mainly aplasia of femoral head) and etiologic aspect (Mendelian inheritance, maternal diseases and teratogenic factors). Unfortunately, we were not able to differentiate these types of limb deficiencies in our data set because it needs a personal check-up due to the low diagnostic reliability of medical doctors in this CA-group (X). However, of the 548 cases with limb deficiencies, 384 (70.1%) had unimelic manifestations, mainly in the upper limb (79.8%). Thus, the major part of our cases may have terminal transverse type with a critical period between 4th and 9th gestational month and vascular disruption was shown to cause the major part of unimelic terminal transverse type of limb deficiencies (McGuirk et al., 2001). The pathogenesis of migraine attacks also involves vascular effects, in addition to dehydration, electrolyte disturbances, etc. (Villalon et al., 2003). Therefore, the possible association between severe maternal migraine during the second and/or third month of gestation and unimelic limb deficiency might be explained by available scientific findings.

The expected number of cases with non-syndromic limb deficiencies is 50 per 100,000 births (X). The estimated occurrence of migraine among pregnant women is 5% and it may associate with 2.5 times higher risk for limb deficiencies. Thus the estimated absolute excess of limb deficiencies may be 6 cases among 100,000 newborn babies which is not a serious public health issue. However, if the possible association between severe migraine and higher risk for limb deficiency would be confirmed, special ultrasound scanning could check the status of limbs of the fetuses at the 20th gestational week.

Previously only the outcomes of pregnancy in women suffering from migraine in a migraine clinic were published without a higher rate of CAs in newborn infants born to mothers with migraine (Wainscott et al., 1978).

In conclusion, our findings indicate that severe migraine of pregnant women associates with a higher incidence of preeclampsia and severe nausea/vomiting but there is no clinically important risk for LBW and PB. However, a higher risk for limb deficiencies was found in infants born to mothers with severe migraine attacks during II and/or III gestational month. The question is whether the recent effective antimigraine drugs can neutralize this teratogenic risk of migraine itself or not.

7.3.3 General Recommendations Regarding to the Treatment of Pregnant Women with Migraine

The general treatment protocol of migraine is partly similar in pregnant and non-pregnant women because the type of treatment is determined mainly the severity of migraine (Diamond, 1990). Partly it is different because the improvement of symptoms and the existence of embryo/fetus should be considered when prescribing possible teratogenic drugs.

In general, migraine improves in pregnant women; therefore several women do not need drug treatment.

If medical help is necessary, the first task is the recommendation of non-pharmacological treatment in pregnant women with improving condition of migraine. Pregnant women can be advised to avoid irregular sleeping habits, avoid missing meals, smoking cessation, and limit their caffeine. In addition, they should be encouraged to avoid their known individual triggering factors (e.g. special foods) and suggest supportive therapy such as regular sleep pattern and meal, massage, relaxation and biofeedback, physical therapy (ice packs), and aerobic exercise. The beneficial effect of non-pharmacological treatment of migraine was shown (Marcus et al., 1998).

However, some pregnant women have severe intractable migraine headaches with symptoms of severe nausea and vomiting, in addition to possible dehydration, therefore they need drug treatments. Triptans are appropriate for this purpose, sometimes supplemented with other analgesic or preventive drugs. Although, caution is always needed when recommending drug therapy to pregnant women. At present the possible teratogenic effect of drugs is often exaggerated. When suggesting medications, both the possible risk and the benefit of drug during pregnancy should be considered.

The teratogenic risks of some recently marketed drugs are unknown and severe migraine may associate with some risk for congenital limb deficiencies. If these exposures occurred during embryogenesis (i.e. in general II and/or III gestational months), then high-resolution ultrasound scanning should be performed to check whether lesions to a specific organ system (particularly limbs) has occurred. If the high-resolution ultrasound is normal (with the 90% sensitivity of the examination), it is reasonable to reassure the pregnant woman that her fetus-baby has no defects. It is also important to mention that folic acid and folic acid containing multivitamin supplementation during the periconceptional period is appropriate for the prevention of not only neural-tube defects (II, III) but about one third of other CAs including terminal transverse type limb deficiencies (III–V, Botto et al., 2004).

7.4 Other Headaches

Headache is a common pathological condition with a wide range of severity and heterogeneous origin. The Headache Classification Subcommittee of the International Headache Society (HCSIHS, 2004) recommended differentiating five categories. Beyond migraine headache, tension, hormone withdrawal, cluster, and medication overuse headaches were classified.

Our plan was to check the possible association of these types of maternal headaches during pregnancy with pregnancy complications, adverse birth outcomes, particularly CAs in their offsprings (VIII). Pregnant women with migraine were evaluated in other studies and these results were summarized in the previous chapter. Here the study of the so-called other headaches is shown but headaches associated to secondary complications of other diseases (such as influenza, sinusitis, glaucoma, severe depression, brain tumor, etc) were excluded from the study

7.4.1 Results of the Study

The case group comprised 22,843 fetuses or newborns with CA, of whom 538 (2.4%) had mothers with headache anytime during the study pregnancy. Out of 38,151 controls without CA, 1,268 (3.3%) had headaches anytime during pregnancy (0.7, 0.6–0.8). Out of 834 malformed controls, 19 (2.3%) had mothers with headache during the study pregnancy (1.0, 0.7–1.6). However, it was not possible to differentiate the categories of headaches beyond migraine without their specification in medical records and/or maternal questionnaire. Most of these headaches may belong to the tension category, but henceforth only "headache" will be mentioned.

The onset of headache according to gestational month was shown in previous Table 7.7. Headache was rarely mentioned in I gestational month; the peak was in III gestational month followed by II and IV gestational months in both case and control mothers

The mean maternal age (24.9 vs. 25.5 year) was lower in mothers with headaches. There was no difference in the marital status and mean birth order (1.7) but the occurrence of headaches was lower in managerial mothers (21.5% vs. 26.7%) and housewives (2.5% vs. 5.4%) with headache than in pregnant women without headache. There was no difference in the use of folic acid and multivitamins between case and control mothers with other headaches.

Case and control mothers with or without headache did not show any difference in the incidence of acute maternal diseases. However, among chronic disorders, chronic hypertension occurred more frequently in both case (4.6% vs. 2.4%) and control (4.2% vs. 1.7%) mothers with headache compared to pregnant women without headache.

Painkiller drugs such dipyrone, aminophenazone (mainly in combination with caffeine, phenacetin, and carbromal), acetylsalicylic acid was used for the treatment of headaches.

Among pregnancy complications, only anemia had a higher incidence in pregnant women with headache (28.7% vs. 16.2%).

Birth outcomes, i.e. gestational age (39.4 week) and birth weight (about 3,280 g) did not show any difference between newborns of pregnant women with or without headache, thus the rate of PB (8.7% vs. 9.2%) and LBW newborns (4.9% vs. 5.7%) was also similar.

Finally, the possible associations between headache and higher risk of different CAs were estimated. The occurrence of headaches in anytime or in II and/or III month of the study pregnancy was compared between case mothers who had offspring with different CAs and control mothers with their matched newborns without CA. There was no higher risk for any CA due to maternal headaches. On the contrary, surprisingly we found that non-migrain headaches have protective effect on some CAs (Table 7.10). However, if hypotension and folic acid use of mothers were considered as confounders, these lower risks disappeared.

7.4.2 Interpretation of Results

Among these categories of headaches, tension-type headache is the most common; its lifetime prevalence in the general population ranges from 30 to 78% (HCSIHS, 2004). Obviously our data set is strongly underascertained regarding to this category of headache. In addition, the higher prevalence of headaches in control mothers than in case mothers is an unusual finding (Table 7.10).

There was only a higher rate of anaemia in pregnant women with headache, and this association may indicate a causal relation. There was no higher risk of adverse birth outcomes (e.g. higher rate of PB) and CA in children of pregnant women with headache.

In conclusion, a higher occurrence of adverse birth outcomes including CA was not found in infants born to mothers with non-migraine headache during early pregnancy.

7.5 Final Conclusions

The evaluation of two chronic common disorders of the nervous system, i.e. epilepsy and migraine, demonstrated that appropriate medical help of pregnant women suffering from these disorders may also have stress-free, healthy pregnancies. However, this goal requires up-to-date knowledge and management, and evidence based recommendations to mothers suffering from these disorders.

References

Abramsky O. Pregnancy and multiple sclerosis. Ann Neurol 1994; 36(Suppl.): 38–41.

Adab N, Tudor SC, Vinten J et al. Common antiepileptic drugs in pregnancy in women with epilepsy. Cochrane Database Syst Rev 2004; (3): CD004848.

Aminoff MJ. Neurologic disorders. In: Creasy RK, Resnik R, Iams JD (eds.) Maternal-Fetal Medicine. 5th ed. Saunders, Philadelphia, 2004. pp. 1165–1191.

Berry RJ, Li Z, Erickson JD et al. Prevention of neural tube defects with folic acid in China. China-US Collaborative Project for Neural Tube Defect Prevention. N Engl J Med 1999; 341: 1485–1490.

Bjerkedahl T, Bahna SL. The occurrence and outcome of pregnancy in women with epilepsy. Acta Obstet Gynecol Scand 1973; 52: 245–248.

Bjekedahl T, CzeizelAE, Goujajrd J et al. Valproic acid and spina bifida. Lancet 1982; 2: 1096 only.

Botto LD, Olney RS, Erickson JD. Vitamin supplements and risk for congenital anomalies other than neural tube defects. Am J Med Genet C 2004; 125C: 12–21.

Dekker G, Sibai B. Primary, secondary and tertiary prevention of preeclampsia. Lancet 2001; 357: 209–215.

Diamond S. Migraine headache prevention and management. Marcel Dekker, New York, 1990.

Diav-Citrin O, Shechtman TW, Freeman RK, Yaffe SJ. Is carbamazepine teratogenic? A prospective controlled study of 210 pregnancies. Neurology 2001; 57: 321–324.

DiLiberti JH, Farndon PA, Dennis NR, Curry CJR. The fetal valproate syndrome. Am J Med Genet 1984; 19: 473–481.

Eldridge RR. Sumatriptan Pregnancy Register. Glaxo Wellcome Inc., Research Triangle Park, NC, 2000.

Esterez M, Gardner KL. Update on the genetics of migraine. Hum Genet 2004; 114: 225–235.

Facchinetty F, Allais G, D'Amico R et al. The relationship between headache and preeclampsia: a case-control study. Eur J Obstet Gynecol Reprod Biol 2005; 121: 143–148.

Fried S, Kozer E, Nulman I et al. Malformation rates in children of women with untreated epilepsy: a metanalysis. Dug Saf 2004; 27: 197–202.

German J, Lowal A, Ehlers KH. Trimethadione and human teratogenesis. Teratology 1970; 3: 349–362.

Giffin NJ, Kowacs F, Libri V. Effect of the adenosine A1 receptor agonist GR79236 on trigeminal nociception with blink reflex recordings in healthy human subjects. Cephalgia 2003; 23: 287–292.

Goadsby PJ. Migraine: diagnosis and management. Intern Med J 2003; 33: 436–442.

Hanson JW, Smith DW. The fetal hydantoin syndrome. J Pediatr 1975; 87: 305–312.

HCSIHS: Headache Classification Subcommittee of the International Headache Society. The International Classification of Headache Disorders. 2nd ed. Cephalgia 2004; 24(Suppl.1): 1–151.

Hemels ME, Einarson A, Koren G et al. Antidepressant use during pregnancy and the rates of spontaneous abortions: a meta-analysis. Ann Pharmacother 2005; 39: 803–809.

Hiilesmaa VK, Teramo K, Granstrom M-L, Bardy AH. Fetal head growth retardation associated with maternal antiepileptic drugs. Lancet 1981; 2: 165–167.

Holmes LB, Harvey EA, Couil BA et al. The teratogenicity of anticonvulsants drugs. N Engl J Med 2001; 344: 1132–1138.

Janz D, Fuchs V. Are anti-epileptic drugs harmful when given during pregnancy? German Med Monog 1964; 9: 20–23.

Jones KL, Johnson KA. Chamber CC. Pregnancy outcome in women treated with phenobarbital monotherapy. Teratology 1992; 45: 452–453.

Kaaja E. Kaaja R, Hiilesmaa V. Major malformations on offspring of women with epilepsy. Neurology 2003; 60: 575–579.

Källen B. Maternal epilepsy, antiepileptic drugs and birth defects. Pathologica 1986; 78: 757–768.

Källen B, Lygner PE. Delivery outcome in women who used drugs for migraine during pregnancy with special reference to sumatriptan. Headache 2001; 41: 351–356.

Knight AH, Rhind EG. Epilepsy and pregnancy: a study of 153 pregnancies in 59 patients. Epilepsia 1975; 16: 99–110.

Koren G, Pastuszak A, Ito S. Drugs in pregnancy. N Engl J Med 1998; 338: 1128–1137.

Kurt AA. Association between migraine and cardiovasculat diseases. Expert Rev Neurother 2007; 7: 1097–1104

Laegread L, Olegard R, Wahlstrom J et al. Abnormalities in children exposed to benzodiazepines in utero. Lancet 1987; i: 108–109.

Laegread L, Hagberg G, Lundborg A. The effect of benzodiazepines in the fetus and the newborns. Neuropediatrics 1992; 23: 18–23.

Lance JW. The pharmacotherapy of migraine. Med J Austr 1986; 44: 85–88.

Lipton RB, Scher AI, Kolodner K. Migraine in the United States: epidemiology and patterns of health care use. Neurology 2002; 58: 885–894.

Lipton RB, Bigal ME, Goadsby PJ. Double-blind clinical trials of oral triptans vs. other classes of acute migraine medication – a review. Cephalgia 2004; 24: 321–332.

Lucas RN. Migraine in twins. J Psychosom Res 1977; 21: 147–156.

MacGregor EA, Brandes J, Eikermann A. Migraine prevalence and treatment: the Global Migraine and Zomitriptan Evaluation Survey. Headache 2003; 43: 19–26.

Marcoux S, Brisson J, Fabia J. Calcium intake from diary products and supplements and the risks of preeclampsia and gestational hypertension. Am J Epidemiol 1991; 133: 1266–1272.

Marcus DA. Migraine in women. Semin Pain Med 2004; 2: 115–122.

Marcus DA, Scharrf L, Mercer S, Turk DC. Nonpharmacological treatment for migraine: incremental utility of physical therapy with relaxation and thermal biofeedback. Cephalgia 1998; 18: 266–272.

Marcus DA, Scharff L, Turk DC. Longitudinal prospective study of Headache during pregnancy and postpartum. Headache 1999; 39: 625–632.

Markowitz S, Saito K, Moskowitz MA. Neurogenically mediated plasma extravasation in dura mater: effect of ergot alkaloids. A possible mechanism of action in vascular Headache. Cephalgia 1988; 8: 83–91.

Massey EW. Migraine during pregnancy. Survey Obstet Gynecol 1977; 32: 693–696.

Mathew Nt. Pathophysiology, epidemiology and impact of migraine. Clin Cornerstone 2001; 4: 1–17.

McGuirk CK, Westage MN, Holmes LB. Limb deficiencies in newborn infants. Pediatrics 2001; 108: e64.

Meadow SR. Anticonvulsant drugs and congenital abnormalities. Lancet 1968; 2: 1296.

Meadow KJ, Baker GA, Browning N et al. Cognitive function at 3 years of age after fetal exposure to antiepileptic drugs. N Engl J Med 2009; 360: 1597–1605.

Meadow K, Reynolds MW, Crean S et al. Pregnancy outcome in women with epilepsy: a systematic review and meta-analysis of published pregnancy registries and cohorts. Epilepsy 2008; 81: 1–13.

Medalie JH. Relationship between nausea and/or vomiting in early pregnancy and abortion. Lancet 1957; 273: 117–119.

Mitchell LE, Adrick NS, Melchionne J et al. Spina bifida. Lancet, 2004; 364: 1885–1895.

Monson RR, Rosenberg L, Harta SC et al. Diphenylhydantoin and selected congenital malformations. N Engl J Med 1973; 289: 1049–1052.

Montouris G. Gabapentin exposure in human pregnancy: results from Gabapentin Pregnancy Registry. Epilepsy Behav 2003; 4: 310–317.

MRC Vitamin Study Research Groups. Prevention of neural tube defect: results of Medical Research Council vitamin study. Lancet 1991; 338: 131–137.

Nakane Y, Okuma T, Takahashi R et al. Multi-institutional study on the teratogenicity and fetal toxicity of antiepileptic drugs. A report of a collaborative study group in Japan. Epilepsy 1980; 21: 663–680.

Narbone MC, Abbate M, Gangemi S. Acute drug treatment of migraine attack. Neurol Sci 2004; 25: S113–S118.

Olesen C, Steffensen FH, Sorensen HT. Pregnancy outcome following prescription for sumatriptan. Headache 2000; 40: 20–24.

Ophoff RA, Terwindt GM, Vergouwe MN. Familial hemiplegic migraine and episodic ataxia type-2 are caused by mutations in the CA^{2+}-channel gene CACNL1A4. Cell 1996; 87: 543–552.

O'Quinn S, Ephross SA, Williams V et al. Pregnancy and perinatal outcomes in migreneurs using sumatriptan: a prospective study. Arch Gynecol Obstet 1999; 263: 7–12.

Poser S, Poser W. Multiple sclerosis and gestation. Neurology 1983; 33: 1422–1427.

Reik L Jr. Headaches in pregnancy. Semin Neurol 1988; 8: 187–192.

Roberts E, Guiband P. Maternal valproate acid and congenital neural tube defects. Lancet 1982; 2: 937 only.

Rosa FW. Spina bifida in infants of women treated with carbamazepine during pregnancy. N Engl J Med 1991; 324: 374–677.

Rosenberg L, Mitchell AA. Lack of correlation of oral clefts to diazepam use during pregnancy. N Engl J Med 1984; 310: 1122 only

Russel MB, Iselius L, Olesen J. Inheritance of migraine investigated by complex segregation analysis. Hum Genet 1995; 96: 726–730.

Russel MB, Hilden J, Sorensen SA, Olesen J. Familial occurrence of migraine without aura and migraine with aura. Neurology 1993; 43: 1369–1373.

Sadovnick AD, Eisen K, Hasimoto SA et al. Pregnancy and multiple sclerosis: a prospective study. Arch Neurol 1994; 54: 1120.

Safra MJ, Oakley GP. Association between cleft lip with or without cleft palate and prenatal exposure to diazepam. Lancet 1975; 2: 478–479.

Sances G, Granella F, Nappi RE. Course of migraine during pregnancy and postpartum: a prospective study. Cephalgia 2003; 23: 197–205.

Saxen I, Saxen L. Association between maternal intake of diazepam and oral clefts. Lancet 1975; 2: 498 only

Shapiro S, Hartz SC, Siskind V et al. Anticonvulsants and prenatal Epilepsy in the development of birth defects. Lancet 1976; 1: 272–275.

Shepard TH, Lemire RJ. Catalog of Teratogenic Agents. 11th ed. Johns Hopkins Univ Press, Baltimore, 2004.

Shunaiber S, Pastuszak A, Schick B. Pregnancy outcome following first trimester exposure to sumatriptan. Neurology 1998; 51: 581–583.

Silberstein SD, Lipton RB. Headache in Clinical Practice. Medical Media, Oxford, 1998. pp. 934–939.

Smithells RW, Sheppard S, Wild J, Schorach CJ. Prevention of neural tube defect recurrence in Yorkshire: final report. Lancet 1989; 2: 498–499.

Stewart WF, Linet MS, Celentano DD. Age- and sex-specific incidence rates of migraine with and without visual aura. Am J Epidemiol 1991; 34: 1111–1120.

Stewart WF, Lipton RB, Celentano DD, Reed ML. Prevalence of migraine Headaches in the United States. J Am Med Ass 1992; 267: 64–69.

Tfelt-Hansen P, Saxena PR. Ergot alkaloids in the acute treatment of migraine. In: Olesen J, Tfelt-Hansen P, Welch KMA (eds.) The Headaches. 2nd ed. Lippincott Williams and Wilkins, Philadelphia, 2000. pp. 399–409.

Tfelt-Hansen P, McEwen J. Nonsteroidal antiinflammatory drugs in the acute treatment of migraine. In: Olesen J, Tfelt-Hansen P, Welch KMA (eds.) The Headaches. 2nd ed. Lippincott Williams and Wilkins, Philadelphia, 2000. pp. 391–397.

Tompson T, Gram L, Siilanpaa M, Johannenssen SI. Epilepsy and Pregnancy. Wrightson Biomedical Publishing Ltd, Hampshire, 1997.

Villalon CM, Centurion D, Valdivia LF. Migraine: pathophysiology, pharmacology, treatment and future trends. Curr Vasc Pharmacol 2003; 1: 71–84.

Wainscott G, Sullivan FM, Volans GN, Wilkinson M. The outcome of pregnancy in women suffering from migraine. Postgrad Med J 1978; 54: 98–102.
Wall VR. Breastfeeding and migraine Headaches. J Hum Lact 1992; 8: 209–212.
Watson JD, Spellacy WN. Neonatal effects of maternal treatment with the anticonvulsant drug diphenylhydantoin. Obstet Gynecol 1971; 37: 881–885.
Weigel MM, Weigel R. Nausea and vomiting of early pregnancy and pregnancy outcomes. An epidemiological study. Br J Obstet Gynecol 1989; 96: 1304–1311.
Wyllie E (ed.) The Treatment of Epilepsy, Principles and Practice. 3rd ed. Lippincott Williams and Wilkins, Philadelphia, 2001.
Zackai EH, Melman WJ, Neiderer B, Hanson JW. The fetal trimethadione syndrome. J Pediatr 1975; 87: 280–284.

Own Publications

I. Kjaer D, Puhó HE, Christensen J, Vestergaard M, Czeizel AE, Sorensen HT, Olsen J. Use of phenytoin, phenobarbitals or diazepam during pregnancy and risk of congenital abnormalities: a case-time control study. Pharmacoepid Drug Safety 2007; 16: 181–188.
II. Czeizel AE, Dudás I. Prevention of the first occurrence of neural-tube defects by periconceptional vitamin supplementation. N Engl J Med 1992; 327: 1832–1835.
III. Czeizel AE, Dobo M, Vargha P. Hungarian cohort-controlled trial of periconceptional multivitamin supplementation shows a reduction in certain congenital abnormalities. Birth Defects Res A 2004; 70: 853–861.
IV. Czeizel AE. Prevention of congenital abnormalities by periconceptional multivitamin supplementation. Br J Med 1993; 306: 1645–1648.
V. Czeizel AE. Reduction of urinary tract and cardiovascular defects by periconceptional multivitamin supplementation. Am J Med Genet 1996; 62: 179–183.
VI. Kjaer D, Puhó HE, Christensen J, Vestergaard M, Czeizel AE, Sorensen HT, Olsen J. Antiepileptic drugs, folic acid and congenital abnormalities – a Hungarian case-control study. Br J Obstet Gynecol 2008; 115: 98–103.
VII. Bánhidy F, Ács N, Puho E, Czeizel AE. Pregnancy complications and delivery outcomes in pregnant women with migraine. Eur J Obstet Gynecol Reprod Biol 2007; 134: 403–409.
VIII. Bánhidy F, Ács N, Horváth-Puho E, Czeizel AE. Maternal severe migraine and risk of congenital limb deficiencies. Birth Defects Res A 2006; 76: 592–601.
IX. Czeizel AE, Ács N, Bánidy F. Migraine in pregnant women (Review). Trends Reprod Biol 2008; 3: 1–8.
X. Czeizel AE, Evans JA, Kodaj I, Lenz W. Congenital Limb Deficiencies in Hungary. Genetic and Teratologic Epidemiologic Studies. Akadémiai Kiadó Budapest, 1994.

Chapter 8
Diseases of the Eye and Adnexa

Our main interest has been the CAs of eyes, here postnatal eye diseases were planned to evaluate in pregnant women. The acute and chronic diseases of eyes are common; nevertheless these pathological conditions were recorded rarely in pregnant women in the dataset of the HCCSCA.

8.1 Interpretation of Data in the HCCSCA

Only two diseases of the eye occurred in the data set of the HCCSCA.

One case affected with ventricular septal defect born to mothers with glaucoma.

Nine pregnant women were reported with severe myopia, 3 delivered malformed cases (ventricular septal defect, hypospadias, and clubfoot, namely talipes equinovarus) and 6 healthy newborns, i.e. controls with the usual gestational age at delivery and birth weight.

N. Ács et al., *Congenital Abnormalities and Preterm Birth Related to Maternal Illnesses During Pregnancy*, DOI 10.1007/978-90-481-8620-4_8,

Chapter 9
Diseases of the Ear and the Mastoid Process

Among the diseases of the ear, otitis media was registered most frequently in the data set of the HCCSCA.

9.1 Otitis Media

This inflammatory disease of ear may be primary clinical entities as acute and chronic serous, mucoid, etc suppurative and nonsupporative disease of the middle ear or secondary complications of other diseases such as measles, influenza, etc.

9.1.1 Results of the Study (I)

Out of 22,843 cases with CA, 58 (0.25%), while out of 38,151 controls without CA, 56 (0.15%) had mothers with medically recorded otitis media in the prenatal care logbook.

The onset of otitis media did not show characteristic distribution according to gestational months, 25 case and 14 control mothers were affected by otitis media in the first trimester of pregnancy. The average duration of otitis media was 3 weeks, and otitis media with its onset in I gestational month continued to II month in all pregnant women.

Pregnant women with otitis media was somewhat younger (25.0–25.3 vs. 25.5 year) but mean birth order was lower (1.7 vs. 1.9) in case but higher (1.8 vs. 1.7) in control mothers. There was no significant difference in the distribution of marital and employment status among study groups. The use of folic acid (48.3% vs. 45.5%) and multivitamins (3.6% vs. 8.6%) was somewhat higher in case mothers than control mothers with otitis media.

The evaluation of maternal diseases showed that only acute diseases of the respiratory system (in case mothers with or without otitis media: 62.1% vs. 9.2%, in control mothers with or without otitis media: 65.5% vs. 9.0%) occurred significantly more frequently. The association of otitis media with acute respiratory diseases is

N. Ács et al., *Congenital Abnormalities and Preterm Birth Related to Maternal Illnesses During Pregnancy*, DOI 10.1007/978-90-481-8620-4_9,

well-known because otitis media is considered as secondary complications of these diseases.

Pregnancy complications did not show difference among the study groups.

After the evaluation of drugs, only medicinal products used for the treatment of otitis media showed a much higher occurrence in pregnant women with otitis media such as ampicillin (67.3% vs. 7.0%), penamecillin (32.7% vs. 6.3%), clotrimazole (8.0% vs. 1.3%), parenteral benzylpenicillin (7.1% vs. 0.3%), and oxytetracycline (6.2% vs. 0.6%). All pregnant women were treated by one or more of the above mentioned drugs. However, only tetracycline was used more frequently by case mothers (5, 8.6%) than control mothers (2, 3.6%). In addition, women with otitis media were treated frequently by antifever-antiinflammatory drugs such as acetylsalicylic acid, paracetamol, and dipyrone as well (63.6% vs. 9.2%).

Birth outcomes were evaluated mainly in control newborns, their mean gestational age at delivery was somewhat longer (39.6 vs. 39.4 week) and it was associated with a somewhat lower rate of PB (7.3% vs. 9.2%). The mean birth weight was larger (3,370 vs. 3,275 g) with a lower rate of LBW newborns (3.6% vs. 5.7%). However, these differences reflected only a trend because they did not reach the level of significance. We may suppose that pregnant women after otitis media had a higher standard of prenatal care (e.g. folic acid and multivitamin use), healthier lifestyle (e.g. lower rate of smokers), and the concomitant antimicrobial treatment might have been effective against the parallel existing frequent vulvovaginitis-bacterial vaginosis which is associated with an increased risk for PB. Thus, these factors may explain the somewhat longer gestational age at delivery and lower rate of PB.

The evaluation of different CA groups including at least 3 cases resulted in an unexpected finding (Table 9.1).

The prevalence of otitis media was compared in case and control pregnant women during the study pregnancy and a higher risk was found in the rate of total CAs explained mainly by the higher rate of CAs of the ears, cardiovascular CAs and the group of other isolated CAs. The highest prevalence of maternal otitis media was found in the group of ear CAs (1.1% vs. 0.1%) and the evaluation of cases with control resulted in a significant association. Most major CA have a critical period in II and/or III gestational months, thus the exposure, i.e. otitis media, was evaluated separately during this time window. Only the risk of CAs of the ears and total CA group was higher, and again the very high risk for ear CAs is noteworthy.

The detailed analysis of 4 cases with CAs of ears and 12 cases with cardiovascular CAs is shown in Table 9.2. Of these 4 cases, 3 had severe CAs of auditory canal and middle ear. The critical period of this CA-group is in II and/or III gestational month and 3 pregnant women were affected with otitis media during this time window. On the other hand their mothers had no other serious disease during the critical period of this CA-group. Out of 12 cases with cardiovascular CAs, only one mother had otitis media in II month of pregnancy, i.e. the critical period of transposition of great vessels.

Table 9.1 Estimation of the risk of otitis media on different CAs in cases compared to matched controls, their mothers were affected with otitis media

		Any time during pregnancy				II–III months			
Study groups	Grand total no.	No.	%	OR[a]	95% CI	No.	%	OR[a]	95% CI
Controls	38,151	55	0.1	Reference		14	0.04	Reference	
CAs of ear	354	4	1.1	**5.5**	**1.6–20.4**	3	0.85	**16.0**	**3.3–71.3**
Cardiovascular CAs	4,479	12	0.3	**3.5**	**1.3–9.7**	4	0.09	6.6	0.7–63.3
Hypospadias	3,038	6	0.2	0.7	0.3–1.8	4	0.13	1.5	0.4–6.1
Poly/syndactyly	1,744	6	0.3	1.9	0.5–6.7	3	0.17	3.1	0.3–30.1
Clubfoot	2,424	6	0.3	1.7	0.6–5.1	2	0.08	3.6	0.3–40.0
Other CAs	10,804	24[b]	0.2	**1.9**	**1.1–3.5**	10	0.09	2.6	0.9–7.2
Total	22,843	58	0.3	**1.8**	**1.2–2.6**	25	0.11	**2.8**	**1.4–5.6**

[a]Adjusted for maternal age, birth order, and employment status.

[b]Cong. hydrocephaly 2, cong. pyloric stenosis 2, undescended testis 2, limb deficiencies 2, torticollis 2, anencephaly 1, spina bifida 1, cleft lip 1, cleft lip + cleft palate, rectal stenosis 1, renal agenesis 1, cystic kidney 1, omphalocele 1, congenital genu varum 1, vaginal atresia 1, indeterminate sex 1, CA of the spine 1, multiple CA 2.

Table 9.2 Data of cases with ear CAs and cardiovascular CAs

	Otitis media (gestational month)	Other diseases	Drug treatments
Ear CAs			
Atresia of auditory canal with fusion of ear ossicles	II–III	–	–
Atresia of auditory canal with microtia	III–IV	Preeclampsia	Dipyrone (III–IV)
Atresia of auditory canal with the absent of membranous labyrinth in the middle ear and organ Corti	III–IV	Tonsillitis (IV)	Xylometazoline (IV–VI) Penamecillin (IV–VI)
Fusion of ear ossicles	VI–VII	Tonsillitis (V–VI)	Xylometazoline (VI–VII)
Cardiovascular CAs			
Transposition of great vessels	VI	–	Ampicillin (VI)
	II–VIII	–	–
	III–IV	Influenza (VIII)	–
Ventricular septal defect	V–VI	Laryngitis (V–IX)	Ampicillin (V), Cefalexin (VI–VII)
	VIII–IX	–	Phenazone tetracain (VIII–IX)
	VIII	Vulvovaginitis (IV)	–
Atrial septal defect, type II	III	Sinusitis (III)	Penamecillin (III)
	VI		–
Endocardial cushion defect	VI	Preeclampsia (VII)	Penamecillin (VI)
	VII	Laryntitis (V)	Benzylpenicillin (V)
Coarctation of aorta	VI	Influenza (VII)	Penamecillin (VI)
Unspecified cardiovascular CA	III	–	Dipyrone (III)

9.1.2 Interpretation of Results

The unexpected higher risk of total CAs and CAs of the ear in the children of pregnant women with otitis media needs explanation. The detailed analysis of cases indicated a possible association of otitis media in pregnant women during II and/or III month with a higher risk of special manifestation of severe ear CAs. This association cannot be explained by the drugs used for the treatment of otitis media. On the one hand the drugs e.g. penamecillin (3), parenteral penicillin (1), ampicillin (4), oxytetracycline (8), cotrimoxazole (19, 20), acetylsalicylic acid (75, 76), paracetamol (77), and dipyrone (81) used frequently for the treatment of otitis media do not cause ear CAs. On the other hand, the frequency of their administration does not show differences between case and control pregnant women with the exception of oxytetracycline. Finally, the mothers of cases with ear CAs were not treated by these drugs during the critical period of this CA-group.

Confounders or chance effect should also be considered, therefore further studies are needed to be done to confirm or reject this association and hypothesis.

Previously in the origin of otitis media a genetic susceptibility was suggested by racial variations because frequency of otitis media is unusually high in American Indians and Australian aborigines and comparatively low in blacks with African origin. This possible genetic predisposition for otitis media was confirmed on the basis of familial aggregation of otitis media, mastoid size, and cholesteatoma (Todd, 1987). Similarly, our hypothesis is that an association may be the anatomic configuration of the middle ear and the auditory canal with a predisposition or higher susceptibility for otitis media. This genetically determined anatomic configuration may also be associated with a higher risk for the developmental errors of the ears.

9.2 Other Diseases

Two pregnant women with deaf-mutes delivered a case with unspecified cardiovascular CA, while another delivered a healthy baby.

Reference

Todd NV. Familial predisposition for otitis media in Apache Indians at Canyon Day, Arizoma. Genet Epidemiol 1987; 4: 25–31.

Own Publication

1. Ács N, Bánhidy F, Puhó HE, Czeizel AE. A possible association between maternal otitis media and ear defect in their offspring. Am J Otolaryng 2010 (in press)

Chapter 10
Diseases of the Circulatory System

Cardiovascular diseases are the leading causes of death in Hungary; more than half of the population dies due to these diseases. Pregnant women are also frequently affected with the different manifestation of this disease group but fortunately the high morbidity is not associated with high mortality.

10.1 Maternal Cardiovascular Adaptation to Pregnancy

There are significant changes in the cardiovascular system during pregnancy (Blanchard and Shabetai, 2004; Monga, 2004; McAnulty et al., 2008). The total blood volume increases steadily during the first trimester and it is increased by almost 50% by the 30th gestational week without any further change in the last weeks of pregnancy. Between 8th and 32nd gestational week, plasma volume increases more intensively (up to 45%) than red blood cell mass (25%). This explains the common "physiologic" anemia of pregnancy, which without iron supplementation may result in low hematocrit (about 33 ml/dL) and hemoglobin (11 g/dL) values.

Heart rate increases gradually throughout pregnancy by 10–20 beats/min, while resting cardiac output rises soon after conception and it is reaching its maximum of 130–145% of the non-pregnant level by the 20th gestational week. This increase in cardiac output is caused mainly by elevated stroke volume in the earlier part of pregnancy while it is caused by the increased heart rate in the second part of pregnancy. There is a hypertrophy in the uterus with endometrial vascularization and the highly vascularised structure of the placenta functions as an arteriovenosus shunt. Furthermore, the enlarged uterus reduces the venous return from the lower extremities.

Blood pressure falls slightly in early pregnancy because systemic vascular resistance decreases until the 20th gestational week, but thereafter it gradually increases till term. The mother's oxygen consumption also increases by 20% within the first half of pregnancy. A further 10% increase in oxygen consumption was also noted by the time of delivery.

N. Ács et al., *Congenital Abnormalities and Preterm Birth Related to Maternal Illnesses During Pregnancy*, DOI 10.1007/978-90-481-8620-4_10,

Arterial compliance of pregnant women is increased. Venous capacitance is also increased with an increase in venous vascular tone. These changes of vascular system are advantageous in maintaining the hemodynamics of a normal pregnancy, but the venous changes partly can explain the higher risk of thromboembolic complications during pregnancy.

The above changes in the cardiovascular system can be satisfactory explained by the effects of the increased levels of circulating reproductive hormones.

Cardiovascular diseases are the leading cause of mortality worldwide; responsible for one-third of all deaths (Vasan et al., 2008). Unfortunately about half of people die due to cardiovascular diseases in Hungary, and the major part of this mortality are caused by hypertension related stroke and coronary artery disease.

10.2 Mitral Stenosis Due to Rheumatic Heart Disease

Rheumatic fever due to streptococcal infection has become rare in Hungary after the introduction of penicillin therapy. The characteristic manifestation of rheumatic heart disease is mitral stenosis. The inflammatory reaction of mitral valve causes stenosis frequently with calcification resulting in enlargement of the left atrium and right ventricle, a diastolic murmur at the cardiac apex, and pulmonary hypertension.

In cases with mitral stenosis pregnancy is dangerous because the increased blood volume, heart rate, and cardiac output raise the left atrial pressure which can cause severe pulmonary congestion with progressive exertional dyspnoe, orthopnea, paroxysmal nocturnal dyspnea, and pulmonary edema sometimes with lethal outcome (Székely et al., 1973).

10.2.1 Interpretation of Data in the HCCSCA

Out of 22,843 cases, 2 had mothers with mitral stenosis, while out of 38,151 controls, also 2 babies were born to mothers with this disease. Both cases were affected by cardiovascular CA: tetralogy of Fallot and unspecified heart CA, while two controls were born on 39th and 41st gestational week with 3,300 and 3,600 g.

10.3 Hypertension

Hypertension is one of the most common chronic conditions which is causing damage in the structure and function of the heart and arteries. It also accelerates the development of arteriosclerosis which leads to myocardial infarction.

In the population blood pressure has normal distribution; therefore there is no obvious natural threshold between normal and pathological blood pressure like in the so-called qualitative (yes or no) diseases (Pickering and Ogedegbe, 2008). Hypertension is frequently neglected due to the lack of obvious symptoms in the early phase of this disease (Hall et al., 2008). At present there is a well-known definition for hypertension following the consensus of experts based on several clinical studies evaluating long term consequences of increased blood pressure. Hypertension is diagnosed if blood pressure exceeds 140/90 mmHg above age 18 measured by the recommended criteria (Rashidi et al., 2008). According to the classification of hypertension by severity, Stage 1 (140–159/90–99 mmHg) and Stage 2 (160/100 or over mmHg) can be differentiated (Pickering and Ogedegbe, 2008).

Another classification of hypertension is based on its origin (Pickering and Ogedegbe, 2008). Primary or essential hypertension occurs in about 95% of patients caused by the interaction of polygenic liability and hazardous environmental factors, while the rest is caused by identifiable causes such as chronic kidney disease, renal artery stenosis, coartation of the aorta, Cushing disease, etc. These hypertensions are classified as secondary hypertension (Hall et al., 2008).

Hypertension can be present before and during pregnancy in 1–5% of women (Rey et al., 1997; Churchill, 2001). During prenatal care of pregnant women with hypertension doctors must consider the possible teratogenic and/or fetotoxic effects of some antihypertensive drugs; therefore, special guidelines are given for controlling blood pressure during pregnancy (Rey et al., 1997; NHBPEWG, 2000; Gifford et al., 2000; Churchill, 2001; Chobanian et al., 2003; JNC7, 2003; Roberts, 2004; Abalos et al., 2007; McAnulty et al., 2008).

A classification system of hypertension in pregnant women prepared by the National Institutes of Health (NIH) differentiated four categories: chronic hypertension, preeclampsia-eclampsia, preeclampsia superimposed upon chronic hypertension, and gestational hypertension (Gifford et al., 2000).

Chronic hypertension in pregnant women is defined as hypertension that is present and observable prior to pregnancy or is diagnosed before the 20th week of gestation. If pregnant women with secondary hypertension, gestational hypertension and preeclampsia are excluded, we may use the term *essential hypertension* (EH) in these pregnant women.

The definition of *gestational hypertension* (GH) is the pregnancy induced hypertension detected first time during pregnancy without proteinuria until the end of pregnancy. In general, gestational hypertension is diagnosed after the 20th gestational week (Roberts, 2004), i.e. after the critical period of most major CAs.

Pregnant women with preeclampsia-eclampsia and with preeclampsia superimposed upon chronic hypertension will be evaluated in a special chapter.

In the group of secondary hypertension only pregnant women with renal diseases having proteinuria and hypertension simultaneously had enough number for evaluation in the HCCSCA and will be evaluated separately among the diseases of urinary tract.

Here pregnant women with EH and GH will be evaluated.

10.3.1 Results of the Study (I, II)

The four main objectives of the study were to evaluate (i) the possible association of maternal EH and GH with pregnancy complications, (ii) with adverse birth outcomes such as PB and/or LBW newborns, (iii) with the risk of CAs in their offspring and (iv) to estimate the efficacy of antihypertensive drugs in the reduction of adverse birth outcomes.

Only pregnant women with prospectively and medical recorded EH or GH in the prenatal maternity logbook were included into the study. The severity of changing hypertension values was evaluated based on related drug treatments. Pregnant women with Stage I hypertension are not recommended to treat with drugs. Dietary modification particularly sodium reduction and more intensive physical activity, in addition to maternal weight control seemed to be enough to control the blood pressure (Rashidi et al., 2008). Thus we assumed that pregnant women with untreated hypertension belonged to the group of Stage 1, while pregnant women with treated hypertension had Stage 2.

The case group consisted of 22,843 malformed newborns or fetuses ("informative offspring"), and 1,030 (4.5%) had mothers with EH during the study pregnancy. Out of 38,151 controls, 1,579 (4.1%) were born to mothers with EH (1.1, 1.0–1.2). Out of 1,030 case mothers with EH, 37 (3.6%), while out of 1,579 control mothers with EH, 57 (3.6%) were not treated probably due to their moderate hypertension, therefore most pregnant women with EH had Stage II hypertension.

The number of case and control pregnant women with GH was 580 (2.5%) and 1,098 (2.9%), respectively. GH was diagnosed after the 20th gestational week in nearly all pregnant women. Out of 580 case mothers, 366 (63.1%), and out of 1,098 control mothers with GH, 441 (40.2%) were treated with antihypertensive drugs.

The main variables of mothers showed a higher mean maternal age due to the larger proportion of women over 30 years in pregnant women with treated EH and GH, but not in untreated women compared to reference group, i.e. pregnant women without hypertension. Pregnant women with treated EH had a somewhat higher socioeconomic status but it was not characteristic for pregnant women with treated GH. The proportion of smokers was 25.4% and 22.2% in case and control mothers with EH, in addition 34.8% and 29.2% of case and control mothers with GH, respectively, while this figure was 18.5% in pregnant women without hypertension. The proportion of hard and regular drinkers did not show significant differences among the study groups. The proportion of folic acid supplementation during pregnancy was larger in pregnant women with EH (58.3%) while it was smaller in pregnant women with GH (48.1%) compared to the reference group (52.3%). A similar trend was seen with multivitamin supplementation. Therefore, pregnant women with EH and GH had different characteristics.

The occurrence of acute maternal diseases (e.g. influenza) did not show significant difference among the study groups. Among chronic diseases, only migraine (4.6% vs. 2.4% in case pregnant women and 4.2% vs. 1.7% in control pregnant women with or without EH) and cardiac dysrhythmias (0.2% in reference group, but 5.0% in case and 4.2% in control mothers) occurred more frequently in pregnant women with EH. The prevalence of migraine was 2.2% in pregnant women with GH.

The first aim of the study was the evaluation of pregnancy complications (except preeclampsia-eclampsia which was excluded from this analysis) in women with EH and GH. The rate of threatened abortion (27.1% vs. 16.5%) and preterm delivery (42.0% vs. 13.2%), in addition to placental disorders (3.4% vs. 1.5%), particularly premature separation of the placenta was significantly higher in women with EH. Placental abruption was much higher in pregnant women with treated EH compared to the reference group. These variables of pregnant women with GH did not differ from the reference values.

Obvious differences were seen in the frequency of drugs used for the treatment of EH and GH in pregnant women. The frequency of drug usage was the following in decreasing order: terbutaline, verapamil, metoprolol, nifedipin, fenoterol, methyldopa in pregnant women with EH, while this order was methyldopa, clopamide, dihydralazine, nifedipin, and metoprolol in pregnant women with GH.

The second aim of the study was the evaluation of birth outcomes of control newborns without CA (Table 10.1).

The mean gestational age at delivery was shorter by 0.5 week and the mean birth weight was lower by 136 g in the treated EH subgroup than in the reference group. On the other hand, the limited number of newborns of untreated pregnant women with EH had longer mean gestational age and larger mean birth weight. In agreement with these quantitative variables, the rate of PB and LBW newborns of pregnant women with treated EH were much higher while lower in the subgroup of untreated women with EH. The mean gestational age was somewhat shorter while mean birth weight were similar between newborns of mother with GH (either treated or not treated) and the reference sample. The rate of PB in pregnant women with GH did not differ from the value of the reference group, while the rate of LBW was marginally higher. Finally, it is worth mentioning the higher rate of twins in the subgroups of pregnant women with treated GH (2.4%) and particularly with treated EH (3.1%) than in the reference group (1.0%).

The third aim of the study was the evaluation of the possible association of pregnant women with EH and the risk of different CAs in their informative offspring (Table 10.2). EH as chronic hypertension started before the conception of the study pregnancy thus all pregnant women with EH were evaluated together.

Two CA-groups, namely oesophageal atresia/stenosis and multiple CAs were associated with higher prevalence of EH in their mothers. Two cases with multiple CA were born to mothers treated with captopril on 39th gestation week but with 2,300 and 2,500 g birth weight. One boy was affected by pectus excavatum and generalized contractures of the lower limb joints born to mothers treated first by oxprenolol, methyldopa, chlortalidone, and nifedipin, and later from IV gestational month with captopril. Another girl was affected with bilateral varus deformities of the feet, congenital dislocation of the hip and skull deformity. Her mother was treated with methyldopa in the early pregnancy and captopril from V gestational months. (This pregnant woman was hospitalized in the last 2 months of pregnancy because of her renal complications.) These two multimalformed cases had oligohydramnios sequence due to the primary kidney lesion (although renal dysgenesis was not notified) with secondary postural deformities and intrauterine growth retardation. The component CAs of other multimalformed cases did not show a characteristic pattern or "syndrome".

Table 10.1 Birth outcomes of newborn infants without CA born to women with EH or GH with or without antihypertensive treatment

Variables	Reference group ($N = 34{,}633$)		EH Without treatment ($N = 57$)		EH With treatment ($N = 1{,}522$)		EH Comparison[a]		GH Without treatment ($N = 441$)		GH With treatment ($N = 657$)		GH Comparison[a]	
Quantitative	Mean	S.D.	Mean	S.D.	Mean	S.D.	*t*	*p*	Mean	S.D.	Mean	S.D.	*t*	*p*
Gestational age (week)	39.4	2.0	**39.9**	1.2	**38.9**	2.2	8.9	**0.0001**	**39.2**	2.0	**39.2**	2.1	2.2	**0.03**
Birth weight (g)	3,279	504	**3,458**	522	3,143	582	8.5	**0.0001**	3,267	520	3,287	578	1.4	0.16
Categorical	No.	%	No.	%	No.	%	OR	95% CI	No.	%	No.	%	OR	95% CI
Twins	330	1.0	1	1.8	47	**3.1**	**3.3**	**2.4–4.5**	6	1.4	16	**2.4**	**2.6**	**1.6–4.3**
PB	3,117	9.0	0	0.0	196	**12.9**	**1.5**	**1.3–1.8**	40	9.1	67	10.2	1.2	0.9–1.5
LBW	1,856	5.4	2	3.5	182	**12.0**	**2.3**	**1.8–2.7**	25	5.7	90	**7.6**	**1.5**	**1.0–2.1**

[a]Comparison of treated pregnant women and the reference group.

Table 10.2 Estimation of associations between congenital abnormalities (CAs) in cases and EH in their mothers during pregnancy in the analysis of cases and their matched controls

		Pregnant women with EH					
		No.	(%)	Crude		Adjusted[a]	
Study groups	Total no.			OR with 95% CI			
Controls	38,151	1,579	4.1	Reference		Reference	
Isolated CA							
Neural-tube defects	1,202	36	3.0	1.0	0.6–1.5	1.0	0.6–1.5
Hydrocephaly, congenital	314	16	5.1	1.3	0.6–2.6	1.3	0.6–2.6
Microcephaly, primary	111	3	2.7	0.9	0.2–3.7	1.2	0.3–5.1
Ear CAs	354	13	3.7	0.9	0.4–1.8	0.9	0.5–1.9
Cleft lip ± palate	1,374	50	3.6	1.1	0.7–1.6	1.1	0.8–1.6
Cleft palate only	601	32	5.3	1.4	0.9–2.4	1.5	0.9–2.5
Cardiovascular CAs	4,480	225	5.0	1.2	0.9–1.4	**1.3**	**1.0–1.5**
Oesophageal atresia/stenosis	217	21	9.7	**2.8**	**1.3–5.9**	**3.1**	**1.4–6.8**
Pyloric stenosis, congenital	241	11	4.6	1.3	0.6–3.0	1.1	0.5–2.7
Intestinal atresia/stenosis	153	13	8.5	2.3	0.9–5.7	2.3	0.9–6.0
Rectal/anal atresia/stenosis	220	15	6.8	1.3	0.6–2.9	1.6	0.7–3.6
Renal a/dysgenesis	126	7	5.6	0.7	0.2–2.0	0.9	0.3–3.0
Obstructive CAs of the urinary tract	343	22	6.4	1.0	0.5–1.9	1.0	0.5–1.9
Hypospadias (without coronal)	3,038	132	4.3	0.9	0.8–1.2	0.9	0.8–1.2
Undescended testis (after 3rd postnatal month)	2,052	77	3.8	0.8	0.6–1.1	0.8	0.6–1.1
Clubfoot	2,424	103	4.2	1.2	0.9–1.5	1.2	0.9–1.6
Poly/syndactyly	1,744	78	4.5	1.0	0.8–1.4	1.0	0.8–1.4
Limb deficiencies	548	21	3.8	1.3	0.7–2.2	1.4	0.8–2.4
CAs of the musculo-skeletal system	594	29	4.9	0.8	0.5–1.3	0.8	0.5–1.3
Exomphalos/ gastroschisis	238	3	1.3	0.3	0.1–0.9	0.3	0.1–1.1
CA of the diaphragm	244	10	4.1	0.8	0.4–1.8	0.8	0.4–1.9
Other isolated CAs	876	36	4.1	1.2	0.8–1.8	1.4	0.9–2.0
Multiple CAs	1,349	77	5.7	**1.6**	**1.1–2.2**	**1.6**	**1.1–2.2**
Total	22,843	1,030	4.5	1.1	1.0–1.2	1.1	1.0–1.2

[a]Adjusted for maternal age, birth order, maternal employment status, and folic acid used during pregnancy.

In addition, there was a borderline increase in the risk of cardiovascular CAs; however, when evaluating these 225 cases we did not find a cluster of any type of cardiovascular CA.

Pregnant women with GH did not show any association with higher risk for CAs.

The fourth aim of the study was to check the efficacy of antihypertensive treatment of pregnant women with EH and GH based on the occurrence of pregnancy complications and adverse birth outcomes. The severe EH which needed antihypertensive treatment associated with a higher risk of threatened abortion and preterm delivery, and also with placental disorders in pregnant women; in addition, they had a higher rate of PB and mostly LBW newborns. GH with and mostly without treatment did not show a higher risk for pregnancy complications and PB, but the rate of LBW somewhat higher.

10.3.2 Interpretation of Results

The prevalence of EH and GH was 4.1% and 2.9% in Hungarian pregnant women, respectively, which is near to the previously published upper values (Rey et al., 1997; Churchill, 2001). Our data also showed that EH and GH occurs more frequently in mothers with advanced age and among smokers. The latter was mainly characteristic for pregnant women with GH. The higher occurrence of migraine in patients with EH is well-known (Hall et al., 2008). Pregnant women with GH had a significantly lower rate of folic acid and multivitamin supplementation. The question is whether these factors may contribute to the origin of GH or not.

Strong associations were found between severe EH and increased risk for some pregnancy complications including threatened abortions, preterm deliveries, and placental disorders. These pregnancy complications may have a causal association with placental dysfunction as a common denominator.

Previously the opinion of experts was that hypertension without preeclampsia had no adverse effect on the fetus (Sibai et al., 1983) although mostly only fetal and perinatal death was evaluated. The above statement was confirmed in GH and untreated, i.e. mild EH in Hungarian pregnant women. However, intrauterine growth retardation was found more frequently in newborn infants of hypertensive women and increases in frequency and severity with increasing maternal blood pressure (Tervila et al., 1973; Rey and Couturier, 1994). This finding was confirmed in our study which demonstrated a 2.2-fold higher risks for LBW newborns in pregnant women with EH. There is an association between hypertension and higher risk of twins, the question is: which is the cause (e.g. two placentas) and which is the consequence?

The study showed that antihypertensive treatment was unable to neutralize the harm caused by EH. Some pregnancy complications and intrauterine growth retardation were related mainly to placental malfunction in pregnant women affected with severe EH. The question is whether the antihypertensive treatment was not appropriate and/or effective, or whether related drug treatments contributed to these adverse effects.

There was a possible association between EH in pregnant women and increased risk for oesophageal atresia/stenosis. The question is whether it is a causal association with EH or could be explained by related drug treatments, lifestyle factors, other or unevaluated confounders, or maybe by chance.

At the interpretation of possible causal associations, we need to consider the possible maternal teratogenic effect of ER. The study of Brazy et al. (1982) was included 29 pregnant women with severe hypertension (diastolic pressure exceeded 110 mmHg in all women) and all were treated with intravenous magnesium sulphate and other antihypertensive drugs. Beyond the intrauterine growth retardation a higher risk of microcephaly (8 infants had head circumferences below the tenth percentile), patent ductus arteriosus, and hypotonia of the skeletal and gut musculature were found. Our study also showed a higher risk for oesophageal atresia/stenosis which may be related to the maldevelopment of gut musculature. In a recent study of Caton et al. (2008) a higher risk of hypospadias was found in children born to pregnant women with hypertension treated with antihypertensive drugs. This finding was confirmed in our study.

The muscular layer of arteries is a target tissue of ES with multifactorial etiology, i.e. the consequence of polygenic-environmental interaction (Pickering and Ogedegbe, 2008; Hall et al., 2008). Most CAs of the gut also have a multifactorial origin with some genetic predisposition which is triggered by environmental actors (Robert et al., 1993). Thus, our hypothesis is that oesophageal atresia/stenosis and EH may have some common genetic predisposition.

Drugs used for the treatment of ES did not indicate any association with these CAs. Initiation of antihypertensive drug therapy is usually considered in pregnant women if systolic blood pressure exceeds 160 mmHg or diastolic pressure exceeds 110 mmHg (Roberts, 1977; Arias and Zamora, 1979; Sibai, 2002). About 96% of our pregnant women were treated with antihypertensive drugs, thus we may consider their condition as Stage 2. At the decision of antihypertensive therapy, drugs must be chosen on the basis of considerations specific to pregnancy.

In pregnant women, in general, methyldopa is the first choice (Sibai et al., 1990). Its safety has been shown in several studies (Shepard and Lemire, 2004; Briggs et al., 2005), in addition, the long term effect of methyldopa was also checked in children without any serious harm (Ounsted et al., 1983). However, this recommendation was not followed in Hungarian pregnant women with EH because methyldopa was only the 4th and 5th most frequently used drug. Direct vasodilators such as hydralazine and beta receptors blockers were found to be also effective and safe (Shepard and Lemire, 2004; Briggs et al., 2005). Our previous study did not indicate the teratogenic and/or fetotoxic effect of calcium receptor antagonists (89). Beyond the above drugs, terbutaline, and fenoterol were used in more than 10% of pregnant women. The teratogenic effect of terbutaline and fenoterol was not indicated by limited human data (Briggs et al., 2005). Mainly these drugs were used for the treatment of pregnant women with EH in Hungary without any detectable teratogenic risk.

However, ACE (angiotensin converting enzyme) inhibitors (Hanssens et al., 1991; Burrows and Burrows, 1998; Cooper et al., 2006) and angiotensin-II-receptor inhibitors/antagonists (Lambot et al., 2001; Martinovic et al., 2001) are contraindicated due to their fetotoxic effect. In our data set 10 pregnant women with EH were treated with captopril, and 2 had malformed offspring, the pattern of their CAs corresponded to the expected oligohydramnios sequence.

Another possible explanation for the association of maternal EH with some specific CAs is unevaluated/unknown confounders. Finally, multiple comparisons may produce non-causal association because significant difference is expected in every 20th estimation due to chance.

The major benefit of antihypertensive therapy is the expected reduction in the incidence of pregnancy complications, particularly preeclampsia-eclampsia and adverse birth outcomes (Arias and Zamora, 1979). (The possible preeclampsia-eclampsia preventive effect of antihypertensive treatment will be evaluated in another study.) The main result of our study is that antihypertensive treatments were not able to prevent the higher occurrence of pregnancy complications and adverse birth outcomes in pregnant women with Stage 2 of EH.

In general, monotherapy is preferred instead of polytherapy (e.g. epileptic pregnant women). However, the polytherapy seems to be more effective in patients with hypertension (Jamerson et al., 2008; Chobanian, 2008) thus it would be necessary to introduce a more effective drug combination in the treatment of pregnant women with severe EH.

In conclusion, a higher interrelated risk of treated EH was found for some pregnancy complications (threatened abortions and preterm deliveries, placental disorders), adverse birth outcomes (LBW and PB), and oesophageal atresia/stenosis.

10.4 Preeclampsia-Eclampsia

Preeclampsia-eclampsia is a frequent and severe complication of pregnancy. In general, preeclampsia-eclampsia is classified as one type of pregnancy-related hypertension (Gifford et al., 2000), although this classification was considered as imperfect as all other classification systems (Roberts, 2004).

The diagnosis of *preeclampsia* (PE) is based on the increased blood pressure accompanied by proteinuria. As the consensus of experts based on several studies, there is a well-known definition of hypertension, namely blood pressure exceeds 140/90 mmHg above age 18 measured by the recommended criteria (Rashidi et al., 2008). It is recommended that gestational blood pressure elevation is defined based on at least two determinations according to the recent international criteria of measurements. Proteinuria is defined as the urinary excretion of 0.3 g protein or greater in 24-h. In general, this value correlate with 30 mg/dL ("1 + dipstick") or greater in a random urine determination (Meyer et al., 1994). Recently experts of the topic strongly recommend the evaluation of a 24-h urine specimen. If that is not feasible, it should be based on a timed collection corrected for creatinine excretion (Gifford et al., 2000). In the past the third symptom of PE was edema, however, edema occurs in too many normal pregnant women, thus edema was declared as an unreliable marker of PE by expert groups (NHBPEWG, 2000; Brown et al., 2000; Chobanian et al., 2003).

On the other hand, it is necessary to differentiate *eclampsia* (E), if the occurrence of seizures in pregnant women with PE cannot be attributed to other causes (Roberts, 2004).

The National Institutes of Health, USA, working group of hypertension on pregnancy classified 4 groups (Gifford et al., 2000): chronic hypertension, PE and E (PE–E), PE *superimposed upon chronic hypertension* (SCH) and gestational hypertension. According to our study design pregnant women with PE–E and PE–E with SCH were included into this study to evaluate the possible association of PE–E and PE–E with SCH with other pregnancy complications, adverse birth outcomes (rate of PB and LBW newborns), and CAs.

Therefore, pregnant women with chronic hypertension diagnosed before conception without proteinuria/albuminuria and with gestational hypertension (blood pressure elevation detected the first time during the study pregnancy without proteinuria) were evaluated in another study (see the previous chapter). The diagnostic criteria of PE–E with SCH were either in women hypertension before conception of the study pregnancy and new onset proteinuria defined as the urinary excretion 0.3 g protein or more in a 24h specimen or in women with hypertension and proteinuria prior to 20 weeks' gestation (Roberts, 2004).

Only pregnant women with medically recorded PE and E in the prenatal care logbook or discharge summaries of hospitalized patients were evaluated.

10.4.1 Results of the Study

The distribution of pregnant women with PE–E is shown in Table 10.3.

Out of 22,843 cases, 739 (3.2%) had mothers with PE–E, and within this group 686 (3.0%) were affected with PE and 53 (0.2%) with E, while 154 (0.7%) pregnant women had PE–E with SCH. Out of 38,151 controls, 1,286 (3.4%) had mothers with PE–E, 1,222 (3.2%) were recorded with PE, and 64 (0.2%) with E. The number of control pregnant women with PE–E with SCH was 269 (0.7%).

The onset of PE–E was recorded rarely in II and IV gestational month, after this there was an increasing trend parallel with gestational months, thus the maximum occurred in the last 2 months.

There was a higher mean maternal age in pregnant women with E (26.2 year) and particularly in the group of PE with SCH (26.4 year) and E with SCH (26.7 year) compared to pregnant women with PE (25.4 year) or to pregnant women without these pregnancy complications (25.4 year). However, the mean birth order was lower in pregnant women with PE (1.6) and E (1.1) than in the reference group (1.8) due to the much larger proportion of primiparae. E occurred more frequently in pregnant women with lower socioeconomic status including many unemployment women. The lifestyle of mothers showed that 10.3% of pregnant women with PE–E were smoker while this figure was 21.3% in pregnant women without PE–E. The occurrence of regular/hard drinkers was about 1% in all study groups.

Among acute maternal diseases, only influenza/common cold (in general secondary complications) occurred more frequently in pregnant women with E (23.4%)

Table 10.3 Distribution of pregnant women with PE and E with or without superimposed upon chronic hypertension (SCH)

Case mothers without PE–E ($N = 22{,}104$)				
PE	without SCH	with SCH	Together	%
No.	554	132	686	
%	80.8	19.2	100.0	92.8
E				
No.	31	22	53	
%	58.5	41.5	100.0	7.2
PE–E				
No.	585	154	739	
%	79.2	20.8	100.0	100.0
Control mothers without PE–E ($N = 36{,}865$)				
PE				
No.	972	250	1,222	
%	79.5	20.5	100.0	95.0
E				
No.	45	19	64	
%	70.3	29.7	100.0	5.0
PE–E				
No.	1,017	269	1,286	
%	79.1	20.1	100.0	100.0

than in pregnant women with PE (17.4%) and in the reference group (18.5%). The prevalence of chronic maternal diseases, including diabetes mellitus and epilepsy, did not show difference among study groups; however, the previously shown association of migraine with preeclampsia was confirmed.

The first aim of the study was the evaluation of other pregnancy complications (Table 10.4).

The rate of threatened abortion (vaginal bleeding with or without permanent uterine spasms) was higher in pregnant women with EP than in pregnant women with E. On the other hand, placental disorders, particularly premature separation of the placenta, i.e. abruptio placentae (10.5%) and polyhydramnios occurred more frequently in pregnant women with E, particularly if it associated with SCH, but not in pregnant women with PE. Threatened preterm delivery occurred more frequently only in pregnant women with PE with SCH, and it was less frequent in pregnant women with E. Finally, the much higher occurrence of edema in pregnancy without mention of hypertension raised the chance of misdiagnosis, although these pregnant women, beyond the lack of hypertension, had no proteinuria/albuminuria as well, therefore it was not possible to diagnose them as preeclamptic pregnant women.

In Hungary, nifedipine and methyldopa were used most frequently for the treatment of hypertension in pregnant women with PE–E during the study period. Dihydralazine and metoprolol were the third and fourth most frequently used drugs among them. Furosemide was frequent in the treatment of pregnant women with E. There was no significant difference in the use of folic acid among the study groups.

The evaluation of adverse birth outcomes resulted in an unexpected finding. The sex ratio did not show difference between the newborns of pregnant women with PE

Table 10.4 Incidence of pregnancy complications during the study pregnancy in the study group

Pregnancy complications	Reference ($N = 36,865$)		Preeclampsia						Eclampsia					
			With SCH ($N = 250$)		Without SCH ($N = 972$)		Together ($N = 1,222$)		With SCH ($N = 19$)		Without SCH ($N = 45$)		Together ($N = 64$)	
	No.	%	No.	%	No.	%	No.	%	No.	%	No.	%	No.	%
Nausea/vomiting, severe	3,733	10.1	25	10.0	104	10.7	129	10.6	3	6.7	3	15.8	6	9.4
Threatened abortion	6,249	17.0	50	20.0	205	21.1	255	20.9	1	5.3	7	15.7	8	12.5
Edema in pregnancy without mention of hypertension	823	2.2	11	4.4	75	7.7	86	7.0	1	5.3	2	4.4	3	4.7
Placental disorders[a]	565	1.5	3	1.2	19	2.0	22	1.8	3	15.8	3	6.7	6	9.4
Gestational diabetes	259	0.7	4	1.6	7	0.7	11	0.9	0	0.0	0	0.0	0	0.0
Threatened preterm delivery	5,260	14.3	55	22.0	125	12.9	180	14.7	2	10.5	4	8.9	6	9.4
Anemia	6,133	16.6	24	9.6	193	19.9	217	17.8	3	15.8	3	6.7	6	9.4

[a]Placenta previa, premature separation of placenta, antepartum hemorrhage.

and the reference group, however, 10% male excess was found in the newborns of pregnant women with E. Twins occurred more frequently in pregnant women with PE with SCH group (2.4% vs. 1.0%).

The mean gestational age at delivery was shorter and the rate of PB was higher in pregnant women with PE with SCH (39.2 week and 11.2%) and particularly with E with SCH (38.6 week and 10.5%) compared to the reference groups (39.4 week and 8.9%). The mean birth weight also showed a significant reduction with a higher rate of LBW newborns of mothers with PE with SCH (3,170 g and 14.0%) and with E with SCH (3,114 g and 15.8%) compared to the reference group (3,278 g and 5.4%). On the contrary, the mean birth weight of newborns of pregnant women with PE exceeded the reference figure (3,316 g) although the rate of LBW newborns was higher (7.6%). The mean birth weight was similar to reference figure in the newborns of mothers with E (3,264 g) with also a higher rate of LBW newborns (13.3%).

Finally the possible association of pregnant women with PE–E and the risk of different CAs in their informative offspring were analyzed (Table 10.5). In general, the onset of PE–E occurred after III gestational month thus all pregnant women with PE–E were evaluated together.

There was no higher risk for total CAs, however, adjusted OR showed a higher risk for renal a/dysgenesis. In the next step we evaluated the offspring of pregnant women with PE with or without SCH separately. Pregnant women with PE without SCH did not associate with a higher risk of any CA-group. However, pregnant women with PE with SCH associated with a higher risk for renal a/dysgenesis and rectal/anal atresia/stenosis in their offspring. This higher rate of renal a/dysgenesis explains the higher rate of this CA-group in pregnant women with PE–E.

10.4.2 Interpretation of Results

The major findings of our study showed that

(i) fever related influenza-common cold occurred more frequently in pregnant women with E,
(ii) the occurrence of placental disorders, particularly abruption of the placenta was more frequent in pregnant women with E,
(iii) there was an unexpected male excess among the newborns of pregnant women with E but not in pregnant women with PE,
(iv) the mean gestational age at delivery was shorter in pregnant women with PE with SCH and E with SCH and it was associated with a higher rate of PB,
(v) there was a reduction of mean birthweight in newborns of mothers with PE with SCH and E with SCH, however, the rate of LBW newborns was somewhat higher in all study groups, particularly with SCH.
(vi) we found an association of maternal PE+H with a higher risk of renal a/dysgenesis and renal/anal atresia/stenosis.

Table 10.5 Estimation of the association between congenital abnormalities (CAs) and PE–E in the analysis of cases and their matched controls

Study groups	Grand total no.	Entire pregnancy				Without SCH				With SCH			
Controls	38,151	1,286	3.4	Reference		1,017	2.7	Reference		269	0.7	Reference	
Isolated CAs													
Neural-tube defects	1,202	20	1.7	0.5	0.3–0.8	19	1.6	0.6	0.4–0.9	1	0.1	0.1	0.0–0.8
Cleft lip ± palate	1,375	27	2.0	0.6	0.4–0.8	23	1.7	0.6	0.4–0.9	4	0.3	0.4	0.2–1.1
Cleft palate only	601	20	3.3	1.0	0.6–1.5	17	2.8	1.1	0.7–1.7	3	0.5	0.7	0.2–2.2
Oesophageal atresia/stenosis	217	7	3.2	1.0	0.4–2.0	4	1.8	0.7	0.3–1.9	3	1.4	2.0	0.6–6.1
Cong. pyloric stenosis	241	7	2.9	0.9	0.4–1.8	4	1.7	0.6	0.2–1.7	3	1.2	1.8	0.6–5.5
Intestinal atresia/stenosis	158	5	3.3	1.0	0.4–2.4	3	1.9	0.7	0.2–2.2	2	1.3	1.8	0.4–7.2
Rectal/anal atresia/stenosis	231	12	5.5	1.7	0.9–3.0	6	2.6	1.0	0.4–2.2	**6**	**2.6**	**3.7**	**1.6–8.5**
Renal a/dysgenesis	126	10	7.9	**2.5**	**1.3–4.7**	6	4.8	1.9	0.8–4.3	**4**	**3.2**	**4.7**	**1.7–12.8**
Obstructive urinary CAs	343	15	4.4	1.3	0.8–2.2	13	3.8	1.4	0.8–2.5	2	0.6	0.8	0.2–3.4
Hypospadias	3,038	117	3.9	**1.2**	**1.0–1.4**	91	3.0	1.1	0.9–1.4	26	0.9	1.2	0.8–1.8
Undescended testis	2,052	70	3.4	1.0	0.8–1.3	56	2.7	1.0	0.8–1.3	14	0.7	1.0	0.6–1.7
Exomphalos/gastroschisis	255	9	3.5	1.6	0.5–2.0	8	3.1	1.2	0.6–2.4	1	0.4	0.6	0.1–4.0
Microcephaly, primary	111	4	3.6	1.1	0.4–2.9	4	3.6	1.4	0.5–3.7	0	0.0	0.0	0.0–0.0
Hydrocephaly, congenital	314	7	2.2	0.7	0.3–1.3	6	1.9	0.7	0.3–1.6	1	0.3	0.4	0.1–3.2
Eye CAs	99	1	1.0	0.3	0.0–2.1	0	0.0	0.0	0.0–0.0	1	1.0	1.4	0.2–10.0
Ear CAs	354	11	3.1	0.9	0.5–1.7	11	3.1	1.2	0.6–2.1	0	0.0	0.0	0.0–0.0
Cardiovascular CAs	4,480	151	3.4	1.0	0.8–1.2	116	2.6	1.0	0.8–1.2	35	0.8	1.1	0.8–1.6
CAs of the genital organs	127	4	3.1	0.9	0.3–2.5	3	2.4	0.9	0.3–2.8	1	0.8	1.1	0.2–8.0
Clubfoot	2,425	73	3.0	0.9	0.7–1.1	56	2.3	0.9	0.7–1.1	17	0.7	1.0	0.6–1.6
Limb deficiencies	548	21	3.8	1.1	0.7–1.8	16	2.9	1.1	0.7–1.8	5	0.9	1.3	0.5–3.2
Poly/syndactyly	1,744	62	3.6	1.1	0.8–1.4	49	2.8	1.1	0.8–1.4	13	0.7	1.1	0.6–1.8
CAs of the musculo-skeletal system	585	24	4.1	1.2	0.8–1.8	22	3.8	1.4	0.9–2.2	2	0.3	0.5	0.1–2.0
Diaphragmatic CAs	244	3	1.2	0.4	0.1–1.1	3	1.2	0.5	0.1–1.4	0	0.0	0.0	0.0–0.0
Other isolated CAs	624	18	2.5	0.8	0.5–1.4	12	1.9	0.7	0.4–1.3	6	1.0	1.4	0.6–3.0
Multiple CAs	1,349	42	3.1	0.9	0.7–1.3	37	2.7	1.0	0.7–1.4	5	0.4	0.5	0.2–1.3
Total	22,843	739	3.2	1.0	**0.9–1.1**	585	2.6	1.0	0.9–1.1	154	0.7	1.0	0.8–1.2

The prevalence of PE and E was 3.20% and 0.17% in pregnant women studied, while the rates of PE with or without SCH were 2.61% and 0.71%, respectively. Thus, the overall prevalence of pregnant women with PE–E, PE with SCH, and E with SCH was 3.4% which is near to the figures of about 4% of pregnancies in other studies (Davies et al., 1970; Roberts, 2004). In addition, PE is expected in 20% of women with prior hypertension (Caritis et al., 1998), the proportion of PE with SCH and E with SCH together was 20.9% in the study.

Advanced maternal age and nulliparity are key risk factors for PE–E mainly without SCH. The previously found lower socioeconomic status of pregnant women with E was confirmed before (Plouin et al., 1986).

When evaluating newborn infants born to mothers with PE–E, the most unexpected finding was the obvious male excess in the group of E. Theoretically there are two explanations for this unexpected finding. (i) A higher rate of early postconceptional selection of female embryos. Unfortunately our data set is not appropriate to measure the rate of miscarriages, but the rate of threatened abortion was lower among them. (ii) The severe form of this pregnancy complication, i.e. E may occur frequently in pregnant women who had male fetuses.

The rate of twin pregnancies was somewhat higher in women with PE, particularly with PE with SCH in agreement with previous findings (Caritis et al., 1998). Other studies focused on the analysis of perinatal mortality of the offspring of pregnant women with PE–E (Lopez-Llear and Horta, 1972; Tervila et al., 1973; Naeye and Friedman, 1979; Plouin et al., 1986; Buchbinder et al., 2002) and higher rates were found mainly explained by placental insufficiency and abruption placentae (Naeye and Friedman, 1979). Our study also showed a higher rate of late fetal death, i.e. stillbirths among cases with CA in mothers with PE–E.

The rate of PB was higher in our analysis, as it was found in another study (Naeye and Friedman, 1979). However, the major risk of fetuses of pregnant women with PE–E is intrauterine growth retardation, particularly in women with PE–E with SCH. There were 2.6- and 2.9-fold higher risks for LBW newborns in pregnant women with PE with SCH and E with SCH. This finding is also in agreement with the results of previous studies (Tervila et al., 1973; Naeye and Friedman, 1979; Plouin et al., 1986; Buchbinder et al., 2002). Intrauterine growth retardation was found more frequently in newborn infants of PE–E and its severity correlated with increasing maternal blood pressure. In addition, a strong association was found between severe E and a higher risk for placental disorders. The decidual vascular changes explain the higher incidence of abruption of the placenta in women with PE–E with SCH (Roberts, 2004). Obviously these pregnancy complications and adverse pregnancy outcomes may have a causal association with the common denominator of placental dysfunction. PE–E is a disorder of placentation and characteristic pathologic changes have preceded the clinical presentation of this disorder.

Initiation of antihypertensive drug therapy is usually considered in pregnant women if systolic blood pressure exceeds 160 mmHg or diastolic pressure exceeds 110 mmHg (Robert and Perloff, 1977; Arias and Zamora, 1979; Sibai, 2002). The major expected benefit of antihypertensive therapy is the reduction of the incidence of PE with SCH (Arias and Zamora, 1979); however, as the results of our study showed, it is not successful in many women.

In general, if drug therapy is necessary in pregnant women, the safety of fetus is an important criterion. Methyldopa is the first choice because its safety has been shown in several materials (Shepard and Lemire, 2004; Briggs et al., 2005), in addition, the long term effect of methyldopa was also checked in children without any serious harm (Ountsted et al., 1983). However, this recommendation was not followed in Hungarian pregnant women because the most frequently used drug was nifedipine. Our previous study did not indicate the teratogenic and/or fetotoxic effect of calcium receptor antagonists (89). The third most frequently used drug, the direct vasodilators hydralazine was also found effective and safe (Shepard and Lemire, 2004; Briggs et al., 2005). However, ACE (angiotensin converting enzyme) inhibitors (Hanssens et al., 1991; Burrows and Burrows, 1998; Cooper et al., 2006) and angiotensin-II-receptor inhibitors/antagonists (Lambot et al., 2001; Martinovic et al., 2001) are contraindicated due to their fetotoxic effect. Magnesium sulphate is the only drug for which there is extensive and compelling evidence of efficacy and safety for the treatment of severe PE and E (The Eclampsia Trial Collaborative Group, 1995; The Magpie Trial Collaborative Group, 2002; Langer et al., 2008). Unfortunately only 9% of Hungarian pregnant women with PE and E were treated with magnesium sulphate during the study period.

Our previous hypothesis regarding the lack of association between PE and CA seemed to be reasonable because the onset of PE is after the first trimester, while most major CAs have their critical period in II and/or III gestational month. However, our hypothesis has not been confirmed. Chronic hypertension started before the conception and continued during the study pregnancy thus this pathological condition may have adverse affect in early pregnancy as well. Our previous study showed an association between maternal chronic-essential hypertension and higher risk for oesophageal atresia/stenosis (I). The combination of PE with SCH associated with another atresia/stenosis of the digestive system. In addition, there was a higher risk for renal a/dysgenesis in this study.

A higher risk for CAs was found in the offspring of pregnant women with PE with SCH. The question is whether the associations of higher risk for renal a/dysgenesis and rectal/anal atresia/stenosis with maternal PE with SCH is causal with, or can be explained by related drug treatments, lifestyle factors, other or unevaluated confounders, or by chance.

When deciding upon antihypertensive therapy, drugs must be chosen on the basis of considerations specific to pregnancy. Beyond the above mentioned drugs, such as methyldopa, hydralazin, beta blockers, and calcium receptor antagonists we did not find any data regarding the teratogenic potential of potassium chlorate and the combination of potassium and magnesium (Shepard and Lemire, 2004). In addition, the use of these drugs was similar in case and control mothers and they were considered as confounders at the calculation of adjusted OR for the risk of CAs. Thus the related drug treatment does not seem to be important in the origin of renal a/dysgenesis and rectal/anal atresia/stenosis.

In conclusion, a higher risk for some pregnancy complications (threatened abortions and placental disorders) and birth outcomes (higher risk of LBW and PB) was found in pregnant women with treated PE–E and PE–H. In addition, our data showed an unexpected male excess among newborn infants born to mothers with E. This unexpected finding needs further studies to confirm or reject this finding which may be important to understand the etiopathogenesis of E. Finally PE with SCH in pregnant women may associate with a higher risk of renal a/dysgenesis and rectal/anal atresia/stenosis.

10.5 Coronary Artery Disease

The incidence of *coronary artery disease* (CAD) is depending on age and sex, thus reproductive aged women have a lower risk for CAD (O'rourke et al., 2008). The term acute coronary syndrome encompasses three different clinical entities: (i) acute myocardial ischemia including ST segment elevation myocardial infarction, (ii) non-ST-segment elevation myocardial infarction and (iii) unstable angina (O'Rourke et al., 2008).

Angina pectoris is the most common manifestation of CAD with causal association with acute myocardial infarction (Hemmingway et al., 2006). Angina pectoris is a clinical syndrome that consists of discomfort or pain in the chest, jaw, shoulder, back, or arm caused by CAD affecting one or more large epicardial arteries. There are 3 different presentations of unstable angina: (a) rest angina or angina with minimal exertion usually lasting at least 20 min, (b) new-onset severe angina, usually defined as occurring within last months and (c) crescendo angina, defined as previously diagnosed angina that has become distinctly more frequent, longer in duration, or more severe in nature (Kim et al., 2008). This unstable angina frequently, but not necessarily, follows a period of classic stable angina pectoris. There are some tests (e.g. electrocardiogram) in patients with suspected stable angina pectoris to establish the diagnosis, but clinical-pathologic studies demonstrated that it is possible to predict the probability of CAD on the basis of simple clinical observations of pain type, age, and sex (O'Rourke et al., 2008).

Typically angina pectoris is precipitated or aggravated by exertion or emotional stress and relieved by nitroglycerin. Thus the standard care for patients with angina pectoris includes oral nitrates and sublingual nitroglycerin (glyceryl-trinitrate), beta blockers, calcium channel blockers, and others depending on other pathological condition (e.g. hypertension, diabetes mellitus). Treatment is also supplemented by an exercise regimen suited to the abilities of patients additional to complete cessation of smoking (Dellegrottaglie et al., 2008).

CAD occurs rarely in pregnant women (Blanchard et al., 2004; McAnulty et al., 2008), thus we have not been able to find papers in the international literature studied the possible association between CAD and related drug treatments in pregnant women and CAs in their offspring based on controlled epidemiological studies.

10.5.1 Results of the Study

The aim of our study was to evaluate the offspring of pregnant women who had previous or present myocardial infarction and angina pectoris during the study pregnancy documented in the prenatal care logbook. CAD related drug treatments were also evaluated.

The case group consisted of 22,843 malformed newborns or fetuses ("informative offspring"), of whom 25 (0.10%) had mothers with CAD. Of these 25 pregnant women, 3 had previous myocardial infarction (one in a diabetic woman) while 22 were affected by angina pectoris (only one pregnant woman was recorded with essential hypertension as well). Out of 22 pregnant women with angina pectoris, 7 had its onset before conception and their angina pectoris continued during pregnancy, in 4 pregnant women until the end of pregnancy. The onset of angina pectoris was reported in III, VII, and VIII gestational months in 4, 4, and 4 pregnant women, while in IV, V, and VI gestational months in 1, 1, and 1 pregnant woman, respectively. Thus, these pregnant women were diagnosed with new-onset angina pectoris.

Among 38,151 controls, 12 (0.03%) were born to mothers with angina pectoris in the study pregnancy. Angina pectoris was combined with cardiac dysrhythmia in one woman. Out of these 12 pregnant women, 6 had the onset of angina pectoris before conception which continued until the end of pregnancy. The new-onset angina pectoris occurred in pregnant woman with the onset in the following months: IV, V, VI, VII, VIII and IX, respectively.

The comparison of maternal data showed a higher mean maternal age (30.3 vs. 25.5 year) due to the larger proportion of women over 30 years (58.2% vs. 19.0%) in the group of pregnant women with CAD compared to pregnant women without CAD. Their mean birth order was also higher (2.4 vs. 1.7).

The evaluation of pregnancy complications did not show significant difference among the study groups.

Among acute maternal diseases, the lower rate of influenza/common cold in pregnant women with CAD (10.8%) compared to pregnant women without CAD (19.7%) is worth mentioning.

Recommended anti-ischemic medications included nitrates for the relief of recurrent angina pectoris followed by calcium channel blockers in Hungary. Of the 25 case mothers, 11, 11 and 3 were treated by nitroglycerin, pentaerythrol-tetranitrate, and isosorbide dinitrate, while out of 12 control mothers, the numbers of these treatments were 5, 5, and 2, respectively. Eight case and 2 control mothers were treated by calcium channel blockers (nifedipine and verapamil). Beta blockers (in 2 case and 6 control mothers) were used rarely. Panangin® was a favored treatment in Hungary; it was used by 12 case and 4 control mothers. Bypass angioplasty revascularization did not occur among them.

There was a somewhat shorter gestational age at delivery (38.8 vs. 39.4 week; $p = 0.3$) in agreement with the higher rate of PB (16.7% vs. 9.2%; 2.0, 0.4–9.0) in newborns infants without CA born to mothers with CAD compared to pregnant women without CAD. The differences in mean birth weight (3,211 vs. 3,276 g; $p = 0.7$) and rate of LBW newborns (8.3% vs. 5.7%; 1.5, 0.2–11.7) between the study groups were not significant.

Three pregnant women with remote myocardial infarction were treated by Nitrosorbid®, in addition to diuretic furosemide and thiazide, their live-born babies

Table 10.6 Estimation of association between maternal angina pectoris during pregnancy and different CAs in their offspring

		Study pregnancy			
Study groups	Total no.	No.	%	OR[a] 95% CI	
Controls	38,151	12	0.03	Reference	
Isolated CA					
Cleft lip ± palate	1,375	6	0.44	**13.3**	**4.9–35.9**
Cleft palate, only	601	2	0.33	**10.5**	**2.3–47.6**
Undescended testis	2,052	2	0.10	3.3	0.7–14.4
Cardiovascular CA	4,480	4	0.09	3.0	0.9–9.4
Clubfoot	2,424	3	0.12	**4.4**	**1.2–15.7**
Poly/syndactyly	1,744	2	0.11	3.8	0.8–17.0
Other isolated	10,167	3[b]	0.03	1.5	0.5–4.8
Total	22,843	22	0.10	**3.7**	**1.8–7.3**

[a]OR adjusted for maternal age, birth order, and maternal employment status.
[b]Cong. hydrocephaly, cong. pyloric stenosis, hypospadias.

had oesophageal atresia, undescended testis, and multiple CA. At the estimation of possible higher risk for CAs, the occurrence of angina pectoris during pregnancy was compared between cases with different CAs and their all matched controls (Table 10.6).

Out of 22 pregnant women with angina pectoris, 6 had cases with cleft lip ± cleft palate and 2 cleft palate only, thus they showed very significant associations with angina pectoris. The occurrence of clubfoot in cases also showed some association with maternal angina pectoris, but this association was based on 3 different CAs (talipes calcaneovalgus, talipes equinovarus and metatarsus varus) and the lower limit of confidence interval was near to 1. We attempted to visit the families of these 8 cases in 2009, but 2 had unknown new addresses. Of the rest 6 case mothers, all were alive but 2 were affected with myocardial infarction after the study period, in addition 4 were hard smoker.

In conclusion 13-fold higher risk for isolated cleft lip ± cleft palate and 10.5-folds higher risk for cleft palate only were found in children of pregnant women with CAD.

10.5.2 Interpretation of Results

The prevalence of CAD was only about 0.1% of pregnant women in the study, because advanced age and male sex are the key risk factors for CAD. Our data also showed that CAD occurs more frequently in mothers with advanced age.

Our data set included 3 pregnant women with previous myocardial infarction. Acute myocardial infarction during pregnancy needs heparin treatment, our patients were treated with Nitrosorbid® and diuretics from the first gestational month, and therefore obviously they had the so-called remote myocardial infarction. Myocardial infarction complicates pregnancies in about 1 in 10,000 (Mabie and Freire, 1995).

The highest incidence appears to occur in the third trimester in multigravid women more than 33 years of age (Roth and Elkayam, 1996).

The main finding of our study is a strong association between maternal angina pectoris and a higher risk for isolated orofacial clefts in their children. Our previous paper showed similar association when analyzing maternal diseases in the origin of isolated orofacial clefts (III). The question is whether it is a causal association with CAD as a possible maternal teratogenic effect, or can be explained by related drug treatments, lifestyle factors, unevaluated confounders or chance.

Isolated orofacial clefts have the multifactorial origin (Marazita, 2002), thus their polygenic predisposition can be triggered by CAD during the critical period of these CAs, i.e. between 7 and 9 gestational weeks (i.e. in II and III months) in cleft lip + palate and 8–14 gestational weeks (i.e. III and IV months) of cleft palate only. Out of 8 case with orofacial cleft, only 4 showed an overlapping between the exposure (angina pectoris and drug treatment) and the critical period of these CAs. Thus obviously this association cannot be explained by CAD as a usual teratogenic factor in the origin of orofacial clefts. If this association is causal, the explanation may be some common genetic origin of CAD and orofacial clefts (Wyszinsky, 2002).

As far as we know the teratogenic potential of nitrates was not checked in controlled human epidemiological studies (Shepard and Lemire, 2004; Briggs et al., 2005), however, animal investigations did not indicate the teratogenic effect of nitroglycerin (Oketani et al., 1981a, b; Sato et al., 1984) and pentaerythritol tetranitrate (Sugawara et al., 1977). Use of nitroglycerin sublingually for angina pectoris during pregnancy without fetal harm has also been reported in a clinical study by Diro et al (Diro et al., 1983). However, in the Collaborative Perinatal Project 7 pregnant women were treated with nitroglycerin and amyl nitrite, 3 with pentaerythritol tetranitrate and 5 with other vasodilators in the first four lunar months (Heinonen et al., 1977). Of these 15 pregnant women, 4 had malformed children which indicated a statistically significant association ($p = 0.02$), however, orofacial cleft did not occur among them. Beta blockers and calcium channel blockers are not classified as human teratogenic drugs (Shepard and Lemire, 2004; Briggs et al., 2005; 89), while Panangin® was not tested from this aspect.

Among confounders, the triggering effect of smoking in the origin of isolated orofacial cleft cannot be excluded. A mild association of maternal smoking with higher risk for orofacial cleft was shown in several studies (Hayes, 2002), including in our validation study. A much higher risk was found in the children of smoker mothers with specific gene polymorphism such as TGFA (Hwang et al., 1995; Shaw et al., 1996; Maestri et al., 1997; Romitti et al., 1999; Christensen et al., 1999), TGFB3, RARA, BCL (Hwang et al., 1995; Shaw et al., 1996; Maestri et al., 1997), MSX1 (Romitti et al., 1999; Boogaard, van den et al., 2008). For example significant interactions were observed between MSX1 allele 4 homozygosity of the child and maternal smoking (2.7, 1.1–6.6) (Boogaard, van den et al., 2008). On the other hand, there is an association of hyperhomocysteinaemia with CAD (Nygerd et al., 1997; Mangoni and Jackson, 2002) and orofacial clefts, although the latter association is controversial (Mills et al., 1999; Blanton et al., 2002).

Another possible explanation for this association is unevaluated/unknown confounders and chance effect, but it is difficult to explain these 13.3- and 10.5-folds risk, respectively, by chance.

Thus, our hypothesis is a gene-environmental interaction in the origin of isolated orofacial cleft based on the common genetic predisposition for both CAD and orofacial cleft and triggering factors, mainly smoking.

10.6 Cardiac Dysrhythmias

Disturbances of the cardiac rhythm can be differentiated into conduction disorders, tachycardia, atrial/ventricular fibrillation, premature beats, extrasystolic arrhythmia, and others including cardiac arrest (Blanchard and Shabetai, 2004). Isolated supraventricular and ventricular extrasystoles are common and no treatment is necessary. However, sustained symptomatic arrhythmia requires treatment which can be pharmacologic or procedural (transcatheter ablation or insertion of an implantable cardiac defibrillator).

Tachyarrhythmias are common during pregnancy and it may the explanation of dizziness, palpitations, and light-headedness (McAnulty et al., 2008). Nevertheless, cardiac arrhythmia that occurs in the absence of organic heart disease is almost always benign and is therefore not an indication for pharmacologic treatment unless the woman finds palpitation intolerable. These experiences may explain that possible association of cardiac dysrhythmias in pregnant women with adverse birth outcomes of their children has not been evaluated/published (Shepard and Lemire, 2004).

There are two manifestations of paroxysmal tachycardia: paroxysmal supraventricular tachycardia and paroxysmal ventricular tachycardia. Supraventricular tachycardias include all tachyarrhythmias that either originate from or incorporate supraventricular tissue in a reentrant circuit (Calkins, 2008).

10.7 Paroxysmal Supraventricular Tachycardia

Paroxysmal supraventricular tachycardia (PSVT) is the most common cardiac arrhythmia in pregnant women (Widerhorn et al., 1992; Lee et al., 1995). PVST is a clinical syndrome characterized by a rapid, regular tachycardia with abrupt onset and termination. About two-thirds of patients with PSVT are caused by atrioventricular nodal reentrant tachycardia. Women are affected twice as often than men. The rest one-third of cases have orthodontic atrioventricular reciprocating tachycardia.

10.7.1 Results of the Study

Pregnant women were recorded with PSVT in the data set of the HCCSCA, thus the aim of our study was to evaluate possible associations between PSVT and birth outcomes, particularly the risk of CAs in their children.

Pregnant women with other conduction disorders, PSVT with other heart diseases (e.g. coronary artery disease, dilated cardiomyopathy, etc) and unspecified paroxysmal tachycardia were excluded from the study, thus we included pregnant women only with PSVT recorded in the prenatal maternity logbook. PSVT related drug treatments and pregnancy complications were also evaluated.

The case group consisted of 22,843 malformed newborns or fetuses ("informative offspring"), of whom 103 (0.45%) had mothers with PSVT. Out of 38,151 controls, 149 (0.39%) were born to mothers with PSVT.

Of the 103 case and 149 control mothers, 45 (43.7%) and 70 (47.0%) had the onset of PSVT before the study pregnancy, i.e. their PSVT was chronic condition. The rest was considered as new onset PSVT without characteristic onset according to gestational months.

There was a higher mean maternal age (26.4 vs. 25.5 year) in pregnant women with PSVT than in pregnant women without PSVT as reference. Their mean birth order was also somewhat higher (1.8 vs. 1.7). Marital and employment status did not show difference among the study groups. Folic acid supplementation during pregnancy was less frequent in case mothers with PSVT (44.7%) than control mothers with PSVT (55.7%) and pregnant women without PSVT (54.4%).

The occurrence of pregnancy complications did not show differences in the study groups.

Among acute maternal diseases, respiratory system was more frequently affected in pregnant women with PSVT (12.1% vs. 9.0%). The evaluation of chronic diseases indicated two strong associations in both case and controls mothers with PSVT. Migraine occurred in 10.7% of case mothers and 14.1% of control mothers with PSVT, while this figure was about 2% in pregnant women without PSVT. The prevalence of essential hypertension was 49.5% in case mothers and 40.9% in control mothers with PSVT while it occurred only 4% in pregnant women without PSVT.

About 20% of case and control mothers with PSVT were treated with the combination of potassium and magnesium (Panangin®). Other medicines belonged to the group of antihypertensive drugs (oxprenolol, verapamil, pindolol, propranolol, metoprolol). In addition, diazepam was also used more frequently by mothers with PSVT (about 25%) compared to pregnant women without PSVT (11%).

The birth outcomes showed a characteristic pattern. The mean gestational age at delivery was 0.3 week shorter in newborn infants born to mothers with PSVT (39.1 vs. 39.4 week) and it was reflected in the higher rate of PB (11.4% vs. 9.2%). However, a similar difference was not seen in mean birth weight, it was practically the same (3,272 vs. 3,276 g). The rate of LBW newborns did also not show significant difference; in fact it was lower in the groups of mother with PSVT (4.7% vs. 5.7%)

Finally the possible association of pregnant women with PSVT and the risk of different CAs in their informative offspring was checked. The occurrence of PSVT was evaluated in II and/or III gestational months and any time during pregnancy. The total rate of cases with CA (1.2, 0.9–1.5) and among specified CA-groups, only 25 cases with cardiovascular CA showed a higher risk (2.1, 1.2–3.7).

In the next step we evaluated the distribution of cardiovascular CAs in 25 cases: ventricular septal defect 12 (48.0%), atrial septal defect, type II 8 (32.0%), endocardial cushion defect 2, coarctation of aorta 2, stenosis of pulmonary valve 1. Of 4,480 cases with cardiovascular CAs in the HCCSCA, 1,656 (37.0%) and 467 (10.4%) had ventricular septal defect and atrial septal defect, type II. Thus the expected number of ventricular septal defect and atrial septal defect, type II was 9.3 and 2.6 on the basis of dataset of the HCCSCA, respectively. In addition, the comparison of PSVT's prevalence in the mothers of cases with these two CAs and their matched controls showed a more obvious association in ventricular septal defect (2.8, 1.4–4.4) and atrial septal defect, type II (5.6, 2.8–14.4).

Finally, maternal PSVT was evaluated only in II and/or III gestational month, i.e. in the critical period of major CAs, including cardiovascular CAs. Of 25 cases with cardiovascular CA, 20 had mothers with PSVT during this time window (1.9, 1.0–5.3). Among these 20 cases, 8 and 7 were affected with ventricular septal defect and atrial septal defect type II, respectively, thus their previously found association with PSVT was strongly confirmed. The risk of total CA was lower during this time window (1.0, 0.7–1.9).

10.7.2 Interpretation of Results

The main finding of the study is that the risk of septal cardiac defects, particularly atrial septal defect, type II was higher in the children of pregnant women with PSVT.

At the interpretation of possible causal association between PSVT and cardiovascular septal CAs, we have to consider the possible maternal teratogenic effect of PSVT, common genetic origin, related drug treatment, confounders and chance effect.

The possible maternal teratogenic effect of PSVT does not seem to be a plausible explanation.

However, the parents without cardiovascular CAs and examined by ECG of 94 cases with ventricular septal defect and 94 matched controls without any defect had a much higher prevalence of incomplete or suspect right bundle branch blocks (18.3% vs. 4.1%; $p < 0.001$) in a previous Hungarian study (IV). These intraventricular conduction disturbances may be subthreshold signs of septal defect therefore PSVT and these cardiovascular CAs may have a common genetic origin.

At the decision of PSVT therapy, drugs must be chosen on the basis of considerations specific to pregnancy, mainly fetus. The main objective of therapy in patients with PSVT is to increase vagal tone in order to inhibit conduction via the atrioventricular node (Atarashi, 2008). Calcium channel blockers such as verapamil are appropriate for this purpose and these drugs are not teratogenic (89). The beta-blockers are antagonists of sympathetic nervous activities, e.g. propranolol, metoprolol, oxprenolol, pindolol, etc are also favourite treatments in these patients because of their beneficial effect for both PSVT and hypertension. However, there is no evidence regarding the human teratogenic effect of these drugs and particularly their cardiovascular CA inducing effect (Briggs et al., 2005, Shepard and Lemire,

2004). In Hungary patients with PSVT were treated frequently benzodiazepines such as diapezam and chlorodiazepoxide. There was no teratogenic potential of diazepam (54) and chlorodiazepoxide (55) in the data set of the HCCSCA. In addition a higher risk of CAs was not found in 112 and 35 women who attempted suicide during pregnancy with extremely large doses of diazepam (25–800 mg) (106) and chlorodiazepoxide (20–300 mg) (107), respectively, in the Budapest Monitoring System of Self-poisoning Pregnant Women.

Other unevaluated/unknown confounders may be also important; in addition multiple comparisons may produce non-causal association.

Two findings are worth mentioning:

(i) There was a higher risk for migraine and mainly for essential hypertension in pregnant women with PSVT. This study confirmed our previous finding which indicated a strong association between migraine and PSVT. Our study design planned to exclude heart diseases related PSVT, but we did not exclude pregnant women with essential hypertension. This study showed a very obvious association between these two maternal conditions, the question is whether PSVT is the cause or it is the consequence of hypertension causing increased load on the heart.

(ii) A shorter gestational age associated with a higher rate of PB in newborn infants born to mothers with PSVT, but the mean birth weight was not smaller and the rate of LBW newborns was not higher. Thus some fetal growth promoting effect cannot be excluded.

The prevalence of pregnant women with PSVT was 0.4–0.5% in Hungarian pregnant women; however, these figures reflected the medically recorded and treated (thus severe) PSVT during the study pregnancy.

About half of the PSVT had an onset prior to the study of pregnancy, but many PSVT manifested during pregnancy, thus pregnancy may be an important causal factor in the new onset PSVT.

Mothers with PSVT were elder in agreement with previous findings (Calkins, 2008). Our pregnant women with PSVT had a somewhat higher occurrence of acute diseases of respiratory system, probable explained by the dysfunction of pulmonary circulation.

In conclusion, a higher risk for cardiovascular septal CAs was found in the children of pregnant women with PSVT, and the rate of PB was higher.

10.8 Extrasystolic Arrhythmia

Five subgroups were separated among patients with extrasystolic arrhythmia on the basis of the localization of premature beats: (i) atrial, (ii) nodal, (iii) supraventricular, (iv) ventricular and (v) unspecified (Blanchard and Shabetai, 2004; Calkins, 2008).

10.8.1 Interpretation of Data in the HCCSCA

Out of 22,843 cases, 8 (0.04%) had mothers with extrasystolic arrhythmia, while out of 38,151 controls, 4 (0.01%) were affected with this type of cardiac arrhythmias. However, it is worth mentioning, that out of 8 cases, 6 were affected with cardiovascular CA (ventricular septal defect 4, atrial septal defect type II 2), in addition, clubfoot and torticollis occurred in 1–1 case. The birth outcomes of 4 controls did not deviate from the Hungarian baseline data.

In conclusion, the cluster of cardiovascular CA in the children of pregnant women with extrasystolic arrhythmia needs further studies.

10.9 Conduction Disorders

Conduction disorders of pregnant women comprises complete or partial atrioventricular blocks, and rarely left or right bundle branch block. High-grade atrioventricular conduction disturbance, particularly when symptomatic, can be treated by artificial pacing. This management does not have any adverse effect on fetal development or fetal heart function (Schroeder and Harrison, 1971). However, it is necessary to diagnose and evaluate cardiac conduction disturbances before conception with full electrophysiological testing and to prepare these women for pregnancy.

10.9.1 Interpretation of Data in the HCCSCA

Out of 22,843 cases, 2 (0.01%) babies with cleft palate and syndactyly on the feet were born to mothers with atrioventricular conduction disturbance. Out of 38,151 controls, 7 newborns (0.02%) had mothers with this pathological condition and all babies were born after the 38th gestational week (4 on the 40th week) with birth weight between 2,900 and 3,950, with a mean of 3,330 g.

In conclusion, conduction disturbance of pregnant women does not result in an increased risk for fetal development.

10.10 Phlebitis, Thrombophlebitis, and Pulmonary Embolism

Among diseases of the veins, here *superficial thrombophlebitis* (STP) of the lower extremities, *deep vein thrombophlebitis* (DVT) of the lower extremities (approximately 70–90% in left leg), and *pulmonary embolism in pregnancy* (PEP) will be discussed. Phlebitis, thrombophlebitis including DVT and PEP is a single disease and are severe complications of pregnancy particularly in postpartum period (Marik and Lauren, 2008). The incidence of venous thromboembolic disease is estimated to 0.76–1.72 per 1,000 pregnancies (Heit et al., 2005; James et al., 2006) which is

4 times higher than in non-pregnant female population. Anticoagulation is the mainstay of therapy for DVT and PEP, but it needs special expertise during pregnancy due to the teratogenic potential of coumarin/warfarin agents (Kerber et al., 1968; Warkany, 1976).

10.10.1 Results of the Study

The aim of our study was to evaluate possible associations between maternal venous diseases of lower extremities and related drug treatment and adverse birth outcomes, particularly the risk of CAs in their children.

The diagnosis of these three forms/stages of venous diseases studied in lower extremities was based on the following criteria:

STP presents a tender, erythematous, indurated lesion in the course of a superficial vein (Wennberg and Rooke, 2008). STP often occurs on varicose veins but the incidence of STP exceeded the incidence of varicose veins of the lower extremities.

DVT is deep vein thrombophlebitis without or with thrombosis diagnosed on the basis of symptoms such as muscle pain, palpable deep linear cord, tenderness, swelling (greater than 2 cm difference between leg circumferences), Homans sign (pain in the calf when the great toe is passively dorsiflexed), dilated superficial veins (Laros, 2004), though these symptoms are non-specific and unreliable (Kahn et al., 2006). Rarely there is a concurrent DVT and STP; these cases were classified as DVT.

PEP covers a wide spectrum of symptoms. Small emboli may go unrecognized by the patients, but tachypnea, dyspnea, pleuritic pain, apprehension, cough, tachycardia, hemoptysis, elevated temperature may help to diagnose pulmonary embolism (Laros, 2004; Konstantinides, 2008).

Other venous thrombosis such as thrombophlebitis migrans, thrombophlebitis of the vena cava, portal vein, renal vein, etc, were excluded from the study.

Only prospectively and medical recorded venous diseases in the medical records were evaluated in the study. STP and DVT related drug treatments and pregnancy complications were also analyzed.

The case group consisted of 22,843 malformed newborns or fetuses ("informative offspring"), of whom 341 (1.49%) had mothers with venous diseases of the lower extremities. PEP occurred in 3 women, 87 pregnant women were specified as DVT in general treated with heparin and/or acenocoumarol (Syncumar), a coumarin derivative, and 251 case mothers were affected with STP without heparin or acenocoumarol treatment.

Out of 38,151 controls, 971 (2.55%) were born to mothers with venous diseases of the lower extremities. PEP occurred only in one woman, 192 were specified having DVT with heparin and/or acenocoumarol treatment and 778 pregnant women were considered to have STP without heparin or acenocoumarol treatment.

The two forms of venous diseases of the lower extremities, i.e. STP and DVT sometimes showed intermediate or continuing conditions in pregnant women, therefore they were evaluated together when analyzing possible association with CAs. Three case mothers and one control mother with PEP were evaluated separately.

Out of 338 case mothers, 91 (26.9%), while out of 970 control mothers, 182 (18.8%) had the onset of STP-DVT before conception, but continued during pregnancy, this condition was considered as chronic. Most of these pregnant women had previous pregnancies. The new onset diseases were recorded mainly after III month with a peak in IV and VI gestational months.

Pregnant women with STP/DVT had a higher mean maternal age (27.9 vs. 25.4 year) due to the larger proportion of women over 30 years. The mean birth order was also higher (2.2 vs. 1.7) with the predominance with birth order 2 or more. Marital status did not show difference among the study groups. However, the proportion of professional women was somewhat larger in pregnant women with STP. Folic acid supplementation during pregnancy was more frequent in pregnant women with STP, but not with DVT. The use of multivitamins was similar among the study groups. The smoking habit was evaluated based on "family consensus" after the home visit of women. Only 3.7% of case women with STP/VDT smoked during the study pregnancy while this figure was 22.0% in case women without STP/VDT.

Among pregnancy complications, only the rate of anemia was higher both in case and control mothers with these venous diseases compared to pregnant women without STP/DVT.

The incidence of acute respiratory disease was somewhat higher in case pregnant women with venous diseases (28.1%) compared to control mothers with STP+VDT (19.8%) and pregnant women without STP+VDT (19.7%). Among chronic diseases, the prevalence of constipation (13.4%, 4.4% and 2.0%) and particularly hemorrhoids (48.8%, 13.5% and 3.6%) showed an interesting pattern in pregnant women with DVT, STP and without STP+VDT, respectively.

The DVT related treatments showed obvious difference between pregnant women with or without these diseases. In Hungary among coumarin derivatives, acenocoumarol (Syncumar) was used for oral treatment of 8 pregnant women. Heparin was available for parenteral treatment, but only 37.8% of case and 28.5% of controls mothers with DVT were treated. These low figures may question the severity or the diagnosis of DVT or it may reflect the previous Hungarian treatment protocol of pregnant women with venous diseases. The treatment of DVT was complemented frequently with the oral treatment of tribenoside and local treatment phenylbutazone.

In addition, Hungarian pregnant women with DVT and particularly STP were treated more frequently by hydroxyethylrutoside (both orally and locally as gel) and a medicinal product containing rutoside and ascorbic acid.

The mean gestational age at delivery was 0.1 week longer in newborn infants born to mothers with STP while it was 0.1 week shorter in the group of pregnant women with DVT than in pregnant women without STP+VDT (39.4 week). There was a lower rate of PB in the newborns of mothers with STP (6.8%) and with VDT (8.3%) than of pregnant women without STP+VDT. A more obvious difference was seen in birth weight, it was 144 and 49 g heavier in the newborns of mothers with STP and DVT, respectively, than in the newborns of pregnant women without STP+VDT (3,273 g) and it resulted in a significant reduction in the rate of LBW in the group of STP (3.6%) but not in the group of VDT (5.2%) compared to the group of pregnant women with STP+VDT (5.7%). Thus these data show some intrauterine growth stimulation in the fetuses of pregnant women with STP and related drug treatments.

Finally, we evaluated the possible associations between STP/DVT in II and III gestational months or any time during pregnancy and the risk for different CAs in their informative offspring. Neither the total rate of cases with CA nor the specified CA-groups showed any increased risk in the children of mothers with STP+DVT.

However, it is worth mentioning that of the 4 women with PEP, 3 had malformed children and two were affected with complex cardiovascular CAs.

Three cases and 5 controls were born to mothers with DVT and coumarin derivative: acenocoumarol (Syncumar) treatments were evaluated separately in detail but the characteristic pattern of "warfarin syndrome" was not observed.

10.10.2 Interpretation of Results

The higher rate of PB and LBW newborns was not found in the children of pregnant women with STP/ DVT; in fact the rate of PB and LBW was lower in newborns of mothers with STP. This unexpected finding may be related to the higher socioeconomic status of mothers, and better prenatal care (which was indicated by the higher use of folic acid) and lifestyle (e.g. lower proportion of smokers and more bed rest).

The risk of CAs was not higher in the children of pregnant women with STP/DVT; again, the total rate of CAs was lower than expected, although 8 pregnant women were treated with acenocoumarol (Syncumar), i.e. warfarin. On the other hand, the 3 malformed children of the 4 women with PEP are worth mentioning.

The STP is usually self-limited with recovery accelerated by rest; elevation of the involved extremity, warm compresses, and certain antiinflammatory agents (Wennberg and Rooke, 2008). The recommended treatment of DVT is active heparin use to prevent clot propagation and pulmonary embolism. Both unfractionated and low-molecular-weight heparin are safe during pregnancy because these chemicals cannot cross the placenta (Shepard and Lemire, 2004), but current guidelines recommend low-molecular-weight heparin (Marik and Lauren, 2008).

The lack of association between maternal STP/DVT and CAs in the study is an indirect proof against the teratogenic effect of drugs used in pregnant women with VDT. However, human teratogenic effect of coumarin/warfarin is widely accepted. Our study seemingly not confirmed it, but 8 pregnant women with acenocoumarol (Syncumar) treatment including 3 cases with the treatment only in I postnatal month were not appropriate for this analysis.

The use of coumarin derivatives (mainly warfarin in other countries) during the first trimester carries a significant risk to the fetus. Only about 70% of pregnancies expected to result in a normal infant (Briggs et al., 2005). Exposure in the 6th–9th gestational weeks induces the specific pattern of CAs called fetal warfarin syndrome including nasal hypoplasia (because of failure of development of the nasal septum) and calcific stippling of the secondary epiphyses (e.g. scoliosis, short proximal limbs and short phalanges), with an incidence up to 25%. The characteristic symptoms of this embryopathy are obvious in the later part of postnatal life (Wesseling et al., 2001). The use of warfarin in the second trimester and early in the third trimester was associated with fetal intracranial hemorrhage and schizencephaly in some studies (Pati and Helmbrecht, 1994; Lee et al., 2003). However, CAs in infants exposed before and after the above mentioned critical period had no proved association with this drug (Briggs et al., 2005). Out of 8 pregnant women in the study, 5 used Syncumar in II and III gestational months, and 2 had different CAs which did not correspond to the specific pattern of fetal warfarin syndrome. However, it is necessary to stress that the cardinal symptoms of fetal warfarin syndrome are not major and well-known CAs, thus a follow–up of these children would be necessary to exclude the diagnosis of this syndrome.

The teratogenic effect of hydroxyethylrutoside was shown in the origin of ocular coloboma (V). As far as we know the teratogenic potential of tribenoside has not been studied (Shepard and Lemire, 2004). The teratogenic effect of phenylbutazone was not found in animal investigations (Larsen and Bredahl, 1966; Schardein et al., 1969), but Kullander and Kallen (1976) reported that 18 women taking phenylbutazone in the first trimester had one miscarriage, 6 minor and one major CA. However, our patients were treated locally with this drug; therefore, a possible teratogenic effect can be excluded.

The lower rate of cases with CA in mothers with STP/DVT needs further explanations. Our hypothesis is based on three facts and/or suppositions. First, a major part of pregnant women with DVT and/or Syncumar treatment are terminated in Hungary due to the higher teratogenic and maternal risks. Second, a higher rate of early fetal death was observed in several studies (Heit et al., 2005; James et al., 2006; Marik and Plante, 2008) and this is a well-accepted clinical experience. These two selection biases may distort the evaluation of live-born babies. Thirdly, the higher level of prenatal care and the more health conscious lifestyle of pregnant women with venous diseases are again worth mentioning.

The prevalence of pregnant women with venous disease was 1.5–2.5% of Hungarian pregnant women, while the prevalence of DVT was 0.4–0.5%, somewhat higher than the figures in other studies (0.08–0.2%) (Heit et al., 2005; James et al., 2006). The incidence of pulmonary embolism was 0.07 per 1,000 in our study. The current estimates of deaths due to pulmonary embolism are 0.01–0.02 per 1,000 in the United States and Europe (Marik and Plante, 2008).

About 20–25% of STP/DVT occurred before the study pregnancy, generally in multiparae, most new onset STP+DVT manifested in the second trimester of pregnancy. Thus pregnancy is an important causal factor in the manifestation of STP/DVT. A meta-analysis showed that two-thirds of DVT occurred in the antepartum period and were distributed equally among all three trimesters (Ray and Chan, 1999). However, 43–60% of pregnancy–related pulmonary embolism appears to occur in the puerperium (Simpson et al., 2001; James et al., 2006).

Mothers with STP+DVT were elder with higher birth order in agreement with previous findings (Laros, 2004; Wennberg and Rooke, 2008). There was a higher risk for anemia in pregnant women with STP/DVT explained mainly by the much higher prevalence of hemorrhoids. In Hungary most anemias during pregnancy are caused by iron deficiency, and about 70% of pregnant women with these diseases were treated with iron products.

In conclusion, a higher risk for CAs, PB and LBW was not found in the children of pregnant women with STP+DVT.

10.11 Varicose Veins of the Lower Extremities

Primary varicosities tend to be familial and occur frequently without other causative events (Wennberg and Rooke, 2008).

Pregnancy induces dilation and proliferation of blood vessels, therefore venous congestion and increased vascular permeability which cause edema of the skin and the subcutaneous tissue, particularly on the vulva and lower legs (Wong and Ellis, 1989). *Varicose veins of lower extremities* (VVLE) often first appear during pregnancy. VVLE was recorded frequently in Hungarian pregnant women; nevertheless, we were not able to find the results of controlled epidemiological studies regarding to possible associations of VVLE in pregnant women with adverse birth outcomes of their children (Shepard and Lemire, 2004). Therefore, the aim of our study was to evaluate possible associations between maternal VVLE and adverse birth outcomes, particularly the risk of CAs in their children.

10.11.1 Results of the Study (VI)

Diagnostic criteria of VVLE were based on the CEAP (clinical manifestation, etiologic factors, anatomic involvement, and pathophysiological feature) classification scheme for lower-extremity venous diseases (Beebe et al., 1996; Eklof et al., 2004): C1 = teleangiectasia or reticular veins, C2 = varicose veins, C3 = edema without skin changes, C4a = skin pigmentation or eczema, C4b = lipodermatosclerosis or atrophie blanche, C5 = healed ulceration, and C6 = active ulceration. Pregnant women with C2 with the following definition: abnormal dilatation and formation of the vena saphena magna, and rarely the vena saphena parva in the lower limbs with the symptoms of burning, bursting, bruised, or aching (Wennberg and Rooke, 2008) were included to the study if VVL was recorded in the prenatal care logbooks. VVLE related drug treatments were also evaluated.

The case group consisted 22,843 malformed newborns or fetuses ("informative offspring") and 332 (1.45%) had mothers with medically recorded and treated VVLL. Out of 38,151 controls, 566 (1.48%) had mothers with VVLL.

Out of 332 case mothers, 91 (27.4%), while out of 566 control mothers, 127 (22.4%) had the onset of VVLE before conception, this condition was considered as chronic. Most of these pregnant women (96%) had previous pregnancies. The new onset VVLE was recorded mainly after II month with a peak in V and VI gestational months.

Pregnant women with VVLE showed a higher mean maternal age (28.3 vs.\break 25.4 year) due to the larger proportion of women with 30 or more years of age and the mean birth order was also higher (2.5 vs. 1.8) than pregnant women without VVLE as reference. Marital status did not show difference among the study groups. The proportion of unskilled workers (with mainly standing working position) was larger in pregnant women with VVLE. Folic acid supplementation during pregnancy was more frequent in pregnant women with VVLE. The use of multivitamins was similar among the study groups.

The rate of anemia (21.4% vs. 16.6%) was higher, while the rate of threatened preterm delivery (12.7% vs. 14.3%) was lower in pregnant women with VVLE.

Among acute maternal diseases, only influenza-common cold (generally with secondary complications) showed some difference. It was less frequent in both case (14.8% vs. 21.8%) and control (15.9% vs. 18.5%) mothers with VVLE than in pregnant women without VVLE. Among chronic diseases, the prevalence of constipation (4.7% vs. 2.0%) and particularly hemorrhoid (18.1% vs. 3.7%) was higher in pregnant women with VVLE.

In Hungary hydroxyethylrutoside (both orally and locally as gel) and a medicinal product containing rutoside and ascorbic acid were used more frequently for the treatment of severe VVLE. Additionally oral tribenoside and local phenylbutazone treatment were used in pregnant women with VVLE. About two-third of pregnant women with VVLE were treated by drugs in the study. Surgical intervention due to VVLE occurred only in 2 pregnant women.

The mean gestational age at delivery (39.4 week) did not show any difference between newborn infants born to mothers with or without VVLE. However, the newborn infants born to pregnant women with VVLE were 74 g heavier (3,349 vs. 3,275 g). In addition, both the rate of PB (7.1% vs. 9.2%) and LBW newborns (3.5% vs. 5.7%) were lower in the group of pregnant women with VVLE compared to children of mothers without VVLE.

Finally, we evaluated the possible association between VVLE and the risk of different CAs in their informative offspring. The occurrence of VVLE in the first trimester (mostly chronic VVLE) and any time during pregnancy was compared between case and control mothers. The total rate of cases with CA (1.0, 0.9–1.1) and any specified CA-group did not show any risk.

However, it is worth evaluating the subgroups of CA-groups including CAs with different manifestations and origin. The groups of musculo-skeletal system CAs had 585 cases. Among those, 82 cases had pectus excavatum. Of these 82 cases, 6 had mothers with VVLE. The percentage figure of pectus excavatum was 0.36% among 22,843 cases with CAs, but of 332 cases with CA born to mothers with VVLE, 6 (1.81%) were affected with pectus excavatum, therefore there is 5 fold higher risk for this CA in the children of mothers with VVLE ($p = 0.002$, after Bonferroni correction 0.03).

10.11.2 Interpretation of the Results

Four findings are worth emphasizing:

(i) Mothers with VVLE were elder with higher birth order, and had a higher rate of unskilled workers in agreement with the findings of previous studies (Kroeger et al., 2004; Kurtz et al., 2001).
(ii) There was a higher occurrence of anemia, constipation, and hemorrhoids in pregnant women with VVLE. The higher prevalence of anemia might have been caused by frequently bleeding hemorrhoids.
(iii) A higher rate of adverse birth outcomes were not found in children of pregnant women with VVLE, in fact, the rate of PB and LBW newborns was lower, and it may be related to better prenatal care which was demonstrated by higher use of folic acid.
(iv) The risk of pectus excavatum was 5 fold higher in the children of pregnant women with VVLE. Pectus excavatum (funnel chest) is a depression deformity of the thorax in which the sternum, usually the lower part, is depressed toward the spine. This condition may be evident at birth, but in the majority of cases it first becomes noticeable when the infant is several months of age (Verhagen, 1969). The severity spectrum of pectus excavatum is wide from the mild manifestation which presents only cosmetic problem, to the severe deformation with impaired ventilator capacity of the lungs and displacement of the heart, therefore needing a surgical intervention. Our cases were selected from HCAR to the HCCSCA within the first three postnatal months; therefore, most cases might have had severe manifestation of pectus excavatum. A certain part of pectus excavatum has autosomal dominant inheritance, but most cases are sporadic.

Hauge and Gundersen (1969) presented a family study of 249 probands with VVLE, and they concluded that multifactorial inheritance seems very probable. Later Matousek and Prerovsky (1974) estimated the heritability of varicose veins as about 50% within its multifactorial origin. The question is whether the possible association of maternal VVLE with the higher risk for pectus excavatum is a causal or can be explained by unevaluated confounders or by chance.

The biological plausibility that maternal VVLE can cause pectus excavatum is minimal. However, both VVLE and pectus excavatum are related to the mesodermal connective tissue, thus they may have common genetic origin. According to the aphorism of Osler: "Varicose veins are the results of an improper selection of grandparents" (Bean and Bean, 1950). Thus, it is possible that the association of VVLE and pectus excavatum is related to the improper selection of parent.

The prevalence of VVLE was 1.5% of Hungarian pregnant women and this figure is much lower than the previously found rate (sometimes 40%) of VVLE in other studies (Evans et al., 1999). However, the prevalence of VVLE in pregnant women depends on age and parity of females, in addition to the diagnostic criteria of VVLE. In our study only severe and treated VVLE were recorded in the prenatal logbook, and this group of mothers may reflect only the tip of the iceberg.

Only one-fourth of VVLE occurred before the study pregnancy, nearly all in multiparae. Most new onset VVLE manifested in the second trimester of pregnancy. The higher risk of VVLE in pregnancy may be related to hormonal changes, arterio-venosus shunts, the mechanical effect of the growing uterus on the abdominal veins, maternal weight gain, and fluid retention (Kroeger et al., 2004). Pregnancy is an important causal factor in the manifestation of VVLE, and it partly explains why VVLE is at least twice as frequent in females compared to males (Wennberg and Rooke, 2008).

The recommended first line therapy of VVLE includes dietary changes, losing weight, smoking cessation, and the education for the proper position of lower. The second line of therapy comprises compressive bandage and some drugs. Drugs used for the treatment of VVLE do not seem to be teratogenic though the teratogenic effect of hydroxyethylrutoside was shown in the origin of ocular coloboma (V). As far as we know, the teratogenic potential of tribenoside has not been studied (Shepard and Lemire, 2004). The teratogenic effect of phenylbutazone was not found in animal investigations (Larsen and Bredahl, 1966; Schardein et al., 1969), but Kullander and Kallen (1976) reported that 18 women taking phenylbutazone in the first trimester had one miscarriage, 6 minor and one major CA. The third line of therapy is sclerotherapy and surgical intervention (ablation of the veins) but it was not recommended for Hungarian pregnant women.

In conclusion, about one-quarter of pregnant women had chronic VVLE. The rest had new onset VVLE. There was no higher risk for adverse birth outcomes in pregnant women with VVLR; in fact, the rate of PB and LBW newborns was somewhat lower. A higher risk for pectus excavatum was found in children born to mothers with VVLE.

10.12 Hemorrhoids

Hemorrhoids are common pathological conditions. External and internal hemorrhoids are differentiated (Weakley, 1983). Hemorrhoids are more frequent in females, particularly in pregnant women (de Swiet, 2002). Nevertheless, this pathological condition is neglected in the handbooks of maternal diseases during pregnancy (Creasy et al., 2004) and in the international literature we did not find any controlled epidemiological study regarding the possible association between adverse birth outcomes including CAs and maternal hemorrhoids (Shepard and Lemire, 2004).

The aim of our study was to fill this vacancy.

10.12.1 Results of the Study

The diagnosis of hemorrhoids is relatively easy (Weakley, 1983). External hemorrhoids consist of a cluster of veins and the overlying, redundant squamous integument at the external brim of the rectal outlet. Secondary aggregates may be found flanking these primary sites to increase the number of external and internal hemorrhoid complexes from the usual three to as many as six. Pain without bleeding is the characteristic symptom produced by these external redundancies. With injury by abnormal bowel movements (diarrhea or constipation), bleeding and painful edema may develop in the overlying skin with or without thrombosis within one or more of the subintegumental hemorrhoidal veins. An internal hemorrhoid consists of a cluster of submucosal veins adjacent to the dentate line. Redundancy of the overlying mucosa produces a prominence immediately within the rectal outlet.

Only prospectively and medical recorded hemorrhoids in the prenatal logbook were evaluated in the study with the related drug treatments.

The case group consisted of 22,843 malformed newborns or fetuses ("informative offspring") and 795 (3.48%) case mothers had medically recorded hemorrhoids. Out of 38,151 controls, 1,617 (4.24%) had medically recorded hemorrhoids in the prenatal maternity logbook (0.8, 0.7–0.9).

Out of 795 case mothers, 276 (34.7%), while out of 1,617 control mothers, 543 (33.6%) had hemorrhoid before the conception which persisted during the study pregnancy. We considered this condition as a *chronic hemorrhoid*, and it occurred mainly in primiparae. In the rest of pregnant women hemorrhoid occurred first in the study pregnancy and this *new-onset* hemorrhoids started mainly between VII and VIII gestation months.

Mean age of pregnant women with hemorrhoid was higher (26.7 vs. 25.4 year) explained by the lower proportion of hemorrhoids in women younger than 20 years (4.1% vs. 8.8%) and by the largest proportion of hemorrhoids in women over 30 years (25.4% vs. 18.8%) than in pregnant women without hemorrhoids. Mean birth order was also somewhat higher (1.9 vs. 1.7) due to the maternal age characteristics. Hemorrhoid occurred more frequently in professional and managerial pregnant women. Folic acid and multivitamin supplementations were more frequent in pregnant women with hemorrhoid particularly in control mothers (57.4% vs. 54.3%).

Anemia showed a much higher rate in pregnant women with hemorrhoid compared to pregnant women without hemorrhoid (24.6% vs. 16.3%).

Among maternal disease, all acute diseases were reported somewhat more frequently in pregnant women with hemorrhoids (Table 10.7).

It is worth mentioning the 2.6–3.4-fold higher occurrences of acute diseases of the digestive system, mainly infectious diarrhea in pregnant women with hemorrhoid (particularly in the group of new onset hemorrhoid). In addition, influenza-common cold (generally with secondary complications) and acute diseases of respiratory system also showed significantly higher occurrence in pregnant women with hemorrhoid. Among chronic disease, about half of the pregnant women with hemorrhoid reported constipation. In addition, varicose veins and venous diseases (superficial thrombophlebitis and deep vein thrombophlebitis with or without thrombosis) in the lower extremities occurred more frequently in pregnant women with hemorrhoid.

In Hungary pregnant women with hemorrhoid were treated mainly by tribenoside (Glyvenol®) and dobesylicum calcium (Doxium®) as oral tablet, the combination

Table 10.7 Incidence of acute maternal disease groups and prevalence of chronic diseases in pregnant women with or without hemorrhoids as reference

	Case mothers				Control mothers			
	Without hemorrhoids		With hemorrhoids		Without hemorrhoids		With hemorrhoids	
	($N = 22{,}048$)		($N = 795$)		($N = 36{,}534$)		($N = 1{,}617$)	
Maternal diseases	No.	%	No.	%	No.	%	No.	%
Acute disease groups								
Influenza – common cold	4,673	21.2	294	37.0	6,614	18.1	447	27.6
Respiratory system	2,010	9.1	108	13.6	3,201	8.8	254	15.7
Digestive system	661	3.0	80	10.1	835	2.3	98	6.1
Urinary tract	1,513	6.9	76	9.6	2,195	6.0	113	7.0
Genital organs	1,602	7.3	74	9.3	2,732	7.5	159	9.8
Others	361	1.6	25	3.1	482	1.3	30	1.9
Chronic diseases								
Diabetes mellitus	76	0.3	4	0.5	68	0.2	6	0.4
Epilepsy	79	0.4	5	0.6	85	0.2	3	0.2
Manic-depression	207	0.9	15	1.9	189	0.5	15	0.9
Migraine	533	2.4	32	4.0	668	1.8	45	2.8
Phlebitis-thrombophlebitis	243	1.1	27	3.4	707	1.9	119	7.4
Varicose veins	281	1.3	51	6.4	448	1.2	118	7.3
Constipation	100	0.5	365	45.9	158	0.4	639	39.5

of phenol + bacterium coli (Reparon®), epinephrine + ephedrine + procaine + others (Hemorid®) as suppository and unguent, epinephrine + chloramphenicol + tetracain + others (Nodicid®), prednisolon + lidocaine + others (Aurobin®) as unguents. However, many supplementary medicinal products as analgesic dipyrone and acetylsalicylic acid, spasmodic drotaverine, laxative senna and antifungal clotrimazole were also used frequently for the treatment of pregnant women with hemorrhoid.

The mean gestational age at delivery between newborn infants of pregnant women with or without hemorrhoid was similar (39.4 week), though the mean birth weight was larger by 67 g in the newborns of mothers with hemorrhoid (3,340 vs. 3.273 g). Thus the rate of LBW newborns was also lower in newborns of mothers with hemorrhoid (4.8% vs. 5.7%). There was a similar trend in the rate of PB (8.5% vs. 9.2%) but this difference did not reach the level of significance.

The possible risk of hemorrhoid for CAs was estimated separately. Hemorrhoid during any time of pregnancy and hemorrhoid in II and/or III gestation month were analyzed in cases with different CA groups and their all matched controls. There was no higher risk for the total group of CAs (0.8, 0.7–0.9) or any particular CA group in the offspring of mothers who were affected by hemorrhoid during any time of pregnancy or in II and III gestational months, i.e. during the critical period of most CAs.

However, the detailed evaluation of other isolated CA group showed that 8 cases had malposition/malrotation of the digestive organs (transposition of small intestine in 4 cases, malrotation of colon in 3 cases, and transposition of stomach in one case). The number of all cases with malposition/malrotation of the digestive organs was 53 (0.23%) in the total group of 22,843 cases with CA, while 8 cases with these CAs represented 1.01% of cases born to 795 mothers with hemorrhoids. However, of 53 cases with malposition/malrotation of digestive organs 8 (15.1%), while out of their 98 matched controls, 3 (3.1%) had mothers with hemorrhoids; this difference shows a significant association with maternal hemorrhoid. ($p = 0.002$. after Boneffroni correction 0.01). All these 8 cases with malposition/malrotation of gut were boy. Familial cases did not occur among these CAs.

10.12.2 Interpretation of Results

A somewhat larger mean birth weight was found in children born to mother with hemorrhoid and it associated with a lower rate of LBW newborns. However, a higher risk of malposition-malrotation-transposition of digestive organs was found in the offspring of mothers with hemorrhoid during pregnancy.

Our study confirmed that pregnant women with hemorrhoid are elder with a higher proportion of multiparae (Weakley, 1983) supporting the previous findings that delivery is a major risk factor in the origin of hemorrhoids. In addition, hemorrhoids occur more frequently in women with higher socioeconomic status and they have better prenatal care including more frequent folic acid/multivitamin supplementation. The question is whether these confounding factors can explain the somewhat higher mean birth weight and lower rate of LBW newborns.

The higher rate of anemia obviously is the secondary complication of hemorrhoids and the higher rate of acute diseases of digestive system and a much higher rate of constipation may associate with a higher risk for hemorrhoids. The higher rate of varicose veins and thrombophlebitis-thrombosis in the lower limbs may have some causal association with hemorrhoids.

About half of hemorrhoids had new onset during the study pregnancy and this finding confirms that pregnancy itself (not only delivery) is a predisposing factor in the origin of hemorrhoids.

Beyond the well-known atresia and stenosis of digestive organs such as pylorus, small and large intestines, rectum/anal canal, the malrotation/malposition of the stomach, small intestine, and colon are differentiated (Minor, 1969). Failure of the bowel to undergo normal migration and attachment on returns from physiological omphalocele to the celomic cavity and simultaneously rotates in a counter clockwise direction around the superior mesenteric pedicle. Eventually the cecum and right colon are fixed to the posterior parietes by the Toldt fusion fascia. If the rotation does not proceed to completion, fixation of the right colon does not occur and the entire intestine is on narrowed pedicle. These defects may be the consequence of the arrest of development during the 10th and 11th week of postconceptional fetal age. Volvulus of the midgut due to short root of mesentery and vascular damage may occur, however, volvulus of the midgut caused by intestinal malrotation was described as an autosomal dominantly inherited CA as well (Carmi et al., 1981; Stalker and Chitayat, 1992).

Our study showed that hemorrhoid in pregnant women associated with a higher risk for malposition/rotation of digestive organs. Both these CAs and hemorrhoids may be related to mesechyma-connective tissues. Thus our hypothesis is not based on the possible teratogenic or triggering effect of maternal hemorrhoid but the common genetic origin of maternal hemorrhoid and these rarely occurring CAs in their children.

There were two important characteristic of the study. On one hand, the diagnosis of hemorrhoid was based on prospective medically recorded data in the prenatal maternity logbook and most pregnant women were treated with drugs indicating the severity of this pathological condition. Thus only severe hemorrhoids were evaluated as the tip of iceberg in our study. On the other hand, both maternal diseases and pregnancy complications showed a higher occurrence in pregnant women with hemorrhoids. The question is whether this phenomenon can be explained by the more cautious medical care (including their more frequent records in the prenatal care logbook) of these pregnant women with more complaints (partly this behavior may explain the higher occurrence of some other maternal diseases based on maternal self-reported information), or these findings reflect a real higher occurrence of other diseases in pregnant women with hemorrhoids due to some interaction of these pathological conditions. However, the better pattern of birth outcomes is an argument against this hypothesis.

The potential teratogenic effect of most frequently used drugs in the treatment of hemorrhoid was not found and it is in agreement with the available scarce data of these drugs (Shepard and Lemire, 2004).

In conclusion, a higher risk for malposition-malrotation of the digestive organs was found in the offspring of pregnant women with hemorrhoid.

10.13 Hypotension

Hypotension is not a disease; it is a symptom of low blood pressure in individuals. In the population blood pressure has normal distribution, thus there is no obvious natural threshold between normal and high/low blood pressure than in the so-called qualitative (yes or no) diseases. Following the consensus of experts, hypotension is diagnosed if blood pressure is 100/70 mmHg or less for adult age 18 years or older measured by the recommended criteria (Rashidi et al., 2008).

Hypotension occurs frequently in Hungarian pregnant women as well; nevertheless we were not able to find any controlled epidemiological study regarding its effect for adverse birth outcomes in the international literature (Shepard and Lemire, 2004). Thus the aims of our study was to evaluate the possible association of maternal hypotension with adverse birth outcomes, particularly the risk of CAs, in addition to pregnancy complications

10.13.1 Results of the Study

Pregnant women with secondary hypotension due to anorexia nervosa, Addison and Simmonds disease, etc and with the so-called orthostatic hypotension were excluded from the study. Only pregnant women with prospectively and medical recorded hypotension in the prenatal maternity logbook were included into the study.

The case group consisted of 22,843 malformed newborns or fetuses ("informative offspring") and 538 (2.4%) had mothers with medically recorded hypotension. Out of 38,151 controls, 1,268 (3.3%) had mothers with hypotension recorded in prenatal care logbook.

Out of 538 case mothers, 262 (48.7%) had the onset of hypotension before conception, this condition was considered as chronic. Out of 1,268 control mothers, 652 (51.4%) were recorded with chronic hypotension. The new onset hypotension started most frequently in III and IV gestational months.

Pregnant women with hypotension had somewhat lower mean maternal age (24.9 vs. 25.5 year) due to the larger proportion of women under age 20 (12.1% vs. 8.5%). However, the mean birth order did not show difference in case and control pregnant women with or without hypotension, respectively. Marital and employment status did also not show characteristic difference among the study groups. The proportion of folic acid supplementation during pregnancy was also similar among the study groups (about 55%) but the use of multivitamins was more frequent in pregnant women with hypotension (13.2% vs. 6.3%).

Pregnancy complications showed characteristic pattern (Table 10.8).

Table 10.8 Incidence of medically recorded pregnancy complications in mothers with or without hypotension

	Case mothers				Control mothers					
	without hypotension		with hypotension		without hypotension		with hypotension		Comparison of case and control mothers with hypotension	
	($N = 22,306$)		($N = 537$)		($N = 36,883$)		($N = 1,268$)			
Pregnancy complications	No.	%	No.	%	No.	%	No.	%		
Nausea-vomiting, sever	1,683	7.5	63	11.7	3,666	9.9	203	16.0	**0.7**	**0.5–0.9**
Threatened abortion	3,393	15.2	108	20.1	6,210	16.8	302	23.8	0.8	0.6–1.0
Preeclampsia-eclampsia	662	3.0	10	1.9	1,143	3.1	18	1.4	1.3	0.6–2.9
Gestational hypertension	575	2.6	0	0.0	1,082	2.9	0	0.0	–	
Placental disorders[a]	287	1.3	7	1.3	575	1.6	17	1.3	1.0	0.4–2.3
Polyhydramnios	205	0.9	7	1.3	180	0.5	11	0.9	1.5	0.6–3.9
Threatened preterm delivery[b]	2,783	12.5	67	12.5	5,803	15.7	183	14.4	0.8	0.6–1.1
Gestational diabetes	140	0.6	1	0.2	261	0.7	9	0.7	0.3	0.0–2.1
Anemia	3,091	13.9	149	27.7	5,992	16.2	364	28.7	1.0	0.8–1.2

[a]Including placenta previa, premature separation of placenta, antepartum hemorrhage.
[b]Including cervical incompetence.

Gestational hypertension did not occur, and the prevalence of preeclampsia-eclampsia was lower, while the occurrence of severe nausea and vomiting, threatened abortion, and particularly anemia was higher in pregnant women with hypotension compared to pregnant women without hypotension.

Among acute maternal diseases, only influenza-common cold (generally with secondary complications) occurred more frequently in both case (29.4% vs. 21.6%) and control (21.6% vs. 18.4%) mothers with hypotension than in pregnant women without hypotension. Among chronic diseases, hemorrhoids were recorded more frequently in case (4.8% vs. 2.4%) and control (5.0% vs. 3.3%) mothers with hypotension. The occurrence of headache in case (2.8% vs. 2.4%) and control (2.8% vs. 1.8%) pregnant women with or without hypotension did not show obvious differences.

The first choice drug for the treatment of hypotensive persons is pholedrine. Nearly half of case (50.2% vs. 2.2%) and control (48.3% vs. 2.4%) pregnant women with hypotension were treated orally by pholedrine drops. Ephedrine was also used more frequently in pregnant women with hypotension.

The mean gestational age was the same (39.4 week) and practically mean birth weight (3,288 vs. 3,275 g) was similar in newborn infants born to mothers with or without hypotension. Both the rate of PB (8.6% vs. 9.2%) and LBW newborns (4.2% vs. 5.7%) was somewhat lower in the group of pregnant women with hypotension but this difference did not reach the level of significance.

Finally, we evaluated the possible association of pregnant women with hypotension and the risk for different CAs in their informative offspring. Out of 23 CA-groups evaluated, 11 included mothers with lower rate of hypotension during pregnancy giving a significant reduction in the total rate of CAs (0.66, 0.59–0.74). However, this lower risk was explained by the parallel use of folic acid/multivitamins in early pregnancy because when this confounder was considered, the lower risk disappeared (0.9, 0.8–1.1).

10.13.2 Interpretation of Results

Most pregnant women with primary hypotension were medically recorded in the prenatal maternity logbook and treated, thus their severe condition may represent the tip of the iceberg.

Three findings are worth emphasizing.

(i) Maternal hypotension is protective against preeclampsia-eclampsia. The opposite trend namely preeclampsia superimposed upon chronic hypertension (Gifford et al., 2000; Roberts, 2004) is well-known.

(ii) There was a higher risk for severe nausea and vomiting, threatened abortion, and anemia in pregnant women with hypotension.

Thus pregnant women with hypotension had a higher occurrence of severe medically recorded and treated nausea/vomiting in the study. Our previous study showed that severe nausea and vomiting in pregnancy resulted in some protective effect for several CAs (VII). Thus, our hypothesis is that there might be some relationship between maternal hypotension and severe nausea/vomiting, and together they may associate with a mild protective effect of some CAs.

There was a higher rate of threatened abortion based on vaginal bleeding and/or permanent uterine spasm in pregnant women with hypotension particularly among case mothers. Unfortunately the occurrence of early fetal deaths (e.g. miscarriages) are not recorded in the HCCSCA, therefore we cannot measure whether the higher risk of threatened abortion is associated with a higher rate of early fetal death. The latter as early prenatal selection of malformed fetuses may explain the lower rate of some CAs at birth.

Our pregnant women with hypotension also had a higher occurrence of anemia which can be explained mainly by their more frequent hemorrhoids, which cause bleeding (Weakley, 1983). In Hungary most anemia during pregnancy is caused by iron deficiency and more than two-third of pregnant women were treated with iron and about one-tenth with micronutrient ("multivitamin") products. However, some relationship between anemia and hypotension cannot be excluded.

(iii) Increased rate of CAs and adverse birth outcomes were not found in the children of pregnant women with hypotension, in fact, the rate of PB and LBW newborns, in addition to the rate of total CA group was lower in the newborns of pregnant women with hypotension due to the parallel use of folic acid/multivitamins.

The prevalence of prospective and medically recorded hypotension was 3.3% in Hungarian pregnant women who later delivered babies without CA, while this rate was 2.4% in the mothers of children with CA. These figures also demonstrate that maternal hypotension seems to have some "beneficial" effect for CAs.

There is a marked early fall in diastolic and systolic blood pressures (about 7 mmHg) due to decreased systematic vascular resistance during pregnancy (Churchill, 2001). This phenomenon explains the new onset hypotension in pregnant women. In our study about half of pregnant women had chronic hypotension with the onset before the study pregnancy and these women were treated by pholedrine and ephedrine.

Some CA groups had a lower risk in the offspring of pregnant women with hypotension and this finding is an important indirect proof against the teratogenic effect of drugs, i.e. pholedrine and ephedrine, used for the treatment of maternal hypotension during pregnancy. To our best knowledge the results of teratogenic investigations regarding pholedrine have not been published (Shepard and Lemire, 2004). Our study did not show any teratogenic potential of pholedrine in the data set of the HCCSCA (94). Heinonen et al. (1977) evaluated 373 offspring of women exposed to ephedrine in the first four lunar months, and 17 offspring were affected with CA, thus the relative risk was 0.98. Werler et al. (1992) did also not find any association between maternal ephedrine use during the first trimester of pregnancy and different CAs.

In conclusion, increased risk for CAs and other adverse birth outcomes was not found in the children of pregnant women with hypotension but this condition modified significantly the incidence of some pregnancy complications.

10.14 Others

10.14.1 Interpretation of Data in the HCCSCA

Acute myocarditis was recorded in one case mother who delivered a boy with cleft lip + palate; one control was born on the 35th gestational week with 2,600 g.

Transient cerebral ischemia was diagnosed in one case mother during the study pregnancy and her live-born case was affected with lethal left heart hypoplasia. One newborn of control pregnant woman was born on the 42nd gestational week with 3,650 g.

Arterial embolism and thrombosis occurred in the mother of one case affected with clubfoot (bilateral talipes equinovarus) while 3 control mothers delivered newborns on the 36th, 39th, and 41st gestational weeks with 1,650, 3,550, and 3,000 g, respectively.

Vulvar varix was recorded in one case mother who had a boy with lethal renal agenesis.

10.15 General Conclusion

After reviewing the international literature, we found it surprising that some very frequent pathological conditions such as hypotension, varicose veins of lower extremities, hemorrhoids, and paroxysmal supraventricular tachycardia have been neglected as prenatal comorbidities, and therefore their possible associations with adverse birth outcomes were absolutely unknown.

The second surprise after the evaluation of cardiovascular diseases was related to their unexpected associations of CAs, e.g. CAD was associated with very high risk of isolated orofacial clefts without known or plausible biological explanation.

Finally, the diseases of the circulatory system are common and determinative for life expectancy and possibly for the outcomes of pregnancy in some cases, therefore they need more attention during prenatal care.

References

Abalos E, Duley L, Steyn DW, Henderson-Smart DJ. Antihypertensive drug therapy for mild to moderate hypertension during pregnancy. Cochrane Databases Syst Rev 2007 update, CD002252.

Arias F, Zamora J. Antihypertensive treatment and pregnancy outcome in patients with mild chronic hypertension. Obstet Gynecol 1979; 53: 489–492.

Atarashi A. Pharmacologic treatment of cardiac arrhythmias. In: van Boxtel CJ, Santoso B, Edwards IR (eds.) Drug Benefits and Risks. IOS Press. Amsterdam, 2008, pp. 599–607.
Bean RB, Bean WB. Sir William Osler Aphorisms From His Bedside Teaching and Writings. Henry Schuman Publications, New York, 1950. p. 142.
Beebe HG, Bergan JJ, Berqvist D et al. Classification and grading of chronic venous disease in the lower limbs: a consensus statement. Eur J Vasc Endovasc Surg 1996. 12: 487–491.
Blanchard DG, Shabetai R. Cardiac disease. In: Creasy RK, Resnik R, Iams JD (eds.) Maternal-Fetal Medicine. Principles and Practice. 5th ed. Saunders, Philadelphia, 2004. pp. 815–843.
Blanton SH, Patel D, Hecht JT et al. MTHFR is not a risk factor in the development of isolated nonsyndromic cleft lip and palate. Am J Med Genet 2002; 110: 404–405.
Boogaard M-JH van den, de Costa D, Krapels IPC et al. The MSX1 allele 4 homozygous child to periconceptional smoking is most sensitive to develop nonsyndromic cleft lip and/or palate. Human Genetics, 2008
Brazy JE, Grimm JK, Little VA. Neonatal manifestations of severe maternal hypertension occurring before the thirty-sixth week of pregnancy. J Pediatr 1982; 100: 265–271.
Briggs GG, Freeman RK, Yaffe SJ. Drugs in Pregnancy and Lactation. 7th ed. Lippincot Williams and Wilkins, Philadelphia, 2005
Brown MA, Lindheimer MD, de Swiet M et al. The classification and diagnosis of the hypertensive disorders of pregnancy : statement from the International Society for the Study of Hypertension in Pregnancy (ISSHP) Hypert Pregnancy 2000; 20: ix
Buchbinder A, Sibai BM, Caritis S et al. Adverse perinatal outcomes are significantly higher in severe gestational hypertension than in mild preeclampsia. Am J Obstet Gynecol 2002; 186: 66–70.
Burrows RF, Burrows EA. Assessing the teratogenic potential of angiotensin-converting enzyme inhibitors in pregnancy. Aust N Z Obstet Gynaecol 1998; 38: 306–311.
Calkins H. Supravenricuar tachycardia: AV nodal reentry and Wolff-Parkinson-White Syndrome. In: Fuster V, Walsh RA, O'Rourke RA, Poole-Wilson P. Hurst's The Heart, 12th ed. McGraw Hill Medical, New York, etc, 2008. pp. 983–1001.
Caritis S, Sibai B, Hauth J et al. Low-dose aspirin to prevent preeclampsia in women at high risk. National Institute of Child Health and Human Development Network of Maternal-Fetal Medicine Units. N Engl J Med 1998; 338: 701–706.
Carmi R, Abeliovich D, Siplovich L et al. Familial midgut anomalies – a spectrum of defects due to the same cause? Am J Med Genet 1981; 8: 443–446.
Caton AR, Bell EM, Druschel CM et al. Maternal hypertension, antihypertensive medication use and the risk of severe hypospadias. Birth Defects Res Part A 2008; 82: 34–40.
Chobanian AV, Bakris GL, Black HR. et al. The seventh report of the Joint National Committee on Prevention, Detection, Evaluation and Treatment of High Blood Pressure: the JNC 7 report. JAMA 2003; 289: 2560–2572.
Chobonian AV. Does it matter how hypertension is controlled? New Engl J Med 2008; 359: 2485–2488.
Christensen K, Olson J, Norgaard-Pedersen B et al. Oral clefts, transforming growth factor alpha gene variants, and maternal smoking: a population-based case-control study in Denmark, 1991–1994. Am J Epidemiol 1999; 149: 248–255.
Churchill D. The new American guidelines on the hypertensive disorders of pregnancy. J Hum Hypertens 2001; 15: 583–585.
Cooper WD, Hernandez-Diaz S, Arbogast PQ et al. Major congenital malformations after first-trimester exposure to ACE inhibitors. N Engl J Med 2006; 354: 2443–2451.
Creasy RK, Resnik R, Iams JD (eds.) Maternal-Fetal Medicine. 5th ed. Saunders Philadelphia, 2004. pp. 1127–1145.
Davies AM, Czaczkes JW, Sadovsky E et al. Toxemia of pregnancy in Jerusalem. I. Epidemiological studies of a total community. Isr J Med Sci 1970; 6: 253–258.
de Swiet EF (ed.) Medical Disorders in Obstetric Practice. 4th ed. Blackwell, Oxford, 2002.

Dellegrottaglie S, Gerschlick AH, Massimo C, Gersch BJ. Pharmacologic therapy for acute coronary syndromes. In: Fuster V, Walsh RA, O'Rourke RA, Poole-Wilson P. Hurst's The Heart. 12th ed. McGraw Hill Medical, New York, etc, 2008. pp. 1405–1425.

Diro M, Beydown SN, Jaranillo B, O'Sullivan MJ, Kieval J. Successful pregnancy in a woman with a left ventricular cardiac aneurysm: a case report. J Report Med 1983; 28: 559–563.

Eklof B, Rutherford RB, Bergan JJ et al. Revision of the CEAP classification for chronic venous disorders: consensus statement. J Vasc Surg 2004; 40: 1248–1252.

Evans CJ, Eowkes FG, Ruckley CV et al. Prevalence of varicose veins and chronic venous insufficiency in men and women in the general population: Edinburgh Vein Study. J Epidemiol Community Health 1999; 53: 149–153.

Gifford R, August P, Cunningham G et al. Report of the National High Blood Pressure Education program Working Group on High Blood Pressure in Pregnancy. Am J Obstet Gynecol 2000; 183: S1–S15.

Hall JE, Granger JP, Hall ME, Jones DW. Pathophysiology of hypertension In: Fuster V, Walsh RA, O'Rourke RA, Poole-Wilson P. Hurst's The Heart. 12th ed. McGraw Hill Medical, New York, etc, 2008. pp. 1570–1609.

Hanssens M, Keirse MJ, Vankelecom F et al. Fetal and neonatal effects of treatment with angiotensin converting enzyme inhibitors in pregnancy. Obstet Gynecol 1991; 78: 128–135.

Hauge M, Gundersen J. Genetics of varicose veins of the lower extremities. Hum Hered 1969; 19: 573–580.

Hayes C. Environmental risk factors and oral clefts. In: Wyszinski DF (ed.) Cleft Lip and Palate. From Origin to Treatment. Oxford University Press, Oxford, 2002. pp. 159–19.

Heinonen OP, Slone D, Shapiro S. Birth Defects and Drugs in Pregnancy. Publishing Sciences Group, Littleton, MA, 1977. pp. 371–373.

Heit JA, Kobbervig CE, James AH et al. Trends in the incidence of venous thromboembolism during pregnancy or postpartum: a 30-year population-based study. Ann Intern Med 2005; 143: 697–706.

Hemmingway H, McCallum A, Shipley M et al. Incidence and prognostic implications of stable angina pectoris among men and women. JAMA 2006; 295: 1401–1411.

Hwang SJ, Beaty TH, Panny SR et al. Association study of transforming growth factor alpha (TGF-alpha) Taq1 polymorphism and oral clefts: indication of gene–environmental interaction in a population-based sample of infants with birth defects. Am J Epidemiol 1995; 141: 329–336.

Jamerson K, Weber MA, Bakris GL et al. Benazepril plus amlodipine or hydrochlorothiazide fro hypertension in high-risk patients. New Engl J Med 2008; 359: 2417–2428.

James AH, Jamison MG, Brancazio LR, Myers MR. Venous thromboembolism during pregnancy and the postpartum period: incidence, risk factors, and mortality. Am J Obstet Gynecol 2006; 194: 1311–1315.

JNC 7. The seventh report of the Joint National Committee on Prevention, Detection, Evaluation and Treatment of High Blood Pressure (JNC 7): the guidelines. Hypertens 2003; 42: 1206.

Kahn NA, Rahim SA, Anand SS et al. Does the clinical examination predict lower extremity peripheral arterial disease? JAMA 2006; 295: 536.

Kerber LJ, Warr OS, Richardson C. Pregnancy in a patient with prosthetic mitral valve. JAMA 1968; 203: 223–225.

Kim MC, Kini AS, Fuster V. Definitions of acute coronary syndromes. In: Fuster V, Walsh RA, O'Rourke RA, Poole-Wilson P. Hurst's The Heart. 12th ed. McGraw Hill Medical, New York, etc, 2008. pp. 1311–1319.

Konstantinides S. Acute pulmonary embolism. New Engl J Med 2008; 359: 2804–2813.

Kroeger K, Ose C, Rudofsky G et al. Risk factors for varicose veins. Int Angio 2004; 23: 29–37.

Kullander B, Kallen B. A prospective study of drugs in pregnancy. Acta Obstet Gynecol Scand 1976; 55: 289–295.

Kurtz X, Lamping DL, Kahn SR et al. Do varicose veins affect quality of life? Results of an international population-based study. J Vasc Surg 2001; 34: 641–648.

Lambot MA, Vermeylen D, Noel JC. Angiotensin-II-receptor inhibitors in pregnancy. Lancet 2001; 357: 1619–1620.

Langer A, Villar J, Kim T, Kennedy S. Reducing eclampsia-related death – a call to action. Lancet 2008; 371: 705–706.

Laros RK. Thromboembolic disease. In: Creasy RK, Resnik R, Iams JD (eds.) Maternal-Fetal Medicine. 5th ed. Saunders, Philadelphia, New Engl J Med 2004. pp. 845–857.

Larsen V, Bredahl E. The embryotoxic effects on rabbits of Monophenylbutazone (Monazen TM) compared with phenylbutazone and thalidomide. Acta Pharmacol Toxicol 1966; 24: 453–455.

Lee HC, Cho Y, Lee HJ et al. Warfarin-associated fetal intracranial hemorrhage: a case report. J Korean Med Sci 2003; 18: 764–767.

Lee SH, Chan SA, Wu TJ et al. Effects of pregnancy on first onset and symptoms of paroxysmal supraventricular tachycardia. Am J Cardiol 1995; 76: 675–678.

Lopez-Llear M, Horta JLH. Perinatal mortality in eclampsia. J Reprod Med 1972; 8: 281–285.

Mabie WC, Freire MV. Sudden chest pain and cardiac emergencies in the obstetric patient. Obstet Gynecol Clin North Am 1995; 22: 19–24.

Maestri NE, Beaty TH, Hetmanski J et al. Application of transmission disequilibrium tests to non-syndromic oral clefts: including candidate genes and environmental exposures in the models. Am J Med Genet 1997; 73: 337–344.

Mangoni AA, Jackson SH. Homocysteine and cardiovascular disease: current evidence and future prospect. Am J Med 2002; 112: 556–565.

Marazita ML. Segregation analyses. In: Wyszinski DF (ed.) Cleft Lip and Palate. From Origin to Treatment. Oxford University Press, Oxford, 2002. pp. 222–233.

Marik PE, Lauren AP. Venous thromboembolic disease and pregnancy. N Engl J Med 2008; 359: 2025–2533.

Marik PE, Plante LA. Venous thromboembolic disease and pregnancy. N Engl J Med 2008; 359: 2025–2033.

Martinovic J, Benachi A, Laurent N et al. Fetal toxic effects and angiotensin-II-receptor antagonists. Lancet 2001; 358: 241.

Matousek V, Prerovsky I. A contribution to the problem of the inheritance of primary varicose veins. Hum Hered 1974; 24: 225–235.

McAnulty JH, Brober CS, Metcalfe J. Heart disease and pregnancy. In: Fuster V, Walsh RA, O'Rourke RA, Poole-Wilson P. Hurst's The Heart. 12th ed. McGraw Hill Medical, New York, etc, 2008. pp. 2188–2202.

Meyer NL, Mercer BM, Friedman SA et al. Urinary dipstick protein: a poor predictor of absent or severe proteinuria. Am J Obstet Gynecol 1994; 170: 137–140.

Mills JL, Kirke PN, Molloy AM et al. Methylenetetrahydrofolate reductase thermolabile variant and oral clefts. Am J Med Genet 1999; 86: 71–74.

Minor CL. Colon, malrotation. In: Rubin A (ed.) Handbook of Congenital Malformations. W.B. Saunders Company, Philadelphia, 1969.

Monga M. Maternal cardiovascular and renal adaptation to pregnancy. In: Creasy RK, Resnik R, Iams JD (eds.) Maternal-Fetal Medicine. 5th ed. Saunders, Philadelphia, 2004, pp. 111–120.

Naeye RL, Friedman EA. Causes of perinatal death associated with gestational hypertension and proteinuria. Am J Obstet Gynecol 1979; 133: 8–12.

NHBPEWG. Report of the National High Blood Pressure Education program Working Group on High Blood Pressure in Pregnancy. Am J Obstet Gyencol 2000; 183: S1–S22.

Nygerd O, Nordehaug JE, Refsum H et al. Plasma homocysteine levels and mortality in patients with coronary artery disease. N Engl J Med 1997; 337: 230–236.

Oketani Y, Mitsuzona T, Ichikawa K et al. Toxicological studies on nitroglycerin (NK-843). 6. Teratologic studies in rabbits. Oyo Yakuri 1981a; 22: 633–48; 737–63. cit. Shepard TH, Lemire RJ, 2004.

Oketani Y, Mitsuzona T, Ichikawa K et al. Toxicological studies on nitroglycerin (NK-843). 8. Teratologic studies in rats. Oyo Yakuri 1981b; 22: 737–51. cit. Shepard TH, Lemire RJ, 2004.

O'Rourke RA, O'Gara PT, Shaw LJ, Douglas JS Jr. Diagnosis and management of patients with chronic ischemic heart disease. In: Fuster V, Walsh RA, O'Rourke RA, Poole-Wilson P (eds.) Hurst's The Heart. 12th ed. McGraw Hill Medical, New York, etc, 2008. pp. 1474–1503.

Ounsted M, Cockburn J, Moar VA et al. Maternal hypertension with superimposed preeclampsia: effects on child development at 7½ years. Br J Obstet Gynecol 1983; 90: 644–650.

Pati S, Helmbrecht GD. Congenital schizencephaly associate with in utero warfarin exposure. Reprod Toxicol 1994; 8: 115–120.

Pickering TG, Ogedegbe G. Epidemiology of hypertension. In: Fuster V, Walsh RA, O'Rourke RA, Poole-Wilson P (eds.) Hurst's The Heart. 12th ed. McGraw Hill Medical, New York, etc, 2008. pp. 1551–1569.

Plouin PE, Chatellier G, Breart G et al. Frequency and perinatal consequences of hypertensive disease of pregnancy. Adv Nephrol 1986; 57: 69–74.

Rashidi A, Rachman M, Wright JT. Diagnosis and treatment of hypertension. In: Fuster V, Walsh RA, O'Rourke RA, Poole-Wilson P (eds.) Hurst's The Heart. 12th ed. McGraw Hill Medical, New York, etc, 2008. pp. 1610–1629.

Ray JG, Chan WS. Deep vein thrombosis during pregnancy and the puerperium: a meta-analysis of the period of risk and leg of presentation. Obstet Gynecol Surv 1999; 54: 265–271.

Rey E, Couturier A. The prognosis of pregnancy in women with chronic hypertension. Am J Obstet Gynecol 1994; 171: 410–415.

Rey E, LeLorier J, Burgess E et al. Report of the Canadian Hypertension Society Consensus Conference. 3. Pharmacologic treatment of hypertensive treatment in pregnancy. Can Med Assoc J 1997; 157: 1245–1254.

Robert E, Mutchinik O, Mastroiacovo P et al. An international collaborative study of esophageal atresia or stenosis. Reprod Toxicol 1993; 7: 405–421.

Roberts JM, Perloff DL. Hypertension and the obstetrician-gynecologist. Am J Obstet Gynecol 1977; 127: 316–322.

Roberts JM. Pregnancy-related hypertension. In: Creasy RK, Resnik R, Iams JD (eds.) Maternal-Fetal Medicine. Principles and Practice. 5th ed. Saunders, Philadelphia, 2004. pp. 859–899.

Romitti PA, Lidral AC, Munger RG et al. Candidate genes for nonsyndromic cleft lip and palate and maternal cigarette smoking and alcohol consumption: evaluation of genotype-environmental interactions from a population-based case-control study of orofacial clefts. Teratology 1999; 59: 39–50.

Roth A, Elkayam U. Acute myocardial infarction associated with pregnancy. Ann Intern Med 1996; 125: 751–755.

Sato K, Taniguchi H, Ohtsuka T et al. Reproductive studies of nitroglycerin applied dermally to pregnant rats and rabbits. Clin Report 1984; 18: 2511–3586.

Schardein JL, Blatz AT, Woosley ET, Kaup DH. Reproductive studies on sodium meclofenamate in comparison to aspirin and phenylbutazone. Toxicol Appl Pharmacol 1969; 15: 46–55.

Schroeder JS, Harrison DC. Repeated cardioversion during pregnancy: treatment of refractory paroxysmal atrial tachycardia during 3 successive pregnancies. Am J Cardiol 1971; 37: 445–446.

Shaw GM, Wasserman CR, Lammer EJ et al. Orofacial clefts, parental cigarette smoking, and transforming growth factor-alpha gene variants. Am J Hum Genet 1996; 58: 551–561.

Shepard TH, Lemire RJ. Catalog of Teratogenic Agents. 11th ed. Johns Hopkins University Press, Baltimore, 2004.

Sibai BM, Abdella TLN, Anderson GD. Pregnancy outcome in 211 patients with mild chronic hypertension. Obstet Gynecol 1983; 61: 571–577.

Sibai BM, Mabie WC, Shamsa R et al. A comparison of no medication versus methyldopa or labetalol in chronic hypertension during pregnancy. Am J Obstet Gynecol 1990; 162:960–967.

Sibai BM. Chronic hypertension in pregnancy. Obstet Gynecol 2002; 100: 369–377.

Simpson EL, Lawrenson RA, Nightingale AL et al. Venous thromboembolism in pregnancy and the puerperium: incidence and additional risk factors from a London perinatal database. Br J Obstet Gynecol 2001; 108: 56–60.

Stalker HJ, Chitayat D. Familial intestinal malrotation with midgut volvulus and facial anomalies: a disorder involving a gene controlling the normal gut rotation? Am J Med Genet 1992; 44: 46–47.

Sugawara T, Uchiyama K, Asano K, Asano O. Toxicological studies on pentaerythritol tetranicotinate (SK-1). VII. Studies on teratogenicity of SK-1 in rabbits. Oyo Yakuri 1977; 14: 903–911. cit. Shepard TH, Lemire RJ, 2004.

Székely P, Turner R, Smith L. Pregnancy and the changing pattern of rheumatic heart disease. Br Heart J 1973; 35: 1293–1303.

Tervila L, Goecke C, Timonen S. Estimation of gestosis of pregnancy (EPH-gestosis) Acta Obstet Gynecol Scand 1973; 52: 235–240.

The Eclampsia Trial Collaborative Group. Which anticonvulsants for women with eclampsia? Evidence from the Collaborative Eclampsia Trial. Lancet 1995; 345: 1455–1463.

The Magpie Trial Collaborative Group. Do women with preeclampsia, and their babies, benefit from magnesium sulfate? The Magpie Trial: a randomized placebo-controlled trial. Lancet 2002; 359: 1877–1890.

Vasan RS, Benjamin EJ, Sullivan LM, D'Agostino, RB. The burden of increasing worldwide cardiovascular disease. In: Fuster V, Walsh RA, O'Rourke RA, Poole-Wilson P. Hurst's The Heart. 12th ed. McGraw Hill Medical, New York, etc, 2008. pp. 17–46.

Verhagen AD. Funnel chest. In: Rubin A (ed.) Handbook of Congenital Malformations. W. B. Saunders Company, Philadephia, 1969. pp. 157–158.

Warkany J. Warfarin embryopathy. Teratology 1976. 14: 205–209.

Weakley FL. Anal and perinatal lesions. In: Farmer RG, Achkar E, Fleshler B (eds.) Clinical Gastroenterology. Raven Press, New York, 1983. pp. 401–407.

Wennberg PW, Rooke TW. Diagnosis and management of diseases of the peripheral arteries and veins. In: Fuster V, Walsh RA, O'Rourke RA, Poole-Wilson P. Hurst's The Heart. 12th ed. McGraw Hill Medical, New York, etc, 2008. pp. 2371–2388.

Werler MM, Mitchell AA, Shapiro S. First trimester maternal medication use in relation to gastroschisis. Teratology 1992; 45: 361–367.

Wesseling J, van Driel D, Heymans HS et al. Coumarins during pregnancy: long-term effect on growth and development of school-age children. Thromb Haemost 2001; 85: 609–613.

Wiederhorn J, Wiederhorn AK, Rahimtoola SH, Elkayam U. WPW syndrome during pregnancy: increased incidence of supraventricular arrhythmias. Am Heart J 1992; 123: 796–798.

Wong RC, Ellis CN. Physiologic skin changes in pregnancy. Semin Dermatol 1989; 8: 7–25.

Wyszinski DF. Locating genes for oral clefts in humans. In: Wyszinski DF (ed.) Cleft Lip and Palate. From Origin to Treatment. Oxford University Press, Oxford, 2002. pp. 255–264.

Own Publications

I. Bánhidy F, Ács N, Puho HE, Czeizel AE. Essential hypertension with related treatment of pregnant women and congenital abnormalities in their offspring – a population-based case-control study. Int J Epidemiol

II. Bánhidy F, Ács N, Puho HE, Czeizel AE. The efficacy of antihypertensive treatment in pregnant women with essential and gestational hypertension: a population-based study. Hypertension Res 2010, (in press)

III. Métneki J, Puho E, Czeizel AE. Maternal diseases and isolated orofacial cleft in Hungary. Birth Defects Res A 2005; 73: 617–623.

IV. Mészáros M, Czeizel AE. ECG-conduction disturbance in the first-degree relatives of children with ventricular septal defects. Clin Genet 1981; 19: 298–301.

V. Vogt G, Puho E, Czeizel AE. A population-based case-control study of isolated ocular coloboma. Ophthal Epid 2005; 12: 191–197.

VI. Bánhidy F, Ács N, Puho HE, Czeizel AE. Varicose veins of lower extremities in pregnant women and birth outcomes of their children – a population-based study. Cent Eur J Publ Health, 2010 (in press).

VII. Czeizel AE, Puho E, Ács N, Bánhidy F. Inverse association between severe nausea and vomiting in pregnancy and some congenital abnormalities. Am J Med Genet 2006; 140A: 453–462.

Chapter 11
Diseases of the Respiratory System

11.1 Respiratory System and Respiratory Function During Pregnancy

The proper function of respiratory system in collaboration with cardiovascular system is extremely important to achieve adequate oxygenation of the fetus; therefore, there are significant changes in the maternal cardio-respiratory system during pregnancy.

First, the anatomic changes of the respiratory system in pregnant women are summarized here (Whitty and Dombrowski, 2004). The level of the diaphragm rises by 4 cm and the transverse diameter of the chest increases by 2 cm, in addition, the so-called subcostal angle increases from 68 to 103°. These changes together with the enlarging uterus result in a decrease in residual volume because lungs are somewhat compressed. However, the decrease of residual lung volume does not associate with decreased ventilation because the excursion of the diaphragm in respiration increases by 1.5 cm.

Although there is no increase in respiratory rate, maternal minute ventilation is increased due to the increase of tidal volume (from 500 to 700 mL in each breath). This hyperventilation results in a compensatory alkalosis and an increase in arterial oxygenation tension in the third trimester of pregnancy. The residual volume is reduced by 20% during pregnancy, but the vital capacity (i.e. the maximum volume of gas that can be expired after a maximum inspiration) does not change during pregnancy.

Second, the oxygen delivery and consumption in pregnancy are also changed partly due to the physiological anemia of pregnancy which results in a reduction in the hemoglobin concentration and arterial oxygen content. Oxygen consumption increases steadily during pregnancy.

Third, when evaluating infectious diseases of respiratory tract we have to consider the immunology of pregnancy. In general, immune function is similar in pregnant and non-pregnant women. However, both T-cell and NK-cell function shows a decrease in pregnant women. Nevertheless, there is no clear trend towards either the suppression or enhancement of systematic immune function during gestation (Silver et al., 2004). However, new studies hypothesize that cellular immune

N. Ács et al., *Congenital Abnormalities and Preterm Birth Related to Maternal Illnesses During Pregnancy*, DOI 10.1007/978-90-481-8620-4_11,

system is weakening while humoral immune system is gaining importance during pregnancy.

Respiratory diseases in pregnancy are differentiated into infectious and non-infectious diseases. Acute infectious diseases of the respiratory system frequently complicate pregnancy. Influenza is a systemic infection with predominance of symptoms of the respiratory system; therefore, this viral disease is evaluated under respiratory tract here in this chapter. The proportion of medically recorded acute respiratory diseases depended on the severity of diseases. As our validation study showed mainly severe acute disease were recorded prospectively in prenatal maternity logbook by medical doctors.

Non-infectious diseases of the respiratory system such as allergic rhinitis (hay fever) and bronchial asthma in general are chronic pathological conditions. (Tuberculosis is discussed in Chapter 2 among infectious diseases.) Most chronic diseases were prospectively and accurately recorded in prenatal maternity logbooks.

11.2 Common Cold

The common cold is a conventional term for mild upper respiratory illnesses caused by different microorganisms mainly by viruses from picornoviridae family (rhinoviruses, echoviruses, coxsackie viruses), influenza, parainfluenza, metapneumovirus, adeno- and respiratory syncytial viruses (Makele et al., 1998). The common cold is manifested such as acute coryza or nasopharingitis with the symptoms of nasal stuffiness and discharge, sneezing, sore throat, and cough, in general without high fever (Heikkinen and Jarvinen, 2003). However, common cold is frequently followed by secondary complications including fever.

11.2.1 Results of the Study (I, II)

The common cold is the most frequently reported maternal disorder during pregnancy in the data set of the HCCSCA. Out of 22,843 cases with CA, 3,827 (16.8%) had mothers who had common cold, while out of 38,151 controls without CA, 5,475 (14.4%) were born to mothers affected with common cold. Finally, out of 834 malformed controls affected by Down syndrome, 144 (17.3%) had mothers with common cold during the study pregnancy. Birth outcomes and pregnancy complications were evaluated in control mothers with common cold, while possible associations of common cold with increased risk for CAs were analyzed by case-controls approach. Finally, the possible etiological factors such as common cold were studied in the origin of congenital cataract.

The seasonal-monthly distribution of common cold showed higher frequency between October and February with a peak in December. The usual duration of common cold without secondary complication was 1 week. However, about two-third of our pregnant women affected by common cold had longer duration due to secondary complications such as sinusitis, otitis media, laryngitis, tracheitis, bronchitis, etc and in general these mothers had fever (and consequently received antipyretic therapy).

The analysis of our pregnant women showed that about 50% of common cold was medically recorded in the prenatal maternity logbook. Major part (57%) of these pregnant women had secondary complications based on longer duration of the disease (2 weeks) and high fever (over 38.5°C). Therefore, data shown here may reflect mainly pregnant women with the secondary complications of common cold.

Common cold was diagnosed in all gestational months with somewhat higher prevalence in III–V gestational months.

Pregnant women with common cold were younger (25.1 vs. 25.5 year) with somewhat lower mean birth order (1.6 vs. 1.7) and higher proportion of professional-managerial employment (43.7% vs. 37.0%) compared to pregnant women without common cold as reference. Among case mothers 21.3% were smoker during pregnancy, but more than half of the mothers quit smoking after common cold.

The evaluation of pregnancy complications showed a higher incidence of anemia (18.9% vs. 16.3%) and a lower incidence of threatened preterm delivery (10.4% vs. 15.0%) in pregnant women with common cold compared to pregnant women without common cold as a reference. The higher rate of anemia was in agreement with the lower intake of iron in pregnant women with common cold.

Table 11.1 summarizes the birth outcomes of newborns without CA born to mothers with or without common cold.

Table 11.1 Data of birth outcomes of newborn infants without CA born to mothers with or without common cold, the latter was used as reference

	Newborn infants born to mothers				
	With (N = 5,475)		Without (N = 32,676)		
Birth outcomes	Common cold				Comparison
Quantitative	Mean	S.D.	Mean	S.D.	$p =$
Gestational age (week)	**39.3**	2.0	39.4	2.1	**0.01**
Birth weight (g)	**3,305**	487	3,271	515	**0.01**
Categorical	No.	%	No.	%	OR (95% CI)
PB	539	**9.8**	2,957	9.1	**1.2 (1.1–1.5)**
LBW	231	**4.2**	1,936	5.9	**0.8 (0.7–0.9)**

On one hand, the somewhat shorter gestational age at delivery and higher rate of PB were in agreement with the symptoms of pregnant women with fever related common cold (i.e. secondary complications). However, a lower rate of threatened preterm delivery was recorded among pregnant women with common cold. On the other hand, there was a somewhat larger birth weight and lower rate of low birthweight newborns in the group of mothers with common cold. At present, our hypothesis for these unexpected findings is that the anxiety caused by the severe but relatively short (2 weeks) common cold resulted in an improved lifestyle (a higher rate of smoking cessation and vitamin use) in the later part, mainly during the third trimester of pregnancy when fetal growth is most dominant.

Antipyretic drugs (acetylsalicylic acid, paracetamol, and dipyrone) and antimicrobial drugs (such as ampicillin, penamecillin, and clotrimazole) were used more frequently by pregnant women who suffered from common cold. However, there was no significant difference in the use of these drugs between case and control mothers with common cold. In addition, the possible teratogenic effect of acetylsalycylic acid (75, 76), paracetamol (77), dipyrone (81), ampicillin (4), penamecillin (3), and clotrimazole (28) have already been evaluated in the data set of the HCCSCA, and only ampicillin showed some association with a higher risk of cleft palate only.

Among pregnancy supplements, the use of folic acid was somewhat lower in case mothers compared to control mothers with common cold (48.6% vs. 52.1%). The intake of vitamin C was much more frequent in mother with common cold than in mothers without common cold.

The main aim of the study was to check possible associations between maternal common cold and increased risk for CAs (Table 11.2).

In the first step, possible associations of maternal common cold (mainly with secondary complications) in II and/or III gestational months with 24 isolated CA groups and 1 multiple CA group were evaluated in case-all matched control analysis and higher risk was found in 8 CA-groups. The group of mixed eye CAs did not show any association with common cold during pregnancy. However, separate analyses of different CA-entities of the eyes revealed an obvious association with congenital cataract. Thus, only this group of eye CAs is shown in Table 11.2.

In the second step, only medically recorded common cold was evaluated to limit the recall bias. The previously shown higher risk of neural-tube defect disappeared in this approach of analysis.

In the third step, all cases were compared with malformed controls (i.e. Down syndrome) with similar recall (bias) and only congenital cataract and cleft lip ± palate demonstrated higher risk.

These analyses clearly demonstrated the importance of methodology in the human studies of teratogenicity and confirmed that maternal recall bias can modify possible associations. In our studies the associations between maternal common cold and congenital cataract or cleft lip ± palate have been demonstrated by all approaches. However, this association was only found if common cold occurred in the critical period of cleft lip ± palate. On the other hand, common cold any time during pregnancy was associated with a higher risk for congenital cataract.

The explanation of these associations might be the high fever since this association could be prevented by antipyretic drug treatment in all 8 groups of CAs (Table 11.2). Therefore, the probable association of maternal complicated common cold with congenital cataract and cleft lip ± palate, and possible association with 6 other CA-groups seem to be preventable by antipyretic drug treatment. Our study previously showed that high fever can induce congenital cataract even after the lens-forming period (III).

Table 11.2 Estimation of the risk of different CAs in informative offspring of pregnant women with common cold (generally with secondary complications) and related treatment in II and/or III gestational months of pregnancy

CA groups/entities	Cases-all matched controls OR (95% CI)	Medically recorded OR (95% CI)	Comparison with malformed controls OR (95% CI)	Antipyretic drugs[a] With OR (95% CI)	Antipyretic drugs[a] Without OR (95% CI)
Isolated CAs					
Neural-tube defects	**1.7 (1.3–2.4)**	1.5 (0.9–2.4)	1.3 (0.9–1.9)	1.0 (0.6–1.7)	**2.4 (1.9–3.0)**
Congenital hydrocephaly	**6.3 (2.7–14.8)**	**3.6 (1.3–9.7)**	1.5 (0.9–2.5)	2.1 (0.7–6.8)	**2.6 (1.7–4.0)**
Congenital cataract[b]	**4.0 (1.7–9.2)**	**3.6 (1.6–8.2)**	**4.0 (2.6–6.2)**	0.6 (0.1–4.0)	**11.1 (5.3–23.3)**
Cleft lip ± palate	**3.2 (2.3–4.3)**	**2.3 (1.5–3.6)**	**1.7 (1.2–2.5)**	1.4 (0.9–2.2)	**2.9 (2.4–3.6)**
Cleft palate only	**2.0 (1.3–3.3)**	**2.3 (1.2–4.1)**	1.1 (0.7–1.8)	1.2 (0.6–2.4)	**1.7 (1.2–2.5)**
Cardiovascular CAs	**1.5 (1.3–1.8)**	**1.5 (1.2–2.0)**	1.0 (0.7–1.3)	1.0 (0.7–1.3)	**1.5 (1.3–1.8)**
Limb deficiencies	**1.7 (1.1–2.7)**	**2.2 (1.1–4.1)**	1.2 (0.8–1.9)	1.2 (0.6–2.3)	**1.8 (1.2–2.6)**
Multiple CAs	**2.1 (1.6–2.9)**	**2.0 (1.4–2.9)**	1.3 (0.9–1.9)	1.3 (0.8–2.0)	**2.0 (1.6–2.6)**
Total	**1.5 (1.4–1.6)**	**1.4 (1.3–1.6)**	1.0 (0.8–1.2)	–	–

[a]Unmatched analysis.
[b]Common cold and influenza were combined.

11.2.2 Interpretation of Results

When evaluating the association of maternal severe complicated common cold with congenital cataract and cleft lip ± palate, in addition to other possible CAs we have to differentiate four possible teratogenic effects: microbial agents, secondary complications with fever, medications, and malnourishment. We did not find any report regarding to the teratogenic effect of microbial agents causing common cold (Roulston et al., 1999). Antipyretic drugs used for the treatment of common cold did not show teratogenic effect (Heinonen et al., 1977) and the lack of teratogenicity of these and other antimicrobial drugs was confirmed in our data set as well (3, 28, 75–77, 81). Severe malnourishment may cause folate deficiency thus indirectly increase the risk for some CAs (Huang et al., 1999). However, most common colds are not so severe and long lasting that it could induce real malnourishment. Therefore, we assume that fever might be the causal factor in the origin of "hyperthermia sensitive CAs". The importance of high fever will be discussed in Part III of this monograph.

Previously Kruppa et al. (1991) found a possible association between anencephaly (the most severe form of neural-tube defects) and maternal common cold, while Zhang and Cai (1993) reported an association between common cold and neural-tube defects, hydrocephalus and cleft lip ± palate.

In conclusion, when evaluating common cold, it is necessary to differentiate the usual common cold (with short duration and without fever) and common cold with secondary complications (i.e. with longer duration and frequently high fever). The gestational age was 0.1 week shorter with a somewhat higher rate of PB, but these differences had no real clinical importance. However, an association between common cold with secondary complications in the critical period of some specific CAs such as cleft lip ± palate, congenital cataract, and possibly other CAs were found. These associations were preventable by antipyretic medications.

11.3 Acute Infectious Diseases of the Respiratory System

Acute infectious diseases of the respiratory system (AIDRS) represent a wide spectrum, and according to ICD-WHO, we differentiate sinusitis, pharyngitis, tonsillitis, laryngitis-tracheitis, bronchitis-bronchiolitis, and pneumonia. As it appeared at the analysis of our data, upper/mild category of AIDRS including sinusitis, pharyngitis, tonsillitis, laryngitis-tracheitis should be separated from lower/severe category of AIDRS comprising bronchitis-bronchiolitis, pneumonia.

AIDRS, particularly uncontrolled or poorly controlled, may cause both maternal and fetal morbity and mortality (Remington and Klein, 1995). Nevertheless, the possible associations of AIDRS with CAs and pregnancy complications have not been frequently studied (Hartert et al., 2003).

11.3.1 Results of the Study (IV, V)

The data set of the HCCSCA included 2,118 cases, 3,455 controls and 92 malformed controls born to mothers with AIDRS during pregnancy. The possible association of AIDRS with CA was checked in case-control approach, while birth outcomes and pregnancy complications in control pregnant women were compared to the reference group, i.e. pregnant women without AIDRS.

The duration of AIDRS was 1.2 ± 0.4 week in pregnant women, although the duration of AIDRS and the proportion of medically recorded diseases depended on the severity of AIDRS (e.g. the latter was nearly 100% in the group of pneumonia). Hospitalization occurred only in pregnant women with pneumonia. AIDRS were recorded more frequently in III gestational month followed by IV and V months. The monthly distribution of AIDRS showed some seasonality; the maximum was found in January followed by February while the minimum occurred in July followed by August.

Pregnant women with AIDRS were somewhat older (26.1 vs. 25.4 year) with the same birth order (1.6) and higher proportion of professional-managerial employment (47.8% vs. 37.1%) than pregnant women without AIDRS.

First, the incidence of pregnancy complications in control pregnant women with or without AIDRS as reference group was compared (Table 11.3). The occurrence of preeclampsia was lower in pregnant women with AIDRS than in pregnant women without AIDRS. However, the group of upper AIDRS category showed association with a somewhat higher incidence of nausea-vomiting in pregnancy (52.4% and 10.7%) than in the groups of lower AIDRS category (48.4% and 6.2%) both according to total (maternal and medical) and medically recorded data. These findings are mentioned because nausea and vomiting in pregnancy seems to have a protective effect for fetal death (Weigel and Weigel, 1989) and CAs (VI). The occurrence of both threatened abortion and preeclampsia-eclampsia reflected a U-shaped severity curve; they showed the highest prevalence in the groups of sinusitis and pneumonia.

Among acute maternal diseases, influenza-common cold (27.2% vs. 17.6%) and diseases of the digestive system (5.2% vs. 2.2%) occurred more frequently in pregnant women with AIDRS than in the reference group. The prevalence of bronchial asthma was also somewhat higher in pregnant women with AIDRS (0.7% vs. 0.4%).

Table 11.4 summarizes the birth outcomes of newborns without CA in pregnant women with or without AIDRS.

Mean gestational age was 0.3 week longer in pregnant women with AIDRS and this finding was in agreement with the lower rate of PB in their babies. The mean birth weight was also 57 grams larger and the rate of LBW newborns was somewhat, marginally significantly lower in newborn infants born to mothers with AIDRS during pregnancy. However, the larger mean birth weight can be explained by the longer mean gestational age at delivery.

Table 11.3 Incidence (%) of medically recorded pregnancy complications in control pregnant women with different groups of acute infectious diseases of the respiratory system and in the reference group (control pregnant women without these disease)

Pregnancy complications	Sinusitis (*N* = 250)	Pharyngitis (*N* = 1,048)	Tonsillitis (*N* = 1,165)	Laryngitis-tracheitis (*N* = 804)	Bronchitis-bronchiolitis (*N* = 398)	Pneumonia (*N* = 182)	Total (*N* = 3,455)[a]		Reference (*N* = 34,696)		Comparison OR (95% CI)
	No.	%	No.	%	No.	%	No.	%	No.	%	
Nausea/vomiting[b]	53.2	50.9	53.6	52.5	48.0	49.5	1,994	51.3	18,175	52.4	1.0 (0.9–1.1)
Nausea/vomiting only severe, treated[c]	8.8	11.2	10.3	11.6	5.0	8.8	329	9.9	3,540	10.2	0.9 (0.8–1.0)
Threatened abortion	20.4	17.5	14.7	18.3	13.1	23.1	573	16.6	5,939	17.1	1.0 (0.9–1.1)
Preeclampsia-eclampsia	9.6	7.5	5.9	7.5	8.0	9.3	254	7.4	2,904	8.6	**0.8 (0.7–0.9)**
Threatened preterm delivery	20.0	12.6	14.5	14.9	5.8	10.4	455	13.2	5,005	14.4	**0.9 (0.8–1.0)**
Placental disorders	2.0	2.4	1.6	2.0	0.3	1.6	58	1.7	534	1.5	1.1 (0.8–1.4)
Poly/oligohydramnios	0.0	1.2	0.9	0.7	0.3	0.1	26	0.8	179	0.5	1.2 (0.8–1.2)
Gestational diabetes	1.2	0.9	0.9	0.5	0.3	0.0	22	0.6	248	0.7	0.9 (0.6–1.4)
Anaemia	14.4	19.1	14.2	19.5	11.3	18.7	553	16.0	5,803	16.7	0.5 (0.8–1.0)

[a]One pregnant woman may have more than one AIDRS.
[b]Based on both retrospective maternal information and prospective medical records.
[c]Based on only prospective medical records.

Table 11.4 Birth outcomes of newborns without CAs of pregnant women with different manifestations of AIDRS or without AIDRS (reference)

	Gestational (week)		PB		Birth weight (g)		LBW newborns	
Different AIDRS	Mean	S.D.	No.	%	Mean	S.D.	No.	%
Sinusitis	39.6	1.7	14	5.6	3,348	489	13	5.2
Pharyngitis	39.6	1.7	61	5.8	3,364	476	36	3.4
Tonsillitis	39.7	1.9	63	5.4	3,340	500	56	4.8
Laryngitis–tracheitis	39.8	1.7	32	4.0	3,349	512	39	4.9
Bronchitis–bronchiolitis	39.1	2.3	49	12.3	3,271	534	26	6.5
Pneumonia	38.9	2.2	28	15.4	3,217	525	16	8.8
Total	39.6	1.9	233	6.7	3,328	503	172	5.0
Mild/upper	39.7	1.8	161	5.5	3,343	496	134	4.6
Severe/lower	39.1	2.3	75	13.0	3,255	528	40	6.9
Total	**39.6**	1.9	233	**6.7**	3,328	503	172	**5.0**
Comparison	**<0.0001**		**0.7 (0.6–0.8)**		**<0.0001**		**0.9 (0.8–1.0)**	
Reference (without AIDRS)	39.3	2.1	3,263	9.4	3,271	512	1,195	5.8

The detailed analysis of these variables in the different groups of AIDRS showed an interesting pattern. There was a significantly shorter mean gestational age and higher rate of PB in lower AIDRS category while upper AIDRS category associated with a longer mean gestational age and lower rate of PB. We did not find significant differences in the mean birth weight and the rate of LBW newborns between upper and lower AIDRS categories at the calculation of adjusted risk figures, i.e. considered confounders (among them gestational age).

We repeated these calculations based only on medically recorded AIDRS and similar associations were found.

Among drugs, antimicrobial (ampicillin, penamecillin) and antipyretic (acetylsalicylic acid, paracetamol, dipyrone) drugs had a more frequent use in mothers with AIDRS, but there was no significant difference in their administration between case and control mothers affected by AIDRS. The use of pregnancy supplements such as folic acid and multivitamins was similar in pregnant women with or without AIDRS, only vitamin C was used more frequently by pregnant women affected by AIDRS.

The association between severe lower category of AIDRS and higher rate of PB is biologically plausible due to the pathological condition of mothers related to fever, drug treatments, etc. However, the association between mild upper category of AIDRS and lower rate of PB births would need further explanation. On one hand we may hypothesize that pregnant women with mild AIDRS later may have more health conscious lifestyle. On the other hand, most pregnant women were treated by antimicrobial drugs and some of them (e.g. ampicillin) may have a beneficial effect on the parallel existing vaginal infections/disease (5) which can induce PB. In addition, paracetamol therapy also associated with a lower risk of PB (78).

The incidence of AIDRS in II and/or III gestational months in pregnant women who later delivered babies with CAs and the incidence of AIDRS in their matched controls did not show significant difference neither when evaluating the total group of CAs nor in any CA-specific group. In the next step we evaluated different groups of AIDRS separately. Tonsillitis did not show an association with the total group of CAs in II and/or III gestational months of pregnancy, but 4 CA-groups/entities showed an association with this fever related maternal diseases. (Table 11.5).

Table 11.5 Estimation of risks of maternal acute infectious diseases of the respiratory system (AIDRS) and tonsillitis in II and/or III gestational months for some CAs

	Cases-matched controls with AIDRS	Cases-matched controls with tonsillitis	With Antipyretic medication	Without Antipyretic medication
CA groups/entities	OR (95% CI)	OR (95% CI)	OR (95% CI)	OR (95% CI)
Isolated CAs				
Neural-tube defects	0.8 (0.6–1.2)	**1.9 (1.4–2.7)**	1.2 (0.6–2.3)	**2.0 (1.4–2.8)**
Congenital cataract	3.0 (0.8–12.0)	**4.4 (1.3–14.0)**	0.6 (0.1–4.0)	**8.6 (4.0–15.1)**
Cleft lip ± palate	1.2 (0.9–1.7)	**1.6 (1.1–2.4)**	0.6 (0.3–1.2)	**1.8 (1.3–2.4)**
Multiple CAs	1.0 (0.8–1.4)	**2.2 (1.3–3.9)**	1.9 (0.8–7.5)	**2.5 (1.9–3.7)**
Total	0.9 (0.8–1.0)	1.2 (0.6–1.4)	–	–

Our validation study showed that 47.7% of pregnant women with tonsillitis had high fever. (The proportion of pregnant women with high fever was lower than 20% in other groups of AIDRS.) The highest OR was found in the group of cases affected with congenital cataract, followed by cases with multiple CA. The other two CA-groups also represented the "hyperthermia sensitive" neural-tube defects and cleft lip ± palate. These data were checked in the subgroups with and without antipyretic drug treatments, and the previously found associations disappeared in the subgroup of pregnant women with antipyretic medications while these risks increased in the subgroup without this treatment. In addition, the tonsillitis-related risk for neural-tube defects and cleft lip ± palate was also reduced by periconceptional folic acid-containing multivitamin supplementation (IV).

Tonsillitis related drug treatments cannot explain the higher risk for the above-mentioned specific CA because the teratogenic effect of ampicillin (4), penamecillin (3), acetylsalicylic acid (75, 76), paracetamol (77), and dipyrone (81) was checked in the data set of the HCCSCA and only ampicillin showed some association with a higher risk for cleft palate only.

11.3.2 Interpretation of Results

Previously mainly pneumonias in pregnant women were only reported in the international literature. Pneumonia is rare during pregnancy, occurring in 1 per

118–2,288 (Whitty and Dombrowski, 2004), our incidence data, 1 in 210 pregnancies, is closer to the upper limit of this range. In most cases pathogens were not identified in our study, however, other studies showed that pneumococcus and *Haemophilus influenza* are the most common identifiable causes of pneumonia in pregnant women (Madinger et al., 1989; Berkovitz and LaSala, 1990). In the lack of comprehensive serologic testing, the true incidence of viral, *Legionella* and mycoplasma pneumonia is difficult to estimate. In our data set aspiration, varicella, and *Pneumocystis carinii* (in HIV patients) pneumonia did not occur.

Preterm delivery was found as a common complication (up to 43%) in pregnant women with pneumonia even after the introduction of antibiotic therapy (Benedetti et al., 1982; Madinger et al., 1989; Berkovitz and LaSala, 1990) with lower mean birth weight (2,770 ± 224 vs. 3,173 ± 99 g) in one study (Madinger et al., 1989). Our recent experiences were better in Hungarian pregnant women affected by pneumonia.

In conclusion, AIDRS during pregnancy have no obvious risk for pregnancy complications. However, severe lower category of AIDRS associated with a higher risk for PB, but the mild upper category of AIDRS seems to indirectly reduce the rate of PB. The latter finding need to be further studied to clarify whether this association is causal or can be explained by unevaluated confounders. Finally, AIDRS during II and III gestational month did not associate with increased risk for CAs. However, the frequently high fever related tonsillitis associated with a higher risk for congenital cataract, neural-tube defects, cleft lip ± palate, and multiple CAs. We may presume that the association between these fever sensitive CA-groups and tonsillitis may be caused by high fever. This hypothesis is supported by the fact that antipyretic medications were able to prevent this risk.

11.4 Pleurisy

Pleurisy, i.e. inflammatory reaction of the pleura often with effusion into the pleural cavity, is caused by infections such as tuberculosis or pneumonia, in addition to chemical toxins or others.

11.4.1 Interpretation of Data in the HCCSCA

Out of 22,843 cases, 8 (0.04%), while out of 38,151 controls, 12 (0.03%) had mothers with medically recorded pleurisy. Of the 8 cases, 2 were affected with hypospadias, while other CAs such as cleft lip + palate, ventricular septal defect, unspecified heart CA, polydactyly, clubfoot and exomphalos occurred in one case. Among 12 controls only one was born on the 30th gestational week with 1,250 g. The mean gestational age at delivery was 38.7 weeks with mean birth weight of 3,311 g in the control group.

11.5 Influenza

Influenza is a highly contagious acute infectious disease of the respiratory system. Influenza is caused by an RNA virus belonging to the Orthomyxoviridae family including A, B and C serotypes, but A and B are responsible for vast majority of influenza. Influenza occurs as an epidemic, generally in winter (Roberts, 1986; Parker and Collier, 1990). In Hungary most epidemic infections are due to influenza A mainly occurring between December and April. The virus is transmitted primarily by respiratory droplets and sometimes by direct contact. The latency period is about 2 days with the range of 1–5 days and the usual duration of influenza is 5 days with high fever, coryza, headache, malaise and cough. However, its clinical spectrum may include life-threatening pneumonia as well. If symptoms persist longer than 5 days, secondary bacterial infections of the respiratory system might stand behind the symptoms (Berkow and Fletcher, 1992).

Pregnant women may have a higher risk for influenza pneumonia, in new pandemics (Kort et al., 1986; Mullooly et al., 1986). For example mortality rate of pregnant women with influenza pneumonia was about 50% in 1918–1919 (Harris, 1919; Freeman and Barno, 1959).

11.5.1 Results of the Study (VII, VIII)

The data set of the HCCSCA included 1,328 cases with CA and 1,838 controls without CA, and this approach was used for the estimation of risk of different CA. In addition the birth outcomes of control newborns and medically recorded pregnancy complications in their mothers were compared to 36,313 pregnant women without influenza as reference group. Finally, the possible role of influenza in the origin of different CAs of the eye was also studied and a higher risk for congenital cataract was found (III).

All pregnant women were affected with influenza during the epidemic periods, and 72% of them were recorded in the prenatal maternity logbook. The onset of influenza according to gestational months did not show any obvious difference with the exception of low incidence in IX month. In our study 91.5% of pregnant women had fever over 38.5°C.

The mean maternal age (25.2 vs. 25.5 year) and birth order (1.6 vs. 1.7) of pregnant women with influenza was somewhat lower than in pregnant women without influenza. The proportion of professionals was somewhat higher among pregnant women with influenza (14.2% vs. 11.3%); in addition, pregnant women with influenza used vitamin C more frequently (9.1% vs. 4.2%). There was no significant difference in the use of folic acid (53.8% vs. 54.5%) and multivitamins (7.6% vs. 6.5%).

There was no difference in the occurrence of other acute infectious and chronic diseases in pregnant women with or without influenza. Penamecillin (19.9%), ampicillin (16.3%), dipyrone (13.4%), and acetylsalicylic acid (12.5%) were used most frequently for the treatment of pregnant women with influenza.

Pregnancy complications did not show a higher incidence in pregnant women affected with influenza.

The birth outcomes of newborn infants without CA born to mothers with influenza or without influenza as reference group during the study pregnancy were analyzed and the results of this evaluation showed unexpected results (Table 11.6).

Table 11.6 Birth outcomes of newborn infants born to pregnant women with influenza or without influenza

	Newborn infants born to pregnant women				
Birth outcomes	with influenza (N = 1,838)		without influenza (N = 36,313)		Comparison
Quantitative	Mean	S.D.	Mean	S.D.	$p =$
Gestational age (week)	39.5	1.9	39.4	2.1	0.12
Birth weight (g)	3,311	492	3,274	512	0.08
Categorical	No.	%	No.	%	OR (95% CI)
PB	147	8.0	3,349	9.2	0.9 (0.8–1.1)
LBW	87	4.7	2,080	5.7	0.9 (0.7–1.1)

No significant differences were seen in quantitative and categorical birth outcomes between babies of mothers who suffered from influenza during their pregnancy and those who were unaffected. It is necessary to mention that influenza occurred rarely in the third trimester of pregnancy, thus our data are not appropriate to study the possible association of maternal influenza during the third trimester with higher risk for PB.

Thus, the short duration of usual maternal influenza during the first and second trimesters of pregnancy does not induce a higher prevalence of adverse birth outcomes.

The major objective of our study was the evaluation of possible associations of maternal influenza in II and/or III months of pregnancy, in the critical period of most major CAs and CAs (Table 11.7). First, all CAs of the eye were evaluated together, however, the analysis of different eye CA-entities showed an association only between maternal influenza and congenital cataract.

Out of the 25 CA-entities, 5 showed an association with maternal influenza: congenital cataract, cleft lip ± cleft palate, cleft palate, neural-tube defects and cardiovascular CAs.

In the next step, we attempted to differentiate cases with the above five "candidate" CAs according to maternal influenza in II and/or III gestational months with or without antipyretic treatment. We did not find the above mentioned associations if maternal influenza was treated by antipyretic medications (Table 11.7).

Finally, we checked the protective effect of high dose (3–6 mg daily) folic acid supplementation in I gestational month (thus including preconceptional time window as well) followed in II gestational month for these 5 candidate CAs

Table 11.7 Estimation of the association (risk) of maternal influenza during II and/or III gestational months of pregnancy with 5 CA groups in cases-matched control analyses

Isolated CA-groups/ entities	Cases-all matched controls OR (95% CI)	Antipyretic medications With OR (95% CI)	Antipyretic medications Without OR (95% CI)
Neural-tube defect	**2.1 (1.5–3.0)**	0.7 (0.3–1.6)	**2.7 (1.8–4.0)**
Congenital cataract	**4.0 (1.7–9.2)**[a]	0.6 (0.1–4.0)	**11.1 (5.3–23.3)**
Cleft lip ± palate	**2.9 (2.2–3.9)**	1.4 (0.8–2.5)	**3.3 (2.4–4.7)**
Cleft palate only	**2.5 (1.6–4.0)**	1.3 (0.6–2.9)	**2.5 (1.4–4.5)**
Cardiovascular CA	**1.8 (1.4–2.2)**	1.4 (0.9–2.1)	**1.7 (1.3–2.2)**
Total	**1.5 (1.3–1.7)**	–	–

[a]During entire pregnancy OR (95% CI): 7.4 (3.9–14.0).

Table 11.8 The estimation of association between maternal influenza during II and/or III months of pregnancy and five candidate congenital abnormalities (CAs) with or without the use of folic acid during I and/or II months of pregnancy

Study groups	All OR (95% CI)	With folic acid OR (95% CI)	Without folic acid OR (95% CI)
Controls	Reference	Reference	Reference
Neural-tube defects	**2.1 (1.5–3.0)**	0.6 (0.1–4.0)	**2.3 (1.6–3.3)**
Congenital cataract[a]	**4.0 (1.7–9.2)**	**3.6 (1.5–8.8)**	**4.1 (1.7–9.3)**
Cleft lip± palate	**2.9 (2.2–3.9)**	1.9 (0.7–5.2)	**3.1 (2.3–4.1)**
Cleft palate only	**2.5 (1.6–4.0)**	1.4 (0.2–10.6)	**2.6 (1.6–4.2)**
Cardiovascular CAs	**1.8 (1.4–2.2)**	**2.0 (1.1–3.7)**	**1.8 (1.4–2.2)**

[a]During entire pregnancy OR (95% CI): 7.4 (3.9–14.0).

(Table 11.8). There was a significant reduction in 3 CAs: neural-tube defects, cleft lip ± palate, and cleft palate only.

11.5.2 Interpretation of Results

Our studies showed the importance of specificity of teratogens as one of the important factor in human teratology. After the evaluation of possible associations between maternal influenza and 25 different CAs, influenza demonstrated an increased risk for 5 CAs. Another important factor in human teratology is the time factor, i.e. critical period of different CAs. The previously mentioned association between maternal influenza and cleft lip ± cleft palate, neural-tube defects, cardiovascular CAs, and cleft palate only was found only if this maternal disease occurred in II and/or III gestational months. Congenital cataract was an exception of this rule: an obvious association was found between the maternal influenza and congenital cataract not only during the critical period of lens development but during the entire pregnancy. Thus, congenital cataract is not only a defect of embryogenesis but it may be connected with the fetal disease of the lens in the second and third trimesters of pregnancy.

It is also necessary to consider and differentiate the possible effects of the pathogens (i.e. influenza viruses), symptoms of the disease (particularly high fever), medications, and the secondary complications such as malnourishment. In the study by Shien and Shiota (1999) influenza viruses did not cross the placenta until late in the gestational period, i.e. after the critical period of CAs. In addition, influenza viruses caused fetal death in pregnant animals but not specific CAs. Thus, we may suppose that influenza viruses are not teratogenic. The different drugs used for the treatment for maternal influenza were evaluated in detail but these medications did not indicate any teratogenic effect. In fact some antipyretic medications showed an "anti-teratogenic" effect in our studies. The hazard of secondary complications of maternal influenza are difficult to exclude, but this hazard exists in the fetuses of all pregnant women and only 5 CAs showed association with maternal influenza. The common factor may be the high fever in the origin of these 5 CA-groups, and this hypothesis is confirmed by the protective effect of antipyretic medications.

Hyperthermia-induced CAs were detected first in animal investigations (Edwards, 1986; Edwards et al., 1995), however, later the evidences for human teratogenicity of high fever have been continuing to accumulate and an association with isolated neural-tube defects, orofacial clefts, cardiovascular CA, and multiple CA was reported is several studies (Tikkanen and Heinonen, 1991; Botto et al., 2001, 2002). The details of these results will be presented in the Part III. However, to our best knowledge, the association of high fever with cleft lip ± palate (IX, II, IV, VII), congenital cataract (III) and multiple CAs (X) were found by us, in addition we delineated the typical pattern of component CAs in high fever related MCA-syndrome (XI).

Previously Botto et al. (2004) showed that the association of maternal fever with some CAs can be reduced by folic acid containing multivitamins. Our previous studies confirmed that the periconceptional high dose folic acid or folic acid containing multivitamin supplementation can also contribute to the prevention of neural- tube defects, oral clefts and cardiovascular CA due to influenza related hyperthermia (125–131).

In conclusion, the short duration of influenza in pregnant women did not increase the risk for pregnancy complications. Our study showed that the appropriately treated pregnant women affected with influenza in the first and second trimester of pregnancy have no higher risk for PB. However, the high fever related influenza in II and/or III gestational month of pregnancy may associate with a higher risk for some "hyperthermia sensitive CAs" such as neural-tube defects, congenital cataract, cleft lip ± palate, cleft palate only, cardiovascular CAs, and multiple CAs. The main finding of our study is that this higher risk for major CA can be prevented by the parallel use of antipyretic medications and folic acid use (XII). Finally, the prevention of seasonal influenza by vaccination in pregnant women is an important and actual challenge.

Among *chronic diseases* with infectious origin only chronic bronchitis was recorded in 10 or more pregnant women.

11.6 Chronic Bronchitis and Emphysema

Chronic bronchitis is considered as the manifestation of *chronic obstructive pulmonary disease* (COPD) frequently associated with emphysema and bronchial asthma, however, the major cause of this disease is smoking.

11.6.1 Interpretation of Data in the HCCSCA

Out of 22,843 cases, 13 (0.06%), while out of 38,151 controls, 16 (0.04%) had mothers with chronic bronchitis. Of these 13 CAs, 4 were affected by cardiovascular CAs such as transposition of the great vessels, ventricular septal defect, persistent ductus arteriosus, and stenosis of the pulmonary artery while 2 cases had hypospadias. Other cases were recorded with atresia of external auditory canal, cleft lip + palate, anal atresia obstructive CA of the urinary tract (stricture of ureter), syndactyly on hands, clubfoot (talipes calcaneovalgus), and multiple CA. The risk of total CAs (1.5, 1.1–2.2) was higher, but chronic bronchitis did not show association with a higher risk of any CA group.

Among 16 control newborns, preterm baby was born only once without LBW newborns, thus their mean gestational age (39.8 week) and birth weight (3,369 g) exceeded the Hungarian baseline figures.

Thus, although risk of total CAs was higher in the offspring of pregnant women with chronic bronchitis, the birth outcomes of their newborns without CA showed a better pattern than the reference sample. Nevertheless, this disease needs further studies.

Chronis bronchitis and *emphysema* frequently have the same etiology, therefore the birth outcomes of two pregnant women with emphysema are mentioned here. One pregnant woman had an affected case with multiple CA while another delivered a healthy baby on the 41st week with 3,400 g.

11.7 Allergic Rhinitis

Allergic diseases occurred in 18–30% of women in childbearing age but recently an increasing trend was found. Thus, allergic conditions and related treatments might cause medical problems in pregnant women as well.

Among allergic disease, *allergic rhinitis* (AR) is also quite frequent during pregnancy (Sibbald, 1993; Mazzotta et al., 1999; Ellegard et al., 2000; Incaudo, 2004).

The seasonal or perennial exposure of atopic individuals to allergens leads to symptoms of sneezing, watery rhinorrhoea, nasal congestion, and itching in patients with AR which may be accompanied by allergic conjunctival reactions (conjunctival itching and lacrimation) or even bronchial hyperresponsiveness. Severe symptoms of AR prevent normal sleep and results in tiredness, thirst, poor concentration, and headache. Uncontrolled symptoms may lead to significant impairment of work productivity, social activities, or school performance. Juniper (1997) stated on the basis of their study that quality of life in AR can be worse than in bronchial asthma.

Obviously the AR-associated symptoms and related drug treatments may have some effects on pregnant women and their fetuses, nevertheless – to our best knowledge – so far the results of controlled epidemiological studies of pregnant women regarding to their risk of pregnancy complications, adverse birth outcomes, and particularly CAs have not been published. These facts motivated us to define the aims of our study.

11.7.1 Results of the Study (XIII)

The preliminary analysis of the data set of the HCCSCA regarding to AR showed that 379 control and 176 case mothers were recorded. However, the diagnosis of AR based on retrospective maternal information was not reliable. The diagnosis of AR was prospectively recorded in the prenatal care logbook in 84% of case mothers and 88% of control mothers, thus we decided to evaluate only these recorded cases. Out of 22,843 cases, 148 (0.65%) had mothers with AR, while 334 (0.88%) control mothers were recorded with AR among 38,151 controls. There was an increasing trend in the prevalence of AR in pregnant women during the study period.

Most pregnant women had AR before their conception; however, about one-third had the onset of AR during the study pregnancy with similar frequency in the first and second trimesters. The onset of AR was rare in the third trimester.

The mean maternal age (26.6 vs. 25.5 year) was higher in pregnant women with AR compared to pregnant women without AR which was used as reference. Nevertheless, their mean birth order was lower (1.4 vs. 1.6). The proportion of professional women (22.5% vs. 11.3%) was much higher among pregnant women with AR. The folic acid supplementation was much more frequent in pregnant women with AR (71.3% vs. 54.5%) and a similar trend was found in the use of multivitamins (12.9% vs. 6.6%).

The evaluation of maternal diseases showed obvious differences between pregnant women with or without AR (Table 11.9).

Among acute diseases, influenza-common cold, acute infectious diseases of the respiratory and digestive system occurred more frequently. However, there was no significant difference in their incidences between case and control mothers with AR. The evaluation of chronic diseases showed a much higher prevalence of bronchial asthma among pregnant women with AR.

Several drugs such as chloropyramine, xylometazoline, budesonide, dimethindene, ketotifene, clemastine, beclomathasone were used for the treatment of pregnant women with AR. All drug treatments were medically recorded and only chloropyramine was used more frequently by case mothers than by control mothers with AR.

There was no difference in the incidence of pregnancy complications between pregnant women with or without AR.

Table 11.9 Diseases in case and control pregnant women with or without AR

	Case mothers				Control mothers			
	Without AR (N = 22,695)		With AR (N = 148)		Without AR (N = 37,817)		With AR (N = 334)	
Diseases	No.	%	No.	%	No.	%	No.	%
Acute infectious disease groups								
Influenza–common cold	4,927	21.7	40	27.0	6,987	18.5	75	22.5
Respiratory system	2,094	9.2	24	16.2	3,404	9.0	51	15.3
Digestive system	723	3.2	19	12.8	902	2.4	31	9.3
Urinary tract	1,570	6.9	12	8.1	2,279	6.0	15	4.5
Genital organs	1,658	7.3	14	9.5	2,860	7.6	25	7.5
Others	378	1.7	8	5.4	500	1.3	12	3.6
Chronic diseases								
Diabetes mellitus	56	0.3	0	0.0	50	0.1	2	0.6
Epilepsy	69	0.3	1	0.7	69	0.2	0	0.0
Asthma bronchiale	505	2.2	6	4.1	737	1.9	22	6.6

Table 11.10 Birth outcomes of newborns without CA of pregnant women with or without AR

Birth outcomes	Mothers without AR (N = 37,817)		Mothers with AR (N = 334)		Comparison	
Quantitative	Mean	S.D.	Mean	S.D.	t	p
Gestational age (week)	39.4	2.1	**39.8**	1.8	2.97[a]	**0.003**
Birth weight (g)	3,275	512	3,344	485	1.63[b]	0.1
Categorical	No.	%	No.	%	$\chi^2 =$	$p =$
PB	3,484	9.2	13	**3.9**	11.26[a]	**0.0008**
LBW newborns	2,154	5.7	14	4.2	1.40[b]	0.24

[a]Adjusted for employment status.
[b]Adjusted for employment status and gestational age at delivery.

Birth outcomes of newborns without CA showed obvious differences in the groups of pregnant women with or without AR (Table 11.10):

The mean gestational age was longer by 0.4 week in the AR group and these findings were reflected in a significant reduction of PB. There was a larger mean birth weight by 69 g, but it can be explained by the longer gestational age at delivery because there was no significant difference in the rate of LBW newborns.

Finally, the risk of different CAs in cases born to mothers with AR during the entire pregnancy or in II and/or III gestational months was estimated by comparing cases to their matched controls. There was no increased risk for the total CA-groups or any CA-group in the offspring of case mothers with AR than in the mothers of their all matched controls. In fact the adjusted OR in the total group of CAs was lower (0.8, 0.6–0.9). However, if folic acid use was considered as confounder, there was no lower risk for the group of total CAs (0.9, 0.8–1.1) and any specified CA-group.

11.7.2 Interpretation of Results

Four main results of the study that are worth discussing:

(i) There is some relationship between AR and some other (mainly respiratory and digestive) diseases in pregnant women (Shaaban et al., 2008).

(ii) AR did not show association with a higher occurrence of pregnancy complications.

(iii) AR was associated with a lower rate of PB probably due to longer gestational age.

A reasonable first hypothesis for the explanation of this association is that pregnant women with AR had a better socioeconomic status and better lifestyle (e.g. higher use of folic acid and multivitamins). Folic acid, mainly in the third trimester may reduce the rate of PB (105) but we did not know it at the time of the study.

Only one study was found in the international literature which showed a similar trend. The mothers of preterm newborns with birth weight below 1,000 g had significantly less medically diagnosed AR (Savilahti et al., 2004). This preventive effect on PB is interesting from the theoretical aspect but needs some explanation. Perhaps the maternal balance between T-helper type 1 (Th1) and type 2 (Th2) cells shifted towards an excess of Th2 cells in pregnant women with AR and it may have a favorable effect on the maintenance of pregnancy.

(iv) There is no higher risk of CA in the offspring of pregnant women with AR. In addition this finding is an important argument against the teratogenic effect of drugs used for the treatment of pregnant women with AR.

In conclusion, pregnant women with AR had no higher rate of pregnancy complications and their offspring did not have a higher risk for any CA. In addition, the newborns of mothers with AR had a somewhat longer gestational age that resulted in a reduction in the rate of PB. AR therefore is not a risk factor for pregnant women.

11.8 Bronchial Asthma

Bronchial asthma (BA) is among the most frequent chronic diseases during pregnancy affecting about 1–2% of pregnant women (Demissie et al., 1998). However, recently BA shows an increasing prevalence among pregnant women as well up to 3.7% or even as high as 8.4% (Schatz, 2001; Murphy et al., 2005). Therefore, approximately 4% of women of childbearing age have a history of physician-diagnosed BA (Whitty and Dombrowski, 2004).

The main symptoms of BA are dyspnoe, coughing, retrosternal chest pain and whistling due do reversible obstructive ventilatory disorder, chronic inflammation, mucosal edema and bronchial hyperresponsiveness. Uncontrolled asthma may lead to arterial hypoxemia or even to life-threatening state of status asthmaticus.

Most studies evaluating the course of BA during pregnancy confirmed that about one-third of patients particularly with severe BA show worsening of the disease during pregnancy (Saunders et al., 1995), while previously mild BA is usually getting better (Schatz et al., 1998). BA requires adequate pharmacology therapy during pregnancy as well (Dombrowski, 1997), thus antiasthmatic drugs are one of the most common reasons for medical treatment in pregnant women. When evaluating fetal development in pregnant women with BA, it is necessary to differentiate the effect of BA, the related drug treatments, and the triggering factors of BA such as allergens, cold air, respiratory viral and bacterial infections, irritants, air pollution, stress, etc. which might induce the acute exacerbation of BA. In 1993 expert group suggested classifying mild, moderate, and severe BA according to symptoms and objective test of pulmonary function (NAEP, 1993)

Previous studies showed an association between chronically poor control of BA and intrauterine growth retardation, LBW newborns, and PB (Kallen et al., 2000; Tan and Thompson, 2000). The latter was not associated with the severity or symptoms of BA, but was associated with the use of medications (Bracken et al., 2003). Recently women with well-controlled asthma during pregnancy, however, have had outcomes as good as in their non-asthmatic counterparts (Tan and Thompson, 2000; Dombrowski et al., 2004). The aim of our study was to check birth outcomes of pregnant women with BA during the study period.

11.8.1 The results of the Study (XIV, XV)

The data set of the HCCSCA included 22,843 cases, and 511 (2.24%) had mothers with BA. Out of 38,151 controls, 757 (1.98%) had mothers with BA. In our data set 88% of pregnant women with BA were recorded prospectively in the prenatal maternity logbooks and/or other medical records. The data of the rest of the pregnant women were based on maternal information, however, the validity of their BA diagnoses was good according to our validation study.

The mean maternal age (25.8 vs. 25.4 year) was somewhat higher, but the mean birth order (1.5 vs. 1.7) was lower in mothers with BA compared to mothers without BA. There was no obvious difference in the distribution of maternal employment status. Also, there was no significant difference in the use of folic acid (56.1% vs. 54.4%). However, the use of calcium, vitamin D, and multivitamins was lower, while the treatment with tocopherol (vitamin E) was higher in pregnant women with BA.

Among acute maternal disorders during pregnancy, only diseases of the respiratory system (12.0% vs. 9.0%) showed a higher incidence in mothers with BA. Among chronic maternal disorders, previous allergic hay fever (32.9% vs. 0.8%) occurred more frequently in pregnant women with BA.

The evaluation of pregnancy complications is showed in Table 11.11.

The incidence of threatened abortions, preeclampsia-eclampsia, and particularly threatened preterm deliveries was higher in mothers with BA than in the mothers without BA.

Table 11.11 The incidence of pregnancy complications in control mothers with or without bronchial asthma (BA)

	Pregnant women				Difference between the two groups	
	Without BA ($N = 37{,}394$)		With BA ($N = 757$)			
Pregnancy complications	No.	%	No.	%	OR	95% CI
Threatened abortion	6,273	16.8	239	31.6	**2.3**	**2.0–2.7**
Nausea-vomiting, severe	3,793	10.1	76	10.0	1.0	0.8–1.3
Preeclampsia-eclampsia	1,128	3.0	33	4.4	**1.5**	**1.0–2.1**
Gestational hypertension	1,066	2.9	19	2.5	0.9	0.6–1.4
Edema in pregnancy	898	2.4	14	1.9	0.8	0.5–1.3
Renal disease without hypertension	338	0.9	11	1.5	1.6	0.9–3.0
Placental disorders[a]	573	1.5	19	2.5	1.7	0.9–2.6
Threatened preterm delivery[b]	5,098	13.6	348	46.0	**5.4**	**4.7–6.2**
Anemia	6,211	16.6	145	19.2	1.2	0.9–1.4
Poly/oligohydramnion	201	0.5	4	0.5	1.0	0.4–2.7
Gestational diabetes	266	0.7	4	0.5	0.7	0.3–2.0
Prolonged pregnancy	497	1.3	11	1.5	1.1	0.6–2.0

[a]Placenta praevia, premature separation of the placenta, antepartum haemorrhage.
[b]Including cervical incompetence.

Drugs were evaluated in two categories. *The first category* includes all antiasthmatic drugs such as fenoterol (53.2% vs. 0.0%), terbutaline (31.8% vs. 10.0%), aminophylline (18.9% vs. 5.7%), ephedrine (17.3% vs. 0.0%), dexamethasone (10.8% vs. 0.7%), salbutamol (10.2% vs. 0.0%), clenbuterol (7.4% vs. 0.0%), and bromhexine (3.2% vs. 2.1%). Some drugs (aminophylline, bromhexine, and terbutaline) were used for other indications as well, e.g. terbutaline is frequently used for the inhibition of uterine contractions in threatened preterm delivery. Inhaled corticosteroids (e.g. budesonide) and short-acting beta-agonist (e.g. carbuterol) were used rarely during the study period. *The second category* of drugs includes other frequently administered drugs (allylestrenol, diazepam, drotaverine, magnesiums) used for the treatment and/or prevention of threatened abortion in Hungary.

When evaluating birth outcomes, a significant change in sex ratio of newborns was found with a nearly 5% male excess in children born to mothers with BA compared to the babies of mothers without BA ($p < 0.0001$).

The birth outcomes of newborn infants without CA born to mother with or without BA are summarized in Table 11.12.

The mean gestational age was 0.6 week shorter in the mothers with BA compared with mothers without BA. The shorter gestational age was obvious in all birthweight groups. The difference was 177 grams in the mean birth weight between live-born babies born to mothers with BA and without BA. Of the 3 gestational age groups, 2 had a lower mean birth weight; the exception was PB group with the practically same birth weight. Both the rate of PB (14.1% vs. 9.1%) and LBW (9.0% vs. 5.6%)

Table 11.12 The distribution of mean gestational age and birth weight in newborn infants born to mothers with (BA) or without bronchial asthma (NO-BA)

Gestational age (week)		36 or less		37–41		42 or more		TOTAL				Gestational age[b]			
Birth weight (g)		BA	NO- BA	BA	NO- BA	BA	NO- BA	BA		NO-BA		BA		NO BA	
								No.	%	No.	%	Mean	S.D.	Mean	S.D.
2,499 or less		40	1,244	28	805	0	51	68	**9.0**	2,100	5.6	35.2	3.1	35.6	3.3
2,500–3,499		66	2,118	402	18,783	23	1,447	491	64.9	22,348	59.8	38.6	1.8	39.1	1.8
3,500 or more		1	28	166	10,608	31	2,310	198	26.2	12,946	34.6	40.2	1.3	40.5	1.1
Total	No.	107	3,390	596	30,196	54	3,808	757	100	37,394	100	**38.8**	2.2	39.4	2.1
	%	14.1	9.1	78.7	80.8	7.1	10.2	100	–	100	–	–	–	–	–
Birth weight[a]	Mean	2,484	2,483	3,220	3,326	3,541	3,617	**3,102**	–	3,279	–	–	–	–	–
	S.D.	487	437	434	430	411	487	520	–	511	–	–	–	–	–

$PB < 0.0001$.
LBW: $p < 0.0001$.
[a]Adjusted for employment status: $p < 0.0001$.
[b]Adjusted for employment status: $p < 0.0001$.

was much higher in the group of mothers with BA. There was no difference in these variables between boys and girls born to mothers with BA.

In the next step, we differentiated control mothers with BA into three groups according to therapy: (i) 401 pregnant women without antiasthmatic therapy who did not receive medication because their doctors did not recommend to use these drugs due to the supposed teratogenic effect and steroid-phobia, (ii) 204 pregnant women with old fashion antiasthmatic treatment and (iii) 152 pregnant women with inhaled steroid treatment. The rate of PB was 17.2, 12.3 and 8.6% in the first, second, and third group with significant differences among these subgroups of pregnant women with BA.

Finally, the risk of different CAs was evaluated in informative offspring of pregnant women with BA. Out of 25 CA groups, clubfoot showed a slightly higher risk (1.5, 1.1–2.2). In addition, cardiovascular CAs (1.4, 1.0–1.8) and multiple CAs (1.6, 1.0–2.6) had marginally increased risk, and these 3 CAs explained the marginal increase in the risk for total CA group (1.2, 1.0–1.3). However, after the evaluation of medically recorded BA in pregnant women, BA only demonstrated a higher risk (1.3, 1.0–2.5) for clubfoot (including mainly deformation type). The deformation type clubfoot is more frequent in premature and/or LBW newborns/infants (XVI, XVII). When these adverse birth outcomes were considered as confounder, this weak association has disappeared.

11.8.2 Interpretation of Results

There are two main findings of the study.

First, there was a shorter gestational age in women with BA and it explains the significantly higher proportion of PB. The lower birth weight and higher proportion of LBW newborns are mainly the secondary consequences of shorter gestational age in newborns of pregnant women with BA.

The old hypothesis of BA effects on fetal development and consequent birth outcomes was hypoxia caused by the exacerbation of BA during pregnancy (Gordon et al., 1970). Acute asthmatic attacks can lead to dangerously low fetal oxygenation; therefore, poor asthma control is associated with adverse birth outcomes. Bracken et al. (2003) explained the higher proportion of PB by drugs used for the treatment of BA during pregnancy. Gestational age was reduced by 2.22 weeks in women treated by oral steroids daily and by 1.11 weeks after theophylline. In the study of Schatz et al. (2004) the use of inhaled beta-agonist, inhaled steroids and theophylline did not increase the risk of CA, PB and LBW newborns, but the use of oral corticosteroids associated with a higher risk with PB and LBW newborns.

On the other hand, some previous reports suggested that BA during pregnancy may provide a risk for the intrauterine development of the fetus (Kallen et al., 2000; Tan and Thompson, 2000; Schatz et al., 1990; Liu et al., 2001). This increased risk (24%) for intrauterine growth retardation occurred in pregnant women with asthmatic attacks and there was a dose-effect (number of asthmatic attacks and degree of LBW) relation (Dombrowski, 1997; Olesen et al., 2001). However, after the use of inhaled steroids in pregnant women with BA, there was no intrauterine fetal retardation (Namazy et al., 2004).

Therefore, recent studies did not show an association between BA and PB and/or LBW after the improved quality of treatment of BA (Hartert et al., 2003; Dombrowski et al., 2004). This finding was confirmed by the results of our study as well. If pregnant women with BA were treated with inhaled steroids, there was no higher risk for PB while untreated pregnant women with BA had a much higher risk for PB. Thus, as ACOG-ACA (2000) stated: the inhaled therapies are the cornerstone of modern treatment of pregnant women with BA. Thus the treatment of BA during pregnancy should be based on inhaled corticosteroids and short-acting beta-agonist, in some cases on inhaled chromones, on anticholinergics, and/or oral leukotriene receptor antagonists, while inhaled long-acting beta-agonists, oral theophylline derivatives, or oral corticosteroids are needed in more severe cases.

The second major finding of our study was that maternal BA during pregnancy and related drug treatment did not associate with a higher risk for CAs and it is an indirect evidence against the teratogenic effect of antiasthmatic drugs as well. Our previous study based on the data set of the HCCSCA showed a very weak teratogenic effect of oral corticosteroids which was not found after their inhaled treatment (70). However, a somewhat higher rate of skeletal CA particularly pectus excavatum was found in children born to mothers with aminophylline treatment (90).

In addition, there were some unexpected findings in our study. The proportion of boys was significantly higher in the newborn infants of mothers with BA compared to mothers without BA. The proportion of threatened abortions was 1.9 times higher in the mothers with BA, but a higher rate of fetal death, in general, associated with a girl excess due to the higher loss of boys. Thus, the expected and observed sex ratio is different and possible association between the sex of the babies and maternal BA needs further evaluations.

The incidence of threatened preterm delivery was also 3.4 times higher in mothers with BA than in mothers without BA, and it may be related to asthmatic attacks. Fortunately, the rate of preterm births was only 1.5 fold in mothers with BA, thus, medical care and medications used for the prevention of preterm births seem to be effective in pregnant women with BA.

Our study confirmed some well-known facts: the higher occurrence of acute infectious diseases of the respiratory system and previous allergic rhinitis in women with BA.

Unfortunately, our findings indicate that the Hungarian old-fashioned protocols of antiasthmatic therapies were not appropriate for the protection of fetal development from the hazard of maternal BA, thus it is necessary to urgently introduce modern therapy of BA during pregnancy as well. Good control of BA is essential for maternal and fetal well-being.

The most important criterion of BA therapy is the prevention of hypoxic episodes in mothers and in their fetuses (Schatz et al., 1990). First, it is necessary to avoid or to control factors that trigger BA. The most effective way to achieve this goal is patient education. The second step is pharmacotherapy in pregnant women with moderate or severe BA including three classes of inhaled anti-inflammatory medications: inhaled corticosteroids, nedocromil sodium and cromolyn sodium (Fanta, 2009).

In conclusion, our findings indicate that inappropriately treated BA can shorten the duration of pregnancy while modern therapeutical guidelines can significantly reduce the risk of adverse birth outcomes in pregnant women with BA.

11.9 Others

Epistaxis, i.e. hemorrhage from nose, was recorded in 4 (0.02) case and 5 (0.01%) control mothers in our data set. Four cases were affected by the absence of the auditory canal and auricle, ventricular septal defect, clubfoot, and multiple CA. All controls were born between 38 and 40 gestational week with a mean birth weight of 3,302 g. However, one girl was born on the 38th week with 2,500 g.

Pneumothorax was recorded in 2 case mothers affected by hypospadias and congenital limb deficiency while 1 control was born on 41st gestational week with 2,900 g.

11.10 Final Conclusions

Diseases of the respiratory system are the most frequent pathological conditions in pregnant women with a high and underestimated risk for adverse birth outcomes such as CA, PB, and LBW of their children. However, the appropriate medical management can reduce these risks drastically, and it is an important task is to use them as wide as possible.

References

ACOG-ACA. The use of newer asthma and allergy medications during pregnancy. The American College of Obstetricians and Gynecologists (ACOG) and The American College of Allergy, A. a. I. A., Ann Allergy Asthma Immunol 2000; 84: 475–480.

Benedetti TJ, Valle R, Ledger W. Antepartum pneumonia in pregnancy. Am J Obstet Gynecol 1982; 144: 412–417.

Berkovitz K, LaSala A. Risk factors associated with the increasing prevalence of pneumonia during pregnancy. Am J Obstet Gynecol 1990; 163: 981–985.

Berkow R, Fletcher AJ. The Merck Manual of Diagnosis and Therapy. 16th ed. Merck and Co Inc, Rahury, NY, 1992.

Botto LD, Olney RS, Erickson JD. Vitamin supplements and the risk for congenital anomalies other than neural tube defects. Am J Med Genet C 2004; 125C: 12–21.

Botto LD, Lynberg MC, Erickson JD. Congenital heart defects, maternal febrile illness, and multivitamin use: a population-based study. Epidemiology 2001; 12: 485–490.

Botto LD, Erickson JD, Mulinare J et al. Maternal fever, multivitamin use and selected birth defects: evidence or interaction. Epidemiology 2002; 13: 620–621.

Bracken MB, Triche EW, Belanger K, Saftlas A, Beckett WS, Leaderes BP. Asthma symptoms, severity, and drug therapy: a prospective study of effects on 2,205 pregnancies. Obstet Gynecol 2003; 102: 739–752.

Demissie K, Breckenbridge MB, Rhoads GG. Infant and maternal outcomes in the pregnancies of asthmatic women. Am J Resp Crit Care Med 1998; 158: 1091–1095.

Dombrowski MP. Pharmacologic therapy of asthma during pregnancy. Obstet Gynecol Clin North Am 1997; 24: 559–574.

Dombrowski MP, Schatz M, Wise R et al. Asthma during pregnancy. Obstet Gynecol 2004; 103: 5–12.

Edwards MJ. Hyperthermia as a teratogen: a review of experimental studies and their clinical significance. Terat Carcinog Mutag 1986; 6: 563–582.

Edwards MJ, Shiota K, Walsh DA, Smith MS. Hyperthermia and birth defects. Reprod Toxicol 1995; 9: 411–425.

Ellegard E, Hellgren M, Karlsson G. The incidence of pregnancy rhinitis. Gynecol Obstet Invest 2000; 49: 98–101.

Fanta CH. Asthma. New Engl J Med 2009; 360: 1002–1014.

Freeman DW, Barno A. Death from Asian influenza associated with pregnancy. Am J Obstet Gynecol 1959; 78: 1172–1175.

Gordon M, Niswanden KR, Berendes H, Kantor AG. Fetal morbidity following potentially anoxigenic obstetric conditions. Am J Obstet Gynecol 1970; 106: 421–429.

Harris JW. Influenza occurring in pregnant women. Am J Med Ass 1919; 72: 978–980.

Hartert TV, Nenzil KM, Mitchel EE et al. Maternal morbidity and perinatal outcomes among pregnant women with respiratory hospitalization during influenza season. Am J Obstet Gynecol 2003; 189: 1705–1712.

Heikkinen T, Jarvinen A. The common cold. Lancet 2003; 361: 51–59.

Heinonen OP, Slope D, Shapiro S. Birth Defects and drugs in Pregnancy. Publishing Sciences Group, Littleton, MA, 1977.

Huang RF, Ho YH, Lin HL et al. Folate deficiency induces a Cell-cycle-specific apoptosis in Hep62 Cells. J Nutr 1999; 129: 25–31.

Incaudo GA. Diagnosis and treatment of allergic rhinitis and sinusitis during pregnancy and lactation. Clin Rev Allergy Immunol 2004; 27: 159–177.

Juniper EF. Measuring health-related quality of life in rhinitis. J Allergy Clin Immunol 1997; 99: S742–S749.

Kallen B, Rydhstroem H, Aberg A. Asthma during pregnancy–a population-based study. Eur J Epidemiol 2000; 16: 167–171.

Kort BA, Cefalo RC, Baker VV. Fatal influenza A pneumonia in pregnancy. Am J Perinatol 1986; 3: 179–182.

Kruppa K, Holmberg PC, Kousma E et al. Anencephaly and maternal common cold. Teratology 1991; 44: 51–55.

Liu S, Wen SW, Demissie K et al. Maternal asthma and pregnancy outcomes: a retrospective cohort study. Am J Obstet Gynecol 2001; 184: 90–96.

Madinger NE, Greenspoon JS, Gray-Ellrodt A. Pneumonia during pregnancy: has modern technology improved maternal and fetal outcome? Am J Obstet Gynecol 1989; 161: 657–652.

Makele MJ, Puhakka T, Ruskanen O et al. Viruses and bacteria in the etiology of common cold. J Clin Microbiol 1998; 36: 539–542.

Mazzotta P, Loebstein R, Koren G. Treating allergic rhinitis in pregnancy. Safety considerations. Drug Saf 1999; 20: 361–375.

Mullooly JP, Barker WH, Nolan TF Jr. Risk of acute respiratory disease among pregnant women during influenza A epidemics. Publ Health Rep 1986; 101: 205–211.

Murphy VE, Gibson PG, Smith R et al. Asthma during pregnancy: mechanism and treament implications. Eur Respir J 2005; 25: 731–750.

NAEP: National Asthma Education Program. Management of Asthma During Pregnancy, Report on the Working Group on Asthma and Pregnancy, September 1993. NIH Publications No. 93-3279.

Namazy J, Schatz M, Long L et al. Use of inhaled steroids by pregnant asthmatic women does not reduce intrauterine growth. J Allergy Clin Immunol 2004; 113: 427–432.

Olesen C, Thrane N, Nielsen GL, Sorensen HT, Olsen J, EuroMAP Group. A population-based prescription study of asthma drugs during pregnancy: changing the intensity of asthma therapy and perinatal outcomes. Respiration 2001; 68: 256–261.

Parker MT, Collier LH. Topley Wilson Principle of Bacteriology, Virology and Immunity. Decker BC, Hamilton, OT, 1990.

Remington JS, Klein JO (eds.) Infectious Diseases in the fetus and newborn Infant. 4th ed. W. B. Saunders, Philadelphia, 1995.

Roberts RB. Infectious Diseases: Pathogenesis, Diagnosis and Therapy. Years Book Medical Publ, Chicago, 1986.

Roulston A, MarCellus RC, Branton PE. Viruses and apoptosis. Ann Rec Microbiol 1999; 53: 577–628.

Saunders B, Porreco R, Sperling W, Kagnoff M, Benenson AS. Perinatal outcomes in the pregnancies of asthmatic women: a prospective controlled analysis. Am J Respir Crit Care Med 1995; 151: 1170–1174.

Savilahti E, Siltanen M, Pekkamen J, Kajosaari M. Mothers of very low birth weight infants have less atopy than mothers of full-term infants, Clin Exp Allergy 2004; 34: 1851–1854.

Schatz M. The efficacy and safety of asthma medications during pregnancy. Semin Perinatol 2001; 25: 145–152.

Schatz M, Zeiger R, Hoffman C et al. Intrauterine growth is related to gestational pulmonary function in pregnant asthmatic women. Kaiser-Permanente Asthma and Pregnancy Study Group. Chest 1990; 98: 389–392.

Schatz M, Harden K, Forsythe A et al. The course of asthma during pregnancy and with successive pregnancies; a prospective analysis. J Allergy Clin Immunol 1998; 81: 12–18.

Schatz M, Dombrowsky MP, Wise R et al. The relationship of asthma medication use to perinatal outcomes. J Allergy Clin Immunol 2004; 113: 1040–1045.

Shaaban R, Zureik M, Soussan D et al. Rhinitis and onset of asthma: a longitudinal population-based study. Lancet 2008; 382: 1049–1057.

Shien JH, Shiota K. Folic acid supplementation of pregnant mice suppresses heat-induced neural-tube defects in offspring. J Nutr 1999; 129: 2070–2073.

Sibbald B. Epidemiology of allergic rhinitis. In: Burr ML (ed.) Epidemiology of Clinical Allergy. Monographs in Allergy. Karger, Basel, 1993. pp. 61–79.

Silver RM, Peltier MR, Branch DW. The immunology of pregnancy. In: Creasy RK, Resnik MD, Iams JD (eds.) Maternal-Fetal Medicine. 5th ed. Saunders, Philadelphia, 2004. pp. 89–109.

Tan KS, Thomson NC. Asthma in pregnancy. Am J Med 2000; 109: 727–733.

Tikkanen J, Heinonen OP. Maternal hyperthermia during pregnancy and cardiovascular malformations in the offspring. Eur J Epidemiol 1991; 7: 628–635.

Weigel MM, Weigel R. Nausea and vomiting o early pregnancy and pregnancy outcome. An epidemiological study. Br J Obstet Gynaecol 1989; 96: 1304–1311.

Whitty JE, Dombrowski MP. Respiratory disease in pregnancy. In: Creasy RK, Resnik MD, Iams JD (eds.) Maternal-Fetal Medicine. 5th ed. Saunders, Philadelphia, 2004. pp. 953–974.

Zhang J, Cai WW. Association of the common cold in the first trimester of pregnancy with birth defects. Pediatrics 1993; 92: 559–563.

Own Publications

I. Bánhidy F, Ács N, Puho HE, Czeizel AE. Pregnancy complications and delivery outcomes of pregnant women with common cold. Cent Eur J Publ Health 2006; 14: 12–16.

II. Ács N, Bánhidy F, Puho HE, Czeizel AE. Population-based case-control study of the common cold during pregnancy and congenital abnormalities. Eur J Epidemiol 2006; 21: 65–75.

III. Vogt G, Puhó E, Czeizel AE. Population-based case-control study of isolated congenital cataract. Birth Defects Res A 2005; 73: 997–1005.
IV. Ács N, Bánhidy F, Puho HE, Czeizel AE. Acute respiratory infections during pregnancy and congenital abnormalities. A population-based case-control study. Cong Anom (Kyoto) 2006; 46: 86–96.
V. Bánhidy F, Ács N, Puho HE, Czeizel AE. Maternal acute respiratory infectious diseases during pregnancy and birth outcomes. Eur J Epidemiol 2008; 23: 29–35.
VI. Czeizel AE, Puho E, Ács N, Bánhidy F. Inverse association between severe nausea and vomiting in pregnancy and some congenital abnormalities. Am J Med Genet 2006; 140A: 453–462.
VII. Ács N, Bánhidy F, Puho HE, Czeizel AE. Maternal influenza during pregnancy and risk of congenital abnormalities in offspring. Birth Defects Res A 2005; 73: 989–996.
VIII. Ács N, Bánhidy F, Puho E, Czeizel AE. Pregnancy complications and delivery outcomes of pregnant women with influenza. J Mat Fetal Neonat Med 2006; 19: 135–140.
IX. Métneki J, Puhó E, Czeizel AE. Maternal diseases and isolated orofacial clefts in Hungary. Birth Defects Res A 2005; 73: 617–623.
X. Czeizel AE, Puho HE, Ács N, Bánhidy F. High fever-related maternal diseases as possible cause of multiple congenital abnormalities: a population-based case-control study. Birth Defects Res A 2007; 79: 544–551.
XI. Czeizel AE, Puho HE, Ács N, Bánhidy F. The delineation of a multiple congenital abnormality syndrome in the offspring of pregnant women with high fever related disorders – a population-based study. Cong Anom (Kyoto) 2008; 48:
XII. Czeizel AE, Ács N, Bánhidy F et al. Primary prevention of congenital abnormalities due to high fever related maternal diseases by antifever therapy and folic acid supplementation. Current Woman's Health 2007; 3: 1–12.
XIII. Somoskövi Á, Brtfay Z, Tamási L et al. Population-based case-control study of allergic rhinitis during pregnancy for birth defects. Eur J Obstet Gynecol Reprod Biol 2007; 131: 21–27.
XIV. Tamási L, Somoskövi Á, Müller V et al. A population-based case-control study on the effect of bronchial asthma during pregnancy for congenital abnormalities of offspring. J Asthma 2006; 43: 81–86.
XV. Ács N, Bánhidy F, Puho E, Czeizel AE. Association between bronchial asthma in pregnancy and shorter gestational age in a population-based study. J Mat Fetal Neonat Medic 2005; 18: 107–112.
XVI. Czeizel AE, Bellyei A, Kranicz J et al. Confirmation of the multifactorial threshold model for congenital talipes equinoivarus. J Med Genet 1981; 18: 99–100.
XVII. Czeizel AE, Tasnady G. Congenital structural talipes equinovarus. In: Czeizel AE, Tasnady G (eds.) Aetiological Studies of Isolated Common Congenital Abnormalities in Hungary. Akadémiai Kiadó, Budapest, 1984. pp. 185–203.

Chapter 12
Diseases of the Digestive System

12.1 Alterations in Gastrointestinal and Liver Functions during Pregnancy

Animal experiments and limited number of human investigations, in addition to clinical experiences suggested that gastrointestinal motility is inhibited during pregnancy due to metabolic and hormonal changes. Particularly the higher level of progesterone mediates this inhibitory effect inducing several digestive symptoms and diseases (Scott and Abu-Hamada, 2004).

The swallowed bolus form the pharynx is transported to the stomach through the motility function (sequential peristaltic contractions) of the *oesophagus* through the relaxed lower oesophageal sphincter. However, the oesophagus must defend itself from the backward transport of gastroduodenal contents, i.e. reflux, because the digested gastroduodenal content may injure the oesophageal mucosa inducing erosive oesophagitis and stricture formation or may associate with their aspiration causing harmful acidic injury in the respiratory system. The peristaltic motility of the oesophagus did not show obvious change during pregnancy, but the resting pressure of lower oesophageal sphincter is reduced parallel with the progression of pregnancy.

There are two important functions of the *stomach*. The first function is related to production of hydrogen ion, gastric acid by the parietal cells in the fundic mucosa of the stomach. The effects of gastric acids have at least three directions: (a) provide the optimal pH for the activation of pepsinogen to pepsin with proteolytic function, (b) induce a hostile environment for pathogenic organisms, and (c) helps the absorption of special nutrients such as ionic iron and ascorbic acid. On the other hand, the adverse effects of gastric acids are also known in the pathogenesis of gastric and/or duodenal ulcers and gastro-oesophageal reflux disease. The second function of the stomach is its motor activity resulting in controlled emptying of the stomach contents. There is a slower gastric emptying with higher residual volume at the end of pregnancy and equivocal changes in acid and pepsin secretion.

The *small intestine* is the major location of digestion and absorption of nutrients. The transit time in the small intestine depends on the activity of the peristaltic movement, and it is slower during pregnancy. Thus the prolonged transit time may have

N. Ács et al., *Congenital Abnormalities and Preterm Birth Related to Maternal Illnesses During Pregnancy*, DOI 10.1007/978-90-481-8620-4_12,

beneficial (such as facilitation of absorption of food components) and unpleasant (bloating and distension) effects during pregnancy.

There are also two important functions of the *colon*. The peristaltic motility function of the colon results in the periodic transfer of luminal contents from the proximal part of colon to the distal part of colon and rectum with periodic evacuation of stool. However, the proximal part of the colon is very important in the electrolyte and water absorption and this function concentrates and desiccates the content of the colon. The colonic motility was found to be reduced in the whole colon with an increased transit time, while sodium and water absorption was increased on the proximal part of the colon in pregnant women and these phenomena may explain the higher occurrence of constipation during pregnancy.

The size of the *liver* and hepatic blood flow do not increase during pregnancy but because cardiac output and blood flow increases to other organs there is a decrease in the relative proportion of cardiac output to the liver. On the other hand, the production of serum proteins, fibrinogen, cholesterol, and transferrin is increased in pregnant women explained by their hormonal, mainly hyperestrogenic state. However, the total serum protein/albumin concentration is diminished by 20% in mid-pregnancy due to expansion of the plasma volume (Joshi et al., 2010).

The symptoms and/or disorders of the digestive system are common in pregnant women (Singer and Brandt, 1991; Fagan, 2002). These maternal disorders can be divided into two groups. The first group includes gastrointestinal disorders specific to pregnancy such as nausea, vomiting, and hyperemesis gravidarum, in addition to intrahepatic cholestatis of pregnancy. The second group comprises gastrointestinal disorders incidental to pregnancy, e.g. dyspepsia, peptic ulcer disease, inflammatory bowel diseases, and constipation (Williamson, 2001; Welsh, 2005).

12.2 Disorders of the Teeth

Diseases of the teeth, mainly severe caries were reported in 6 case mothers and 12 control mothers, obviously these numbers indicate a very significant underascertainment of this disease group, thus is not appropriate for analysis.

12.3 Periodontal Diseases

This group of diseases includes gingivitis, periodontitis, other periodontal diseases (such as epulis), disease of the jaws, stomatitis, glossitis, etc.

12.3.1 Results of the Study (I)

The case group of the HCCSCA included 22,843 cases and among them 21 (0.09%) children with CA had mothers with *periodontal disease in pregnancy* (PDP). Out of 38,151 controls, 17 (0.04%) newborn infants were born to mothers affected with PDP. (One control with her mother affected with erytroplakia was omitted from this analysis). There was a shorter mean gestational age (38.9 vs. 39.4 week) and somewhat lower mean birth weight (3,244 vs. 3,276 g) in 17 control children but only one was born as preterm baby (5.9% vs. 9.2%). Obviously this low number of children is not appropriate for analysis.

Among maternal diseases, acute diseases of respiratory system occurred more frequently in case (19.0%) and control (23.5%) mothers with PDP than in 60,956 pregnant women without PDP (9.1%). Of these 4 case mothers, 2 were affected with tonsillitis and 2 with pharyngitis, while of these 4 control mothers, 2 had pharyngitis, 1 tonsillitis and 1 sinusitis. Chronic diseases such as diabetes mellitus, epilepsy, etc, did not show different prevalence in the study groups.

Of 21 case mothers, 15 (71.4%) were treated with antimicrobial drugs (ampicillin 5, doxycycline 3, penamecillin 2, clindamycin 2, cephalosporins 2, metrodinazole 1), while of 17 control mothers, 15 (88.2%) had antimicrobial drug treatment (ampicillin 5, penamecillin 3, doxycycline 3, metrodinazole 2, cephalosporins 2). In addition 15 case and 11 control mothers were treated with analgesic drugs, mainly dipyrone. There was no significant difference in the frequency of different drug treatments between case and control mothers with PDP.

However, of the 21 cases, 6 (28.6%) were affected with cleft lip ± palate and it means a very obvious association with PDP (10.7, 4.2–27.3). Cleft palate only occurred in 2 cases (7.9, 1.8–34.2). Four cases had hypospadias (3.0, 1.0–9.0) while cardiovascular CAs and poly/syndactyly were recorded in 2–2 cases. The rest 5 cases were affected with different CAs such as oesophageal stenosis, anal atresia, undescended testis, primary microcephaly, multiple CA (renal agenesis + CA of ear + atrial septal defect, type II).

Thus a very obvious association was found between the higher risk for isolated orofacial clefts and PDP. Four cases had hypospadias, but the critical period of hypospadias is in III and/or IV gestational month, and only one case with hypospadias was born to mother with PDP during this time window. However, it is worth focusing this analysis to PDP during II and/or III gestational month, the critical period of most major CAs. We found again a much higher risk of cleft lip ± palate based on 4 cases (15.9, 4.7–53.5). There was only one case with cleft palate only. Two cases with poly/syndactyly had mothers with PDP during this time window and it resulted in a marginally higher risk (5.9, 1.0–28.2). However, one case with polydactyly had a father with similar CA, thus it is better to exclude this familial case from this analysis.

The data of 8 cases with isolated orofacial clefts are shown in Table 12.1. These data are based mainly on the data set of the HCCSCA, but we attempted to visit the mothers of these cases at home in 2009, thus e.g. their lifestyle habit was evaluated based on the personal interview of mothers and their family members living together and finally the so-called "family consensus" was accepted. We were not able to visit one mother due to new unknown address.

Two cases with cleft palate only were female and it is important to mention that both had mothers with PDP in the critical period of this CA, i.e. in IV and/or V gestational month. The mother of one case with cleft palate only was treated with ampicillin and this case had a brother affected with cleft palate though their parents were not affected with visible palatal defect.

Table 12.1 Birth year of cases with cleft lip ± palate and cleft palate only, in addition the diagnosis of periodontal disease in pregnancy (PDP), related drug treatments, other diseases and other drug treatment in their mothers during the gestational month (roman numbers) of the study pregnancy

		Cases									
Birth year	Isolated orofacial clefts	Sex	Gestational age (week)	Birth weight (g)	PDP	PDP related treatment	Other diseases	Other treatments	Age of mother (father) (year)	Birth order	Lifestyle
1985	Cleft palate	F	39	3,200	Acute periodontitis (IV)	Ampicillin (IV)	Nausea/vomiting (I–II) Iron deficiency anemia (VI–IX)	Iron (VI–IX)	28 (28)	3[a]	Sm (15/day)
1995	Cleft palate	F	38	3,680	Chronic periodontitis (I–III)	Dipyrone (I–III)	Tonsillitis (I–III) Nausea/vomiting (I–III) Common cold (VIII)	Dipyrone (VIII) Vitamin B6 (I–III)	25 (28)	2	Sm (10/day)
1985	Cleft lip, bilateral + cleft palate[b]	M	40	3,200	Periodontitis (I–IX)	Penamecillin (I–II) Dipyrone (I–II)	Orofacial herpes (IV) Cervical incompetence (IX)	Multivitamin (I–III) Diazepam (IX)	29 (27)	1	?
1993	Cleft lip, bilateral + cleft palate	M	36	2,300	Ginginitis (V–IX)	–	Threatened abortion (III) Cervical incompetence (IV–IX)	Aminophylline (IX) Oxytocin (IX)	22 (20)	3	Sm (20/day) regular drinker
1994	Cleft lip, left + cleft palate	F	41	3,550	Acute periodontitis (I–II)		Appendicitis (IV)	Folic acid (I–IX) Calcium (IV–IX) Iron (I–IX)	21 (22)	2	Sm (10/day)
1995	Cleft lip, bilateral + cleft palate	M	35	2,700	Acute periodontitis (II–III)	Cefaclor (II–III) Aminophenazone + phenacetine + aethylmorphin (II–III)	–	Folic acid (VII–IX) Iron (VII–IX)	20 (22)	1	Sm (25/day)

Table 12.1 (continued)

		Cases									
Birth year	Isolated orofacial clefts	Sex	Gestational age (week)	Birth weight (g)	PDP	PDP related treatment	Other diseases	Other treatments	Age of mother (father) (year)	Birth order	Lifestyle
1996	Cleft lip, left	F	40	3,150	Acute periodontitis (IV–V)	Dipyrone (IV–V)	Nausea/vomiting (I–II) Vulvovaginitis (VI) Tonsillitis (VII)	Ampicillin (VII) Paracetamol (VII) Multivitamin (VIII–IX) Iron (VIII–IX)	20 (30)	1	Sm (10/day) at present
1996	Cleft lip, left + cleft palate	F	40	3,700	Acute periodontitis (II)	Cefalexin (II) Dipyrone (II)	–	Folic acid (II–III) Iron (II–IX) Vitamin D (II–IX)	29 (42)	3	No sm

M, male; F, female; Sm, smoker.

[a]The mother of this case had new unknown address.

[b]One brother is affected with cleft palate though parents have not visible palatal defect.

Of 6 cases with cleft lip ± palate (3 males, 3 females), only one was affected with cleft lip, the rest 5 cases had cleft lip + cleft palate. Familial case did not occur. To our best knowledge, related drug treatments and other maternal diseases in case mothers and their related drug treatments (diazepam was used in IX month in one pregnant woman while ampicillin in VII month in another case mother) have no teratogenic potential.

All mothers were younger than 30 years, of 7 case mothers visited at home, 6 were smoker and 5 smoked surely during the study pregnancy.

12.3.2 Interpretation of Results

Thus a strong association between PDP and a higher risk for isolated orofacial clefts in their children, the question is whether it is a causal association, or can be explained by related drug treatments and lifestyle factors, unevaluated confounders or by chance.

Thus at the interpretation of possible causal association, we have to consider the possible maternal teratogenic effect of PDP. Isolated orofacial clefts have the multifactorial origin, thus their polygenic predisposition may be triggered by PDP during the critical period of these CAs, i.e. between 7 and 9 gestational weeks (i.e. in II and III months) in cleft lip ± palate and 8–14 gestational weeks (i.e. III and IV months) of cleft palate only. Of 8 cases with orofacial cleft, 6 showed an overlapping between the exposure (PDP) and the critical period of these CAs.

Drugs used for the treatment of PDP do not seem to be teratogenic at the comparison of case and control mothers. Tetracyclines are in the list of human teratogenic drugs (Shepard and Lemire, 2004). Our study confirmed the teratogenic effect of oxytetracyclines (8) but doxycycline did not show teratogenic effect (9). In addition, these drugs were not used by the mothers of cases with isolated orofacial clefts. Ampicillin associated with a higher risk for cleft palate only in our previous population-based case-control study (4.2, 1.4–16.3) (4), and one case with cleft palate only had mothers with treatment of ampicillin in IV gestational month. However, this case was familial. Penamecillin (3), clindamycin (14) and cephalosporins such as cefaclor and cefalexin (11) did not associate with a higher risk of any CA in our previous studies. A weak association was found between oral treatment of metroninazole and a higher risk of cleft lip ± palate, but it was not confirmed in the adjusted case-matched control comparison (41, 42), in addition the vaginal metrodinazole treatment did not have any association with this CA (43). There was no mother with metrodinazole and clindamycin treatment in the group of cases with isolated orofacial cleft. The most frequently used analgesic drug, dipyrone had no teratogenic potential (81).

The lifestyle, mainly smoking of case mothers who delivered later children with isolated orofacial cleft seems to be important. On the one hand the smoking habit of pregnant women with PDP was more frequent than in mothers without PDP (much higher than the usual 20% in Hungarian pregnant women). In addition, of 8 cases with orofacial cleft, 5 had mothers who smoked during the study pregnancy. One mother with cleft lip + palate was not visited at home, and one mother did not smoke during the study pregnancy. A higher risk of acute respiratory diseases of mother with PDP may also be associated with their more frequent smoking habit. Previously a mild association of maternal smoking with higher risk for orofacial cleft was shown in several studies, however, a much higher risk was found in the children of smoker mothers with specific gene polymorphism such as TGFA, TGFB3, RARA, BCL, MSX1 (I). These gene polymorphisms result in a higher risk for isolated orofacial clefts, but we did not find any report regarding gene polymorphisms which showed a higher risk for PDP. Nevertheless at present our hypothesis for this possible association is a common genetic predisposition for PDP in pregnant women and for isolated orofacial clefts in their children triggered by smoking habit in pregnant women.

Some previous case-control studies suggested a higher risk for PB in children born to mothers with periodontal diseases (Offenbacher et al., 1996; Jeffcoat et al., 2001). One potential explanation for this association is an intrauterine infection caused by gingival crevice organisms by way of maternal bacteremia and transplacental passage (Offenbacher et al., 1998). However, another study was not able to prove the increased intrauterine bacterial colonisation behind histological chorioamnionitis (Goepfert et al., 2004). Thus the biological pathway underlying the relation between periodontal disease and PB remains elusive (Goldenberg et al., 2008).

In conclusion, an unexpected 16 folds higher risk for isolated cleft lip ± palate and 8 folds higher risk for cleft palate only were found in the children of pregnant women with PDP. These findings are considered as signals which need confirmation or rejection in other studies.

12.4 Nausea and Vomiting in Pregnancy

Nausea and vomiting in pregnancy (NVP) is a collection of symptoms of nausea alone, or nausea in combination with vomiting that begins early in pregnancy before the 20th week of gestation and is not associated with primary maternal diseases such as gastrointestinal infections (Biggs, 1975; Flaxman and Sherman, 2000). Morning sickness is not an appropriate term because symptoms generally occur throughout the day, not just in the morning, and sickness refers pathology, whereas about two-thirds of pregnant women experience NVP (Einarson et al., 1986).

In general, NVP is a typical pregnancy complication; nevertheless, NVP is discussed among the pathological conditions of the digestive system.

Several studies showed that women with NVP had a lower risk of miscarriage than women who did not experience NVP (Medalie, 1957; Petitti, 1986; Weigel and Weigel, 1989). Studies concerning the possible association between NVP and CAs are inconsistent (Yerushalmy and Milkovich, 1965; Milkovich and van den Berg, 1976; Kullander and Kallen, 1976; Klebanoff and Mills, 1986). In addition, other adverse birth outcomes such as PB have not been evaluated in the newborn infants of mothers with NVP. Thus, the objectives of our studies were to check the possible association of NVP with PB and LBW, in addition to CAs.

12.4.1 Results of the Study (II–IV)

Out of 22,843 cases with CA, 1,713 (7.5%) had mothers with medically recorded NVP in the prenatal maternity logbooks during the study pregnancy, while NVP diagnosis was based on maternal information in 10,721 (46.9%), and either in prenatal maternity logbook or in maternal questionnaire information in 10,906 (47.7%) pregnant women. Out of 38,151 controls, 3,777 (9.9%) had mothers with medically recorded NVP, while 19,192 (50.3%) were reported by mothers, giving a sum of 20,013 mothers with NVP (52.5%). Finally, out of 834 malformed controls, 61 (7.3%) had mothers with medically recorded, while 376 (45.1%) mothers had self-reported NVP, resulting in 389 mothers with NVP in this group (46.6%). Most NVP recorded in the prenatal maternity logbook were reported by the mothers in the questionnaire as well.

Three categories of NVP were differentiated:

(i) mild NVP based on retrospective maternal information, they were rarely treated by antiemetics (7.0% of case and 8.2% of control mothers),
(ii) severe NVP based on prospective medical records with or without maternal information and all pregnant women were treated by antiemetics,
(iii) very severe NVP, i.e. hyperemesis gravidarum with intractable vomiting, resulting in dehydration, ketosis and significant weight loss of 5% or more. These women needed hospitalization and intensive treatment including infusion. Hyperemesis gravidarum occurred in 0.1% of case and 0.2% of control mothers.

Table 12.2 shows the comparison of prevalence of mild, severe, and very severe NVP and in mothers who had cases with different CA-groups, and in mothers who delivered controls without CA as referent and in malformed control mothers with Down syndrome offspring.

There was a severity dependent association between NVP and total CA group. In addition, mild and severe NVP associated with a lower risk for 3 and 10 CA-groups, respectively. The number of cases with different CAs was too small for the evaluation in the very severe NVP group. Malformed controls compared with controls showed also a lower OR in the category of severe NVP.

After these findings we excluded pregnant women with mild NVP from the analysis, because the ascertainment of mild NVP was based only on retrospective self-reported information from the mother depending on the individual sensitivity of pregnant women. Pregnant women with very severe NVP were also excluded due to the low number of cases, previous selection (pregnancy was terminated in several women due to very severe NVP) and the intensive treatment in hospitals.

Thus, medically recorded and treated severe NVP were evaluated in detail, without mentioning "severe" henceforth.

NVP earliest started in I gestational month, more exactly in the fourth postmenstrual week. The peak of frequency of NVP in II month, thereafter the frequency declined (Figure 1). After the 20th week NVP was rare (2.5% in the case and 2.6%

Table 12.2 Risk of different CA-groups in cases born to mother with different degree of NVP

	Mild NVP		Severe NVP		Very severe NVP	
Study groups	OR[a]	95% CI	OR[a]	95% CI	OR[a]	95% CI
Controls	1.00	–	1.00	–	1.00	–
Cases with isolated CAs						
Neural-tube defects	0.89	0.80 –1.01	**0.80**	**0.65 –0.98**	–	–
Cleft lip ± palate	0.91	0.82–1.02	**0.68**	**0.55–0.83**	0.30	0.04–2.16
Cleft palate only	0.87	0.74–1.03	**0.72**	**0.53–0.98**	–	–
Oesophageal atresia/stenosis	0.90	0.68–1.18	0.72	0.43–1.21	–	–
Congenital pyloric stenosis	0.86	0.66–1.12	0.96	0.62–1.48	–	–
Intestinal atresia/stenosis	0.88	0.64–1.22	1.14	0.69–1.89	–	–
Rectal/anal atresia/stenosis	0.93	0.71–1.22	0.91	0.57–1.44	1.89	0.26–13.6
Renal a/dysgenesis	0.86	0.58–1.27	0.56	0.24–1.27	4.02	0.55–29.1
Obstructive CAs of the urinary tract	0.85	0.71–1.02	**0.46**	**0.30–0.69**	–	–
Hypospadias	0.93	0.86–1.00	**0.71**	**0.62–0.82**	0.41	0.13–1.29
Undescended testis	**0.89**	**0.81–0.98**	**0.65**	**0.54–0.77**	0.81	0.30–2.20
CAs of the abdominal wall	0.89	0.69–1.16	0.93	0.60–1.44	–	–
Microcephaly, primary	0.76	0.52–1.13	1.13	0.62–2.05	–	–
Congenital hydrocephaly	0.80	0.64–1.01	0.65	0.42–1.02	1.32	0.18–9.51
CAs of the eye	0.72	0.47–1.09	0.38	0.14–1.04	–	–
CAs of the ear	0.91	0.73–1.12	0.75	0.51–1.11	1.17	0.16–8.43
Cardiovascular CAs	**0.92**	**0.86–0.98**	**0.71**	**0.63–0.80**	0.93	0.48–1.78
CAs of the genital organs	0.79	0.55–1.14	0.72	0.36–1.42	–	–
Clubfoot	0.94	0.86–1.02	**0.73**	**0.62–0.85**	0.86	0.35–2.11
Limb deficiencies	0.88	0.74–1.05	0.77	0.57–1.06	–	–
Poly/syndactyly	0.98	0.89–1.08	**0.70**	**0.58–0.85**	0.71	0.23–2.25
CAs of the musculo-skeletal system	0.79	0.59–1.04	1.28	0.85–1.93	1.97	0.27–14.2
CAs of the diaphragm	0.96	0.74–1.24	0.82	0.52–1.29	–	–
Other isolated CAs	0.90	0.79–1.04	1.21	0.98–1.48	0.92	0.23–3.72
Multiple CAs	**0.89**	**0.80–0.99**	**0.70**	**0.57–0.86**	–	–
Total CAs	**0.91**	**0.88 –0.94**	**0.74**	**0.70–0.78**	**0.58**	**0.39–0.86**

[a]Crude unmatched OR.

in the control group). Among these 142 pregnant women five had chronic gastrointestinal diseases. I gestational month had a higher occurrence of NVP in the control group than in the case group. The mean duration of NVP was 2.0 ± 1.9 and 2.7 ± 2.0 months in case and control pregnant women, respectively ($p < 0.0001$).

Mean maternal age was lower in the group of NVP (24.6 vs. 25.5 year) due to the higher proportion of young pregnant women (less than 25 years) (56.0% vs. 46.1%). This association is reflected in the lower mean birth order as well (1.4 vs. 1.6). The

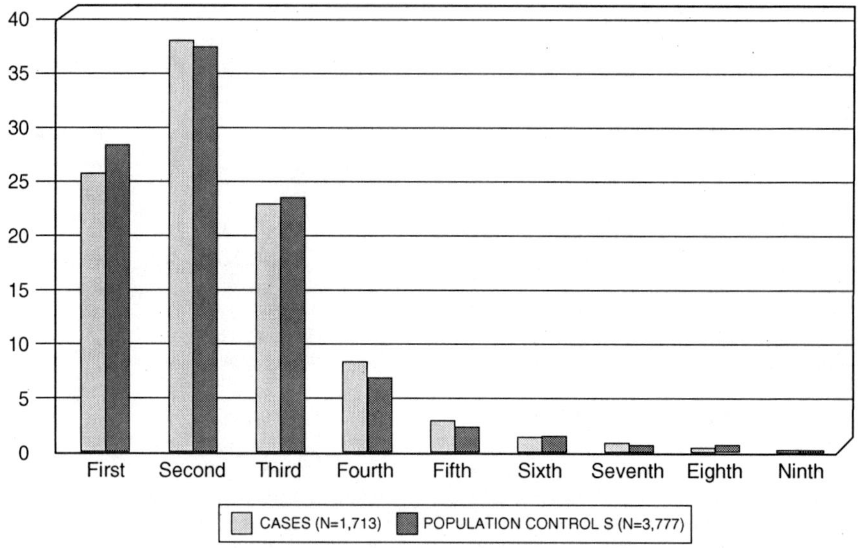

Fig. 12.1 Incidence of severe nausea and vomiting in pregnancy according to gestational months in the case mothers with congenital abnormality-affected offspringand in population control mothers with newborn infants without congenital abnormalities.

proportion of professional women was somewhat smaller, while the proportion of skilled workers was larger in control mothers with NVP.

Among other pregnancy complications, the rate of threatened abortion (20.6% vs. 14.6%) and threatened preterm delivery (19.1% vs. 14.6%) was higher in control mother with NVP than in control mothers without NVP.

The incidence of influenza/common cold (0.87, 0.79–0.98) and acute diseases of the genital organs (0.86, 0.75–0.95) was somewhat lower in pregnant women with NVP. Among chronic maternal disorders, only peptic ulcer and dyspepsia together occurred somewhat more frequently in mothers with NVP (1.1%) than in mothers without NVP (2.5, 1.8–3.6).

As it was mentioned previously all pregnant women with NVP were treated by one of the 3 antiemetics used in Hungary: vitamin B6, dimenhydrinate, thiethylperazine. Other drugs did not show difference between pregnant women with NVP and without NVP. Among pregnancy supplements, folic acid was used more frequently by women with NVP (58.5%), particularly by control mothers (59.7%), than by control women without NVP (51.9%), and by case mothers (48.9%).

The mean gestational age was 0.3 weak longer in the newborns without CA of pregnant women with NVP compared with the figure of newborns infants born to mothers without NVP ($p < 0.0001$), thus the rate of PB (6.4% vs. 9.5%) was also lower in newborns of pregnant women with NVP (0.76, 0.65–0.89). The mean birth weight was only 16 g larger in live-born babies born to mothers with NVP ($p = 0.54$), and the difference in the rate of LBW newborns (5.0% vs. 5.8%) was also not significant (0.90, 0.85–1.42).

However, it is necessary to mention that there was a lower proportion of males by 5% among newborn infants born to mothers with severe NVP ($p < 0.0001$). There was no difference in the proportion of boys in the different gestational age groups in mothers with NVP, while a slight increase was seen parallel with advanced gestational age in pregnant women without NVP. A similar increasing trend of boys was found according to increasing birthweight groups in both study groups. The point is that the lower proportion of boys in all gestational age and birthweight groups was characteristic for newborn infants of pregnant women with NVP compared to pregnant women without NVP.

The prevalence of NVP in the mothers of cases with different CA groups and their all matched controls were compared and adjusted OR were used as the best estimate (Table 12.3).

Out of 25 CA-groups, 5 CA groups such as cleft lip ± cleft palate, cleft palate only, renal a/dysgenesis (but based only on 6 cases), obstructive CAs of the urinary tract, and cardiovascular CAs showed a significantly lower risk. These five CA-groups have their critical period between II and IV gestational month. However, out of 25 CA groups, 22 had lower OR than 1 and it was reflected in the adjusted OR of the total CA group: 0.74, 0.68–0.79. Only two CA-groups had OR above 1, and the critical period of congenital pyloric stenosis and primary microcephaly is after IV gestational month. OR was 1.0 in one CA-group (CAs of the ear). Malformed control group compared to control group showed only an OR lower than 1.0 but the difference was not significant.

It is worth evaluating the possible association between NVP and different CA risk in males and females, separately (Table 12.3). Three CA-groups showed similar pattern in both sexes, while the group of renal a/dysgenesis had too low number for evaluation. However, the possible "protective" effect of NVP for "cleft palate only" was seen only in females (and this trend was characteristic for cleft lip ± palate as well), while NVP showed an association with lower prevalence of limb deficiencies in males.

Thus the major findings of pregnancy/birth outcome analyses of pregnant women can be summarized in the following points:

(1) There is a lower rate of early fetal death, i.e. miscarriages.
(2) There is lower proportion of males among their newborns.
(3) Newborns of pregnant women with NVP had a somewhat longer gestational age and lower rate of PB.
(4) There is a lower risk of some CAs and it results in a significant reduction in the total rate of CAs.

12.4.2 Interpretation of Results

NVP is the most common pregnancy complication. In the United States 64 ± 14% of women experienced NVP symptoms as compared to 75 ± 12% in the United Kingdom and 62 ± 10% in other countries (Weigel and Weigel, 1989; Einarson

Table 12.3 Estimation of risk for different CAs in cases of mothers with NVP compared with their matched controls without CAs

	Males		Females		Total			
CA groups	OR[a]	95% CI	OR[a]	95% CI	No.	%	OR[b]	95% CI
Cases with isolated CAs								
Neural-tube defects	0.69	0.39–1.22	0.82	0.52–1.28	97	8.1	0.77	0.54–1.08
Cleft lip± palate	**0.62**	**0.40–0.95**	**0.39**	**0.23–0.64**	95	6.9	**0.50**	**0.37–0.70**
Cleft palate only	0.73	0.33–1.65	**0.50**	**0.25–0.99**	44	7.3	**0.53**	**0.32–0.89**
Oesophageal atresia/stenosis	1.09	0.28–4.26	1.07	0.21–5.47	16	7.4	0.99	0.37–2.63
Congenital pyloric stenosis	1.89	0.79–4.49	3.20	0.13–77.3	23	9.5	1.89	0.83–4.27
Intestinal atresia/stenosis	1.18	0.30–4.64	0.30	0.06–1.44	17	11.1	0.58	0.22–1.49
Rectal/anal atresia/stenosis	1.27	0.51–3.15	0.30	0.04–2.29	20	9.1	0.80	0.36–1.75
Renal a/dysgenesis	0.13	0.01–1.43	0.03	0.00–1.09	6	5.8	**0.23**	**0.06–0.96**
Obstructive CAs of the urinary tract	**0.29**	**0.14–0.63**	**0.29**	**0.10–0.81**	24	4.8	**0.32**	**0.18–0.58**
Hypospadias	0.84	0.67–1.04	–	–	221	7.3	0.83	0.67–1.03
Undescended testis	0.81	0.61–1.07	–	–	136	6.6	0.81	0.61–1.07
CAs of the abdominal wall	0.77	0.21–2.85	0.53	0.15–1.84	22	9.2	0.86	0.39–1.90
Microcephaly, primary	8.19	0.39–173.5	2.55	0.50–12.9	12	11.0	2.48	0.65–9.42
Congenital hydrocephaly	1.75	0.72–4.23	0.55	0.12–2.49	21	6.7	0.98	0.49–2.00
CAs of the eye	0.59	0.05–7.80	6.45	0.40–103.9	4	4.0	0.91	0.18–4.60
CAs of the ear	1.10	0.41–2.94	0.87	0.26–2.88	27	7.6	1.01	0.48–2.09
Cardiovascular CAs	**0.72**	**0.56–0.92**	**0.65**	**0.51–0.83**	324	7.2	**0.68**	**0.57–0.81**
CAs of the genital organs	1.31	0.03–62.3	0.53	0.12–2.35	9	7.3	0.73	0.21–2.48
Clubfoot	0.83	0.61–1.14	0.74	0.51–1.06	179	7.4	0.79	0.62–1.02
Limb deficiencies	**0.40**	**0.20–0.78**	1.17	0.55–2.48	43	7.9	0.65	0.40–1.06
Poly/syndactyly	0.87	0.61–1.24	0.70	0.44–1.10	125	7.2	0.79	0.60–1.05
CAs of the musculo-skeletal system	0.74	0.32–1.70	0.78	0.24–2.60	26	12.4	0.66	0.33–1.30
CAs of the diaphragm	0.59	0.23–1.52	0.54	0.16–1.77	20	8.2	0.58	0.28–1.20
Other isolated CAs	0.74	0.46–1.20	0.68	0.41–1.15	106	11.7	0.73	0.52–1.04
Multiple CAs	0.73	0.48–1.10	0.98	0.59–1.63	96	7.1	0.81	0.59–1.12
Total CAs	**0.78**	**0.70–0.86**	**0.67**	**0.59–0.77**	1,713	7.5	**0.74**	**0.68–0.79**
Total controls	Reference		Reference		3,777	9.9	Reference	
Total malformed controls	0.73	0.39– 1.39	0.87	0.49–1.52	61	7.3	0.82	0.54–1.24

[a]ORs are adjusted for maternal age, birth order, maternal employment status, use of antiemetics (including vitamin B6), and pregnancy supplements (folic acid, multivitamins).

et al., 1996b). However, NVP encompasses a continuum from slight food aversion, heartburn and mild nausea to extreme nausea and vomiting, known as hyperemesis gravidarum. Most NVP causes only heartburn and mild nausea with some dietary aversions and cravings (Flaxman and Sherman, 2000), while very severe NVP occurs in less than 1% of pregnancies (Fairweather, 1968; Tsang et al., 1996).

In the data set of the HCCSCA, 47.7% of case mothers (40.1% mild, 7.5% severe and 0.1% very severe), 52.5% of control mothers (42.4 mild, 9.9% severe and 0.2% very severe), and 46.6% of malformed control mothers (39.1% mild, 7.3% severe and 0.0% very severe) had NVP. However, only prospectively medically recorded and treated severe NVP was evaluated in this study.

The findings of our study showed a longer gestational age at delivery which associated with a lower rate of PB. Similar experiences were published by Brandes (1967), Klebanoff et al. (1985) and Ananth and Rao (1993). However, Jarnfelt-Samsioe et al. (1983), Tierson et al. (1986), Weigel and Weigel (1989), and Chin (1989) did not find significant differences between the rate of PB of newborns of pregnant women with or without NVP. On the other hand, Brandes (1967), Little (1979), Tierson et al. (1986) reported a lower rate of LBW newborns of mothers with NVD, although others did not find difference in this variable in pregnant women with or without NVP (Jarnfeldt-Samsioe et al., 1985; Weigel and Weigel, 1989; Ananth and Rao, 1993; Gadsby et al., 1980). These differences can be explained partly by the different study design (e.g. the different severity of NVP was not separated).

The most important finding of our study suggests an inverse association between *severe* NVP and risk of some CAs and severe NVP associated with 26% protective effect against the occurrence of total CAs. In addition, a somewhat later onset and shorter duration of severe NVP were found in the mothers of cases with CA compared with their controls without CA.

Yerushalmy and Milkovich (1965) reported that women with NVP were less likely to bear children with major CAs than women who did not experience NVP. Others did not find an association between NVP and CAs (Milkovich and van den Berg, 1976; Petitti, 1986; Klebanoff and Mills, 1986; Weigel and Weigel, 1989), while Kullander and Källen (1976) found a higher rate of CAs in children born to mothers with NVP than in babies of mothers without NVP.

Some studies focused on specific CAs. Ferencz et al. (1983) and Boneva et al. (1999) found that NVP was associated with a reduced risk for cardiovascular CAs and it was confirmed by our findings. Our preliminary study showed that severe NVP provided some protective effect for isolated oral clefts (III), and it was confirmed by the final analysis of the data set of HCCSCA (IV), although Saxen (1975) and Golding et al. (1983) found no association between NVP and oral clefts. Our recent findings indicate a significant protective effect of NVP for obstructive CAs of the urinary tract and renal a/dysgenesis as well. Kricker et al. (1986) found a higher rate of limb deficiencies in children born to mothers with NVP, while our study showed a lower occurrence of this CA-group in males. In our study many other CAs had a lower OR than 1.0 and it explains that severe NVP associates with 26% protective effect against the occurrence of total CAs.

The possible causal association between severe NVP and the reduction of some CAs needs explanation.

We cannot exclude that women with medically recorded NVP had a better and/or more frequent prenatal care (due to better socio-economic status, more health conscious, etc.) with a better record of pregnancy complications and these factors resulted in a higher incidence of NVP compared to other pregnant women. However, this information bias was considered at the calculation of adjusted risk figures.

The possible CA-protective effect of antiemetic drugs is also worth attention (Golding et al., 1983). Our previous case-control study regarding the teratogenic potential of vitamin B6 showed a protective effect for cardiovascular CAs (0.9, 0.7–0.9) (73). Vitamin B6 (i.e. pyridoxine) was used very frequently (60%) in pregnant women with NVP; however, the effect of this antiemetic vitamin was considered as confounder. Out of 22,843 cases, 914 (4.0%) had mother with dimenhydrinate treatment, while out of 38,151 controls, 1,726 (4.5%) were born to mothers who were treated with this antiemetic drug (71). There was no higher risk for total CAs (0.9, 0.8–1.0) or any CA-groups in children born to mothers with oral dimenhydrinate treatment in II and III gestational months. In fact there was a lower risk for obstructive CA of the urinary tract in children of mothers treated with dimenhydrinate in the first trimester of pregnancy. (However, when evaluating these data we did not consider the possible preventive effect of NVP in pregnant women with dimenhydrinate treatment.) Finally, we summarize the case-control teratologic study of thiethylperazine treatment (72). Out of 22,843 cases, 411 (1.8%), while out of 38,151 controls, 746 (2.0%) mothers were treated by oral thiethylperazine and/or suppository. There was no higher risk for total CA groups; however, the separate analysis of different CA-groups showed a somewhat higher risk for cleft lip ± cleft palate in children born to mothers with thiethylperazine treatment during the first trimester of pregnancy (2.0, 1.0–4.0). However, a lower risk for cleft lip ± cleft palate was found in children of pregnant women with severe NVP. (Doxylamine-dicyclomine, i.e. Bendectin® was not used in Hungary.)

There are several hypotheses for the explanation of the possible preventive effect of NVP on adverse pregnancy/birth outcomes. One of them is related to bacterial infections, particularly Helicobacter pylori in women with NVP (Pirisi, 2001). Our data did not indicate a higher frequency of acute infectious diseases of the digestive system, although gastrointestinal disorders were recorded somewhat more frequently in pregnant women with NVP. However, almost all individuals who are infected with H. pylori are asymptomatic.

An old hypothesis regarding the possible protective effect of NVP on adverse pregnancy/births outcomes was based on the supposition that some food may pose potential danger to embryos thus NVP protects the embryo by causing pregnant women to physically expel and subsequently avoid foods and foodborne pathogenic microorganisms that contain teratogenic and abortifacient toxic chemicals (Tierson et al., 1985; Hook, 1987; Profet, 1988; Sherman and Flaxman, 2002).

We favor the next hypothesis which explains the beneficial effects of NVP for pregnancy outcomes by larger placenta (Huxley, 2000), a higher blood level of human chorionic gonadotropin (Kaupilla et al., 1984; Masson et al., 1985; Appierto et al., 1996) and estrogens (Jarnfelt-Samsioe et al., 1983; Masson et al., 1985) in pregnant women with NVP and this hormonal milieu may have a protective effect for some CAs. In addition, higher estrogen concentration during pregnancy induces a hyperacuity of the olfactory system to odors which may be the primary stimulus for NVP (Furneaux et al., 2001).

Another important argument for the above two hypotheses is that the peak of NVP occurs from the 5th to 10th gestational week, which corresponds to the organ-forming period when embryonic susceptibility to teratogens is most obvious and when the level of human chorionic gonadotropin is the highest. Thus, this hormonal hypothesis may explain the protective effect of NVP both for early fetal loss, i.e. spontaneous abortion and CAs.

However, in general, there is an opposite association between fetal loss and CAs because very severe CAs are selected prenatally as fetal loss and this decreases the prevalence of CAs at birth. Among newborn infants without CA born to mothers with NVP, the proportion of males was smaller than in babies born to mothers without NVP, and the so-called protective effect of NVP for CAs was somewhat more obvious in females (32%) than in males (22%) in our study; however, this difference was not significant. On the other hand, if NVP is associated with higher level of estrogen, we might expect an increased risk for CAs such as hypospadias (Briggs, 1982), but we found a somewhat lower incidence of hypospadias.

Our hypothesis is based on two further observations: (i) malformed controls including Down syndrome caused by trisomy 21 before conception also showed some, although not significant association with NVP (adjusted OR: 0.82, 0.54–1.24), but (ii) a similar association was not seen in two CAs with critical period after "the NVP period". Vigorous embryo-placenta unit – as "parasite" of maternal organism – can induce NVP, while pathological conditions such CAs or destruction of embryo-placenta unit reduce this effect and may associate with CAs and fetal death.

Physiological and genetic factors may have a role in the origin of NVP but this unpleasant pregnancy complication may indicate the benefit of early fetal development. NVP is associated with reduced occurrence of miscarriages, but not late fetal death, i.e. stillbirths (Chin, 1989).

A 26% lower occurrence of total CAs in cases born to mothers with severe NVP and particularly the association between the significant reduction in the prevalence of some specific CAs at birth and NVP may have some far-reaching implementations. On one hand, the possible relation between severe NVP and reduction of some CAs may contribute to better understanding of the pathogenesis of CAs. On the other hand, when evaluating drugs or other exposures during pregnancy, severe NVP should be considered as a confounding factor. Finally, as Sherman and Flaxman (2002) stated: "Knowledge that NVP indicates the functioning of a woman's defense system, rather than a bodily malfunction, may reassure patients and enable health care providers new ways of minimizing the uncomfortable symptoms."

12.5 Dyspepsia and Gastro-Oesophageal Reflux Disease

Dyspepsia is a complex of symptoms originating from the upper gastrointestinal tract, including *gastro-oesophageal reflux disease* (GORD) (Heading, 1991; Van Zanten et al., 2000; Van Zanten, 2009). Dyspepsia itself was defined as pain and discomfort centered in the upper abdominal (epigastric) judged by the physician to originate in the upper gastrointestinal tract. GORD is defined as the abnormal reflux of acidic gastric content into the oesophagus with the cardinal symptom of heartburn. Dyspepsia might be accompanied by symptoms of GORD, such as regurgitation, heartburn, nausea, and bloating. Some experts argue that GORD has to be considered separately from dyspepsia. However, a broad definition of dyspepsia including heartburn and GORD makes clinical sense in medical care (Van Zanten et al., 2000; Van Zanten, 2009).

Dyspepsia and GORD are among the most common gastrointestinal diagnoses; their prevalences are estimated between 14 and 20% in adults (Nebel et al., 1976; Heading, 1999; Camilleri et al., 2005). Patients with severe dyspepsia are treated by antacids, H_2-receptor antagonists, and proton-pump inhibitors (DeVault and Castelli, 2005; Armstrong et al., 2005; Kahrilas et al., 2008a, b).

Dyspepsia is particularly common in the second part of gestation; 21% of pregnant women complained about heartburn daily, 52% at least once a month and as many as 80% of pregnant women complained at least once in the third trimester (Nagler and Spiro, 1961; Olans and Wolf, 1975). Dyspepsia with or without GORD during pregnancy may be related to conditions that can favor the manifestation of this gastrointestinal disease-group which is symptomatic but without overt oesophagitis due to the limited period of gestation.

12.5.1 Results of the Study (V)

The aim of our study was to check the possible associations between different CAs, adverse birth outcomes and maternal dyspepsia with related drug treatments in the population-based data set of the HCCSCA.

The selection of pregnant women with dyspepsia had three steps:

First, we differentiated dyspepsia including heartburn and GORD from other pathological conditions such as hiatal hernia, eosinophilic oesophagitis, achalasia, diffuse oesophageal spasm (Williamson, 2001; Welsh, 2005; Vakil et al., 2006); pregnant women with the these diagnoses were excluded from the study.

In the second step, two groups of dyspepsia were differentiated according to the source of diagnosis and information: (i) prospectively and medically recorded dyspepsia in the prenatal maternity logbook and (ii) dyspepsia based on retrospective maternal information. The symptoms of dyspepsia are wide and their perception is subjective, in addition, our validation study showed that the symptoms/diagnosis of gastritis, "excess gas" and some functional disorders of the upper gastrointestinal system were frequently confused by mothers in the questionnaire. Therefore, we decided to evaluate only prospectively and medical recorded dyspepsia including heartburn and GORD in the prenatal maternity logbook.

The case group consisted of 22,843 malformed newborns or fetuses ("informative offspring"), of whom 175 (0.77%) had mothers with medically recorded dyspepsia. Out of 38,151 controls, 270 (0.71%) were born to mothers with dyspepsia. However, the analysis of these pregnant women with dyspepsia showed two different groups. One group included pregnant women with dyspepsia at the first visit of prenatal care that had "chronic" dyspepsia, in general with the onset before conception (about 96%) which continued during pregnancy at least in II and III gestational months, i.e. in the critical period of most major CAs. Another group comprised pregnant women with dyspepsia diagnosed after III gestational month. In the third step of selection, pregnant women with newly diagnosed dyspepsia (heartburn and GORD) during the study pregnancy were excluded from the study.

Thus finally, as the third step of selection, we evaluated 148 (0.65%) case and 214 (0.56%) control mothers with *severe chronic dyspepsia* (SCD) treated by drugs (1.2, 0.9–1.4). Of these 148 cases, 122 (82.4%), while out of 214 controls, 158 (73.8%) had mothers with recorded diagnosis of GORD. When symptoms of SCD are typical and the patients respond to therapy, there is no problem with the validity of diagnosis (Kahrilas, 2008); therefore, endoscopy and IgG antibody-titer assay for the status of H. pylori are not necessary.

The mothers of cases with SCD had a higher mean maternal age (26.3 vs. 25.5 year) than mothers without SCD, but the mean birth order (1.8) did not show difference compared to pregnant women without SCD. There was no difference in marital status among the study groups, but SCD occurred more frequently in professional, managerial, and skilled worker pregnant women.

The evaluation of pregnancy complications showed that 21.0% of pregnant women with SCD had threatened abortion while this figure was 16.4% in pregnant women without SCD.

The occurrence of acute and chronic maternal diseases did not show difference among the study groups.

All pregnant women with SCD were treated with antacids (92%) and/or H_2-receptor antagonists (11%), particularly cimetidine, while the proportion of these drugs was less than 2% in case and control mothers without SCD. In addition, spasmodic drotaverine (20%) and analgesic dipyrone (16%) were also used frequently for the treatment of SCD in Hungary.

Among vitamin supplements, the use of folic acid (49.3% vs. 49.4%) was similar by case mothers with or without SCD while control mothers with SCD used folic acid more frequently (62.1%) than control pregnant women without SCD (54.4%). The use of multivitamins was more frequent in case (8.8%) and control (10.7%) mothers with SCD than in case (5.8%) and control (6.6%) pregnant women without SCD.

Birth outcomes of newborns without CA (i.e. controls) are showed in Table 12.4.

The mean gestational age at birth was longer in mothers with SCD than in mothers without SCD. This difference was reflected in the lower rate of PB. There was

Table 12.4 Birth outcomes of newborns without CA born to mothers with or without severe chronic dyspepsia (SCD)

	Newborns born to mother					
Variables	With SCD		Without SCD		Comparison	
Quantitative	Mean	S.D.	Mean	S.D.	*t*	*p*
Gestational age (week)	**39.7**	1.7	39.4	2.0	2.2	**0.03**
Birth weight (g)	3,317	505	3,275	511	1.2	0.23
Categorical	No.	%	No.	%	OR (95% CI)	
PB	9	**4.2**	3,487	9.2	**0.4 (0.2–0.8)**	
LBW newborns	10	4.7	2,157	5.7	0.8 (0.4–1.5)	

no significant difference in the mean birth weight and in the rate of LBW newborns born to mothers with or without SCD.

The prevalence of SCD during early pregnancy including II and III gestational months was compared between cases with different CAs and their all matched controls. There was no difference in adjusted OR (1.2, 0.9–1.4) when comparing total CA rate. However, at the evaluation of cases with different CA, one CA-group, namely cases with isolated rectal/anal atresia/stenosis had mothers with significantly higher rate of SCD (4.3, 1.7–10.5) based on 5 cases. After the so-called Bonferoni correction, the *p* value was 0.0015.

12.5.2 Interpretation of Results

Our findings confirmed the results of previous studies that dyspepsia including heartburn and GORD, i.e. SCD occurs more frequently in mothers with advanced age (Sullivan, 1983; Williamson, 2001; Dent et al., 2005) and in higher socioeconomic status. Pregnant women with SCD had better family planning attitude (e.g. higher use of folic acid and multivitamin supplementation) which may explain the longer gestational age and lower rate of PB of their newborn infants compared to the babies of pregnant women without SCD.

Recommended treatment for mild dyspepsia includes lifestyle modifications: avoidance of acidic and other irritative foods (such as citrus fruits, tomatoes, onions, spicy foods), and foods that cause gastric reflux (fatty or fried foods, coffee, tea, chocolate, mint, alcoholic beverages), avoidance of eating within 3 hr before bedtime, smoking cessation, reduction of overweight or obesity, elevation of head-of-bed during the sleep, etc (Johnson and DeMeester, 1981; Mahadevan and Kane, 2006; Kahrilas, 2008). If pregnant women have severe dyspepsia previously antacids, histamine-2-receptor antagonists (such as cimetidine), and proton-pump inhibitors (e.g. omeprazole) have been recommended (Misiewicz, 1973; Mahadevan and Kane, 2006; Thukral and Wolf, 2006; Kahrila et al, 2008a, b). Reducing the acidity of gastric fluid ameliorates reflux symptoms and allows oesophagitis to heal. The potential teratogenic effect of these drugs, including cimetidine and omeprazole was not found (Garbis et al., 1999; Kallen, 2001); nevertheless, omeprazole was classified as category C (no adequate human studies or adverse fetal effects in animals found). Hungarian pregnant women with SCD were treated frequently with the spasmodic drotaverine (83) and analgesic dipyrone (81); our previous studies did not show their teratogenic potential.

The prevalence of SCD was only about 0.6% of pregnant women in our study. It is much lower than previously published prevalence of dyspepsia and/or GORD in pregnant women (Nagler and Spiro, 1961; Olans and Wolf, 1975; Nebel et al., 1976). The high incidence of dyspepsia and/or GORD during pregnancy is explained by the transient lower oesophageal sphincter relaxation and by the abdomino-thoracic pressure gradient due to the enlarging uterine fundus, which is getting more prevalent in each trimester as pregnancy progresses (Van Thiel and Wald, 1981). However, we evaluated pregnant women with dyspepsia with the onset before conception which needed drug treatment recorded in the prenatal care logbook, i.e. SCD.

The main result of the study showed a possible association between maternal SCD and 4 fold higher risk for isolated rectal/anal atresia/stenosis in their children. We strictly differentiated cases with isolated and multiple rectal/anal atresia/stenosis, which is important because about 70% of this CA-group is associated with other CA. The question is whether it is a causal association, or can be explained by related drug treatments, unevaluated confounders, or by chance.

Rectal/anal atresia/stenosis has the multifactorial origin; therefore, the polygenic predisposition of this CA can be triggered by environmental factors such as SCD in the critical period of this CA, i.e. in the 7th gestational week (Briard et al., 1975). In addition, there is a well-know pathogenetical relationship between oesophageal atresia/stenosis and rectal/anal atresia/stenosis, the best evidence for this common background is VACTERL-association. An abnormality of circular smooth muscle of lower oesophageal sphincter was shown (Richter and Castell, 1982) as a major cause of GORD. Similar anal sphincter dysplasia (Zorsi et al., 1991) or internal anal sphincter myopathy (Kamm et al., 1991; Celik et al., 1995) are known with genetic origin. Thus we may suppose that functional postnatal anomalies and CA of oesophageal and/or anal sphincters have some common genetic predisposition explaining the possible association of rectal/anal atresia/stenosis in the children of mothers with SCD.

Drugs used for the treatment of SCD do not seem to be teratogenic as we discussed previously. Another possible explanation for this association is unevaluated/unknown confounders. Finally, multiple comparisons may produce non-causal association; however, this association was significant after Bonferoni correction as well.

In conclusion, 4 folds higher risk for isolated rectal/anal atresia/stenosis was found in the children of pregnant women with SCD which needs further study to confirm or to reject this finding.

12.6 Gastritis and Duodenitis

This group of diseases is neglected in the well-known handbooks of maternal-fetal medicine (e.g., Scott and Abu-Hamda, 2004), although *acute gastritis and duodenitis* (AGD) are frequently associated with symptoms of pregnant women and sometimes differential-diagnosis might cause problems.

12.6.1 Interpretation of Data in the HCCSCA

Out of 22,843 cases, 67 (0.29%) had mothers with AGD, while out of 38,151 controls, 78 (0.20%) were born to mothers with AGD. The onset of AGD was during the study pregnancy; the peak was in II and IV gestational months. Most AGD were reported by mothers; the lack of medical recorded AGD in the prenatal maternity logbook is an important argument against the severity of AGD.

Mean maternal age (26.0 vs. 25.5 year) was somewhat higher with an excess of professional-managerial employment status (53.9% vs. 38.5%). Among pregnancy complication only the higher incidence or severe nausea-vomiting in pregnancy (19.2% vs. 10.1%) is worth mentioning. The evaluation of acute diseases showed a higher incidence of influenza-common cold (30.8% vs. 18.4%) and acute diseases of the respiratory system (17.9% vs. 9.0%) and the urinary tract (12.8% vs. 7.3%) in pregnant women with AGD. Among chronic diseases prevalence of hemorrhoids (10.3% vs. 4.2%) was higher in pregnant women with AGD.

The evaluation of drug treatment showed a much higher frequency of aluminum hydroxide and magnesium carbonate (Tisacid®), aluminum hydroxide, magnesium hydroxide and sorbitol combination (Almagel®), clioquinol and spasmodic drotaverine in pregnant women with AGD.

The birth outcomes of newborns without CA born to mother with or without AGD did not show clinically important difference. Mean gestational age at delivery was 0.1 week longer (39.5 vs. 39.4 week) while mean birth weight was 41 g larger (3,317 vs. 3,276 g) in newborns of pregnant women with AGD. These figures associated with a lower rate of PB (6.4% vs. 9.2%) and LBW newborns (5.1% vs. 5.7%).

The occurrence of AGD during pregnancy was compared between cases with different CAs and their all matched controls. A marginally higher risk for total CAs (1.4, 1.0–2.0) was found explained mainly by the higher risk for congenital hydrocephalus in 3 cases (4.7, 1.5–15.0), rectal/anal atresia/stenosis in 3 cases (6.4, 2.0–20.5), and clubfoot in 10 cases (2.0, 1.0–3.9). However, of the 3 cases with rectal/anal atresia/stenosis, only one had mother with AGD in the critical period (i.e. II month) of this CA-group. In addition, the AGD occurred after III gestational month in all 3 pregnant women of cases with congenital hydrocephalus, i.e. after its critical period. Of the 10 cases with clubfoot, 8 had mothers with AGD also after III month and most of the clubfoot was deformation type with the critical period during the last months of pregnancy. Thus this marginally increased risk needs further studies.

12.7 Peptic Ulcer Disease

An ulcer is a defect of the mucosal layer of the gastrointestinal tract. In order to be diagnosed as an ulcer the defect must be greater than 0.5 cm^2 and must involve the full thickness of the mucosa and reach the muscularis mucosa layer. Most ulcers are single and most commonly appear in the stomach or the duodenum. They are called *peptic ulcer disease* (PUD) because release of pepsin and acid causes autolysis of the mucosa (Achkar, 1983). The primary cause of PUD is the upset of balance of acid and pepsin secretion. Multiple factors influence acid secretion and mucosal defense (Grossman, 1981).

The diagnosis of uncomplicated PUD generally is based on presenting symptoms such as epigastric burning pain in an empty stomach often awakening the patient. The pain usually can be relieved by food or antacids (Scott and Abu-Hamda, 2004). PUD is a common pathological condition in adult people, mainly affecting men between age 20 and 50, but it may occur in pregnant women as well (Welsh, 2005). Nevertheless, as far as we know the possible association between PUD in pregnant women and CAs in their offspring has not been evaluated in controlled epidemiological studies (Shepard and Lemire, 2004). Sometimes the usual treatment of PUD (Fleshler and Achkar, 1981; Grossman et al., 1981) may cause problems in pregnant women due to the possible teratogenic and/or fetotoxic effect of related drug treatments (Mahadevan and Kane, 2006; Thukral and Wolf, 2006).

12.7.1 Results of the Study

The population-based data set of the HCCSCA was appropriate for the study of possible association between maternal PUD with related drug treatments and CAs or other adverse birth outcomes.

The case group consisted of 22,843 malformed newborns or fetuses ("informative offspring"), of whom 48 (0.21%) had mothers with previously diagnosed PUD. Out of 38,151 controls, 104 (0.27%) were born to mothers with previously diagnosed PUD.

However, of the 48 case mothers, 20 (41.7%), while out of 104 control mothers, 58 (55.8%) had medically recorded active PUD during the study pregnancy in the prenatal maternity logbook: In the rest (i.e. 28 case mothers and 46 control mothers), we were unable to state that the previously diagnosed PUD was active during the study pregnancy on the basis of retrospective self-reported maternal information. Therefore, finally we decided to evaluate only medically recorded and active PUD during the study pregnancy in 20 (0.09%) case and 58 (0.15%) control mothers (0.6, 0.3-0.9). The number of pregnant women with gastric and duodenal ulcer was 13: 7 among case and 45:13 among control mothers.

Out of 20 case mothers, 19 (95.0%) had PUD in I gestational month; therefore, the onset of PUD was before conception, while one pregnant woman had the onset of PUD in III gestational month. Out of 58 control mothers, 50 (86.2%) had the onset of PUD in I gestation month. In addition, 4, 2, and 2 pregnant women had the onset of PUD in III, IV, and V gestational months, respectively. There was no significant difference in the onset of PUD according to the gestational months between the two study groups.

The main variables of mothers showed a higher mean maternal age (27.6 vs. 25.4 year) and mean birth order (2.2 vs. 1.7) in pregnant women with PUD compared to the reference group. There was no difference in marital status among the study groups but PUD occurred less frequently in professional pregnant women.

Among pregnancy complications, only anemia occurred more frequently in pregnant women with PUD (26.9% vs. 17.8%).

Acute and chronic maternal diseases did not show difference in their prevalence among the study groups.

Mainly 4 drugs were used for the treatment of PUD in Hungarian pregnant women: aluminum hydroxide, magnesium hydroxide and sorbitol (Almagel®), aluminum hydroxide and magnesium carbonate (Tisacid®) (together 56.4%), spasmodic drotaverine (28.2%), and analgesic dipyrone (17.9%). In addition, atropine, cimetidine, sucralfate, and some other drugs were used rarely for the treatment of PUD.

Among vitamin supplements the use of folic acid was less frequent by case pregnant women with PUD (47.4%) compared to case women without PUD (52.5%) while folic acid use was similar in control mothers (53.5% vs. 54.5%) with or without PUD.

The birth outcomes of newborns without CA born to mother with or without PUD did not show clinically important differences. The mean gestational age at delivery was 0.1 week longer while the mean birth weight was 34 g larger in the newborns of pregnant women with PUD. There was no significant in the rate of PB (3.5% vs. 9.2%) and LBW newborns (5.2% vs. 5.7%) between the two subgroups.

The occurrence of PUD during pregnancy was compared between cases with different CAs and their all matched controls. There was no higher risk for total CA; in fact, adjusted OR was significantly lower, i.e. 0.6, 0.3–0.9. However, if folic acid was considered as confounder, the previously found "protective effect" of PUD disappeared (0.8, 0.7–1.1). In addition, we did not find a higher risk for any CA group in the offspring of pregnant women with PUD.

12.7.2 Interpretation of Results

PUD is more frequent in elder multiparous pregnant women with a somewhat lower socioeconomic status. Additionally, our data showed a lower level of family planning attitude (i.e. lower use of folic acid supplementation) and rare new-onset PUD during pregnancy. Nevertheless, only the higher rate of anemia in pregnant women with PUD may indicate the adverse effect of PUD. Bleeding occurs during the course of PUD in 15–25% of patients with duodenal ulcer and in 10–15% of patients with gastric ulcer (Chin and Weckesser, 1951; Fry, 1964). Unfortunately, we had no information regarding to the origin of PUD, although almost 100% of patients have

H. pylori in their stomach, and 15% of those carrying H. pylori will eventually have peptic ulceration (Welsh, 2005).

The prevalence of PUD evaluated was only about 0.1% in pregnant women in our study, although 5–10% of adult people have PUD (Welsh, 2005). However, PUD is more frequent in males, particularly duodenal ulcer (2–3 folds) (Achkar, 1983). In addition, 72% of our pregnant women with PUD were younger than 30 years old and we selected only pregnant women with medically recorded active and severe PUD during the study pregnancy. Finally, prior data indicated that pre-existing PUD improves or disappears in almost 90% of pregnant women (Clark, 1953; Welsh, 2005). The explanations for the beneficial effect of PUD during pregnancy are increased prostaglandins that have a protective effect on the gastric mucosa, dietary alterations (e.g. an increase in milk), healthier lifestyle (cessation of smoking), and better medical care. On the other hand, mild PUD (particularly gastric ulcer) is generally underdiagnosed in pregnant women (Welsh, 2005).

Recommended treatment for PUD includes – beyond smoking cessation, diet with regular meals, and avoidance of symptom-producing foods, and more rest – three levels of drugs (Achkar, 1983; Mahadevan and Kane, 2006; Thukral and Wolf, 2006): (a) acid suppression by interfering with various phases of secretion, such as H2-receptor blockers, (ii) acid neutralization with antacids, e.g. the combinations of aluminum hydroxide, magnesium hydroxide/carbonate, (iii) drugs, acting on injured tissue such as sucralfate, prostaglandins, bismuth, etc.

In Hungary, antacids were used most frequently for the treatment of pregnant women with PUD during the study period. The potential teratogenic effect of aluminum was checked in animal experiments and their results showed that aluminum exposure is unlikely to pose risk for CAs (Borak and Wise, 1998). Heinonen et al. (1977) did not find increased incidents of CAs among the offspring of 141 women treated by magnesium sulphate during pregnancy. Rudnicki et al. (1991) used intravenous therapy of magnesium hydroxide in 27 pregnant women and no adverse effect was found in their newborns. Aluminum- and magnesium-containing antacids belong to the non-absorbed alginate-containing drugs. Sucralfate is also an aluminum salt of a sulphated disaccharide that inhibits pepsin activity and protects against ulceration. Its mucosal protective effect is based on aluminum hydroxide because sucralfate is not absorbed in significant amounts from the gastrointestinal tract. In a surveillance study of Michigan Medicaid recipients conducted between 1885 and 1992 involving 229,101 completed pregnancies, 138 newborns had been exposed to sucralfate during the first trimester. A total of 5 (2.7%) major CAs were observed (8 expected and there was no higher risk for 6 CA groups studied. Thus these data do not support an association between sucralfate and CAs (Rosa, 1993). Among H2 receptor blockers, cimetidine, famotidine, and ranitidine were used. Omeprazole was marketed only the last years of the study period. The findings of human teratologic studies showed that these acid-suppressing and proton pump blocker drugs did not associate with a higher risk for CAs (Ruigomez et al., 1999; Kallen, 2001; Garbis et al., 2005; Lalkin et al., 1998). In addition a regimen of the so-called triple therapy: proton pump inhibitor, amoxicillin, and clarithromycin are used for the treatment of *H. pylori* infection during pregnancy. Both amoxicillin (6) and clarithromycin (Einarson et al., 1998a) are safe during pregnancy. Our previous studies did not show any teratogenic potential of drotaverine [83] and dipyrone [81] use during pregnancy.

Nearly all pregnant women with PUD were treated during pregnancy in our study, and there was no teratogenic (CA-inducing) effect of related drugs treatments. Thus the secondary results of our study show the lack of teratogenic effect of drugs used for the treatment of PUD.

In conclusion, a higher occurrence of CAs or any other adverse birth outcomes was not found in the offspring of mothers with PUD and related treatment during pregnancy. Thus women with treated PUD during pregnancy have a good chance to have healthy babies

12.8 Appendicitis

Acute appendicitis is the most common non-obstetric cause of acute abdominal pain leading to exploratory laparatomy during pregnancy, even though its incidence may be less common in pregnant women than in the general population. The incidence of appendicitis is estimated approximately 1 in 1,500 deliveries (Scott and Abu-Hamda, 2004).

The rate of fetal death was found higher, particularly if perforation has occurred or pregnant women had the so-called negative appendectomy (i.e., the lack of appendectomy after the diagnosis of appendicitis) (McGory et al, 2007). However, previously a higher rate of CAs was not found in babies born to mothers with appendectomy during pregnancy in the Swedish registry (Mazze and Kallen, 1991).

12.8.1 Results of the Study (VI)

Out of 22,843 cases, 21 (0.09%), while out of 38,151 controls, 25 (0.07%) had mothers with appendicitis/appendectomy during the study pregnancy (1.4, 0.7–2.6). Thus our study did also not indicate a higher risk for the total group of CAs. Acute appendicitis was diagnosed more frequently between III and V gestational months and in general was followed by open appendectomy within 1 week.

The mean maternal age (23.7 vs. 25.5 year) and birth order (1.4 vs. 1.8) was lower in mothers with appendicitis/appendectomy than in mothers without appendicitis/appendectomy.

Birth outcomes did not show significant differences: mean gestational age (39.5 vs. 39.4 year, $p = 0.73$) and birth weight (3,302 vs. 3,276 g, $p = 0.63$), rate of PB (8.0% vs. 9.2%, 0.9, 0.2–3.7) and LBW newborns (4.0% vs. 5.7%, 0.9, 0.1–7.3).

However, cases affected by primary microcephaly were associated with the appendicitis/appendectomy of their mothers during pregnancy (26.6, 6.1–115.1), although this association was based only on 2 cases, thus the effect of chance cannot be excluded. The data of these 2 cases are presented here.

A 3,750 g (90th percentile) girl with a length of 58 cm (90th percentile) and a head circumference of 29 cm (5 percentile) was born at the 43rd gestational week. Her forehead was narrow and occiput flattened. No other birth defects or cerebral lesions were found after her birth. The mother was a 28-year-old healthy clerk who was a smoker (10 cigarettes/day). The father was a 31-year-old disabled man collecting disability pension because of an accident; he was a regular drinker and smoker (20 cigarettes/day). The family history of this couple was negative and their 3 previous children, with birth weights of 3,050–3,300 g, were healthy. The study pregnancy was unplanned, the mother had anemia, and she had iron and folic acid supplementation after her first prenatal visit in the 10th gestational week. Acute appendicitis was diagnosed in the 14th gestational week, but surgical intervention was postponed to 30th gestational week because of the reluctance of physicians to conduct surgery during pregnancy. At the time of surgery, a gangrenous and ruptured appendicitis with generalized peritonitis was found. In III–VII month of gestation, the mother had a common cold complicated by secondary pneumonia.

The second case was a 1,900 g (3rd percentile) girl with a length of 47 cm (3rd percentile) and a head circumference of 30 cm (3rd percentile) born at the 38th gestational week. Other than her microcephaly, no birth defects were found. The mother was a healthy 20-year-old radiologic assistant. The father was a 23-year-old healthy skilled worker. Neither parent drank alcohol or smoked. Their family history was negative for genetic diseases and birth defects. The mother previously had one induced abortion owing to social reason. This pregnancy was planned but she underwent a Lash procedure, because of cervical incompetence before conception. Because of a threatened abortion (minimal vaginal bleeding and uterine contractions) in the 9th week of gestation, the mother was treated with promethazine, magnesium, folic acid, multivitamin, iron, vitamins D and E, and iron. Acute appendicitis was diagnosed in the 16th week of gestation but surgical intervention was postponed to 24th week at the request of the mother. She was treated with ampicillin and conservative physical methods (bed rest with cold compress). At the time of surgery, ruptured appendix with peritoneal abscess was found. After surgical intervention, she had gastrointestinal atonia treated with 0.5 mg neostigmine by intramuscular administration 3 times/day for 5 days.

Fetal toxoplasmosis, cytomegalovirus, and rubella effects were excluded in both cases with microcephaly; and neither infant had evidence of craniostenosis or other defects.

12.8.2 Interpretation of Results

Birth outcomes of pregnant women with appendicitis did not show significant difference from the reference sample. However, a higher rate of appendicitis was found among primary microcephalic cases based only on 2 cases but very similar pathological process. The critical period of primary microcephaly is between the 10th and 20th gestational weeks. Acute appendicitis was diagnosed in the 14th and 16th gestational weeks in the mothers of previously presented 2 cases, but the surgical intervention was postponed to 30th and 24th gestational weeks, i.e., by 16 and 8 weeks, respectively, due to the reluctance of physicians to conduct surgery during pregnancy and/or the request of pregnant women. Thus the causal association with inadequately treated maternal appendicitis cannot be excluded in these cases. In addition, we were unable to find any other possible causes (e.g. infections or drugs) in the origin of microcephaly in these two cases.

The diagnosis of appendicitis in pregnant women becomes more difficult with the progress of pregnancy. Cunningham and McCubbin (1975) did not find delay in the diagnosis in the first trimester, in contrast to delays occurring in 18% in the second trimester and 75% in the third trimester. This delay in the diagnosis associated with a higher incidence of complications such as perforation. The right lower quadrant pain is the most common symptom in all three trimesters (Mourad et al., 2000). Recent studies showed the safety of laparoscopic appendectomy in all three trimesters of pregnancy (Lyass et al., 2001).

The rate of appendectomy during pregnancy was 1 in 936 in Sweden (Mazze and Kallen, 1989, 1991) and 1 in 5,955 in Hungary. To the best of our knowledge the incidence of appendicitis does not differ significantly between the two populations, thus we suggest that the drastic difference in the rate of appendectomy reflects the different attitude of medical doctors regarding to surgery during pregnancy. The course of appendicitis in these two pregnant women suggests an important warning: complications of appendicitis ensuing from delaying surgery may have a role in the origin of primary microcephaly.

Thus, the classical statement of Babler (1908): "the mortality of appendicitis is the mortality of delay", might be supplemented with the notion that the risk to fetuses in pregnant women with appendicitis is the delay of surgical intervention.

In conclusion, appendicitis followed by urgent appendectomy had no risk for the fetal development according to birth outcomes evaluated. However, the secondary complications of appendicitis due to the delay of surgical intervention may increase the risk of primary microcephaly during second trimester. Thus, we believe it is prudent to recommend appendectomy for pregnant patients promptly after the diagnosis of appendicitis

12.9 Ulcerative Colitis

Ulcerative colitis (UC) is primarily a mucosal disease always involving the rectum and extending proximally in a continuous fashion, sometimes involving the entire colon. The main symptoms of UC are diarrhea often with bleeding and some degree of abdominal pain (Scott and Abu-Hamda, 2004).

UC occurs in women of childbearing age as well; therefore the risk of adverse pregnancy and birth outcomes has been subject to research during the last decades. However, these studies included patients with UC in general without appropriate controls, sometimes UC and Crohn disease were not differentiated or different types of CAs were not separated within the total group of CAs. CAs cannot be regarded as a single homogeneous outcome because exposure to a teratogen does not uniformly increase the rates of all CAs, but rather tends to increase rates of specific CAs. Thus the objective of our case-control study was to evaluate the possible adverse effects of UC for the fetal development and particularly its role in the origin of different CAs in the population-based dataset of the HCCSCA.

12.9.1 Results of the Study (VIII)

The case groups consisted of 22,843 informative offspring with CA, of whom 71 (0.3%) had mothers with UC. Among 38,151 controls without CA, 95 (0.2%) had mothers with UC. Of the 71 case mothers, 60 (84.5%) and of the 91 control mothers, 66 (69.5%) had prospectively and medically recorded UC in the prenatal maternity logbook. All pregnant women had the onset of UC before conception. High proportion of pregnant women was treated mainly by sulfasalazine and promethazine.

The mean maternal age (25.9 vs. 25.5 year) and birth order (1.6) did not show significant differences between pregnant women with or without UC; however, the sulfasalazine treatments (10.5% vs. 0.4%) and promethazine (25.3% vs. 15.8%) of pregnant women with UC.

There was no significant difference in the occurrence of acute and other chronic maternal disease between pregnant women with or without UC. Among pregnancy complications, only anemia occurred more frequently in pregnant women with UC (19.9% vs. 15.7%).

Table 12.5 summarizes the most important data of birth outcome of controls without CA.

There was a shorter gestational age which associated with a much higher rate of PB. However, there was no clinically important difference in the mean birth weight and the rate of LBW newborns; in fact the latter was lower in babies born to mothers with UC.

The risk of total CAs in informative offspring of mother with UC was not higher (1.3, 0.9–1.8). However, higher risk for congenital limb deficiencies (6.2, 2.9–13.1),

Table 12.5 Birth outcomes of newborn infants born to mothers with or without UC

	Pregnant women					
	Without UC		With UC			
Birth outcomes	($N = 38{,}056$)		($N = 95$)		Comparison	
Quantitative	Mean	S.D.	Mean	S.D.	*t*	*p*
Gestational age (week)	39.4	2.1	**38.7**	2.3	3.2	**0.0001**
Birth weight (g)	3,276	511	3,249	511	0.5	0.61
Categorical	No.	%	No.	%	OR	95% CI
PB	3,478	9.1	18	**18.9**	2.3	**1.4–3.9**
LBW newborns	2,163	5.7	4	4.2	0.7	0.3–2.0

obstructive CAs of the urinary tract (3.3, 1.1–9.5) and multiple CAs (2.6, 1.3–5.4) was found.

The evaluation of 8 cases with congenital limb deficiencies showed that only one limb was affected in all cases, 6 occurred in upper limbs and 2 in lower limbs. Their estimated diagnosis was terminal transverse type and this type of congenital limb deficiencies is caused by vascular disruption of the limb buds.

Four cases were affected by obstructive CAs of the urinary tract; hydronephrosis occurred in 2 children due to stricture of the ureterovesical junction. However, the third case was familial; the father also had obstructive CA of the urinary tract which needed surgery. Therefore, we excluded this case and after this exclusion, the previously mentioned higher risk disappeared for obstructive CA of the urinary tract.

The distribution of component CAs in 9 cases with multiple CA is worth our attention:

1. Conjoined twin A: cleft lip with cleft palate, cardiovascular CA (common ventricle), limb deficiency in upper limbs, and syndactyly in lower limbs.
2. Conjoined twin B: cleft lip with cleft palate, omphalocele
3. Cleft lip with cleft palate, cardiovascular CA (cor triatriatum), CA of the diaphragm with lung hypoplasia and dextrocardia, absence of the external auditory canal causing impairment of hearing.
4. Cardiovascular CA (unspecified), CA of the ear, polydactyly in upper limbs
5. Congenital limb deficiency in lower limbs, double kidney with double pelvis, hemivertebrae
6. Anal atresia with pseudohermaphroditism
7. Congenital hydrocephalus, Hirschsprung's disease
8. Congenital hydrocephalus, microcephalus, CA of the cauda equine, talipes equinovarus
9. Omphalocele with mesenterium commune.

On the one hand, among these multimalformed children, we had a conjoined twin pair (its occurrence is extremely rare: 1 in 75,000 births), 3 cleft lip with cleft palate (but 2 occurred on the monozygotic conjoined twins), 3 cardiovascular CA (each different), 2 limb deficiencies, and 2 ear CAs. Thus, no characteristic pattern of CAs was found in these children. On the other hand, if we calculate with the monozygotic twins as one subject (because they were the product of one conception) and we exclude No. 9, because mesenterium commune may be the secondary consequence of omphalocele, the previously found higher risk disappears.

12.9.2 Interpretation of Results

Thus, finally only a higher risk for unimelic limb deficiencies seems to be important from clinical aspect among the children of mothers with UC during the study pregnancy. The question is whether this association is causal, or connected with related drug treatment, other confounders, or influenced by chance.

Most pregnant women with UC were treated with sulfasalazine. Its active moiety is 5-amino salicylate which joins to sulfapyridine by an azo-linkage. The drug is broken by colonic bacteria into its component parts and salicylate works locally within the colonic lumen and exerts an anti-inflammatory effect through inhibition of both the cyclooxygenase and lipoxygenase pathways of arachidonic acid metabolism (Stenson, 1995). Sulfasalazine and its metabolite, sulfapyridine, readily cross the placenta, and their fetal concentrations are approximately the same as maternal concentrations. In addition sulfasalazine can inhibit absorption and metabolism of folate; therefore, such supplements should be prescribed for these patients. This method was followed in Hungary and we did not find any teratogenic potential of sulfasalazine (18). In addition, there was no higher risk for neural-tube defects (1.4, 0.5–3.8). In Hungary promethazine is used frequently in pregnant women for the treatment of threatened abortion and preterm delivery without any harm for fetal development (74). Patients with UC had a lower proportion of smokers and drinkers than pregnant women without UC. However, more data are needed to determine whether this association is causal or influenced by chance.

Finally, it is worth comparing our findings with the results of previous studies. In the cohort study by Fedorkow et al. (1989), the crude risk of CAs was increased 4-fold in children of pregnant women with both UC and Crohn disease together. Out of 98 exposed mothers, 4 (4.1%) children were affected with CA. (spina bifida, pyloric stenosis, hypospadias and trisomy18). Mogadam et al. (1981) conducted a cohort study in pregnant women with UC but they did not provide any risk estimates for CAs. The cohort study of Dominitz et al. (2002) showed a 3.8-fold risk for CAs in children born to mothers with UC, of the 107 exposed pregnant women, 8 (7.5%) had children affected with undescended testis, obstruction of the renal pelvis, congenital subluxation of the hip, omphalocele, a multiple CA caused by chromosomal aberration, and one unspecified CA. Thus previous studies did not find any association between maternal UC and a higher risk for limb deficiencies which might be explained by the obvious differences in the samples, study designs and evaluations from our approach.

In conclusion, our study indicates a higher risk for PB and limb deficiencies in the children of pregnant women with UC.

12.10 Crohn Disease

Another manifestation of inflammatory bowel diseases is Crohn disease which may involve any region of the gastrointestinal tract but colon and terminal ileum are most frequently affected. The major pathological process is the transmural granulomatous inflammation which causes abdominal pain, diarrhea, and bleeding sometimes with fistulous complications. Most frequently rectovaginal fistula occurs.

12.10.1 Interpretation of Data in the HCCSCA

In the data set of the HCCSCA only 9 controls and 3 cases had mothers with Crohn disease. These figures compared to the number of ulcerative colitis indicate an underascertainment of pregnant women with Crohn disease. The explanation may be the confusion of its diagnosis with ulcerative colitis; in addition, the symptoms of Crohn disease are less predictable. Thus the data of recorded pregnant women with Crohn disease are not appropriate for analysis.

12.11 Constipation

Constipation is one of the most frequent pathological conditions which affect 11–38% of pregnant women (Welsh, 2005); however, some clinical reports mentioned the complaints of constipation in over half of pregnant women (Fagan, 2002). Constipation is not a crucial issue during pregnancy; therefore, the occurrence of constipation as pregnancy-related problem is often neglected in the medical community (Scott and Abu-Hamad, 2004; Sauvat, 2007). This view is supported by the lack of appropriate epidemiological studies in this field (Shepard and Lemire, 2004).

Constipation is defined as the infrequent passage of hard stool. However, previously extreme definitions were used for this pathological condition. For example "Any patients who strains to defecate and does not pass at least one stool daily without effort is constipated" (Painter, 1980) or another extreme definition was "everyone should have at least one bowel movement a week" (Owen, 1983). Recently constipation has been defined by a frequency of spontaneous stools of less than 2 or 3 per week (Fagan, 2002). According to the study of Drossman et al. (1982) slightly more than 4% of adult people had fewer than two stools per week without subjective complaints.

Sometimes the management of constipation by diet is not enough, and drug treatment may be necessary. The possible teratogenic and/or fetotoxic effect of related drug treatments may cause a dilemma in clinical practice (Jewel and Young, 1998; Mahadevan and Kane, 2006; Thukral and Wolf, 2006).

12.11.1 Results of the Study (IX)

The objective of our study was to evaluate the possible association between maternal constipation with related drug treatments and adverse pregnancy outcomes, particularly CAs in the data set of the HCCSCA.

If pregnant women had constipation as the secondary consequence of other diseases, such as the symptoms of irritable bowel syndrome, Hirschsprung's disease, hiatal hernia, diverticular disease, malignant diseases, etc. were excluded from the study because the aim was to evaluate pregnant women with the so-called functional or idiopathic constipation.

There is no standard definition of constipation in the Hungarian clinical practice. As it appeared at the preliminary evaluation of our pregnant women with functional constipation, two groups could be differentiated: (i) prospectively and medically recorded constipation in the prenatal maternity logbook, thus the diagnosis was made by medical doctors and these pregnant women were treated with appropriate drugs and (ii) constipation based on retrospective maternal information. These pregnant women were rarely treated by laxative drugs, mainly lactulose. The spectrum of constipation is wide and the perception of symptoms is subjective, therefore we decided to evaluate only the first group, i.e. medically recorded and treated *severe constipation* (SC) during pregnancy.

The case group consisted of 22,843 malformed newborns or fetuses ("informative offspring"), of whom 465 (2.0%) were reported by mothers to have constipation but only 78 (0.34%) were medically recorded. Out of 38,151 controls, 797 (2.1%) were reported with constipation, but only 144 (0.38%) were medically recorded. We evaluated only 78 case and 144 control mothers with medically recorded SC (0.9, 0.6–1.3).

Out of 78 case mothers, 38 (48.7%), while out of 144 control mothers, 60 (41.7%) had SC in the first gestational weeks, thus the onset of this pathological condition was before conception. We considered this condition as a *chronic* disease because its symptoms were continued during the entire pregnancy as well. In another group, constipation occurred first in the study pregnancy and the highest frequency of the onset of this *new-onset* constipation fell between III and V gestational months. The new onset constipation may be related to several factors during pregancy: (i) the common oral iron therapy during pregnancy which may exacerbate constipation, (ii) poor oral fluid intake due to nausea and vomiting during pregnancy, (iii) increased transit time due to slower gastrointestinal movement (explained by higher production of progesterone) (iv) and alteration in diet. SC had long duration during pregnancy, and nearly all worsened due to rectosigmoid pressure from the gravid uterus in the third trimester.

Pregnant women with SC had a higher mean maternal age (26.6 vs. 25.4 year) due to the larger proportion of women in the age group of 30 and more years but a lower mean birth order (1.6 vs. 1.7) due to the higher proportion of primiparae (58.3% vs. 47.7%) compared to mothers without SC. There was no difference in marital status among the study groups but SC was more frequent in professional and managerial pregnant women.

The incidence of different pregnancy complications showed obvious differences in pregnant women with or without SC. Here the data of 144 control pregnant women with SC are shown (Table 12.6).

Thus there was a higher occurrence of threatened abortion and preterm delivery, severe nausea and vomiting, and a much higher incidence of anemia in pregnant women with SC.

Among acute diseases, only vulvovaginitis and bacterial vaginosis were more frequent in pregnant women with SC (15.3% vs. 7.6%, 2.2, 1.4–3.5), and these mothers were treated during pregnancy. Among chronic diseases, only the prevalence of hemorrhoid was 10-fold more frequent in pregnant women with SC than in pregnant women without SC (33.3% vs. 3.3%, 14.5, 10.2–20.6).

There was an obvious difference in the distribution and frequency of drugs used for SC and/or hemorrhoids between the study groups, The oral treatment of

Table 12.6 Pregnancy complications of pregnant women with or without severe constipation (SC)

Pregnancy complications	Without SC ($N = 38{,}007$)		With SC ($N = 144$)		Comparison	
	No.	%	No.	%	OR	95% CI
Nausea-vomiting, severe	3,838	10.1	31	21.5	**2.1**	**1.5–2.7**
Threatened abortion	6,466	17.0	46	31.9	**2.3**	**1.6–3.2**
Preeclampsia-eclampsia	3,204	8.4	17	11.8	1.5	0.9–2.4
Threatened preterm delivery	5,417	14.3	43	29.9	**2.6**	**1.8–3.7**
Placental disorders[a]	587	1.5	5	3.5	2.3	0.9–5.6
Poly/oligohydramnios	205	0.5	0	0.0	–	–
Gestational diabetes	269	0.7	1	0.7	1.0	0.1–7.0
Anemia	6,250	16.4	106	73.6	**14.2**	**9.8–20.5**

[a]Including placenta previa, premature separation of the placenta, antepartum haemorrhage.

senna and phenolphthalein was used most frequently for the treatment of SC, while two suppositories: Reparon® (Bacterium coli + phenol) and Hemorid® (ephedrine + epinephrine + procaine + camphor + choralhydrate + menthol) were the most common medications for local treatment of hemorrhoids. Only the use of phenolphthalein showed a higher frequency in case mothers compared to control mothers with SC (4.0, 2.4–18.2).

Among pregnancy supplements, mainly iron (83.3% vs. 70.1%) was used more frequently by pregnant women with SC compared to pregnant women without SC. However, folic acid (64.6% and 54.4%) and multivitamins (10.4% vs. 6.6%) were also used more frequently by pregnant women with SC than without SC.

The evaluation of birth outcomes (Table 12.7) resulted in an unexpected finding: there was a more obvious male excess among newborns of mothers with SC than

Table 12.7 Birth outcomes of newborn infants born to mothers with or without severe constipation (SC)

Variables	Without SC ($N = 38{,}007$)		With SC ($N = 144$)		Comparison
Quantitative	Mean	S.D.	Mean	S.D.	
Gestational age, week[a]	39.4	2.0	**39.8**	1.9	t=2.2, p=**0.03**
Birth weight, g[b]	3,276	511	3,275	516	$t = 1.6, p = 0.11$
Categorical	No.	%	No.	%	OR (95% CI)
Males	24,693	65.0	106	**73.6**	**1.5 (1.0–2.2)**
PB[a]	3,490	9.2	6	**4.2**	**0.5 (0.2–0.9)**
LBW[b]	2,161	5.7	6	4.2	1.1 (0.4–2.9)

[a]Adjusted for maternal age, birth order, maternal employment status, and drug use.

[b]Adjusted for maternal age, birth order, maternal employment status, drug use, and gestational age.

in the babies of mothers without SC; the latter corresponded to the usual sex ratio in the data set of the HCCSCA. However, the male excess was found only in the subgroup of 60 pregnant women with chronic SC (80.0%) compared to 84 pregnant women with new onset SC (66.7%) (2.2, 1.1–4.1, $p = 0.01$).

The mean gestational age was significantly longer in babies born to mothers with SC compared to the reference group. There was no difference in the mean birth weight between the two study groups. The rate of PB was lower in the group of mothers with SC, while the rate of LBW newborns was also somewhat lower, but this difference was far from the level of significance.

First the occurrence of SC during the entire pregnancy was considered when evaluating CAs. The adjusted OR for the total CA group was 1.0 (0.7–1.3) and there was no higher risk for any CA group. In the second step, pregnant women with SC were evaluated only during the first trimester and there was no higher risk in any CA group either.

12.11.2 Interpretation of Results

Our study resulted in four main findings.

First, the prevalence of anemia was much higher in pregnant women with SC explained partly with their high occurrence of hemorrhoids.

Second, there was a male excess in the newborns of mothers with chronic SC but not in the newborns of pregnant women with new onset SC.

Third, the gestational age was longer and it associated with a lower rate of PB of newborn infants born to mothers with SC. However, the longer gestational age did not associate with a larger birth weight, and it may indicate some delay in intrauterine growth.

Fourth, a higher risk for total or any CA group was not found in the offspring of mothers with SC and related drug treatment during pregnancy.

At the interpretation of these results, it is necessary to stress that we evaluated pregnant women with SC because our study design was based on the dose-effect relation concept of human teratology. Thus if there is no teratogenic (CA-inducing) effect of SC, we may neglect this effect in pregnant women with less severe functional constipation. The prevalence of SC was 0.3–0.4% in our pregnant women, although 11–38% of pregnant women reported constipation in other studies (Welsh, 2005). We have three further arguments for SC in our pregnant women: (i) their constipation was medically recorded in the prenatal maternity logbook; (ii) nearly one third were affected by hemorrhoids as well; and (iii) all pregnant women had third line therapy.

The recommended first line therapy includes increased fiber and fluid intakes, regular defecation, and increased exercise. The second line of therapy comprises osmotic laxatives such as magnesium hydrochloride ("milk of magnesium", which mobilizes fluid within the gut volume) and lactulose (which exerts its effect in the colonic lumen). The third line therapy is based on stimulant medications, such as senna (Jewell and Young, 1998; Williamson, 2001; Tytgat et al., 2003; Welsh, 2005;

Mahadevan and Kane, 2006; Thukral and Wolf, 2006). All pregnant women with SC were treated by senna (about 90%) and/or phenolphthalein (about 10%) in Hungary.

Previously the possible teratogenic effect of senna drugs was studied only in rats and rabbits without any teratogenic effect (Mengs, 1986). Senna is one of the strongest stimulant laxatives, containing two stereoisomers: sennosides A and B. These compounds do not appear to be absorbed in the small intestine but are broken by colonic bacteria of large bowel to monoanthrone, a glycone structure. The latter stimulates colonic motility and may interfere with water and sodium reabsorption within 8–12 h. Occasionally senna drugs take 24 h to produce stool evacuation. Our recent population-based case-control study indicated the lack of teratogenicity of senna (93).

However, our previously mentioned data showed a higher occurrence of phenolphthalein treatment in case mothers compared to control mothers with SC and it may show its possible teratogenic risk for CA. Phenolphthalein is diphenylmethane derivative laxative that acts as a stimulant on the colon and take at least 6 h to produce a fecal evacuation. We found only one epidemiological study regarding to the use of phenolphthalein during pregnancy conducted by Heinonen et al. (1977). The study did not show any increase in the prevalence of CAs among the offspring of 806 women who took this laxative during pregnancy. Therefore, we decided to conduct a case-control study to check the teratogenic potential of phenolphthalein in II and III month of gestation (92). There was no higher risk for total CA group (1.2, 0.9–1.8), but the detailed analysis of the group of "Other isolated CA" showed an association of phenolphthalein treatment with a higher risk of Hirschsprung's disease. Out of 35 cases with Hirschsprung's disease, 4 (11.4%) born to mothers with phenolphthalein treatment, while 64 matched controls had no mothers with this treatment ($p = 0.01$).

The much higher rate of anemia (most caused by iron deficiency in Hungary) may be related to the well-known association between constipation and hemorrhoids, i.e. frequent bleeding in pregnant women. Most pregnant women with anemia were treated by iron.

The excess of males among newborn infants born to mothers with chronic SC needs some discussion. There was a male excess in the reference group as well, explained by the study design (see Subchapter 1.5.1). However, a significantly higher proportion of males were found among newborns in the subgroup of pregnant women with chronic SC than in the reference group and in the subgroup of new onset SC. Theoretically, there may be two explanations for this unexpected finding. (i) A higher rate of early postconceptional selection of female embryos. Unfortunately, our data set is not appropriate to measure the rate of miscarriages, but this hypothesis does not seem to be plausible. (ii) Chronic SC may modify pH of vaginal fluid and the less acidic vaginal pH may prefer the transfer of spermatozoa including Y chromosome (Jaffe et al., 1987). This hypothesis may be supported by the somewhat higher rate of vulvovaginitis or bacterial vaginosis in pregnant women with SC.

The findings of the study showed that SC was more frequent in elder primiparae who had better socioeconomic status and a higher standard of prenatal care (e.g.

folic acid and/or multivitamin supplementation). The latter characteristics of these mothers may explain their longer gestational age and lower rate of PB. The delayed intrauterine growth of fetus in pregnant women with SC would also need further studies, but the rate of LBW newborns was not higher, and this finding is against the severe intrauterine fetal growth retardation. On the other hand, a higher rate of threatened abortion and preterm delivery, in addition to severe nausea and vomiting was recorded in pregnant women with SC. The question is whether it may have a causal association with SC in the mothers, or only medical doctors considered these pregnancies at high risk with these labels. The observed birth outcomes seem to confirm the latter speculation. However, the higher rate of severe nausea and vomiting in pregnancy may have some causal association with SC (Williamson, 2001; Welsh, 2005).

In conclusion, SC during pregnancy associates frequently with anemia due to hemorrhoids but there is no higher risk for adverse birth outcomes. In fact the rate of PB was lower and a higher occurrence of CAs was not found in the offspring of mothers with SC treated mostly by senna. The unexpected finding, i.e. male excess among babies born to mothers with chronic SC needs further studies.

The maternal disorders of the *liver and the biliary system* can also be divided into two groups (Joshi et al., 2010). The first group includes disorders specific to pregnancy, e.g. intrahepatic cholestatis of pregnancy. The second group comprises liver and biliary system disorders incidental to pregnancy, e.g. cholecystitis-cholelithiasis (Williamson, 2001).

12.12 Intrahepatic Cholestasis of Pregnancy

Intrahepatic cholestasis of pregnancy (IHCP) is a rare disease with an incidence of 1 in 100 to 1 in 1000 pregnant women; nevertheless, IHCP is the most common pathological liver disease unique to pregnancy (Landon, 2004). The typical symptom of IHCP is progressive pruritus, especially of the palms and soles of pregnant women followed rarely by jaundice several weeks later with elevated serum bile acids occurring in the second half (usually from week 25) of pregnancy. However, the increase of direct bilirubin is mild, rarely exceeding 5 mg/dL. There is an increased risk for stillbirth and PB, thus the perinatal mortality is higher. The proposed mechanism for intrauterine fetal death was that the bile acid taurocholate impaired cardiomyocyte function (Williamson et al., 2001).

12.12.1 Interpretation of Data in the HCCSCA

IHCP occurred in 2 case mothers and 7 control mothers. One case was affected by anencephaly, while another one was affected by tetralogy of Fallot. Out of 7 controls, 4 had LBW although the mean gestational age was only slightly shorter (39.1 vs. 39.4 week). The mean birth weight (2,466 vs. 3,276 g) was much lower indicating intrauterine growth retardation. Three control mothers and no case mother were treated with ursodeoxycholic acid (Mazella at al., 2001).

12.13 Cirrhosis of Liver

Liver cirrhosis is defined as the histological development of regenerative nodules surrounded by fibrous bands in response to chronic liver injury which leads to portal hypertension and end-stage liver disease (Schuppan and Afdhal, 2008). Liver cirrhosis is rare in pregnant women because most women with this disease have oligomenorrhea and infertility (Landon, 2004). The origin of liver cirrhosis is worth differentiating into two main groups: the secondary consequence of viral hepatitis (the latter disease group is discussed among infectious diseases) or chronic non-viral hepatitis due to autoimmune conditions, alcohol abuse, drug or toxin-induced injury. Liver cirrhosis is associated with an increased risk for PB and perinatal mortality.

12.13.1 Interpretation of Data in the HCCSCA

The data base of the HCCSCA included 2 controls and one case with giant kidney. One control was born on the 33rd gestational week with 1,880 g while another was born on the 37th gestational week with 2,960 g.

12.14 Cholecystitis

Although the onset of cholecystitis is rare during pregnancy (Welsh, 2005), acute cholecystitis is the second most common cause of acute abdomen during pregnancy, occurring in 1 in 1,600–10,000 pregnancies (Landon, 2004; Augustin and Majerovic, 2007). The treatment of cholecystitis may cause problems in pregnant women due to the possible teratogenic and/or fetotoxic effect of related drug treatments (Holzbach, 1983; Mahadevan and Kane, 2006; Thukral and Wolf, 2006). As far as we know, the possible association between cholecystitis in pregnant women and adverse birth outcomes, particularly CAs in their offspring has not been evaluated in case-control epidemiological studies.

12.14.1 Results of the Study (X)

Cholecystitis was classified according to acute and chronic cholecystitis without mention of calculus (gallstones). The symptoms of cholecystitis cover a wide spectrum such as nausea, vomiting, dyspepsia, intolerance of fatty foods, and acute onset of a colic or stabbing pain that begins over the midepigastrium or right upper abdominal quadrant and radiates to the back. If the acute cholecystitis is not complicated, symptoms and signs usually subside gradually within 2–3 days (Landers et al., 1987; Landon, 2004). Cholelithiasis is the cause of cholecystitis or common secondary complication in over 90% of cases (Kammerer, 1979), but our plan was to evaluate pregnant women with cholecystitis without the diagnosis of cholelithiasis. If pregnant women were affected with cholelithiasis and cholecystitis, these pregnant women were evaluated among the patients with cholelithiasis. In addition, postcholecystectomy syndrome and cholangitis were also excluded from this study group.

We decided to evaluate only medically recorded cholecystitis because the perception of the symptoms of this disease is subjective, and because we were unable to differentiate cholecystitis with or without cholelithiasis during the study pregnancy on the basis of maternal self-reported information.

The case group consisted of 22,843 malformed newborns or fetuses ("informative offspring"), of whom 109 (0.48%) had mothers with medically recorded cholecystitis. Out of 38,151 controls, 145 (0.38%) were born to mothers with cholecystitis (1.3, 1.0–1.6).

Out of 109 case and 145 control mothers with cholecystitis, only 10 (9.2%) and 19 (13.1%) had surgical intervention, i.e. cholecystectomy during the study pregnancy, respectively.

Cholecystitis was diagnosed in I gestational month in 37% of pregnant women which continued at least in II gestational month in all pregnant women. The onset of cholecystitis occurred during the study pregnancy in 63% of pregnant women. This new onset cholecystitis occurred during II and III gestational months in 25 case mothers and 25 control mothers. Therefore, 57% of pregnant women were affected with cholecystitis during II and/or III gestational month. The duration of cholecystitis was between 1 week and 9 months, however, the mean was 2.4 months. The duration of cholecystitis therefore was much longer than the expected 2–3 days (i.e. less than 1 week) of acute cholecystitis. Some pregnant women reported on fever as well; therefore, we suppose that most of our pregnant women had *complicated cholecystitis* (CC).

Mean maternal age of pregnant women with CC (27.1 vs. 25.4 year) was higher than pregnant women without CC due to the larger proportion of elder (30 or more years old) women with CC. Mean birth order (2.0 vs. 1.7) was also higher in pregnant women with CC. There was no significant difference in marital and employment status among the study groups.

Folic acid supplementation as the indicator of prenatal care's standard was less frequent in mothers with CC (41.7%), particularly in case mothers (33.9%) compared to pregnant women without CC (52.6%).

Among other acute and chronic maternal diseases, only migraine occurred more frequently in pregnant women with CC (5.9% vs. 2.1%).

Most pregnant women with CC had three kinds of treatment. The first group included specific medicinal products for the treatment of pregnant women with CC in Hungary such as Bilagit® (phenolphthalein + papaverine + methenamine + menthol + sodium choleinicum; 23.9%), Pancreatin® (lipase + protease + amylase, 7.3%), and Almagel® (aluminium-magnesium hydroxide; 5.5%). The second group of these drugs comprised of spasmodic drotaverine (35.8%) and analgesic dipyrone (22.9%), in addition to acetylsalicylic acid (14.7%). Antibiotics such as ampicillin (13.8%) and penamecillin (6.4%) belonged to the third group.

The first objective of our study was to evaluate the occurrence of pregnancy complications in pregnant women with CC. Only the incidence of preeclampsia-eclampsia (16.6%) was higher in pregnant women with CC compared to pregnant women without CC (8.3%).

The second objective of our study was to evaluate pregnancy/birth outcomes of pregnant women affected with CC. The mean gestational age at delivery (39.1 vs. 39.4 week) was 0.3 week shorter in babies born to mother with CC compared to the reference group. The rate of PB (11.0% vs. 9.2%) was somewhat higher in the group of mothers with CC. The difference in the mean birth weight (3,293 vs. 3,276 g, i.e. 17 g excess) in the group of mothers with CC was not important from clinical aspect, nevertheless the rate of LBW newborns (9.0% vs. 5.7%) was higher in the group of mothers with CC.

The prevalence of CC during the entire pregnancy and particularly in II and/or III gestational month was compared between cases with different CA groups and their all matched controls. CC during any time of pregnancy did not pose increased risk for total CA or any CA group. However, when evaluating CC only in II and/or III gestational months, we found a higher risk for neural-tube defect (OR: 2.7, 1.2–6.1) based on 6 cases.

Of the 6 cases with neural-tube defects, 3 anencephaly and 3 had spina bifida aperta. The critical period of neural-tube defects is the 6th gestational week, i.e. in II gestational month. Of the 6 cases, all 6 mothers had exposure of CC in II gestational month. Of these 6 pregnant women, only one was supplemented with folic acid from the 4th and 5th gestational month, but nobody used folic acid containing multivitamins.

12.14.2 Interpretation of Results

Three main findings of the study are worth discussing, but it is important to stress that our pregnant women were affected by CC, i.e. severe complicated cholecystitis.

First, the incidence of preeclampsia-eclampsia was higher in pregnant women with CC compared to pregnant women without CC. This association can be explained partly by the involvement of liver in this pregnancy complication.

Second, there was a somewhat shorter gestational age in pregnant women with CC and it was associated with an increased rate of PB.

Third, maternal CC during II month of gestation associated with a higher risk for neural-tube defects. We were not able to find any previous report regarding to this association between cholecystitis and neural-tube defects (Elwood et al., 1992).

When analyzing this association between CC and neural-tube defects, the maternal-teratogenic effect of CC itself, the causes of CC (i.e. the microbial agents), related drug treatments, other confounders and chance effect should be considered.

Our and other studies indicated an association between neural-tube defects and high fever during the critical period of this CA (XV). The high fever is not characteristic for cholecystitis, but some pregnant women with CC reported on fever in their study pregnancy. We did not find any data regarding the possible association between the microbial causes of cholecystitis and neural-tube defects (Elwood et al., 1992). Drugs might have a role in the origin of neural-tube defects, particularly folate antagonists such as cotrimoxazole (Hernadez-Diaz et al., 2000; 19, 20) but their use is not recommended in pregnancy, therefore these drugs were not used frequently in the treatment of our pregnant women with CC. The most frequently used drug for the treatment of pregnant women with CC was drotaverine, however, this drug was found to be safe in pregnancy (83). In addition, we evaluated CC related drugs as confounders in the calculation of adjusted OR.

Our previous intervention trials showed an obvious protective effect of folic acid-containing multivitamins during the periconceptional period for the first occurrence of neural-tube defects (125, 131). The use of folic acid and folic acid-containing multivitamins was less frequent in case mothers; we, therefore, evaluated these supplementations as confounders in the study.

Our hypothesis for the explanation of possible association between CC and neural-tube defects is based on the observation that our pregnant women were not treated adequately; therefore, most of them had chronic inflammation with secondary complications and some had high fever. Therefore, the possible association between CC in early pregnancy and a higher risk for neural-tube defects can be explained by high fever. Our previous studies showed that this fever related risk for CA is preventable by antipyretic drug therapy (XV), but the small number of cases born to mothers with CC was not appropriate to check this possible benefit in the study.

The incidence of acute symptomatic biliary tract diseases during pregnancy ranges from 0.05 to 0.3% (Printen and Ott, 1978; Basso et al., 1992). The figure of CC was 0.42% in the study, i.e. somewhat higher than expected because our samples included chronic cholecystitis as well.

The new onset of CC can be explained by the physiological changes in pregnant women. On one hand, the amount of biliary sludge is increased during pregnancy as a result of delayed gallbladder emptying and a higher gallbladder residual volume (Behar, 1999). These changes are explained mainly by the higher production of progesterone during pregnancy. Progesterone induces smooth muscle relaxation of the gallbladder (Braverman et al., 1980); therefore gallbladder volume is increased in pregnant women (Axelrod et al., 1994).

Our study confirmed the prior study which showed that pregnant women with CC are usually elder with a higher proportion of multiparae (Basso et al., 1992). There was no difference in the socioeconomic status of pregnant women with CC or without CC; however, the folic acid supplementation as an indicator of prenatal care's standard was less frequent among pregnant women with CC. The proportion of surgical interventions was much lower in the Hungary than in recent international studies (Hiatt et al., 1994; Lu et al., 2004).

Thus, we recommend active treatment in pregnant women with cholecystitis primary with the combination of antimicrobial and antipyretic drugs and secondary with surgical management to prevent CC with possible maternal-teratogenic effect for the offspring. In addition, there is a strong indication for periconceptional folic acid/multivitamin supplementation in pregnant women with cholecystitis.

In conclusion, a higher risk for PB and neural-tube defects was found in the children of pregnant women with complicated cholecystitis.

12.15 Cholelithiasis (Gallstone Disease)

Cholelithiasis or gallstone disease is another common pathological condition of the biliary system. Patients with cholelithiasis can be differentiated into two main groups: "*silent*", i.e. asymptomatic gallstones and *symptomatic* cholelithiasis with biliary colic presenting with sudden onset pain typically located at the epigastric area or right upper quadrant. The intensity of the pain usually remains severe and steady for up 3–5 h, although in nearly half of the patients the duration was less than 1 h. If the pain is prolonged more than 5 h and it remains severe with prominent sign of abdominal tenderness associated with fever and systematic symptoms, acute cholecystitis must be suspected (Landon, 2004).

12.15.1 Results of the Study (X)

Obviously the data set of the HCCSCA included pregnant women with *symptomatic cholelithiasis (SC)* with or without cholecystitis and the aim of the study was the evaluation of pregnancy complications of these pregnant women and the adverse birth outcomes, particularly CAs in their offspring. We decided to evaluate only medically recorded SC in the prenatal maternity logbook partly because the perception of the symptoms of SC is subjective; and partly because we were unable to differentiate previous and present SC during the study pregnancy on the basis of maternal self-reported information.

The case group consisted of 22,843 malformed newborns or fetuses ("informative offspring"), of whom 62 (0.27%) had mothers with medically recorded SC. Out of 38,151 controls, 119 (0.31%) were born to mothers with SC (0.9, 0.6–1.3).

Out of 181 pregnant women with SC, 26 (14.4%) had cholecystectomy during the study pregnancy.

Out of 181 pregnant women with SC, 101 (55.8%) were affected by SC in I gestational month and its symptoms continued at least in II gestational months in all pregnant women. We considered this condition as a *chronic* disease. Thus SC occurred first in the study pregnancy of 80 women and this *new-onset* SC showed a characteristic gestational time pattern with a peak between II and IV gestation months (77.5%). The duration of SC was between 1 week and 9 months, however, the mean was 3.3 months in pregnant women during the study pregnancy.

Mean maternal age (26.5 vs. 25.4 year) and birth order (2.2 vs. 1.7) was higher in pregnant women with SC compared to pregnant women without SC. There was no significant difference in marital and employment status among the study groups. Folic acid and multivitamin supplementations as the indicator of prenatal care was similar in pregnant women with or without SC.

Among acute maternal diseases, only the acute diseases of the respiratory system were more frequent in pregnant women with SC (16.8%) compared to mothers without SC (9.0%). We checked the different diseases within this group (sinusitis, pharyngitis, tonsillitis, laryngitis-tracheitis, bronchitis-bronchiolitis, and pneumonia) but specific cluster was not found. Among chronic diseases, essential hypertension (3.4% vs. 0.6%), varicose veins of the lower extremities (3.4% vs. 1.5%), thrombophlebitis (5.9% vs. 2.4%), hemorrhoids (15.1% vs. 3.3%), and dyspepsia-heartburn-gastro-oesophageal reflux (2.5% vs. 0.4%) occurred more frequently in pregnant women with SC than in pregnant women without SC.

Most pregnant women with SC had three kinds of treatment. The first group included specific pharmaceutical products for the treatment of pregnant women with CC in Hungary such as Cholagol® (magnesium salicylicum + menthol + pimenta radicis curcumae; 6.5%), and Bilagit® (phenolphthalein + papaverine + methenamine + menthol + sodium choleinicum; 25.8%). The second group of these drugs comprised spasmodic drotaverine (40.3%) and analgesic dipyrone. Antibiotics such as ampicillin (14.5%) and penamecillin (9.7%) belonged to the third group. Some other drugs were used for the treatment of other maternal pathological condition, e.g. senna (9.7%).

The first objective of the study was to check the possible association of SC in pregnant women with a higher risk for pregnancy complications. The frequency of different pregnancy complications was similar in pregnant women with SC or without SC.

The second objective of our study was to evaluate pregnancy/birth outcomes of pregnant women with SC or without SC. The mean gestational age (39.4 week) was similar in mothers with SC and without SC; however, the rate of PB (6.7% vs. 9.2%) was lower in the group of mothers with SC. The difference in the mean birth weight (i.e. 23 g excess) in the live-born babies of mothers with SC was not important from clinical aspect, but the rate of LBW newborns (3.4% vs. 5.7%) was lower in the group of mothers with SC.

The prevalence of SC during the entire pregnancy and particularly in II and/or III gestational months was compared between cases with different CA groups and their all matched controls. There was no higher risk for total CA or any CA group in mothers affected by SC. We evaluated case and control mothers with SC separately during II and/or III gestational months and significant risk was not found for total CA or any CA group.

12.15.2 Interpretation of Results

The incidence of biliary tract disease during pregnancy ranges from 0.05 to 0.3% (Printen and Ott, 1978; Basso et al., 1992). The incidence figure of SC was 0.30% in our study. Our study confirmed that pregnant women with SC are elder with higher proportion of multiparae (Swisher et al., 1994).

The new onset SC can be explained by three factors. (i) The higher production of progesterone during pregnancy may induce smooth muscle relaxation of the gallbladder which promotes stasis of bile and increases the risk of cholelithiasis and subsequently of cholecystitis (Behar, 1999). (ii) The elevated level of estrogens during pregnancy increases the lithogenicity of the bile, which further increases the risk for SC (Braverman et al., 1980). (iii) Gallbladder in pregnant women shows a decrease in the emptying rate and an increase in residual volume after emptying (Axelrod et al., 1994). On the other hand, the elevated level of estrogens during pregnancy inhibits gallbladder contraction with retention of cholesterol crystals, the precursor for stone formation (Bennion and Grundy, 1978). These changes promote stasis of the bile and increase the lithogenicity of the bile resulting in a higher risk for cholelithiasis and subsequently for cholecystitis. In conclusion, approximately 15% of women over 35 have asymptomatic gallstones (Scott, 1992).

Medical versus surgical management of SC was debated (Lee et al., 2000; Lu et al., 2004). Oral chenodeoxycholic acid and ursodeoxycholic acid are used for the treatment of SC (Thistle and Hoffmann, 1973; Iser et al., 1975). Their use is recommended in pregnancy (Shepard and Lemire, 2004).

There was a low proportion of surgical intervention in our pregnant women with SC. Our finding reflects the previous view of Hungarian physicians which preferred a delay in operation after delivery (VII). Owing to the high incidence of fetal loss, early studies recommended medical management of SC and the delay of the operation until after delivery (Greene et al., 1963). However, recently the previous strategy has been modified. If there is no recovery after conservative dietary and spasmolytic drug treatment, cholecystectomy is recommended (Sung et al., 2000; Cosenza et al., 1999) based on four arguments: (i) Non-operative management of SC increases the risk of gallstone pancreatitis up to 13% (Scott, 1992) which causes fetal loss in 10–20% of cases, in addition, other life-threatening complications such as perforation, peritonitis, sepsis may occur. (ii) Non-operative management has also been associated with the higher occurrence of miscarriages and preterm deliveries compared to patients who underwent cholecystectomy (McKellar et al., 1992). (iii) Surgery as a primary treatment can reduce the use of medications and the frequent recurrence rate (Curet, 2000). (iv) The recent progress in the two surgical procedures, i.e. laparoscopic and open cholecystectomy during pregnancy did not appear to be associated with increased complications (Graham et al., 1998; Glasgow et al., 1998; Simmons et al., 2004).

In conclusion, SC was combined frequently with other chronic maternal diseases, however, higher risk for adverse birth outcomes, including PB and CAs was not found in the newborn infants of pregnant women with SC.

12.16 Cholangitis

Cholangitis is a chronic cholestatic disease of unknown etiology characterized by fibrosis and inflammation of the intra- and extrahepatic bile ducts. This pathological process explains its term, primary sclerosing cholangitis, which is leading to biliary cirrhosis, hepatic failure, and ultimately death (Landon, 2004).

12.16.1 Interpretation of Data in the HCCSCA

There were 10 controls and 9 cases that had mother with reported/recorded cholangitis. Out of 9 cases, 3 had cardiovascular CAs (ventricular septal defect, patent ductus arteriosus, unspecified), 2 clubfoot, 1–1 oesophageal stenosis, anal atresia, hypospadias, and unimelic limb deficiency on the upper limb. Controls had a lower mean birth weight (3,006 vs. 3,276 g) with the usual mean gestational age (39.4 week) therefore some delay in the intrauterine growth of the fetuses should be considered.

12.17 Pancreatitis

The incidence of pancreatitis during pregnancy has ranged from 1 in 1,066 to 1 in 3,300 pregnancies (Landon, 2004), thus the range of expected numbers of pregnant women with pancreatitis is between 18 and 57, but the recorded number was 8 in the HCCSCA. Thus this disorder is either underreported or less frequent in the Hungarian pregnant population. In general, pancreatitis is associated with gallstones mostly in the third trimester of pregnancy. The major symptoms of acute pancreatitis are epigastric pain which may radiate to the flanks or shoulders along with abdominal tenderness. These symptoms require appropriate laboratory investigations to confirm the diagnosis. There are internationally accepted guidelines for the management of acute pancreatitis (UK Working Party, 2005). However, acute pancreatitis resolves spontaneously within several days in 90% of pregnant women.

12.17.1 Interpretation of Data in the HCCSCA

Four cases born to mothers with pancreatitis had cleft lip and palate, pseudohermaphroditism, clubfoot, and polydactyly on the hands. Out of 4 control mothers, 2 were affected by acute, and 2 were affected by chronic pancreatitis, the birth outcomes of their newborns were within the normal range.

12.18 Hernias

Hernias such as inguinal or ventral are classified among the diseases of the digestive system in the ICD.

12.18.1 Interpretation of Data in the HCCSCA

Inguinal hernia occurred in 17 control mothers and 3 case mothers. The children of case mothers were affected by ventricular septal defect, coarctation of the aorta and talipes equinovarus. PB did not occur among 17 controls, and their mean birth weight was 3,402 g.

All ventral hernias were the secondary complications of previous surgical interventions. The children of 4 case mothers were affected by coarctation of the aorta, unspecified cardiovascular CA, and macrodactyly, while among 4 controls, 2 were born as preterm baby.

12.19 Final Conclusions

The occurrence of the diseases of the digestive system is very frequent during pregnancy if we include 'nausea and vomiting in pregnancy' and constipation. Nevertheless, these pathological conditions have not been studied appropriately before; therefore, our investigations resulted in some unexpected findings, e.g. CA protective effect of nausea and vomiting in pregnancy or male excess among the newborns of pregnant women with chronic constipation. These findings may be important both from practical and theoretical aspect; therefore, they require further studies for confirmation or rejection.

References

Achkar E. Peptic ulcer disease. In: Farmer RG, Achkar E, Fleshler B (eds.) Clinical Gastroenterology. Raven Press, New York, 1983. pp.221–235.

Ananth CV, Rao PSG. Epidemiology of nausea and vomiting of pregnancy and its relation to fetal outcome in a rural area. J Tropic Pediat 1993; 39: 313–317.

Appierto U, Subrizi DA, Minozzi M, Unfer V. Nausea, vomiting and thyroid; function before and after induced abortion in normal pregnancy. Clin Exp Obstet Gynecol 1996; 23: 18–20.

Armstrong D, Marshall JK, Chiba N et al. Canadian Consensus Conference on the management of gastroesophageal reflux disease in adults – update 2004. Can J Gastroenterol 2005; 19: 15–35.

Augustin G, Majerovic M, Non-obstetrical acute abdomen during pregnancy. Eur J Obstet Gynecol Reprod Biol 2007; 131: 4–12.

Axelrod A, Fleischer D, Strack LL et al. Performance of ERCP fro symptomatic choledocholithiasis during pregnancy: techniques to increase safety and improve patient management. Am J Gastroenterol 1994; 89: 109–112.

Babler EA. Perforative appendicitis complicating pregnancy. JAMA 1908; 51: 1310–1312.

Basso L, McCollum P, Darling M et al. A study of cholelithiasis during pregnancy and its relationship with age, parity, menarche, breastfeeding, dysmenorrhoea, oral contraception and maternal history of cholelithiasis. Gynecol Obstet 1992; 175: 41–46.

Behar J. Clinical aspects of gallbladder motor function and dysfunction. Curr Gastroenterol Rep 1999; 1: 91–94.

Bennion LJ, Grundy SM. Risk factors for the development of cholelithiasis in man. N Engl J Med 1978; 299: 1161–1167, 1221–1227.

Biggs JS. Vomiting in pregnancy. Causes and management. Drugs 1975; 9: 299–306.

Boneva RS, Moore CA, Botto L, Wong LY, Erickson JD. Nausea during pregnancy and congenital heart defects: a population-based case-control study. Am J Epidemiol 1999; 149: 717–725.

Borak J, Wise SJP. Does aluminium exposure of pregnant animals lead to accumulation in mothers or their offspring? Teratology 1998; 57: 127–129.

Brandes JM. First-trimester nausea and vomiting as related to outcome of pregnancy. Obstet Gynecol 1967; 30: 427–433.

Braverman DZ, Johnson ML, Kern F Jr. Effect of pregnancy and contraceptive steroids on gallbladder function. N Engl J Med 1980; 302: 362–364.

Briard ML, Feingold J, Kaplan J. Epidemiologie et genetique des malfomations ano-rectales. J Genet Hum 1975; 23(Suppl. 242): 29–35.

Briggs MH. Hypospadias, androgen biosynthesis and synthetic progestogens during pregnancy. Int J Fertil 1982; 27: 70–72.

Camillcri M, Dubois D, Coulie B et al. Prevalence and socioeconomic impact of functional gastroenterological disorders in the United States: results from the US Upper Gastrointestinal Study. Clin Gastroenterol Hepatol 2005; 3: 543–552.

Celik AF, Katsinelos P, Read NW et al. Hereditary proctalgia fugax and constipation: report of a second family. Gut 1995; 6: 581–584.

Chin RKH. Antenatal complications and perinatal outcome in patients with nausea and vomiting-complicated pregnancy. Eur J Obstet Gynecol Reprod Biol 1989; 33: 215–219.

Chin AB, Weckesser EC. Acute hemorrhage from peptic ulceration: analysis of 322 cases. Ann Intern Med 1951; 34: 339–351.

Clark DH. Peptic ulcer in women. Br Med J 1953; 1: 1254–1257.

Cosenza CA, Saffari B, Jabbour N et al. Surgical management of biliary gallstone disease during pregnancy. Am J Surg 1999; 178: 545–548.

Cunningham FG, McCubbn JH. Appendicitis complicating pregnancy. Obstet Gynecol 1975; 45: 415–419.

Curet MJ. Special problems in laparoscopic surgery: previous abdominal surgery, obesity, pregnancy. Surg Clin North Am 2000; 80: 1093–1110.

Dent J, El-Serg HB, Wallander MA et al. Epidemiology of gastroesophageal reflux disease: a systematic review. Gut 2005; 54: 710–717.

DeVault KR, Castelli DO. Updated guidelines for the diagnosis and treatment of gastroesophageal reflux disease. Am J Gastoenterol 2005; 100: 190–220.

Domonitz JA, Young JC, Boyko EJ. Outcomes of infants born to mothers with inflammatory bowel disease: a population-based cohort study, Am J Gastroenterol 2002; 97: 641–648.

Drossman DA, Sandler RS, McKee DC, Lovitz AJ. Bowel patterns subjects not seeking health care. Gastroenterology 1982; 83: 529–534.

Einarson A, Schick B, Addis A et al. A prospective controlled multicentre study of clarithromycin in pregnancy. Teratology 1998a; 57: 188 only.

Einarson A, Koren G, Bergrman U. Nausea and vomiting in pregnancy: a comparative European study. Eur J Obstet Gynecol Reprod Biol 1998b; 76: 1–3.

Elwood JM, Little J, Elwood JH. Epidemiology and Control of Neural Tube Defects. Oxford University Press, Oxford, 1992.

Fagan EA. Disorders of the liver, biliary system and pancreas. Disorders of the gastrointestinal tract. In: de Swiet EF (ed.) Medical Disorders in Obstetric practice. 4th ed. Blackwell, Oxford, 2002.

Fairweather DV. Nausea and vomiting in pregnancy. Amer J Obstet Gynecol 1968; 102: 135–175.

Fedorkow DM, Persaud D, Nimrod CA. Inflammatory bowel disease: a controlled study of late pregnancy outcome. Am J Obstet Gynecol 1989; 160: 998–1001.

Ferencz C, Rubin JD, Loffredo CA, Magee CA (eds.) Perspectives in Pediatric Cardiology. Epidemiology of congenital heart disease. Future Publishing Co. Inc., New York, 1983; 4: 169–180.

Flaxman SM, Sherman PW. Morning sickness: a mechanism for protecting mother and embryo. Q Rev Biol 2000; 75: 113–148.

Fleshler B, Achkar E. An aggressive approach to the medical management of peptic ulcer disease. Arch Intern Med 1981; 141: 848–851.

Fry J. Peptic ulcer: a profile. Br Med J 1964; 2: 807–812.

Furneaux EC, Langley-Evans AJ, Langley-Evans SC. Nausea and vomiting of pregnancy endocrine basis and contribution to pregnancy outcomes. Obstet Gynecol Surv 2001; 56: 755–782.
Gadsby R, Barnie-Adshead AM, Jagger C. Pregnancy nausea related to women's obstetric and personal histories. Acta Obstet Gynaecol Scand 1980; 59: 495–497.
Garbis H, Elefant E, Diav-Citrin O et al. Pregnancy outcome after exposure to ranitidine and other H2-blockers. A collaborative study of the European Network of Teratology Information Service. Am J Epidemiol 2005; 150: 476–481.
Glasgow RE, Visser BC, Harris HW et al. Changing management of gallstone disease during pregnancy. Surg Endosc 1998; 12: 241–246.
Goepfert AR, Jeffcoat M, Andrews WW et al. Periodontal disease and upper genital tract inflammation in early spontaneous preterm birth. Am J Obstet Gynecol 2004; 104: 777–783.
Goldenberg RL, Culhane JF, Iams JD, Romero R. Epidemiology and causes of preterm birth. Lancet 2008; 371: 75–84.
Golding J, Vivian S, Baldwin JA. Maternal anti-nauseants and clefts of lip and palate. Hum Toxicol 1983; 2: 63–73.
Graham G, Baxi L, Tharakan T. Laparoscopic cholecystectomy during pregnancy: a case series and review of the literature. Obstet Gynecol 1998; 53: 566–574.
Greene J, Rogers A, Rubin L. Fetal loss after cholecystectomy during pregnancy. Canad Med Ass 1963; 88: 576–577.
Grossman MI (ed.) Peptic ulcer. In: A Guide for the Practicing Physician. Year Book, Chicago, 1981.
Grossman MI, Kurata JH, Rotter JL et al. Peptic ulcer: new therapies, new diseases. Ann Intern Med 1981; 95: 609–627.
Heading RC. Definition of dyspepsia. Scand J Gastroenterol Suppl 1991; 182: 1–6.
Heading RC. Prevalence of upper gastrointestinal symptoms in the general population: a systematic review. Scand J Gastroenterol Suppl 1999; 231: 3–8.
Heinonen OP, Slone D, Shapiro S. Birth Defects and Drugs in Pregnancy. Publishing Sciences Group Inc., Littleton, MA, 1977.
Hernandez-Diaz S, Werler MM, Walker AM, Mitchell AA. Folic acid antagonists during: pregnancy and the risk of birth defects. N Engl J Med 2000; 343: 1608–1914.
Hiatt JR, Hiatt JC, Williams RA et al. Biliary disease in pregnancy: strategy for surgical management. Am J Gastroenterol 1994; 89: 109–112.
Holzbach RT. Gallstones: pathophysiology, complications, and approach to treatment. In: Farmer RG, Achkar E, Fleshler B (eds.) Clinical Gastroenterology. Raven Press, New York, 1983; pp. 447–463.
Hook EB. Dietary cravings and aversions during pregnancy. Am J Clin Nutr 1987; 31: 1355–1362.
Huxley RR. Nausea and vomiting in early pregnancy: its role in placental development. Obstet Gynecol 2000; 95: 779–782.
Iser JH, Dowling RH, Mok HYI, Bell GD. Chenodeoxycholic acid treatment of gallstones: a follow-up report and analysis of factors influencing response to therapy. N Engl J. Med 1975; 293: 378–383.
Jaffe SB, Jewelewicz R, Wahl E, Khatamee MA. A controlled study for gender selection. Fertil Steril 1987; 56: 254–258.
Jarnfelt-Samsioe A, Samsioe G, Velinder GM. Nausea and vomiting in pregnancy – a contribution to its epidemiology. Gynecol Obstet Invest 1983; 16: 221–225.
Jarnfelt-Samsioe A, Erickson B, Waldenstrom J, Samsioe G. Some new aspect on emesis gravidarum. Gynecol Obstet Invest 1985; 19: 174–186.
Jeaffcoat MK, Geurs NC, Reddy MS et al. Periodontal infection and preterm birth: results of a prospective study. J Am Dent Assoc 2001; 132: 875–880.
Jewell DJ, Young G. Interventions for treating constipation in pregnancy. Cochrane Database Syst Rev 1998; 3: CD 001142.
Johnson LF, DeMeester RT. Evaluation of elevation of the head of the bed, bethanechol, and antacid foam tablets on gastroesophageal reflux. Dig Dis Sci 1981; 26: 673–680.

Joshi D, James A, Quaglia A et al. Liver disease in pregnancy. Lancet 2010; 375: 594–605.
Kahrilas PJ. Gastroesophageal reflux disease. N Engl J Med 2008; 359: 1700–1707.
Kahrilas PJ, Shaheen NJ, Vaezi M et al. AGAI medical position statement: management of gastroesophageal reflux disease. Gastroenterology 2008a; 135: 1383–1391.
Kahrilas PJ, Shaheen NJ, Vaezi M. AGAI technical review: management of gastroesophageal reflux disease. Gastroenterology 2008b; 135: 1392–413.
Kallen BAJ. Use of omeprazole during pregnancy – no hazard demonstrated in 955 infants exposed during pregnancy. Eur J Obst Gynecol Reprod Biol 2001; 96: 63–68.
Kamm MA, Hoyle CHV, Burleigh DE et al. Hereditary internal anal sphincter myopathy causing proctalgia fugax and constipation: a newly identified condition. Gastroenterology 1991; 100: 805–810.
Kammerer W. Nonobstetric surgery during pregnancy. Med Clin North Am 1979; 63: 1157–1164.
Kauppila A, Heikinheimo M, Lohela H, Ylikorkala O. Human chorionic gonadotropin and pregnancy-specific beta-1-glycoprotein in predicting pregnancy outcome and in association with early pregnancy vomiting. Gynecol Obstet Invest 1984; 18: 49–53.
Klebanoff MA, Koslowe PA, Kaslow R, Rhoads GG. Epidemiology of vomiting in early pregnancy. Obstet Gynecol 1985; 66: 612–616.
Klebanoff MA, Mills YL. Is vomiting during pregnancy teratogenic? Br Med J 1986; 292: 724–726.
Kricker A, Ellio AJ, Forrest J, McCredie J. Congenital limb deficiency: maternal factors in pregnancy. Aust N Zeel J Obstet Gynecol 1986; 26: 272–275.
Kullander S, Källen B. A prospective study of drugs and pregnancy. II. Anti-emetic drugs. Acta Obstet Gynecol Scand 1976; 55: 105–111.
Lalkin A, Loebstein R, Addis A et al. The safety of omeprazole during pregnancy: a multicenter prospective controlled study. Am J Obstet Gynecol 1998; 179: 727–730.
Landers D, Carmona R, Cromblehome W, Lim R. Acute cholecystitis in pregnancy. Obstet Gynecol 1987; 69: 131–133.
Landon MB. Diesease of the liver, biliary system, and pancreas. In: Creasy RK, Resnik, R, Iams JD (eds.) Maternal Fetal medicine. 5th ed. Saunders. Philadelphia, 2004. pp. 1127–1145.
Lee S, Bradley JP, Mele MM et al. Cholelithiasis in pregnancy: surgical versus medical management. Obstet Gynecol 2000; 95: S70–S71.
Little RE, Hook EB. Maternal alcohol and tobacco consumption and their association with nausea and vomiting during pregnancy. Acta Obstet Gynaecol Scand 1979; 25: 15–17.
Lu EJ, Curet MJ, El-Sayed YY, Kirkwod KS. Medical versus surgical management of biliary tract disease in pregnancy. Am J Surg 2004; 188: 755–759.
Lyass S, Pikarsky A, Eisenberg VH et al. Is laparoscopic appendectomy safe in pregnant women? Surg Endos 2001; 15: 377–379.
Mahadevan U, Kane S. American gastroenterological association institute technical review on the use of gastrointestinal medications in pregnancy. Gastroenterology 2006; 131: 283–311.
Masson GM, Anthony F, Chau E. Serum chorionic gonadotropin (hCG), schwangerschaftsprotein 1 (SP1), progesterone and oestradiol levels in patients with nausea and vomiting in early pregnancy. Br J Obstet Gynaecol 1985; 92: 211–215.
Mazze RI, Kallen B. Reproductive outcome after anesthesia and operation during pregnancy: a registry study of 5,405 cases. Am J Obstet Gynecol 1989; 161: 1178–1185.
Mazze RI, Kallen B. Appendectomy during pregnancy: a Swedish registry study of 778 cases. Obstet Gynecol 1991; 77: 835–840.
Mazzella G, Rizzo N, Azzaroli F et al. Ursodeoxycholic acid administration in patients with cholestatis of pregnancy: effects on primary bile acids in babies and mothers. Hepatology 2001; 33: 504–508.
McGory ML, Zingmond DS, Tillou A et al. Negative appendectomy in pregnant women is associated with a substantial risk of fetal loss. J Am Coll Surg 2007; 205: 534.
McKellar DP, Anderseon CT, Boynton CJ, Peoples JB Cholecystectomy during pregnancy without fetal loss. Surg Gynecol Obstet 1992; 174: 465–468.

Medalie JH. Relationship between nausea and/or vomiting in early pregnancy and abortion. Lancet 1957; 273: 117–119.
Mengs U. Reproductive toxicological investigation with sennosides. Arzneim Forsch 1986; 36: 1355–1358.
Milkovich L, van den berg BJ. An evaluation of teratogenicity of certain antinauseant drugs. Am J Obstet Gynecol 1976; 125: 244–248.
Misiewicz JJ. Symposium on gastroesophageal reflux and its complications. 4. Pharmacology and therapeutics. Gut 1973; 14: 243–246.
Mogadam M, Dobbins WO, Korelitz BI et al. Pregnancy in inflammatory bowel disease: effects of sulfasalazine and corticosteroids on fetal outcome. Gastroenterol 1981; 80: 72–76.
Mourad J, Elliott JP, Erickson L et al. Appendicitis in pregnancy: new information that contradicts long-held clinical beliefs. Am J Obstet Gynecol 2000; 182: 1027–1030.
Nagler R, Spiro HM. Heartburn in late pregnancy: manometric studies of esophageal motor function. J Clin Invest 1961; 40: 954–970.
Nebel OT, Fornes MF, Castell JL. Symptomatic gastroesophageal reflux: incidence and precipitating factor. Digest Dis Sci 1976; 21: 953–957.
Offenbacher S, Katz V, Fertik G et al. Periodontal infections as a possible risk factor for preterm low birth weight. J Periodontol 1996; 67: 1103–1113.
Offenbacher S, Jared HL, O'Reilly PG et al. Potential pathogenic mechanisms of periodontitis associated pregnancy complications. Ann Periodontol 1998; 3: 233–250.
Olans LB, Wolf JL. Gastroesophageal reflux in pregnancy. Gastrointest Endosc Clin North Am 1975; 82: 699–703.
Owen FJ, Sr. Constipation. In: Farmer GR, Achkar E, Fleshler B (eds.) Clinical Gastroenterology. Raven Press, New York, 1983. pp. 61–6.
Painter NS. Constipation. Practitioner 1980; 224: 387–391.
Petitti DB. Nausea and pregnancy outcome. Birth 1986; 13: 223–226.
Pirisi A. Meaning of morning sickness still unsettled. Lancet 2001; 357: 1272.
Printen KJ, Ott RA. Cholecystectomy during pregnancy. Am J Surg 1978; 44: 432–434.
Profet M. The evolution of pregnancy sickness as protection to the embryo against Pleistocene teratogens. Evol Theor 1988; 8: 177–190.
Richter JE, Castell DO. Gastroesophageal reflux: pathogenesis, diagnosis, and therapy. Ann Intern Med 1982; 97: 93–103.
Rosa F: personal communications,1993. In: Briggs GG, Freeman RK, Yaffe SJ (eds.) Drug in Pregnancy and Lactation. 7th ed. Lippincott Williams Wilkins. Philadelphia, 2004; pp. 14949–1450.
Rudnicki M, Frolich A, Rasmussen WF, McNair P. The effect of magnesium on maternal blood pressure in pregnancy-induce hypertension. A randomized double-blind placebo-controlled trial. Acta Obstet Gynecol Scand 1991; 70: 445–450.
Ruigomez A, Rodrigez LAG, Cattaruzzi C et al. Use of cimetidine, meprazole, and ranitidine in pregnant women and pregnancy outcomes. Am J Epidemiol 1999; 150: 476–481.
Sauvat F. Diagnosis of constipation in children. Ann Nestlé 2007; 65: 63–71.
Saxen I. Epidemiology of cleft lip with or without cleft palate. An attempt to rule out chance correlations. Br J Prev Soc Med 1975; 29: 103–110.
Schuppan D, Afdhal NH. Liver cirrhosis. Lancet 2008; 371: 838–851.
Scott LD. Gallstone disease and pancreatitis in pregnancy. Gastroenterol Clin North Am 1992; 21: 803–815.
Scott LD, Abu-Hamda E. Gastrointestinal disease in pregnancy. In: Creasy RK, Resnik R, Iams JD (eds.) Maternal-Fetal Medicine. Saunders, Philadelphia, 2004. pp. 1109–1126.
Shepard TH, Lemire RJ. Catalog of Teratogenic Agents. 11th ed. Johns Hopkins University Press. Baltimore, 2004.
Sherman PW, Flaxman SM. Nausea and vomiting of pregnancy in an evolutionary perspective. Am J Obstet Gynecol 2002; 186(Suppl. 5): S190–S197.

Simmons DC, Tarnasky PR, Rivera-Alsina ME et al. Endoscopic retrograde cholangiopancreatography (ERCP) in pregnancy without the use of radiation. Am J Obstet Gyencol 2004; 190: 1467–1469.

Singer AJ, Brandt LJ. Pathophysiology of the gastrointestinal tract during pregnancy. Am J Gastroeneterol 1991; 86: 1695–1699.

Stenson WF. Inflammatory bowel disease. In: Yamada T (ed.) Textbook of Gastroenterology. 2nd ed. JB Lippincott, Philadelphia, 1995. pp. 1748–1806.

Sullivan BH Jr. Heartburn and regurgitation. In: Farmer EG, Achkar E, Fleshler B (eds.) Clinical Gastroenterology. Raven Press, New York, 1983. pp. 13–15.

Sung HP, Hinerman PM, Steiner H et al. Laparoscopic cholecystectomy and interventional endoscopy for gallstone complications during pregnancy. Surg Endosc 2000; 14: 267–271.

Swisher S, Schmidt P, Hunt K et al. Biliary disease during pregnancy. Am J Surg 1994; 168: 576–579.

Thistle JB, Hoffmann AF. Efficacy and specificity of chenodeoxycholic acid therapy for dissolving gallstones. N Engl J Med 1973; 289: 655–659.

Thukral C, Wolf JL. Therapy insight: drugs for gastrointestinal disorders in pregnant woman. Nat Clin Pract Gastroenterol Hepatol 2006; 3: 256–266.

Tierson FD, Olsen CL, Hook EB. Influence of cravings and aversions on diet in pregnancy. Ecol Food Nutr 1986; 17: 117–129.

Tsang IS, Katz VL, Wells SD. Maternal and fetal outcomes in hyperemesis gravidarum. Int J Gynecol Obstet 1996; 55: 231–235.

Tytgat GW, Heading RC, Muller-Lissners AR et al. Contemporary understanding and management of reflux and constipation in general population and pregnancy: a consensus meeting. Aliment Pharmacol Ther 2003; 18: 291–301.

UK Working Group Party on Acute Pancreatitis. UK guidelines for the management of acute pancreatitis. Gut 2005; 54 (Suppl.): 1–9.

Vakil N, van Zanten SV, Kahrilas P et al. The Montreal definition and classification of gastroesophageal reflux disease: a global evidence-based consensus. Am J Gastroenterol 2006; 101: 1900–1920.

Van Thiel DH, Wald A. Evidence refuting a role for increased abdominal pressure in the pahogeness of the heartburn associated with pregnancy. Am J Obstet Gynecol 1981; 140: 420–425.

Van Zanten VSJ, Floot N, Chiba N et al. for the Canadian Working Group. An evidence-based approach to the management of patient with dyspepsia in the era of Helicobacter pylory. Canad Med Ass J 2000; 162(Suppl. 12): S3–S23.

Van Zanten VSJ. Dyspepsia and reflux in primary care: rough DIAMOND of a trial. Lancet 2009; 373: 187–188.

Weigel MM, Weigel R. Nausea and vomiting of early pregnancy and pregnancy outcome. An epidemiological study. Br J Obstet Gynaecol 1989; 96: 1304–1311.

Welsh A. Hyperemesis, gastrointestinal and liver disorders in pregnancy. Curr Obstet Gynaecol 2005; 15: 123–131.

Williamson C. Gastrointestinal disease. Best Practice and Research Clinical Obstetrics and Gynaecology 2001; 15(5): 937–952.

Williamson C, Gorelik J, Eaton BM et al. The bile taurocholate impairs rate cardiomyocyte function: a proposed mechanism for intra-uterine fetal death in obstetric cholestasis. Clin Sci 2001; 4: 363–370.

Yerushalmy J, Milkovich L. Evaluation of the teratogenic effects of medicine in man. Am J Obstet Gynecol 1965; 93: 553–562.

Zorzi A, Schinzel A, Hirsig J. Analsphinkterdysplasia als Ursache chronischer Defekationsstörungen: eine klinische und genetische Studie. Schweiz Med Wschr 1991; 121: 1567–1575.

Own Publications

I. Bánhidy F, Ács N, Puho HE, Czeizel AE. Possible association of periodontal infectious diseases in pregnant women with isolated orofacial clefts in their children: a population-based case-control study. Birth Defects Res Part A, 2010 (in press).

II. Czeizel AE, Puhó E. Association between severe nausea and vomiting in pregnancy and lower rate of preterm birth. Paediat Perinatal Epid 2004; 18: 253–259.

III. Czeizel AE, Sárközi A, Wyszynski DF. Protective effect of hyperemesis gravidarum for isolated oral clefts. Obstet Gynecol 2003a; 101: 737–744.

IV. Czeizel AE, Puho E, Ács N, Bánhidy F. Inverse association between severe nausea and vomiting in pregnancy and some congenital abnormality. Am J Med Genet 2006; 140A: 453–462.

V. Ács N, Bánhidy F, Puho HE, Czeizel AE. A possible association between maternal dyspepsia and congenital rectal/anal atresia/stenosis in their children: a population-based case-control study. Acta Obstet Gynecol 2009; 88: 1017–1023.

VI. Ács N, Bánhidy F, Czeizel AE. Primary microcephaly in two children born to mothers with complicated appendicitis or late appendectomy during pregnancy. Birth Defects Res A: 2009.

VII. Czeizel AE, Pataki T, Rockenbauer M. Reproductive outcome after exposure to surgery under anesthesia during pregnancy. Arch Gynecol Obstet 1998; 261: 193–199.

VIII. Norgard B, Puho E, Pedersen L et al. The risk of congenital abnormalities in children born to women with ulcerative colitis: a population-based case-control study. Amer J Gastroenterol 2003; 98: 2006–2010.

IX. Ács N, Bánhidy F, Puho HE, Czeizel AE. No association between severe constipation with related drug treatment in pregnant women and congenital abnormalities in their offspring – a population-based case-control study. Cong Anom, 2010 (in press).

X. Ács N, Bánhidy F, Puho HE, Czeizel AE. Possible association between symptomatic cholelithiasis-complicated cholecystitis in pregnant women and congenital abnormalities in their offspring – a population-based case-control study. Eur J Obstet Gynecol Reprod Biol 2009; 143: 152–155.

XI. Czeizel AE, Ács N, Bánhidy F et al. Primary prevention of congenital abnormalities due to high fever related maternal diseases by antifever therapy and folic acid supplementation. Curr Women's Health Rev 2007; 3: 1–15.

Chapter 13
Diseases of the Skin and Subcutaneous Tissue

There are numerous changes in the skin due to the hormonal and physical changes in pregnancy like pigmentary alterations (chloasma), vascular changes (varicosity) and connective tissue alterations (striae) (Rapini, 2004). Here dermatological diseases reported to the HCCSCA are evaluated.

13.1 Atopic Dermatitis

Atopic dermatitis is an allergic skin disease with the symptoms of pruritic eczematous skin lesions. Similar to other allergic diseases, there is a strong familial predisposition. In addition, atopic dermatitis frequently associated with allergic rhinitis, asthma bronchiale, or food allergies. The chronic atopic dermatitis can worsen (52%) or improve (24%) during pregnancy (Kemmett and Tidman, 1991).

13.1.1 Interpretation of Data in the HCCSCA

Out of 22,843 cases with CA, 80 (0.35%), while out of 38,151 controls without CA, 91 (0.24%) had mothers with atopic dermatitis. However, the diagnosis of this disease was based on maternal information in all pregnant women. Out of 80 case mothers, 38 (47.5%) and of 91 control mothers, 32 (35.2%) were affected by atopic dermatitis before conception and it continued during pregnancy. However, more than half of the case mothers and two-third of the control mothers had new onset atopic dermatitis during the study pregnancy.

There was no difference in the mean maternal age but mean birth order was somewhat lower (1.6 vs. 1.7) in pregnant women with atopic dermatitis. Beyond the higher incidence of influenza-common cold (39.2% vs. 19.5%), the more common occurrences of allergic rhinitis, asthma bronchiale, and other respiratory diseases were characteristic (15.8% vs. 9.1%).

The atopic dermatitis was appropriately treated in 8 (10.0%) case mothers and in 9 (9.9%) control mothers according to maternal information.

N. Ács et al., *Congenital Abnormalities and Preterm Birth Related to Maternal Illnesses During Pregnancy*, DOI 10.1007/978-90-481-8620-4_13,

The mean gestational age was much shorter (38.9 vs. 39.4 week) and it associated with a higher rate of PB (13.2% vs. 9.2%). The reduction in mean birth weight (3,234 vs. 3,276 g) was moderate but is resulted in a higher rate of LBW newborns (9.9% vs. 5.7%). However, the latter figures were related to the shorter gestational age as well.

There was a higher risk of total CAs (1.5, 1.1–2.0) explained mainly by the higher risk of 5 cases with congenital limb deficiencies (3.9, 1.6–9.5) and 4 cases with CAs of the musculo-skeletal system (2.9, 1.1–7.9). However, CAs of the skeletal system were different: severe depression in skull, craniosynostosis, torticollis, pectus excavatum. All of these abnormalities belong to the group of deformation.

In conclusion, atopic dermatitis in pregnant women associated with a higher risk for PB, congenital limb deficiencies, and deformation type musculoskeletal CAs. However, most pregnant women with atopic dermatitis were not treated appropriately because of the anxiety of teratogenic potential of drugs. In addition the recall bias may be important in the evaluation of higher risk for congenital limb deficiencies and deformations. Nevertheless, these findings need further studies.

13.2 Psoriasis

Psoriasis is a papulosquamous skin disease sometimes associated with arthritis or other complications. The prevalence of psoriasis is 1–3% in the general population. In the study of Dunna and Finlay (1989) psoriasis remained unchanged in 43%, improved in 41% and worsened in 14% of pregnant women.

13.2.1 Interpretation of Data in the HCCSCA

Out of 22,843 cases, 18 (0.08%) had mothers with psoriasis, while out of 38,151 controls, 40 (0.10%) were born to mothers with psoriasis during the study pregnancy. The diagnosis of psoriasis in about 90% of pregnant woman was based on maternal information. The onset of psoriasis was before conception in 88.9% of case mothers and 90.0% of control mothers.

The mean maternal age and birth order, in addition to marital and employment status did not show differences between pregnant women with or without psoriasis. The evaluation of pregnancy complications revealed a much higher rate of threatened abortion (31.0% vs. 16.4%) and preeclampsia-eclampsia (8.6% vs. 3.0%). About 90% of pregnant women were treated by topical corticosteroids and/or oral psoralen combined with ultraviolet A light (PUVA).

The mean gestational age was longer (39.7 vs. 39.4 week) thus the rate of PB was lower (2.5% vs. 9.2%) in the newborns of pregnant women with psoriasis. The mean birth weight was also larger (3,368 vs. 3,276 g) and LBW did not occur among 40 newborns. There was no higher risk of total CA (0.8, 0.4–1.3) or in any specific CA group. The distribution of 18 CAs was the following: hypospadias 5 (1.6,

0.6–4.0), clubfoot 3, poly/syndactyly 2, multiple CA 2, neural-tube defect 1, undescended testis 1, obstructive CA of the urinary tract 1, ear CA 1, cardiovascular CA 1, branchial cyst 1.

In conclusion, the treatment of psoriatic pregnant women was effective and harmless indicated by the better pattern of birth outcomes and that is an important argument against the teratogenic potential of drugs used for the treatment of psoriasis during the study period.

13.3 Pruritus

Pruritus means generalized itching but it is a symptom which may be the sign of several diseases such as pruritus gravidarum, PUPP (pruritic urticarial papules and plaques of pregnancy, previously called as polymorphic eruption of pregnancy or toxemic rash of pregnancy or late-onset prurigo of pregnancy). Experts stressed the importance the differentiation of these skin diseases with cholestasis of pregnancy (Roger et al., 1994). The onset of priritus gravidarum is in early pregnancy, while PUPP generally started in the last trimester. Up to 14% of pregnant women complain of itching (Rapini, 2004).

13.3.1 Interpretation of Data in the HCCSCA

Out of 22,843 cases, 8 (0.04%) had mothers with pruritus, while out of 38,151 controls, 25 (0.07%) were born to mothers with this dermatological symptom. The diagnosis of pruritus was based on maternal information in all pregnant women. Of the 8 case mothers, 7 were manifested in I and II gestational month, thus the diagnosis may be pruritus gravidarum. Out of 25 control mothers, only 14 were manifested in early pregnancy, the rest occurred in the last trimester.

The mean maternal age and birth order did not show obvious differences between pregnant women with or without pruritus. The incidence of threatened abortion was higher in pregnant women with pruritus (27.3% vs. 16.4%). Among acute maternal diseases, the influenza-common cold (42.4% vs. 19.5%) and the infections of the respiratory system (21.2% vs. 9.1%) occurred more frequently in pregnant women with pruritus.

The mean gestational age at delivery (39.3 vs. 39.4 week) and birth weight (3,273 vs. 3,276 g) was similar but the rate of PB was much higher (16.0% of 9.2%) based on 4 preterm babies. The rate of LBW newborns (4.0% vs. 5.7%) was also similar.

There was no increased risk found for the group of total CAs (0.4, 0.1–1.1). The distribution of 8 CAs was the following: congenital hydrocephalus 2 (9.8, 2.3–41.5), cardiovascular CAs 2, hypospadias 1, undescended testis 1, clubfoot 1, CA of the diaphragm 1. Although the birth prevalence of congenital hydrocephalus showed some association with maternal pruritus in early pregnancy, it was based only on 2 cases.

13.4 Allergic Urticaria

Allergic urticaria is triggered by several environmental factors, mostly by drugs.

13.4.1 Interpretation of Data in the HCCSCA

Out of 22,843 cases, 95 (0.42%) were born to mothers with urticaria during the study pregnancy. Among 38,151 controls, 187 (0.49%) had mothers with allergic urticaria. Out of 94 case mothers, 11 (11.7%), while out of 187 control mothers, 19 (10.2%) had medically documented urticaria in the prenatal maternity logbook. All medically recorded allergic urticarias were drug related adverse side effects. About half of maternally reported urticarias were also drug induced allergic reactions, one-third was related to other factors such as cosmetics, chemicals, plants, etc. The etiology was unknown in the rest of the mothers.

There was no difference in the mean maternal age and birth order between pregnant women with or without allergic urticaria but it occurred more frequently in pregnant women with higher socioeconomic status based professional and managerial employment (53.5% vs. 38.5%). The incidence of pregnancy complications was not higher among pregnant women with allergic urticaria, but some acute and chronic maternal diseases occurred more frequently: influenza-common cold (38.9% vs. 19.5%), respiratory system's disease (13.2% vs. 9.1%), migraine (5.7% vs. 2.1%).

Most pregnant women with allergic urticaria were treated by oral antihistamines such as chloropyramine, cyproheptadine, diphenhydramine, cetirizine, loratidine, and calcium derivatives.

The mean gestational age was the same (39.4 week) in babies born to mothers with or without allergic urticaria with similar mean birth weight (3,294 vs. 3,276 g). The rate of PB (7.0% vs. 9.2%) and LBW newborns (5.3% vs. 5.7%) did also not show significant differences.

There was no higher risk for total CAs (0.8, 0.7–1.1) or in any specific CA group. Out of 95 cases, 3 had cleft palate only (1.0, 0.3–3.2) and 6 cases were affected by cleft lip $\pm$ cleft palate (0.9, 0.4–2.0). We mentioned the data of these two CA-groups here in detail because previously an increased risk for cleft palate was reported after the use of diphenhydramine during pregnancy in one study (Hale and Pomeranz, 2002). We did not find the above mentioned association in our data set.

In conclusion, allergic drug reactions cover a wide spectrum from Quincke's edema to different forms (giant, papulosa, pigmentosa) of urticaria; however, the main result of our analysis is that well treated allergic urticaria during pregnancy is not associated with increased risk for adverse birth outcomes.

13.5 Others

Carbuncle and furuncle occurred in mothers of 1 case and 2 controls. This case was affected by atrial septal defect, type II, while the two controls were both born on the 39th gestational week with 2,610 and 2,750 g, respectively.

Lymphadenitis was recorded in 3 case and 3 control mothers. These cases were affected by anal atresia, hypospadias, and polydactyly on the hands, while controls were born on 39th, 39th, 41st gestational week with 3,150, 3,150, and 3,650 g.

Erythema nodosum occurred in one case mother and her son was affected with transposition of the great vessels and in one control mother who delivered a girl on the 36th gestational week with 2,600 g. This skin disease is characterized by tender nodules on the anterior lower legs, usually caused by drug reactions, an infection, mostly streptococcal pharyngitis, sometimes coccidiomycosis, sarcoidosis, or inflammatory bowel disease.

Alopecia was reported by 2 case mothers and one control mothers. One girl of case mother was affected by congenital stenosis of the aortic valve, while another boy had cleft lip. The control mother delivered a girl on the 40th gestational week with 3,850 g.

Chronic ulcer of the skin occurred in one case mother (her daughter was affected with lethal hypoplastic left heart) and one control mother (she delivered a boy on the 38th gestational week with 3,850 g).

13.6 General Conclusions

Our experience based on the data set of the HCCSCA is that the skin disorders of pregnant women are often neglected during prenatal care because these pathological conditions were very rarely recorded in the prenatal care logbook.

References

Dunna SE, Finlay AY. Psoriasis improvement during and worsening after pregnancy. Br J Dermatol 1989; 120: 584.

Hale EK, Pomeranz MK. Dermatologic agents during pregnancy and lactation. An update and clinical review. Int J Dermatol 2002; 41: 197–203.

Kemmett D, Tidman MJ. The influence of the menstrual cycle and pregnancy on atopic dermatitis. Br J Dermatol 1991; 125: 59–61.

Rapini RP. The skin and pregnancy. In: Creasy RK, Resnik R, Iams JD (eds.) Maternal-Fetal Medicine. 5th ed. Saunders, Philadelphia, 2004. pp. 1201–1211.

Roger D, Vaillant L, Fignon A et al. Specific pruritic disease of pregnancy: a prospective study of 3192 pregnant women. Arch Dermatol 1994, 130: 734–739.

Chapter 14
Diseases of the Musculoskeletal System and Connective Tissue

The diseases of the musculoskeletal system cover a wide range of pathological conditions; here diseases recorded in the HCCSCA are shown. Most connective tissue disorders belong the group of autoimmune disease with a common denominator of persistent, uncontrolled, immunologically mediated tissue damage of the joints, skin, kidney, blood vessels, etc (Hankins and Suarez, 2004). The major explanation of different autoimmune diseases such as rheumatoid arthritis or systemic lupus erythematosus is that the immune system loses its ability to discriminate between self and non-self cells. There is a predominance of autoimmune disease among women, during pregnancy some of these diseases improve or worsen, in addition most of these diseases exacerbate after delivery, during the postpartum period.

14.1 Rheumatoid Arthritis

Rheumatoid arthritis (RA) is a systematic chronic inflammatory disease with the manifestation of symmetric polyarthritis of the small joints of the hands and feet. About 1% of the population is affected by RA. There is a female predominance among patients (2:1 to 4:1) with a frequent onset during childbearing age, thus pregnant women might also be affected. However, there is a well-known beneficial effect of pregnancy on RA: improvement of symptoms usually occurs in the first trimester and increases as pregnancy progresses (Ostensen, 1999).

RA belongs to the group of autoimmune diseases with a moderate recurrence risk (about 5%) in first degree relatives (I). Chronicity and remissions are characteristics of the natural history of RA with progressive erosive synovitis leading to fibrosis, ankylosis, and joint deformities (Klareskog et al., 2008).

14.1.1 Interpretation of Data in the HCCSCA

Out of 22,843 cases, 36 (0.16%) had mothers with RA, while out of 38,151 controls, 68 (0.18%) were born to mothers with RA. RA was not documented in the

N. Ács et al., *Congenital Abnormalities and Preterm Birth Related to Maternal Illnesses During Pregnancy*, DOI 10.1007/978-90-481-8620-4_14,

prenatal maternity logbook in most cases, thus their data were based on maternal information. The onset of RA was prior to conception in all cases.

Mean maternal age (29.0 vs. 25.5 year) and birth order (2.3 vs. 1.7) was higher in pregnant women with RA than in pregnant women without RA. There was no difference in their socioeconomic status.

Among pregnancy complications, the higher rate of anemia (30.9% vs. 16.6%) is worth mentioning possibly explained by the higher prevalence of hemorrhoids (19.1% vs. 4.2%). The incidence of influenza-common cold (29.8% vs. 19.5%) was more frequent in pregnant women with RA. Other acute diseases did not show higher incidence. However, among chronic diseases, diabetes mellitus (4.8% vs. 0.6%), migraine (7.7% vs. 2.1%), and thrombophlebitis (7.7% vs. 0.3%) also occurred more frequently in pregnant women with RA compared to reference group.

Non-steroidal anti-inflammatory drugs (NSAIDs) such as diclofenac and naproxen were the most frequently used drugs; however, dipyrone was also common in the treatment of RA (23.1% vs. 5.4%). Indomethacin treatment was recorded in 3 case mothers and 1 control mother; methotrexate was not used in pregnant women.

The mean gestational age at delivery was somewhat longer (39.5 vs. 39.4 week) and the mean birth weight was 134 g larger (3,409 vs. 3,275 g). The rate of PB was lower (4.4% vs. 9.2%) but the rate of LBW newborns was uneffected (5.9% vs. 5.7%).

The risk of total CA was not higher in the offspring of pregnant women with RA (0.9, 0.6–1.3). The distribution of CAs was the following: cardiovascular CA 8, hypospadias 5, clubfoot 5, cleft lip ± palate 3, undescended testis 3, poly/syndactyly 3, obstructive CA of the urinary tract 2, multiple CA 2, while other 5 CAs occurred only once.

In conclusion, RA during pregnancy does not associate with a higher risk for adverse birth outcomes, and these findings provide an indirect proof against the teratogenicity of the above mentioned drugs used for the treatment of RA in pregnant women.

14.2 Intervertebral Disc Disorders (Lumbago)

This pathological condition is caused by the development of prolapsed lumbar intervertebral disks. Most disk lesions involve the lumbar-5 and sacral-2 roots. The symptoms and signs of lumbar disk protrusion during pregnancy are similar to those occurring in non-pregnant women, i.e. radicular and low back pain in general with segmental motor and sensory disturbance in the limbs. Pregnancy is one etiologic factor in the origin of prolapsed lumbar intervertebral disks and it explains that the onset of this disorder occurs commonly during pregnancy (O'Connel, 1960) because the postural and mechanical stresses, in addition to drastic hormonal changes render the lumbar intervertebral disks more vulnerable in pregnant women.

14.2.1 Interpretation of Data in the HCCSCA

Out of 22,843 cases, 41 (0.18%) had mothers with lumbago, while out of 38,151 controls, 80 (0.21%) were born to mothers with lumbago. Out of 41 case mothers, only 6 (14.6%), while out of 80 control mothers, 10 (12.5%) had medically recorded intervertebral disc disorders in the prenatal maternity logbook. Therefore, the diagnosis of lumbago was based on maternal information in the questionnaire in the case of most pregnant women.

The onset of lumbago was stated prior to conception in 15 (36.6%) case mothers and 27 (33.8%) control mothers. In general, the localization of intervertebral disc disorders was not mentioned, and lumbago or discopathy diagnoses were only given in the questionnaire.

The mean maternal age (27.7 vs. 25.5 year) and birth order (1.9 vs. 1.7) was higher in pregnant women with lumbago without characteristic employment status.

Among pregnancy complications, the rate of threatened abortion was higher (25.0% vs. 17.0%) while the incidence of threatened preterm birth was lower (12.5% vs. 14.3%). The prevalence of diabetes mellitus (4.1% vs. 0.6%) and thrombophlebitis (5.0% vs. 0.4%) was more frequent in pregnant women with lumbago compared to pregnant women without lumbago as reference. The most commonly used drugs were the anti-inflammatory-analgesic dipyrone (32.2% vs. 5.4%), lidocain (19.8% vs. 0.1%), and tolperison (16.5% vs. 0.1%).

The mean gestational age at delivery was longer (40.0 vs. 39.4 week) and the mean birth weight was 163 g larger (3,438 vs. 3,275 g) in the newborns of pregnant women with lumbago. These figures were reflected in the lower rate of PB (3.8% vs. 9.2%) and LBW newborns (1.3% vs. 5.7%).

The risk of total CAs was not higher in the offspring of pregnant women with lumbago (0.9, 0.6–1.2). The distribution of CAs followed the total prevalence of different CA-groups: cardiovascular CA 8 (different types), undescended testis 4, clubfoot 4, poly/syndactyly 4, hypospadias 3, neural-tube defect 2, cleft lip ± palate 2, eye CA 2, multiple CA 2, while 10 CAs occurred only once. Only 2 cases with rare eye CA showed association with maternal lumbago (9.8, 2.4–40.5), however, these CAs were different (microphthalmia, coloboma).

In conclusion, lumbago during pregnancy does not associate with a higher risk for adverse birth outcomes, in fact, the longer gestational age and larger birth weight associated with a lower rate of PB and LBW newborns. The explanation of these beneficial effects may be the recommended bedrest of pregnant women, particularly in the second half of pregnancy.

14.3 Rheumatism, Myalgia, Neuralgia

Sometimes only symptoms such as *rheumatism, myalgia, and neuralgia* (RMN) were reported by mothers of cases and controls in the data set of the HCCSCA. Our plan was to evaluate all registered pregnant women, thus we did not want to exclude them from this analysis; however, they were combined into this heterogeneous group without mentioning the cause or disease.

14.3.1 Interpretation of Data in the HCSSCA

Out of 22,843 cases, 28 (0.12%) were born to pregnant women with RMN, while out of 38,151 controls, 33 (0.09%) had mothers with RMN. These symptoms were reported by mothers in the questionnaire, nobody had medically recorded diagnosis/symptom in the prenatal maternity logbook. The onset of RMN happened prior to conception only in 5 (17.9%) case mothers and 7 (21.2%) control mothers. RMN started during pregnancy in the rest of the pregnant women.

The mean maternal age (28.3 vs. 25.5 year) and mean birth order (2.0 vs. 1.7) was higher in pregnant women with RMN. When evaluating pregnancy complications, acute, or chronic diseases, we did not find any pathological condition with higher frequency in pregnant women with RMN. The spectrum of related drug treatments was similar to pregnant women with RA.

The mean gestational age (39.6 vs. 39.4 week) and birth weight (3,353 vs. 3,276 g) was higher, but the rate of PB (9.1% vs. 9.2%) were similar and the rate of LBW newborns (12.1% vs. 5.7%) was higher in pregnant women with RMN.

The risk of total CAs (1.4, 0.9–2.3) or any specific CA-group was not higher in the offspring of pregnant women with RMN. The distribution of 28 CAs was the following: clubfoot 5, cardiovascular CAs 4, undescended testis 3, multiple CA 3, neural-tube defects 2, cleft palate only 2, poly/syndactyly 2, while the other 7 CAs occurred once in cases.

14.4 Pain in Hip Join

Pain in hip joint occurs commonly during pregnancy because the postural and mechanical stresses, in addition, drastic hormonal changes induce alteration in hip join; therefore, this part of the body becomes more vulnerable in pregnant women.

14.4.1 Interpretation of Data in the HCCSCA

Out of 22,843 cases, 6 (0.03%) had mother with this pathological condition. It is worth mentioning that all 6 cases were boys affected by congenital stenosis of the pulmonary artery, congenital aneurysm of the cerebral vessels, oesophageal stenosis, congenital pyloric stenosis and hypospadias. Out of 38,151 controls, 10 (0.03%) were born to mother with pain in hip joint and their gestational age was between 36 and 42 weeks with 3,144 g mean birth weight. Preterm and low birth weight newborn did not occur among them.

14.5 Others

Systemic lupus erythematosus (SLE) is multisystem autoimmune disease with serious skin, musculoskeletal, renal, and cardiovascular symptoms. SLE affects mostly women during the reproductive years (female to male ratio is 9:1). There is increased risk of fetal death (both miscarriages and stillbirths), PB, and intrauterine growth retardation in the pregnancies of women with SLE. There are 2 controls with some intrauterine retardation (these boys were born on 38th and 39th gestational weeks with 2,800 and 2,890 g) and 1 case boy affected by renal agenesis in the data set of the HCCSCA.

Ankylosing spondylitis (AS), previously it was called as Bechterew's disease. AS is a chronic inflammatory disease of the spine ascending from the sacroiliac joints encompassing the entire spine and flattening the lumbar curvature. The onset of AS is generally in young adults (ages 15 and 40 years) with insidious low backache. AS worsened in one-third of pregnant women and improved in another third. The treatment of AS is similar to the treatment of RA. In the data set of the HCCSCA there is one control born on 36th gestational week with 2,800 g and 2 cases affected with ventricular septal defect and hypospadias, respectively.

Acquired scoliosis and kyphosis were recorded in 4 controls born on term with adequate birth weight and 2 cases with ventricular septal defect and unspecified cardiovascular CA in the data set of the HCCSCA without mentioning any cause.

14.6 Final Conclusions

After the discussion of pregnant women with musculoskeletal diseases, three notes seem to be necessary. (i) Unfortunately these diseases were reported by the mothers nearly in all pregnant women; therefore, the validity of diagnosis and symptoms is questionable. (ii) There was no higher risk of CA in the offspring of pregnant women with these diseases despite the fact that retrospective maternal information is burdened by the strong recall bias in case-control studies. (iii) The longer gestational age at delivery is characteristic of pregnant women with musculoskeletal diseases and this phenomenon needs further studies.

References

Hankins GD, Suarez VR. Rheumatologic and connective tissue disorders. In: Creasy RK, Resnik R, Iams JD (eds.) Maternal-Fetal Medicine. 5th ed. Saunders, Philadelphia, 2004. pp. 1147–1163.

Klareskog L, Catrina AI, Paget S. Rheumatoid arthritis Lancet 2008; 373: 659–676.

O'Connel JEA. Lumbar disc protrusions in pregnancy. J Neurol Neurosurg Psychiatry 1960; 23: 138–141.

Ostensen M. Sex hormone and pregnancy in rheumatoid arthritis and systemic lupus erythematosus. Ann NY Acad Sci 1999; 876: 131–143.

Own Publication

I. Siró B, Czeizel AE. Genetic counseling in patients with rheumatoid arthritis. (Hungarian with English abstract) Az Orvostudomány Aktuális Problémái 1988; 58: 79–81.

Chapter 15
Diseases of the Urinary Tract

The International Classification of Diseases (WHO) combined the diseases of the urinary tract and genital organs into the "Diseases of the genitourinary system"; nevertheless we prefer to split the diseases of these two organs into different chapters.

15.1 Maternal Renal Adaptation to Pregnancy

Here only the structural changes of the urinary tract will be summarized (Monga, 2004). Kidney length increases by 1 cm while kidney volume increases by 30% during pregnancy. These changes of the size and weight of the kidneys are caused by an increase in vascular and interstitial volume. However, there is a more drastic change in the urinary collection system, because caliceal and ureteral dilatation occurs in about 85% of pregnant women. This caliceal dilatation is 3 times (15 vs. 5 mm) more pronounced on the right side due to dextrorotation of gravid uterus and the location of the right ovarian veins that crosses the ureter. Therefore, physiological hydronephrosis and hydroureter is explained by the compression of the ureters by the enlarging uterus and ovarian vein plexus. The ureteral tone also progressively increases as a result of mechanical obstruction; however, ureteral peristalsis is not changing in pregnant women.

The diseases of the urinary tract are differentiated into infectious and non-infectious, and acute or chronic categories. The above dilatation of the urinary collecting system and urinary stasis are important factors behind the increased prevalence of ascending urinary tract infections. Infectious diseases of the urinary tract therefore frequently complicate pregnancy partly due to the previously mentioned striking alterations in renal structure, tubular function, and volume homeostatis in pregnancy caused by hemodynamic and hormonal changes. The growing uterus also has a direct effect for the urinary tract. Finally, the neighborhood of the urethra and vagina can explain the common occurrence of urogenital infections.

Certain diseases of the urinary tract including kidney may cause a complication of pregnancy or may be only an independent, concomitant disease (MacKey, 1963;

N. Ács et al., *Congenital Abnormalities and Preterm Birth Related to Maternal Illnesses During Pregnancy*, DOI 10.1007/978-90-481-8620-4_15,

Sims, 1971; Heptinstall, 1983; Davidson and Lindheimer, 2004). However, the diseases of the kidney are considered to belong to the common pathological conditions in pregnant women.

Most chronic diseases of the kidney were prospectively and medically recorded in prenatal maternity logbooks. The proportion of medically recorded acute diseases depended on the severity of the diseases.

15.2 Glomerulonephritis

In general the term *glomerulonephritis* (GN) encompasses a range of immune-mediated disorders causing inflammation within the glomerules or other compartments of the kidney (Levey et al., 2000). With chronic GN patients are more prone to develop superimposed preeclampsia or hypertensive crises (Davidson and Lindheimer, 2004).

The topic of GN and pregnancy was evaluated and discussed several times (e.g. Fairley et al., 1973), however, we did not find any publication regarding to possible associations between GN and CAs (Shepard and Lemire, 2004), however all other aspects of GN were discussed thoroughly in the literature (Chadban and Atkins, 2005). Acute poststreptococcal GN is a very rare complication of pregnancy and if it occurs late in pregnancy, it can be misdiagnosed as preeclampsia (Davidson and Lindheimer, 2004).

The aim of our study was to check possible associations between maternal GN and pregnancy complications, in addition to adverse birth outcomes, particularly CAs in the offspring.

15.2.1 Results of the Study (I)

Among pregnant women recorded and/or reported with different kidney diseases, only mothers with GN and/or nephritis with the onset before the study pregnancy (3 or more months) (Levey et al., 2000) were included into the study. GN is a subject of confusion among health-care workers (Chadban and Atkins, 2005) because GN may have multiple etiological, pathological, clinical descriptions and/or classification. We attempted to consider the latter approach, i.e. nephritis syndrome, rapidly progressive GN, nephrotic syndrome, and chronic GN was included in the group of GN evaluated in the study, if it occurred during the first trimester of the study pregnancy. The persistent proteinuria was the principal marker of kidney damage in this group of kidney diseases. However, generally the precise diagnosis based on histological or other data was not available.

Pregnant women who had essential hypertension, infections of the urinary tract, nephrolithiasis, lupus nephropathy, acute or chronic renal failure, renal sclerosis, renal osteodystrophy, nephronoptosis, cystic kidney diseases, gestational proteinuria and microscopic hematuria (Brown et al., 2005) or kidney diseases with the onset during the study pregnancy were excluded from this analysis.

The case group consisted of 22,843 malformed newborns or fetuses ("informative offspring"), of whom 309 (1.35%) had mothers with GN, while out of 38,151 controls, 479 (1.26%) were born to mothers with GN (1.1, 0.9–1.3).

Out of 309 case and 479 control mothers, 243 (78.6%) and 373 (77.9%) had medically recorded GN in the prenatal maternity logbooks. Four case and six control mothers with GN were hospitalized during the study pregnancy.

The onset of GN was after the first trimester of pregnancy in 5 case and 4 control mothers. They were excluded from this analysis. Thus, all pregnant women had GN with its onset before the conception of the study pregnancy and lasted during the first trimester.

The mean maternal age (24.2 vs. 25.5 year) and birth order (1.5 vs. 1.7) were lower in pregnant women with GN than in pregnant women without GN. Thus mothers with GN were younger with a higher proportion of primiparae (62.6% vs. 47.5%). The distribution of employment status showed some difference explained mainly by lower proportion of professionals (8.4% vs. 11.5%) and higher proportion of skilled and semiskilled workers (51.2% vs. 45.7%).

Out of 309 case and 479 control mothers with GN, 96 (31.1%) and 128 (26.7%) had no other diseases during the study pregnancy, respectively. Among other acute maternal diseases, only the incidence of infections of the urinary tract 11.8% vs. 6.0% (2.1, 1.7–2.6) and genital organs 9.5% vs. 7.5% (1.3, 1.0–1.7) was higher in pregnant women with GN than in pregnant women without GN. The prevalence of chronic maternal diseases (such as diabetes mellitus, epilepsy) was similar in the study groups.

There was no difference in the distribution and frequency of drugs used by case or control mothers with GN.

The incidence of pregnancy complications showed some differences between pregnant women with or without GN (Table 15.1).

The incidence of preeclampsia-eclampsia and anemia was higher in mothers with GN than in mothers without GN.

The birth outcomes of controls without CA born to mothers with or without GN showed important differences (Table 15.2).

There was a shorter mean gestational age and a higher rate of PB of newborns born to mothers with GN but these differences were not reflected in mean birth weight or in the proportion of LBW.

The evaluation of cases with different CAs and their all matched controls is summarized in Table 15.3.

The risk of total CA group was not higher, but the higher prevalence of GN in pregnant women associated with a higher risk for only one CA-group: isolated intestinal atresia/stenosis. There was no positive family history in these 5 cases with isolated intestinal atresia/stenosis and GN was medically recorded in the prenatal maternity logbook of these pregnant women.

Table 15.1 Incidence of pregnancy complications in mothers with or without GN

	Mothers				Comparison	
	Without GN ($N = 37{,}672$)		With GN ($N = 479$)		Of case and control mothers with GN	
Pregnancy complications	No.	%	No.	%	OR	95% CI
Threatened abortion	6,438	17.1	74	15.5	0.9	0.7–1.2
Placental disorders[a]	583	1.6	9	1.9	1.2	0.8–1.5
Preeclampsia-eclampsia	2,863	7.6	48	10.0	**1.3**	**1.1–1.8**
Nausea-vomiting, severe	3,827	10.2	42	8.8	0.9	0.5–1.5
Threatened preterm delivery[b]	5,387	14.3	73	15.2	1.1	0.5–1.5
Polyhydramnios	189	0.5	2	0.4	0.8	0.4–1.4
Olygohydramnios	14	0.0	0	0.0	–	–
Gestational diabetes	266	0.7	4	0.8	1.1	0.4–2.4
Anemia	6,210	16.5	146	30.5	**1.8**	**1.6–2.6**

[a]Including placenta previa, premature separation of the placenta, antepartum hemorrhage.
[b]Including cervical incompetence.

Table 15.2 Mean gestational age and birth weight, in addition to the rate of PB and LBW newborns without CA born to mothers with or without GN

	Newborns without CA born to mothers					
Birth outcomes	With GN (N=479)		Without GN (N=37,672)		Comparison	
Quantitative	Mean	S.D.	Mean	S.D.	t	p
Gestational age (week)	39.1	2.2	39.4	2.0	**2.7**	**0.007**[a]
Birth weight (g)	3,252	477	3,276	512	0.6	0.53[b]
Categorical	No.	%	No.	%	OR with 95% CI	
PB	71	14.8	3,425	9.1	**1.7**	**1.3–1.2**[a]
LBW newborns	29	6.0	2,138	5.7	0.8	0.5–1.1[b]

[a]Adjusted for maternal age and employment status, birth order and use of pregnancy supplements during pregnancy.
[b]Adjusted for maternal age and employment status, birth order, use of pregnancy supplements and gestational age.

The group of multiple CA included 20 cases but multimalformed offspring did not have intestinal atresia/stenosis.

15.2.2 Interpretation of the Results

We examined the possible association between maternal GN during the study pregnancy and pregnancy complications, in addition to adverse birth outcomes including different CAs in their offspring. Three findings of the study are worth emphasizing:

Table 15.3 Estimation of risks for different CAs in cases and all matched controls born to mothers with GN during the study pregnancy

	Grand total	GN		
Study groups	*N*	No.	%	Adjusted OR (95% CI)[a]
Isolated CAs				
Neural-tube defects	1,202	17	1.4	0.6 (0.3–1.0)
Cleft lip ± palate	1,375	14	1.0	0.9 (0.5–1.9)
Cleft palate only	601	10	1.7	2.2 (0.8–5.8)
Oesophageal atresia/stenosis	217	3	1.4	3.3 (0.3–34.7)
Congenital pyloric stenosis	241	4	1.7	1.4 (0.4–5.6)
Intestinal atresia/stenosis	158	5	3.2	**6.8 (1.3–37.4)**
Rectal/anal atresia/stenosis	231	2	0.9	–
Renal a/dysgenesis	126	2	1.9	2.8 (0.2–36.2)
Obstructive urinary CAs	343	2	0.6	0.6 (0.1–4.0)
Hypospadias	3,038	32	1.1	0.7 (0.5–1.2)
Undescended testis	2,052	32	1.6	1.3 (0.8–2.1)
Exomphalos/gastroschisis	255	4	1.6	0.7 (0.2–2.4)
Microcephaly, primary	111	3	2.7	0.9 (0.2–4.4)
Congenital hydrocephaly	314	8	2.5	1.8 (0.6–5.5)
Ear CAs	354	7	2.0	0.7 (0.2–1.8)
Cardiovascular CAs	4,480	50	1.1	1.0 (0.6–1.4)
CAs of the genital organs	127	3	2.4	0.9 (0.2–5.0)
Clubfoot	2,424	34	1.4	1.0 (0.6–1.6)
Limb deficiencies	548	11	2.0	1.7 (0.7–4.6)
Poly/syndactyly	1,744	22	1.3	0.8 (0.4–1.4)
Diaphragmatic CAs	244	6	2.5	6.5 (0.8–55.4)
Other isolated CAs	1,309	18	1.4	1.2 (0.6–2.2)
Multiple CAs	1,349	20	1.5	1.2 (0.7–2.3)
Total cases	22,843	309	1.4	1.0 (0.9–1.2)
Total controls	38,151	479	1.3	Reference

[a]Matched OR adjusted for maternal employment status and use of antimicrobial drugs any time during pregnancy.

(1) A higher incidence of preeclampsia-eclampsia and anemia. The well-known association of renal diseases with preeclampsia (MacGillirray, 1958; Altchek et al., 1968; Kincaid-Smith and Fairley, 1976; Katz et al., 1980) was confirmed in our study. In addition, we found a higher prevalence of anemia during the study pregnancy with GN without any reasonable explanation.
(2) Shorter gestational age and higher rate of PB was noticed in infants born to mothers with GN. Mothers with GN were younger and had a higher proportion of primiparae. Their employment also indicated a somewhat lower socioeconomic status. These confounders may associate with a higher risk of PB, however, at the calculation of adjusted OR they were considered. The rate of threatened preterm delivery did not show any difference.

(3) A higher prevalence of GN was found only in one CA group, i.e. isolated intestinal atresia/stenosis. The association of GN and intestinal atresia/stenosis was unexpected because it has not been mentioned in the international literature before (Davidson and Lindheimer, 2004). The question is whether this possible association is causal or explained by biases, confounders, or by chance. The role of possible biases might be limited because all cases with isolated intestinal atresia/stenosis were born to mothers with prospectively and medically recorded GN during the first trimester of the study pregnancy. In addition, the effect of confounders particularly related drug treatment was taken into consideration at the calculation of adjusted OR in our matched case-control approach. Previously a higher risk of infantile pyloric stenosis in infants exposed to nalidixic acid was observed (24); however, there was no mother treated by nalidixic acid within the 5 cases with intestinal atresia/stenosis. Nevertheless, the effect of other unknown or residual confounders cannot be excluded. Finally, multiple comparisons between maternal diseases and various CA-groups may produce a chance association in every 20th analysis.

Congenital intestinal atresia and stenosis is defined as total or partial obstruction of the intestine at any level (ileum is the most common site followed by duodenum and jejunum, colon is the least common) due to the lack or narrowing of the lumen in the fetus. Cases with isolated congenital hypertrophic pyloric stenosis, anal/rectal stenosis, or atresia, and with multiple CAs associated with intestinal atresia/stenosis (e.g., cases with Down syndrome), in addition to other CAs of the digestive system such as abnormal fixation, malrotation, duplication, diverticulum, etc. were excluded and evaluated separately. The etiology of isolated intestinal atresia and stenosis is probably similar but not well-known. In general, isolated intestinal atresia/stenosis does not associate with other CAs beyond intestinal atresia/stenosis. Multiple intestinal atresia may have autosomal recessive inheritance (Dallaire and Perreault, 1974). Jejunal atresia (the so-called apple peel syndrome) due to obliteration of the superior mesenteric artery (Mishalany and Najjar, 1968), duodenal atresia (Fonkalsrud et al., 1969) and intestinal pseudoobstruction due to neuronal disease (Tanner et al., 1976) were not recognized in these cases. However, most isolated intestinal atresia/stenosis is thought to be the result of fibrosis following intrauterine ischemia, i.e. vascular disruption. There are morphological and immunological evidence of coagulopathy in renal complications of pregnancy (Seymour et al., 1976, Chadban and Atkins, 2005). Therefore, our hypothesis is that the pathomechanism of isolated intestinal atresia/stenosis in cases born to mothers with GN might be explained by the vascular lesion of the intestinal tract.

The absolute risk for isolated intestinal atresia/stenosis related to GN is small. The expected number of cases with this CA is 16 per 100,000 births (see in Part I of the monograph). The estimated prevalence of GN during pregnancy is 1.3% and it may associate with 7 fold increased risk for isolated intestinal atresia/stenosis. Thus, the estimated absolute excess number of isolated intestinal atresia/stenosis may be 1.5 cases among 100,000 newborn babies.

In general, GN is underdiagnosed and undertreated (Levey et al., 2006), although the evidence of kidney damage based on proteinuria, low calculated glomerular filtration rate, or the combination of these features may help us to have an appropriate diagnosis of GN (Chadban and Atkins, 2005). GN is more frequent in males and there is an increase in its prevalence with age (Chadban and Atkins, 2005; Levey et al., 2006). If we consider these facts, the 1.3% prevalence of pregnant women with GN did not indicate an underascertainment.

In conclusion, a higher occurrence of PB and intestinal atresia/stenosis was found in the offspring of mothers with GN. However, the association between maternal GN and intestinal atresia/stenosis in their children was based only on 5 cases, therefore, this finding is considered only as a signal and further studies are needed to confirm or reject this possible association.

15.3 Urinary Tract Infections

The urinary tract represents one of the most common sites of bacterial infections, particularly in women (Roberts, 1986; Hart and Weisholtz, 1986, Parker and Collier, 1990; Davidson and Lindheimer, 2004). According to the epidemiological studies, 10–15% of the adult female population is affected with *urinary tract infection* (UTI) at some time in their lifetime (Hart and Weisholtz, 1986). UTI is one of the most frequent complications in pregnant women because pregnancy is considered as an important risk factor for UTI (Andriole, 1975). Several previously mentioned changes in the urinary tract predispose to UTI during pregnancy mostly from the third gestational month, particularly in primiparae (Monga, 2004). The changes above allow bacteria, mainly *Escherichia coli*, additional to Enterobacter, Klebsiella, Pseudomonas, and Proteus species to ascend to the upper tract.

Previously an association between UTI (including significant bacteriuria) and higher rate of PB/LBW newborns was shown in several studies (Kass, 1960; Hart and Weisholtz, 1986, II). Bacteriuria occurs in about 5% of pregnant women, usually appears during the first trimester and predisposes to the development of acute pyelonephritis, associated with LBW and PB (Kass, 1960). However, previously published results on UTI and PB/preterm delivery require cautious interpretation because of statistical methodological problems (O'Neil et al., 2003). On the other hand, kidney diseases in pregnant women are frequently associated with pregnancy complications (Davidson and Lindheimer, 2004).

Up to date, no association between UTI and CAs has been found or published (Shepard and Lemire, 2004). However, as an exception to the rule, in the study of Wilson et al. (1998) UTI was found to be an attributable risk factor (6.4%) for atrial septal defect.

Our study was planned to evaluate pregnancy complication in pregnant women with UTI, in addition to the relative risk for CAs or other adverse birth outcomes in the offspring of mothers affected by UTI and treated by related drugs during pregnancy.

15.3.1 Results of the Study (III, IV)

Three diagnoses of UTI were accepted for our evaluation:

(i) Urinary tract infection based on the so-called *significant or true bacteriuria* (i.e. more than 100,000 bacteria/mL) diagnosed by quantitative bacterial culture of fresh midstream urine collected after cleaning the urethral region and measured in two consecutive urine specimens (Davidson and Lindheimer, 2004, V, VI). This laboratory investigation was performed in most pregnant women with any symptoms of genital infections mainly fluor, bacterial vaginosis, vulvovaginitis, etc. at the time of prenatal visits. The main purpose of laboratory investigation in pregnant women with "true bacteriuria" examination was the identification and quantification of bacteria. Mainly *E. coli*, Enterobacter, Klebsiella, Pseudomonas and Proteus agents were identified in the urine and appropriate treatment was given to each patient. There are two forms of true bacteriuria: (i) symptomatic UTI and (ii) asymptomatic covert bacteriuria, i.e. without the symptoms of UTI, but often with the symptoms of infections of the lower genital tract.

(ii) *Acute cystitis*, or lower UTI. The diagnosis was based on the symptoms of the inflammation of the bladder produces typical symptoms such as dysuria, urgency, and frequency with or without suprapubic tenderness.

(iii) *Acute pyelonephritis*, or upper UTI. Formerly it was called pyelitis of pregnancy; however, the parenchyma of the kidney is also involved, so recently the term pyelonephritis is used (Davidson and Lindheimer, 2004). The typical symptoms include fever and flank tenderness/plain with or without accompanying symptoms of cystitis.

Several pregnant women showed progression of UTI and always the most severe diagnosis was used in the evaluation.

The above three forms of UTI were evaluated in the study if UTI was diagnosed during the study pregnancy. If UTI occurred before the conception of the study pregnancy or the diagnosis was chronic cystitis or pyelonephritis, pregnant women were excluded from this analysis. Of course, pregnant women with other diseases of the urinary tract, such as glomerulonephritis, nephritis, calculus of kidney/ureter, vesicoureteric reflux, etc. were also excluded from the study.

Out of 22,843 cases with CA, 1,542 (6.75%). pregnant women were affected by UTI during pregnancy, while out of 38,151 controls without CAs, 2,188 (5.74%) had mothers who suffered from UTI during pregnancy (1.2, 1.1–1.3). The OR of the analysis of UTI in II and/or III months of pregnancy was 1.2 (1.0–1.4).

Out of 1,542 case mothers, 1,277 (82.8%), while out of 2,188 mothers, 1,969 (90.0%) had prospectively and medically recorded UTI in prenatal maternity logbooks and about 95% of these UTI were reported by mothers as well. Out of 2,640 non-respondent case mothers evaluated after the home visit, 181 (6.7%) had UTI during the study pregnancy and only 12 (6.6%) reported high fever (over 38.5°C)

Table 15.4 Incidence and distribution of different manifestations/diagnoses of urinary tract infections during the study pregnancy

Different groups of urinary tract infections	Case group		Incidence	Control group		Incidence
	No.	%	%	No.	%	%
True bacteriuria with symptoms of genital infections	1,250	81.1	5.47	1,767	80.8	4.63
Acute cystitis	149	9.7	0.65	178	8.1	0.47
Acute pyelonephritis	143	9.3	0.63	243	11.1	0.64
Total	1,542	100.0	6.75	2,188	100.0	5.74

due to UTI. Of these 12 pregnant women, 8 had acute pyelonephritis. Of the 800 control mothers visited at home, 50 (6.3%) had UTI. Finally, we evaluated medically recorded and maternal reported UTI together.

The distribution of different manifestations of UTI is shown in Table 15.4. The group of mothers with true bacteriuria had an obvious predominance. The reason for bacterial testing of the urine was to recognize and prevent lower genital infections in pregnant women.

The occurrence of UTI according to gestational months depended on the type of UTI. Most true bacteriuria was diagnosed at the first visit in the prenatal care clinics. Most pregnant women with acute cystitis and pyelonephritis were recorded in III–IV and VII gestational month, respectively. However, there was no significant difference in the onset of UTI by the gestational months between the case and control groups.

The mean maternal age (24.6 vs. 25.5 year) and mean birth order (1.6 vs. 1.7) was somewhat lower in pregnant women with UTI than in pregnant women without UTI as reference group. Thus pregnant women were somewhat younger with a higher proportion of primiparae (57.5% vs. 47.1%). The proportion of unmarried women did not show obvious differences but the proportion of professional-managerial women (34.0% vs. 38.2%) was lower in pregnant women with UTI. The use of folic acid was somewhat lower in case mothers (49.0%) than in control mothers (53.6%) with UTI (0.8, 0.7–0.9). Similar pattern was found at the use of folic acid during the periconceptional period (i.e. I and II gestational month). However, control mothers without UTI used more frequently folic acid during pregnancy.

Among case and control mothers with UTI, 469 (35.3%) and 537 (29.2%) had no other diseases during the study pregnancy, respectively. The occurrences of other acute infectious maternal diseases are shown in Table 15.5.

Three acute diseases showed some associations with UTI in pregnant women. The association of UTI and digestive system's diseases can be explained by the higher prevalence of enteritis in these pregnant women. The higher occurrence of urinary tract diseases was explained mainly by glomerulonephritis and particularly kidney stones. The prevalence of kidney stones (0.27% vs. 0.75%; 2.8, 1.9–4.2)

Table 15.5 Occurrence of other acute and chronic diseases in control pregnant women with or without urinary tract infections (UTI)

	Pregnant women					
	Without UTI (N = 35,963)		With UTI (N = 2,188)		Comparison	
Maternal diseases	No.	%	No.	%	OR	95% CI
Acute						
Influenza – common cold	6,651	18.5	410	18.7	1.0	0.9–1.1
Respiratory system	3,250	9.0	205	9.4	1.0	0.9–1.2
Digestive system	868	2.4	71	3.2	**1.4**	**1.1–1.7**
Urinary tract[a]	113	0.3	20	0.9	**2.9**	**1.8–4.7**
Genital organs[b]	2,680	7.5	211	9.6	**1.3**	**1.1–1.5**
Others	488	1.4	24	1.1	0.8	0.5–1.2
Chronic						
Diabetes mellitus	44	0.1	8	0.4	**2.4**	**1.3–4.4**
Epilepsy	74	0.2	3	0.1	0.7	0.2–2.1
Others	5,603	15.6	334	15.3	1.0	0.9–1.1

[a]Without UTI.
[b]Without fluor, vaginosis, or vulvovaginitis because these patients were included into the group of significant bacteriuria.

was higher in pregnant women with UTI compared to mothers without UTI. Acute infections of genital organs associated with UTI because fluor, bacterial vaginosis, and vulvovaginitis, i.e. infections of the lower genital organs were not excluded. Thus mild infectious diseases of lower genital organs like vulvovaginitis and bacterial vaginosis occurred in more than 90% of pregnant women with UTI justifying bacterial examination of urine in these cases. Among chronic maternal diseases insulin dependent diabetes mellitus was more frequent in mothers with UTI.

Among frequently used drugs, urinary tract antiseptics: nitrofurantoin (32.0% vs. 31.0%) and nalidixic acid (9.5% vs. 10.0%), antimicrobial drugs: ampicillin (31.3% vs. 33.0%), cefalexin (8.4% vs. 7.6%), and sulfamethoxazole + trimethoprim (7.2% vs. 8.1%), in addition to drugs for genital infectious diseases: clotrimazole (12.1% vs. 12.9%) and metronidazole (9.5% vs. 6.3%) showed a higher frequency in mothers with UTI compared to pregnant women without UTI. However, the use of these drugs did not show significant differences between case and control mothers with UTI during II and/or III gestational months.

One of the main objectives of our study was the evaluation of pregnancy complications in pregnant women with UTI (Table 15.6).

Three pregnancy complications: polyhydramnios, preeclampsia-eclampsia, and anemia were more frequent in mothers with UTI compared to mothers without UTI.

Second main objective of the study was the analysis of birth outcomes (Table 15.7).

Table 15.6 Incidence of pregnancy complications in control mothers with or without UTI

	Pregnant women					
	Without UTI ($N = 35{,}963$)		With UTI ($N = 2{,}188$)		Comparison	
Pregnancy complications	No.	%	No.	%	OR	95% CI
Threatened abortion	6,124	17.0	388	17.7	1.1	0.9–1.2
Placental disorders[a]	559	1.6	33	1.5	1.0	0.7–1.4
Preeclampsia-eclampsia	2,988	8.3	233	10.7	**1.3**	**1.1–1.5**
Nausea, vomiting, severe	3,642	10.1	227	10.4	1.0	0.9–1.2
Threatened preterm delivery[b]	5,161	14.4	299	13.7	0.9	0.8–1.1
Polyhydramnios	170	0.5	21	1.0	**2.0**	**1.3–3.2**
Oligohydramnios	13	0.0	1	0.1	1.3	0.2–9.7
Prolonged pregnancy	482	1.3	26	1.2	0.9	0.6–1.3
Gestational diabetes	255	0.7	15	0.7	1.0	0.6–1.6
Anemia	5,946	16.5	410	18.7	**1.2**	**1.0–1.3**

[a]Including placenta previa, premature separation of the placenta, antepartum hemorrhage.
[b]Including cervical incompetence.

The figures of no UTI group correspond well to the Hungarian newborn population in the study period. The mean gestational age was somewhat shorter in newborn infants born to mothers with UTI compared to mothers without UTI as a reference group. The mean birth weight was slightly smaller in the babies of mothers with UTI. However, this statistical significant difference was caused by 0.1 week and 27 g which are clinically not significant. The rate of PB was higher in the group of mothers with UTI but the similar trend in the proportion of LBW did not reach the level of significance.

Table 15.7 Main birth outcomes of 2,188 newborn infants without CA born to mothers with urinary tract infections (UTI) and 35,963 newborn infants without CA born to mothers without UTI as reference

	UTI group		No UTI group		Comparison	
Quantitative	Mean	S.D.	Mean	S.D.	t	p
Gestational age (week)[a]	39.3	2.2	39.4	2.0	**2.1**	**0.04**
Birth weight[b] (g)	3,251	513	3,278	511	**2.4**	**0.02**
Categorical	No.	%	No.	%	OR	with 95% CI
PB[a]	228	10.4	3,268	9.1	**1.2**	**1.0–1.3**
LBW newborns[b]	146	6.7	2,021	5.6	1.1	0.9–1.4

[a]Adjusted for maternal employment status and use of vitamin supplements during pregnancy.
[b]Adjusted for maternal employment status, use of vitamin supplements during pregnancy, and gestational age.

Table 15.8. Birth outcomes according to the different group (severity) of UTI

Different group of UTI	No.	%	Gestational age (week) Mean	S.D.	PB No.	%	Birth weight (g) Mean	S.D.	LBW No.	%
True bacteriuria with symptoms of genital infection	1,767	80.8	39.3	2.2	190	10.8	3,250	509	115	6.5
Acute cystitis	178	8.1	39.4	2.0	14	7.9	3,302	558	11	6.2
Acute cystopyelitis	171	7.8	39.2	2.0	16	9.4	3,237	506	13	7.6
Acute pyelonephritis	72	3.3	39.1	2.1	9	12.5	3,141	520	8	11.1
Total	2,188	100.0	39.3	2.2	228	10.4	3,251	513	146	6.7

We studied the possible correlation between severity of UTI including cystitis, cystopyelitis, pyelonephritis and mean gestation age and birth weight (Table 15.8).

There was an obvious association between the severity of the UTI and the proportion of PB and LBW newborns. The exception is true bacteriuria which was connected with genital infections of pregnant women with a high rate of PB but a low rate of LBW newborns. Thus PB inducing effect of true bacteriuria is associated with the infections of the genital organs in our study.

We evaluated the PB-preventive effect of different drugs in mothers with UTI as well (Table 15.9)

Antimicrobial drugs such as ampicillin, cefalexin, and cotrimoxazole seemed to be very effective in the prevention of PB in mothers with UTI, while the so-called urinary tract antiseptics such as nitrofurantoin and nalidixic acid did not show any preventive effect. It is worth mentioning that pregnant women with UTI and appropriate antimicrobial treatment had a lower rate of PB (7.4%) than the high PB rate of the Hungarian pregnant population (9.1%) during the study period.

Finally, cases with different CA-groups were compared with their matched controls according to the prevalence of UTI during II and/or III months of pregnancy, i.e. in the critical period of most major CAs. UTI in pregnant women did not show increased risk for the total CAs or any CA groups. This finding was also confirmed by the evaluation of only medically recorded UTI cases (data not shown).

We compared the expected number of different subgroups of cardiovascular CAs based on the data set of the HCCSCA and observed number of cases with different cardiovascular CAs (including atrial septal defect, type II) in the newborn infants born to mothers with UTI during II and/or III gestational months. We did not find any difference.

Finally, the different manifestations of UTI were evaluated separately with possible associations of CAs; however, no severity dependant effect of UTI was found.

Table 15.9 Rate of PB (%) in newborns of mothers with different manifestation of UTI and with or without antimicrobial drugs such as ampicillin, cefalexin, and cotrimoxazole or urinary tract antiseptics such as nitrofurantoin and nalidixic acid treatment

		Ampicillin, cefalexin, cotrimoxazole								Nitrofurantoin-Nalidixic acid							
		No			Yes					No			Yes[b]				
		PB			PB			Comparison		PB			PB			Comparison	
Urinary tract infections	*N*	*N*	No.	%	*N*	No.	%	OR[a]	95% CI	*N*	No.	%	*N*	No.	%	OR[a]	95% CI
True bacteriuria	1,767	948	128	13.5	819	62	7.6	**0.6**	**0.3–0.9**	1,075	102	9.5	692	88	12.7	**1.3**	**1.1–1.3**
Cystitis	178	97	10	10.3	81	4	4.9	0.5	0.1–5.1	143	9	6.3	45	5	11.1	1.8	0.8–2.6
Cystopyelitis-pyelonephritis	243	154	17	11.0	98	8	8.2	0.7	0.4–2.1	144	16	11.1	108	9	8.3	0.8	0.4–2.1
Together	2,188	1,199	155	12.9	998	74	7.4	**0.6**	**0.4–1.0**	1,362	127	9.3	845	102	12.1	**1.3**	**1.1–1.5**

[a]Adjusted for maternal age, birth order, employment status, other maternal diseases, and drug treatments.
[b]Without ampicillin, cefalexin or clotrimazole treatment.

15.3.2 Interpretation of Results

Our study resulted in three important findings.

First, maternal UTI showed an association with polyhydramnios and preeclampsia. It is a generally accepted hypothesis that renal diseases are associated with a higher risk for preeclampsia (Kincaid-Smith and Fairley, 1976; Katz et al., 1980; Hepintstall, 1983). The possible association between polyhydramnios and UTI was also found (Naeye, 1979). The slightly higher rate of anemia might be explained by the somewhat lower socioeconomic status of mothers with UTI.

Second, there is an association between the severity of UTI and shorter gestational age of newborns together with a higher rate of PB. However, the most important message of this study is that major part of PB is preventable by antimicrobial drugs such as ampicillin, cefalexin, and cotrimoxazole and their beneficial effect can explain the low rate of PB in mothers with UTI. This effect of ampicillin (5) and clotrimazole (29, 30) was shown previously in the data set of the HCCSCA.

True bacteriuria may be a marker for low socioeconomic status and sexually transmitted diseases which are associated with PB and/or LBW. Our study confirmed the previous findings that UTI in pregnant women associate with a higher rate of PB, but it depends on the severity of maternal diseases and the efficacy of treatment. Up to 30% of mothers develop acute pyelonephritis if true bacteriuria goes untreated; meanwhile, antibiotic treatment is able to reduce the risk of pyelonephritis and the related increased risk for PB in pregnant women (Fan et al., 1987). However, treated pyelonephritis during pregnancy does not appear to predispose to higher risk for PB or LBW (Smaill, 2001) and this finding was confirmed in lower UTI as well in our study.

Only a small number of women acquired UTI during pregnancy (Norden and Kass, 1968; Trembath and Rijhsinghani, 2002), UTI in unplanned pregnancies often goes untreated and it partly explains the higher rate of PB in these pregnant women (Yaris et al., 2004). As our Hungarian experiences showed, the preconceptional or early postconceptional screening is necessary in women with symptoms of infections of the genitourinary system followed by an effective treatment to prevent increased risk for PB (VII, VIII).

Third, there was no association between maternal UTI and higher risk for CAs in their offspring.

Some specific infections caused by rubella, varicella, cytomegaloviruses, Treponema pallidum, Toxoplasma gondii, etc during pregnancy have been associated with CAs and/or fetal diseases. However, the effects of these microbial agents during pregnancy are well-known but the possible association of some common infections such as UTI with CAs was rarely studied, therefore its consequences remained unknown. Because of the relatively high occurrence of UTI during pregnancy, even a minimally increased risk for CA or other adverse pregnancy outcomes might have important consequences at the population level.

The analysis of maternal UTI was focused on different specific CAs because teratogens can cause specific CAs without affecting the overall rate. We did not find any association between UTI and related drug treatments during II and/or III month of pregnancy and CAs, including atrial septal defect. Therefore, we were unable to confirm the finding of Wilson et al. (1998). These authors evaluated the attributable fractions for 8 different cardiovascular CAs in the Baltimore-Washington Infant Study from 1981 to 1989. UTI had a small relative risk of 1.6 for atrial septal defect, but the large percent exposed (20.3%) resulted in an extra attributable fraction of 6.4%. In our study the expected number of atrial septal defect, type II was 6.3 while the observed number was 3 among newborn infants born to mothers who had UTI during II and/or III gestational month (p=0.30).

Our findings may indicate the lack of teratogenicity of microorganisms causing UTI and related drug treatments. The teratogenic potential of these drugs were also checked in the data set of the HCCSCA in separate studies. Nitrofurantoin (22), nalidixic acid (24), cefalexin (11), clotrimazole (28), and vaginal metronidazole (42, 43) were not associated with increased risk for any CA group. However, sulfamethoxazole+trimethoprim=cotrimoxazole (19, 20) treatment was associated with a higher risk for cardiovascular CAs and multiple CAs. The use of ampicillin associated slightly with a higher risk for cleft palate (4), and oral treatment of metronidazole associated with a higher risk for cleft lip ± palate (41). However, these associations were weak and were not confirmed in this study due to the limited number of pregnant women treated by these drugs.

Asymptomatic significant bacteriuria caused mostly by *E. coli* was found in 5.9% of the Hungarian reproductive aged female population (V), in 6.4% of pregnant women (VI), and in 14.0% of pregnant women with preterm deliveries (II). In our study the incidence of asymptomatic significant bacteriuria with the symptoms of genital infections during pregnancy was 6.8 and 5.7% in case and control mothers, respectively. These figures are within the range of asymptomatic significant bacteriuria (2–10%) according to the international literature (Davidson and Lindheimer, 2004).

The occurrence of cystitis and pyelonephritis in pregnant women was found in about 1 and 2% in other studies (Davidson and Lindheimer, 2004). Our figures were somewhat lower (0.8 and 1.1% in the control group) because mostly only severe UTIs were recorded in the prenatal maternity logbook.

In our study UTI occurred mainly in younger primiparae with lower socioeconomic status. UTI frequently associated with infections/diseases of the lower genital organs, probably because genital infections were the main indications of laboratory examinations of the urine in our data set. Among other maternal diseases only kidney stones had an association with UTI because kidney stones may predispose to UTI during pregnancy as well.

In conclusion, our study showed that maternal UTI increases the incidence of preeclampsia-eclampsia, polyhydramnion, and the rate of PB, however, available antimicrobial drugs provide an effective protection for these adverse complications of pregnancies. In addition, higher occurrence of CAs was not found in the offspring of mothers with UTI and related drug treatments during II and/or III months of pregnancy; therefore, early treatment of UTI is strongly recommended.

15.4 Kidney Stones

Urolithiasis, i.e. urinary tract stones, particularly nephrolithiasis, i.e. *kidney stones* (KS) is a common diagnosis, but not a disease (Moe, 2006). KS are known to develop due to various metabolic and environmental-nutritional factors including hypercalciuria, hyperoxaliuria, hyperuricosuria, hypocitraruria, and low urine volume (Pak, 1998; Borghi et al., 1996). About 80% of KS are composed of calcium salts which usually occur as calcium oxalate and less commonly as calcium phosphate (Moe, 2006). Clinicians should understand that KS can be a mere sentinel of an underlying disease and they should do their best to detect that disease. The occurrence of primary bladder stones had reduced considerably in developed countries (Moe, 2006), thus practically urolithiasis corresponds to the KS in Hungary.

The three main diagnostic criteria of KS are microscopic hematuria, recurrent urinary tract symptoms, and the laboratory diagnosis of pyelonephritis. The presence of two of these criteria indicates the diagnosis of KS in a substantial proportion of pregnant women (Bucholz et al., 1998). Ultrasonography may be useful to confirm the diagnosis of KS but less efficient in detecting very small calculi. The diagnosis of small calculi may need intravenous urography as well.

Initially the management of KS symptoms should be conservative with adequate hydration, appropriate antibiotic and pain relief, and analgesic/spamolytic therapy. Surgical intervention is rarely needed because of the relatively benign history of KS with uncomplicated calcium stones.

The yearly incidence of KS was estimated to be about 0.5% in Europe and North America, while the lifetime risk of KS was about 10–15% (Pak, 998). In addition, the prevalence of KS increased from 3.2 to 5.2% in the USA between 1976 and 1994 (Stamatelon et al., 2003). KS are largely a recurrent pathological condition with a relapse rate of 50% in 5–10 years (Trinchieri et al., 1999). The higher recurrence risk is related to young age of onset, dietary factors, positive family history, and infection stones, etc. (Pak, 1998; Curhan et al., 2004; Moe, 2006).

KS may occur in pregnant women, however, as far as we know, the possible association between KS and CAs has not been studied (Shepard and Lemire, 2004). Thus, we decided to estimate the risk for CAs and other adverse birth outcomes in the offspring of mothers affected by KS during pregnancy.

15.4.1 Results of the Study (IX)

The case group consisted of 22,843 fetuses or newborn infants ("informative offspring") with CA. 69 (0.30%) mothers were affected by KS, while out of 38,151 controls without CAs, 147 (0.39%) had mothers with KS (0.8, 0.6–1.0). All pregnant women had KS; and other manifestations of urolithiasis were not reported. Out of 69 case mothers, 62 (89.9%) and out of 147 control mothers, 141 (95.9%) had medically recorded KS in the prenatal maternity logbooks. Therefore, the proportion of maternal self-reported KS was somewhat larger in the case group (p=0.08).

Table 15.10 Distribution of the onset of kidney stones according to gestational months

Gestational months	Case group		Control group	
	No.	%	No.	%
I	22[a]	31.9	40[a]	27.2
II	2	2.9	4	2.7
III	5	7.3	8	5.4
IV	7	10.1	17	11.6
V	6	8.7	24	16.3
VI	10	14.5	15	10.2
VII	11	15.9	18	12.2
VIII	4	5.8	12	8.2
IX	2	2.9	9	6.1
Total	69	100.0	147	100.0

[a] 18 case and 28 control pregnant women had recurrence of KS in II and III gestational months as well.

The distribution of the onset of KS during the study pregnancy is shown in Table 15.10.

The very high proportion of KS in I gestational month reflects the onset of KS before conception with the recurrence of KS during the study pregnancy. In addition, the onset of KS occurred frequently between IV and V months of pregnancy both in case and control groups. The monthly prevalence of KS did not show significant difference between the two study groups.

The mean maternal age (25.5 vs. 25.7 year) was somewhat lower in pregnant women with KS compared to pregnant women without KS as reference although their mean birth order (1.7) was similar. KS was more frequent among professionals (18.4% vs. 11.4%) and skilled workers (35.4% vs. 30.6%), while it was less frequent in managerial (21.1% vs. 26.6%) and semiskilled workers (10.2% vs. 15.2%). There was no difference in the administration of folic acid and multivitamin supplementation between case and control groups.

Among case and control mothers with KS, 14 (20.3%) and 22 (15.0%) had no other diseases during the study pregnancy, respectively. The occurrence of other maternal diseases was similar in the study groups, except the urinary tract infections from true bacteriuria to pyelonephritis (16.7% vs. 6.4%) which were more frequent in pregnant women with KS (2.9, 2.0–4.2; $p<0.001$). Chronic maternal diseases including insulin dependent diabetes mellitus and epilepsy showed similar occurrences in the study groups.

Mainly antispasmodic drotaverine (42.0% vs. 41.5%) and papaverine (8.7% vs. 5.4%), in addition to analgesic dipyrone (23.2% vs. 25.2%) were used for the treatment of case and control pregnant women with KS. In addition, the occurrence of antimicrobial ampicillin (23.2% vs. 20.4%) and cefalexin (5.8% vs. 1.4%), antifungal clotrimazole (7.3% vs. 13.6%), urinary tract antiseptics nitrofurantoin (11.6% vs. 6.1%) and nalidixic acid (2.9% vs. 6.1%) were used more frequently in these pregnant women. Specific drug treatments in pregnant women with KS were used rarely and only hydrochlorothiazide (2.9% vs. 2.7%) had a higher occurrence in

Table 15.11 Birth outcomes of newborn infants without congenital abnormalities (the so-called controls) born to mothers with or without kidney stones (KS)

	Mothers				Comparison			
	Without KS ($N = 8{,}004$)		With KS ($N = 147$)		Unadjusted		Adjusted	
Variables of Newborns								
Quantitative	Mean	S.D.	Mean	S.D.	*t*	*p*	*t*	*p*
Gestational age (week)	39.4	2.0	39.5	1.9	0.7	0.48	0.5^a	0.60
Birth weight (g)	3,276	511	3,387	537	**2.6**	**0.008**	$\mathbf{2.3^b}$	**0.02**
Categorical	No.	%	No.	%	OR	95% CI	OR	95% CI
PB	3,488	9.2	8	5.4	0.6	0.3–1.2	0.6^a	0.3–1.2
LBW	2,158	5.7	9	6.1	1.1	0.6–2.1	1.5^b	0.7–3.2

[a]Adjusted for maternal age, maternal employment status, use of pregnancy supplements, and sex.
[b]Adjusted for maternal age, maternal employment status, use of pregnancy supplements, sex, and gestational age.

pregnant women with KS. However, the use of these drugs was similar in case and control mothers with KS.

Pregnancy complications did not show difference between the study groups except preeclampsia-eclampsia with a higher incidence in the case group 14.5% vs. 7.8% (2.0, 1.0–3.9). Similar difference was not seen in the control group (8.2% vs. 8.4%).

The data of birth outcomes are shown in Table 15.11.

Mean gestational age was 0.1 week longer in newborn infants born to mothers with KS than in babies of mothers without KS, while mean birth weight was significantly larger by 111 g in newborns who had mother with KS. However, the rate of PB was somewhat lower while the rate of LBW newborns was similar to newborn infants born to mothers with KS compared to the newborns of pregnant women without KS.

There was no CA-group associated with a higher prevalence of maternal KS during the first trimester of pregnancy or anytime during pregnancy in case mothers compared to their matched controls.

15.4.2 Interpretation of Results

As far as we know it is the first controlled epidemiologic study to check the possible associations between maternal KS during pregnancy and adverse birth outcomes particularly different CAs.

We did not find any association between CAs and KS during the first trimester of pregnancy. This finding is an important argument against the possible teratogenic effect of drugs used for the treatment of pregnant women with KS (Laerum and

Larsen, 1984, Ellinger et al., 1997). The teratogenic potential of drotaverine (83), dipyrone (81), cefalexin (11), clotrimazole (28), nitrofurantoin (22), and nalidixic acid (24) were checked in the data set of the HCCSCA without increased risk for any CA. Only ampicillin (4) was associated with a slightly higher risk for cleft palate.

In addition, pregnant women with KS had no higher rate of other adverse birth outcomes such as PB or LBW. In fact, the mean birth weight of children born to mothers with KS was larger by 111 g which does not seem to be important from clinical aspect. This association may be related to the somewhat longer gestational age likely due to the effect of antifungal clotrimazole (29, 30), ampicillin (5), and spasmodic drugs (83).

The study confirmed the well-known association between KS and urinary tract infections. On one hand, the so-called "infection" stones of struvite (magnesium ammonium phosphate) (Gettman and Segura, 1995) or carbonate apatite is caused by recurrent urinary infection due to the altered urine pH and/or underlying anatomic predisposition (Moe, 2006). On the other hand, lesions in the urinary tract caused by KS may also predispose for infections.

Finally, there was a higher risk for preeclampsia-eclampsia in case mothers with KS but not in control mothers with KS. Thus KS, fetal defect and preeclampsia triad may have some association and this phenomenon needs further evaluations.

The observed prevalence of KS in Hungarian pregnant women was about 0.3–0.4% and it is much lower than in the general population (Moe, 2006, Stamatelon et al., 2003) but corresponds well to the figure of other pregnant populations between 0.03 and 0.35% (Butler et al., 2000). KS are more common in men than in women throughout adult life (Soucie et al., 1994) due to the protective effect of estrogens (Heller et al., 2002).

In conclusion, the higher occurrence of adverse birth outcomes such as PB, LBW newborns and particularly CAs was not found in the offspring of mothers with KS during pregnancy.

15.5 Chronic Kidney Diseases with Secondary Hypertension

The first step in hypertension classification is the differentiation of primary and secondary hypertension. Among the causes of secondary hypertension the biggest group is related to renal diseases (Pickering and Ogedegbe, 2008). These renal causes are heterogeneous caused by chronic kidney diseases (including IgA nephropathy, polycystic kidney disease, etc.), renal artery stenosis, obstructive uropathy, etc. Chronic kidney diseases are very harmful for the arteries because they pose an increased risk for atherosclerosis. Uremia in general is accelerating atherogenesis and the remodeling of the arteries and increases arterial wall rigidity. Therefore, renal hypertension is malignant and it is associated with a markedly increased risk for cardiovascular and end-stage renal diseases.

15.5.1 Interpretation of Data in the HCCSCA

Out of 22,843 cases, i.e. fetuses or newborn infants with CA, 34 (0.15%) had mothers with *renal diseases related secondary hypertension* (RDRSH). Out of 38,151 controls without CAs, 49 (0.13%) newborns had mothers with RDRSH. Out of 34 case mothers, 26 (76.5%) and out of 49 control mothers, 31 (63.3%) had medically recorded RDRSH in the prenatal maternity logbooks. Only half of these pregnant women had specified diagnosis of RDRSH such as nephritis, nephropathy, small kidney, polycystic kidney disease, obstructive uropathy, etc.

The mean maternal age (25.0 vs. 25.5 year) was somewhat lower in pregnant women with RDRSH than in pregnant women without RDRSH and their mean birth order was also somewhat lower (1.6 vs. 1.7). There was no obvious difference in marital and employment status among study groups. There was a lower rate of folic acid administration (46.4% vs. 49.4% in the case and 50.4% vs. 54.5% in the control group) in pregnant women with RDRSH. Similar trend was seen in the use of multivitamins as well.

The incidence of acute disease groups did not show difference among study groups. However, out of 34 case mothers, 4 (11.8%), while out of 49 control mothers, 8 (16.3%) were diabetic.

Mainly antihypertensive (methyldopa, nifedipin) and urinary tract antiseptic (nitrofurantoin, nalidixic acid) drugs were used for the treatment of pregnant women with RDRSH.

Among pregnancy complications, anemia was recorded more frequently in pregnant women with RDRSH (22% vs. 15%).

Mean gestational age (39.3 vs. 39.4) was 0.1 week shorter in newborn infants born to mothers with RDRSH but it associated with a higher rate of PB (13.0% vs. 9.1%). The mean birth weight (3,268 vs. 3,276 g) and the rate of LBW newborns (6.7% vs. 5.7%) were nearly similar.

The comparison of cases with different CA-groups and their matched controls according to the prevalence of maternal RDRSH during pregnancy did not show a higher risk for total CA group (1.1, 0.9–1.1) or any CA-group.

Thus this severe group of maternal diseases did not associate with a higher risk for adverse birth outcomes likely due to the early phase of RDRSH.

15.6 Other Renal Diseases

Only one control without CA was born on the 41st week within 3,700 g to mother affected with *nephroptosis*.

Two cases with unspecified heart CA and congenital pyloric stenosis had mothers with *vesicoureteric reflux*.

Other chronic renal disease such as diabetic nephropathy, systemic lupus erythematosus were not recorded in the data set of the HCCSCA. The explanation of the lack of pregnant women with acute renal failure due to preeclampsia-eclampsia or pyelonephritis can be explained by the interruption of pregnancies in these very severe diseases.

15.7 Final Conclusions

The interaction between kidney diseases and pregnancy is strong and in general risky. For example the frequent UTI associated with a higher risk of PB and LBW. However, as our data showed antimicrobial drugs provide an effective preventive therapy for these adverse complications of pregnancies. Thus the necessary early treatment of UTI and other kidney diseases are strongly recommended.

References

Altchek A, Albright NL, Sommers SC. The renal pathology of toxemia of pregnancy. Obstet Gynecol 1968; 31: 555–560.

Andriole VT. Urinary tract infection in pregnancy. Urol Clin N Am 1975; 2: 485–499

Borghi L, Meschi T, Amato F, Brigant A, Novarini A, Giannini A. Urinary volume, water and recurrences in idiopathic calcium nephrolithiasis: a 5 year randomized prospective study. J Urol 1996; 155: 839–844.

Brown MA, Holt JL, Mangos GJ et al. Microscopic hematuria in pregnancy: relevance to pregnancy outcomes. J Kidney Dis 2005; 45: 667–673.

Bucholz N-P, Biyabani MR. Urolithiasis in pregnancy – a clinical challenge. Eur J Obstet Gynecol Reprod Biol 1998; 80: 25–28.

Butler EL, Cox SM, Eberts EG et al. Symptomatic nephrolithiasis complicating pregnancy. Obstet Gynecol 2000; 96: 753–756.

Chadban SJ, Atkins R. Glomerulonephritis. Lancet 2005; 365: 1797–1806.

Curhan GC, Willett WC, Knight EL, Stampfer MJ. Dietary factors and risk of incident kidney stones in younger women: Nurses' Health Study II. Arch Intern Med 2004; 164: 885–891.

Dallaire L, Perreault G. Hereditary multiple intestinal atresia. Birth Defects Orig Art Ser X 1974; 10(4): 259–264.

Davidson JM, Lindheimer MD. Renal disorders. In: Creasy RK, Resnik MD, Iams JD (eds.) Maternal-Fetal Medicine. 5th ed. Saunders, Philadelphia, 2004. pp. 901–923.

Ellinger B, Pak CY, Citron JT, Thomas C, Adams-Huet B, Vangessel A. Potassium-magnesium citrate is an effective prophylaxis against recurrent calcium oxalate nephrolithiasis. J Urol 1997; 158: s2069–2073.

Fairley KF, Whitworth JA, Kincaid-Smith P. Glomerulonephritis and pregnancy. In: Kincaid-Smith P, Mathew TH, Becker ELC (eds) Glomerulonephritis: Morphology, Natural History, and Treatment. Wiley, New York, 1973. pp. 997–1011.

Fan YD, Pastorek JG, Miller JM Jr, Mulvey J. Acute pyelonephritis in pregnancy. Am J Perinatol 1987; 4: 324–326.

Fonkalsrud EW, de Lorimer AA, Hays DM. Congenital atresia and stenosis of the duodenum. Pediatrics 1969; 43: 79–83.

Gettman MT, Segura JW. Struvite stones: diagnosis and current treatment concepts. J Endocrinol 1995; 13: 653–658.

Hart CC, Weisholtz SJ. Urinary tract infections. In: Roberts RB (ed). Infectious Diseases. Pathogenesis, Diagnosis and Therapy. Year Book Medical Publ., Chicago, 1986. pp. 73–96.

Heller H, Sakhaee K, Moe OW, Pak CY. Etiological role of estrogen status on renal formation. J Urol 2002; 168: 1923–1927.

Heptinstall RH. Renal diseases in pregnancy. In: Heptinstall RH (ed.) Pathology of Kidney. 3rd ed. Little, Brown and Co., Boston, 1983. pp. 963–991.

Kass EH. Bacteriuria and pyelonephritis of pregnancy. Arch Intern Med 1960; 105: 42–46.

Katz AI, Davison JM, Hayslett JP, Singson E, Lindheimer MD. Pregnancy in women with kidney diseases. Kidney Int 1980; 18: 192–196.

Kincaid-Smith P, Fairley KF. The differential diagnosis between preeclamptic toxemia and glomerulonephritis in patients with proteinuria during pregnancy. In: Lindheimer MD, Katz AI, Zuspan FP (eds.) Hypertension in Pregnancy. Wiley, New York, 1976. pp. 157–171.

Laerum E, Larsen S. Thiazide prophylaxis of urolithiasis: a double blind study in general practice. Acta Med Scand 1984; 215: 383–389.

Levey AS, Coresh J, Balk E et al. National kidney foundation practice guidelines for chronic kidney disease: evaluation, classification and stratification. Ann Intern Med 2006; 139: 137–147.

MacGillirray I. Some observations on the incidence of pre-eclampsia. J Obstet Gynecol 1958; 65: 536–540.

MacKey EV. Pregnancy and renal disease: a ten-year survey. Aust NZ J Obstet Gynecol 1963; 3: 21–26.

Mishalany HG, Najjar FB. Familial jejunal atresia: three cases in one family. J Pediat 1968; 73: 753–755.

Monga M. Maternal cardiovascular and renal adaptation to pregnancy. In: Creasy RK, Resnik MD, Iams JD (eds.) Maternal-Fetal Medicine. 5th ed. Saunders, Philadelphia, 2004. pp. 111–120.

Moe OW. Kidney stones: pathophysiology and medical management. Lancet 2006; 367: 333–344.

Naeye RL. Causes of the excessive rates of perinatal mortality and prematurity in pregnancies complicated by maternal urinary tract infections. N Engl J Med 1979; 300: 819–823.

Norden CW, Kass EH. Bacteriuria of pregnancy – a critical appraisal. Ann Rev Med 1968; 19: 431–440.

O'Neill MS, Hertz-Picciotto I, Pastore LM, Wetherley BD. Have studies of urinary tract infection and pregerm delivery used the most appropriate methods? Paediat Perinat Epidemiol 2003; 17: 226–233.

Pak CY. Kidney stones. Lancet 1998; 351: 1797–1801.

Parker MT, Collier LH (eds.). Topley Wilson Principles of Bacteriology, Virology and Immunity. Decker BC, Philadelphia, 1990.

Pickering TG, Ogedegbe G. Epidemiology of hypertension. In: Fuster V, Walsh RA, O'Rourke RA, Poole-Wilson P (eds.). Hurst's the Heart. 12th ed. McGraw Hill Medical, New York, etc, 2008. pp. 1551–1569.

Roberts RB (ed.). Infectious Diseases: Pathogenesis, Diagnosis and Therapy. Year Book Medical Publ., Chicago, 1986.

Seymour AE, Petracco OM, Clarkson AR et al. Morphologic and immunological evidence of coagulopathy in renal complications of pregnancy. In: Lindheimer MD, Katz AI, Zuspan FP (eds.) Hypertension in Pregnancies. Wiley, New York, 1976. pp. 139–145.

Shepard TH, Lemire RJ. Catalog of Teratogenic Agents. 11th ed. Johns Hopkins Univ Press, Baltimore, 2004.

Sims EAH. The kidney in pregnancy. In: Strauss MB, Welt LG (eds.) Diseases of the Kidney. 2nd ed. Little, Brown and Co., Boston, 1971. pp. 1155–1211.

Smaill F. Antibiotics for asymptomatic bacteriuria in pregnancy. Cochrane Database Syst Rev 2001; CD 000490.

Soucie JM, Thun MJ, Coates RK, McClellan W, Austin H. Demographic and geographic variability of kidney stones in the United States. Kidney Int 1994; 46: 893–895.

Stamatelon KK, Francis ME, Jones CA, Nyberg LM, Curhan GC. Time trends in reported prevalence of kidney stones in the United States: 1976–1994. Kidney Int 2003; 63: 1817–1823.

Tanner MS, Smith B, Lloyd JK. Functional intestinal obstruction due to deficiency of argyrophil neurones in the myenteric plexus: familial syndrome presenting with short small bowel, malrotation, and pyloric hypertrophy. Arch Dis Child 1976; 51: 837–841.

Trembath DG, Rijhsinghani A. Possible maternal inheritance of common obstructive urinary tract infections and two sons with posterior urethal valves. J Reprod Med 2002; 47: 962–964.

Trinchieri A, Ostini F, Nespoli R, Rovera F, Zanetti G. A prospective study of recurrence rate and risk factors for recurrence after a first renal stone. J Urol 1999; 162: 27–30.

Wilson PD, Loffredo CA, Correa-Villasenor A, Ferencz C. Attributable fraction for cardiac malformations. Am J Epidemiol 1998; 148: 414–423.

Yaris F, Kadioglu M, Kesim M et al. Urinary tract infections in unplanned pregnancies and fetal outcome. Eur J Contracept Reprod Health Care 2004; 9: 141–146.

Own Publications

I. Ács N, Bánhidy F, Puho HE, Czeizel AE. A possible association between maternal glomerulonephritis and congenital intestinal atresia/stenosis – a population-based case-control study. Eur J Epidemiol 2007; 22: 557–564.

II. Czeizel AE, Hancsok M, Ormay L, Philipp G. The connection between significant bacteriuria during pregnancy and premature births (Hungarian with English abstract). Orv Hetil 1967; 108: 101–102.

III. Bánhidy F, Ács N, Puhó E, Czeizel AE. Pregnancy complications and birth outcomes of pregnant women with urinary tract infections and related drug treatments. Scand J Infect Dis 2007; 37: 390–397.

IV. Bánhidy F, Ács N, Puho HE, Czeizel AE. Maternal urinary tract infection and related drug treatments during pregnancy and risk of congenital abnormalities in the offspring. Br J Obstet Gynaecol 2006; 113: 1465–1471.

V. Czeizel AE, Berecz M, Gerőfi J, Vándor K, Domány Z. Study of asymptomatic significant bacteriuria in a population section of Budapest (Hungarian with English abstract). Orvosi Hetilap 1968; 109: 1985–1987.

VI. Czeizel AE, Hancsok M, Margitay Becht D, Ormay L, Berecz M, Tarján G. Incidence of significant bacteriuria during pregnancy (Hungarian with English abstract). Orvosi Hetilap 1967; 108: 684–686.

VII. Czeizel AE. Ten years experience in periconceptional care. Eur J Obstet Gynecol Reprod Biol 1999; 84: 43–49.

VIII. Czeizel AE, Dobó M, Dudás I, Gasztonyi Z, Lantos I. The Hungarian Periconceptional Service as a model for community genetics. Commun Genet 1998; 1: 252–259.

IX. Bánhidy F, Ács N, Puho HE, Czeizel AE. Maternal kidney stones during pregnancy and adverse birth outcomes, particularly congenital abnormalities in the offspring. Arch Gynecol Obstet 2007; 275: 481–487.

Chapter 16
Diseases of the Genital Organs

The female genital organs undergo dramatic changes during pregnancy. These changes are crucial for the intrauterine development of the fetus, prevention of spontaneous abortion and preterm delivery, and the timely initiation of labor at term (Monga and Sanborn, 2004).

The weight of a nonpregnant uterus is ranging between 40 and 70 g with a volume capacity of 10 mL. The weight of the pregnant uterus at the end of gestation is 1,100–1,200 g with an average volume capacity of 5 L. There is an increase in the number of myometrial cells in the early pregnancy while in the second half of the pregnancy the size of the cells is increasing tremendously. The increase in the size of the uterus associated with 10-fold increase in uterine blood flow. The cervix primarily contains fibrous connective tissue combined with 10–15% of smooth muscle cells. The structure of cervix is also extensively changing during pregnancy resulting in progressively softening and shortening of the cervix.

The vagina is also changing during pregnancy: vaginal mucosa is thickening meanwhile there is an enlargement of the papillae; in addition, the vascularity of the vagina, fallopian tubes, and ovaries also shows increases. The ovulation is stopped in the ovaries; corpus luteal function is decreasing after the 5th postconceptional week because the placenta surpasses the production of necessary progesterone.

The more intensive vascularity of the female genital organs parallel with the immunological changes in the maternal body may contribute to some diseases, mainly infections during pregnancy.

16.1 Pelvic Inflammatory Diseases

The ICD (WHO) classification started with the main code of "Inflammatory disease of the ovaries, the uterus, the fallopian tubes, pelvis cellular tissue, and the peritoneum", but recently the term pelvic inflammatory disease is used for this disease group.

N. Ács et al., *Congenital Abnormalities and Preterm Birth Related to Maternal Illnesses During Pregnancy*, DOI 10.1007/978-90-481-8620-4_16,

Pelvic inflammatory disease is a clinical diagnosis of acute or chronic infections/diseases of the upper genital tract. As far as we know the possible association between *acute pelvic inflammatory disease* (APID) in pregnant women and CAs in their offspring has not been analyzed in case-control epidemiological studies. The objective of our study was to evaluate this possible association.

In general, APIDs were recorded as acute salpingitis or adnexitis in the prenatal maternity logbook or hospital discharge summaries as a first episode during study pregnancies. Thus chronic pelvic inflammatory diseases, i.e. pregnant women with any previous history of pelvic inflammatory diseases were excluded from the study.

The symptoms of APID are fever, cervical discharge, bilateral adnexal and cervical motion tenderness with laboratory indication of infection such as elevated count of white blood cells and sedimentation rate (Gjonaess, 1982; Stacey et al., 1992). APID is frequently associated with cervicitis and/or vulvovaginitis, therefore pregnant women with APID and these associated conditions were also included to the study. However, vulvovaginitis and bacterial vaginosis without APID, abscess of Bartholin's gland and vulva, gonococcal and syphilitic infections were excluded from the study.

16.1.1 Results of the Study (I)

Out of 22,843 cases with CA, 87 (0.38%) had mothers with the diagnosis of APID including 2 endometritis, 20 salpingitis, and 65 adnexitis. Among 38,151 controls, 158 (0.41%) mothers were affected with APID including 2 endometritis, 30 salpingitis, and 126 adnexitis. However, the diagnosis was based only on retrospective maternal information in 18 case and 26 control mothers, generally after the first trimester. Thus, we decided to evaluate only 69 (0.30%) case mothers and 132 (0.35%) control mothers with prospectively and medically recorded APID in the prenatal maternity logbook and/or hospital discharge summary. Therefore, pregnant women with APID based only on maternal information were excluded from the study.

The diagnosis of APID was recorded at the first visit in prenatal care clinics during II and III gestational month in most pregnant women; therefore the onset of APID occurred early in pregnancy. The duration of APID was shorter than a month, but all APID with their onset in I gestational month continued into II gestational month. The onset of medically recorded APID was after the first trimester in 2 case mothers and in 4 control mothers. These pregnant women were also excluded from the study. Thus, finally the medically recorded diagnoses of APID during II and/or III gestational months were evaluated in 67 (0.29%) case mothers and 128 (0.34%) control mothers.

Eight case mothers with APID were visited at home, and 5 (62.5%) reported high fever (over 38.5°C) due to their APID during pregnancy.

Mean maternal age (25.0 vs. 25.5 year) was somewhat lower, while birth order (1.8 vs. 1.7) was somewhat higher in pregnant women with APID than in pregnant women without APID as reference. Marital and employment status did not show significant difference between the study groups.

There was no difference in the use of folic acid during pregnancy between case (47.8%) and control (48.4%) mothers with APID, but their combined occurrence (48.2%) was lower than in pregnant women without APID (54.4%). The folic acid-containing multivitamin supplementations during pregnancy showed similar occurrence (3.5–6.0%) in the study groups. We evaluated periconceptional supplementation of folic acid and multivitamins separately; about one-tenth of the above pregnant women used both of them in I gestational month.

When evaluating other acute diseases in pregnant women with or without APID, the incidence of two groups of diseases showed some differences. The incidence of acute infectious diseases of the urinary tract was much more frequent in case and control pregnant women with APID together (16.4%) than in pregnant women without APID (6.0%) (3.1, 1.9–4.9). In addition, the incidence of influenza-common cold (the latter generally together with secondary complications) was also higher in pregnant women with APID (26.7%) compared to pregnant women without APID (18.5%) (1.6, 1.1–2.4). However, the incidence of these and other diseases did not show difference between case and control pregnant women with APID.

The prevalence of chronic maternal diseases such as diabetes mellitus and epilepsy did not show significant differences among study groups.

Antimicrobial-antifungal drugs such as ampicillin (15.6% vs. 6.9%), clotrimazole (18.8% vs. 8.0%), metronidazole (16.4% vs. 3.7%), oxytetracycline (6.3% vs. 2.8%), penamecillin (8.6% vs. 5.9%), sulfamethoxazole+trimethoprim (7.0% vs. 1.1%) were used more frequently in pregnant women with APID compared to pregnant women without APID. In addition, drugs used for the treatment of threatened abortion and preterm delivery such as allylestrenol (25.8% vs. 14.0%), diazepam (22.7% vs. 10.8%), drotaverine (18.0% vs. 9.1%), and promethazine (21.9% vs. 15.9%) were also used more frequently by pregnant women with APID. However, only ampicillin (29.9% vs. 15.6%, 2.3, 1.1–4.7) and dipyrone, an analgesic drug (20.9% vs. 6.3%; 4.0, 1.6–10.0) was used more frequently by case mothers than control mothers with APID.

Among pregnancy complications, the incidence of threatened abortions (25.6% vs. 16.4%) and preterm deliveries (19.5% vs. 13.2%), in addition to placental disorders (4.1% vs. 1.5%) were more frequent in pregnant women with APID. However, there was no significant difference between the pregnancy complications of case and control mothers with APID.

Table 16.1 shows the birth characteristics of cases and controls.

Mean gestational age (39.1 vs. 39.4 week; $p = 0.17$) was 0.3 week shorter and mean birth weight (3,207 vs. 3,276 g; $p = 0.13$) was 69 g smaller in newborns of mothers with APID compared to babies born to mothers without APID. The rate of PB (14.1% vs. 9.1%; 1.6, 0.9–2.7) and LBW (8.6% vs. 5.7%; $p = 1.6$, 0.8–2.9) was somewhat higher in newborns of mothers with APID. However, we have to remember that APID occurred in early pregnancy.

The possible associations between APID and CAs were evaluated in 12 CA groups including at least 3 cases (Table 16.2).

Table 16.1 Birth characteristics of control newborns without CAs who had mothers with acute pelvic inflammatory disease (APID)

	Newborns of pregnant women			
Variables	with APID (*N*=128)		without APID (*N*=38,023)	
Quantitative	Mean	S.D.	Mean	S.D.
Gestational age at delivery (week)	39.1	2.2	39.4	2.0
Birth weight (g)	3,207	569	3,276	511
Categorical	No.	%	No.	%
PB	18	14.1	3,478	9.1
LBW newborns	11	8.6	2,156	5.7

Table 16.2 Estimation of risks for total and different CA groups in cases and their all matched controls of pregnant women with APID during II and/or III gestational months

	Grand total	APID		
Study groups	No.	No.	%	Adjusted OR[a] with 95% CI
Isolated CAs				
Neural-tube defects	1,202	5	0.4	1.2 (0.4–4.0)
Cleft lip ± palate	1,375	5	0.4	1.4 (0.4–4.7)
Oesophageal atresia/stenosis	217	3	1.4	1.1 (0.2–5.9)
Obstructive urinary CAs	343	3	0.9	4.5 (0.4–46.4)
Hypospadias	3,038	9	0.3	0.9 (0.4–2.0)
Undescended testis	2,052	3	0.2	0.4 (0.1–1.3)
Cardiovascular CAs	4,480	18	0.4	**2.6 (1.2–5.4)**
Clubfoot	2,424	3	0.1	0.6 (0.2–2.2)
Poly/syndactyly	1,744	3	0.2	0.5 (0.2–1.9)
Other isolated CAs	4,619	11[b]	0.2	0.7 (0.2–2.9)
Multiple CAs	1,349	4	0.3	1.1 (0.3–3.9)
Total cases	22,843	67	0.3	0.95 (0.70–1.29)
Total controls	38,151	128	0.3	Reference

[a]Matched OR adjusted for maternal age, employment status, birth order, other maternal diseases and drug uses, and folic acid supplementation.
[b]Cong. hydrocephaly, ear CA, macrostomia, horseshoe kidney, rectal atresia, pseudohermaphroditism, limb deficiency, pectus excavatum, rib CA, torticollis, and gastroschisis.

All mothers were affected by APID in II and/or III months of pregnancy and only cases with cardiovascular CAs had mothers with a higher rate of APID during pregnancy.

In the next step, we compared the expected numbers of different types of cardiovascular CAs based on the total data set of the HCCSCA and the observed numbers in our study (Table 16.3).

Table 16.3. Expected and observed number of different types of cardiovascular CAs in cases born to mothers with APID in II and/or III gestational months

	Expected		Observed	
Types of cardiovascular CA	%	No.	No.	p
Common truncus	0.7	0.0	0	–
Transposition of the great arteries	3.4	0.6	0	0.43
Tetralogy of Fallot	1.9	0.3	1	0.20
Ventricular septal defect	34.9	6.3	4	0.26
Atrial septal defect, type II	**10.3**	**1.9**	**8**	**<0.0001**
Hypoplastic left heart	2.6	0.5	0	0.47
Patent ductus arteriosus	3.9	0.7	0	0.39
Coarctation of the aorta	2.6	0.5	0	0.47
Other CAs of the aorta/aortic valves	2.0	0.4	0	0.52
CAs of the pulmonary artery/valves	5.9	1.1	1	0.92
Other specified cardiovascular CAs	3.9	0.7	0	0.39
Unspecified cardiovascular CAs	27.9	5.0	4	0.60
Total	100.0	18.0	18	1.00

Atrial septal defect, type II showed a 4.2-fold increase. Out of their 8 mothers, 2 were also affected by common cold with secondary complication, 1 with influenza and 1 with recurrent orofacial herpes in the 4th, 7th, 6th, and 8th gestational week, respectively. One pregnant woman with influenza later was visited at home and according to her recall, her fever exceeded 40°C. In addition, two pregnant women were treated with ampicillin (in gestational month IV and V), co-trimoxazole (sulphametoxazole + trimethoprim) (in gestatational month I), and sulfonamides (in gestational month VII).

16.1.2 Interpretation of Results

This population-based case-control study showed a higher risk for cardiovascular CAs, particularly atrial septal defect type II in the newborns of pregnant women with APID during II and/or III gestational months.

The observed rate of pregnant women with APID corresponded well to the published rates published in international publications (e.g. Westron, 1980). Our study confirmed the well-known association between APID and acute infectious diseases of the urinary tract (cystitis, pyelitis, and pyelonephritis) and showed a higher risk for placental disorders in pregnant women with APID.

Previously a possible association between the genitourinary infections or promiscuity and gastroschisis was suggested (Werler et al., 1992; Torfs et al., 1994) but our data set had only one case with gastroschisis.

When evaluating the possible association between APID in pregnant women and cardiovascular CAs in their offspring, the effect of APID itself (e.g. fever), the causes of APID (i.e. the microbial agents), related drug treatments, other confounders, and chance effect should be considered.

Miettinen et al. (1970) found a secular trend in the prevalence of coarctation of the aorta explained by seasonal changes of virus infections. Tikkanen and Heinonen (1994) reported an association between upper respiratory tract infection during the first trimester of pregnancy and hypoplastic left heart syndrome. The Baltimore Washington Infant Study found an association between maternal urinary tract infections and some types of cardiovascular CAs, such as heterotaxies, transposition of the great vessels and atrial septal defects (Ferencz et al., 1997). Finally some studies indicated an association between cardiovascular CA and high fever during the critical period of these CAs (Tikkanen and Heinonen, 1991; Botto et al., 2001; II–V). Thus the common denominator of these findings may be the high fever because the teratogenic effect of high fever/hyperthermia is well-established (III).

We did not find any data regarding to the possible association between the microbial causes of APID and cardiovascular CAs.

The drugs have a role in the origin of cardiovascular CAs (Kallen and Olausson, 2003), particularly cotrimoxazole (Hernandez-Diaz et al., 2000; 19, 20), some types of sulfonamides (17), and oxytetracycline (8). However, only two drugs: ampicillin and dipyrone were used more frequently by case mothers with APID compared to control mothers with APID. Both ampicillin (4) and dipyrone (81) were evaluated in the HCCSCA and they did not demonstrate any cardiovascular CA inducing effect. In addition, we evaluated APID related drugs as confounders when calculating the adjusted OR. Only one of the above-mentioned drugs was used for the treatment of APID in pregnant women who later delivered babies with atrial septal defects type II and this drug was cotrimoxazole in I gestational month of pregnancy, i.e. before the critical period of this CA.

Our previous intervention trials showed some protective effect of folic acid – containing multivitamins during the periconceptional period for cardiovascular CAs (128, 129, 131). We therefore evaluated these supplementations as confounders, but there was no difference in their use between case and control mothers with APID.

Our hypothesis is that the cause of the possible association between APID in early pregnancy and a higher risk for cardiovascular CAs particularly atrial septal defect, type II may be the high fever which is characteristic for APID. Our previous studies showed that this fever related risk is preventable by antipyretic drug therapy (III); therefore it is necessary to combine antimicrobial and antipyretics in the treatment of APID in pregnant women.

In conclusion, our population-based case-control study showed an association between APID in early pregnancy and an increased risk for cardiovascular CAs, particularly atrial septal defect type II. This finding is considered only as a signal and further studies are needed to confirm or reject this association.

16.2 Vulvovaginitis and Bacterial Vaginosis

Lower genital tract infections such as vulvovaginal infections are among the most common reasons why women seek help of medical doctors and are the most frequent diseases during pregnancy (Yarberry-Allen et al., 1986). The associations between antenatal infection/inflammation of the lower genital tract and fetal tissue injuries particularly in the origin of preterm premature rupture of membranes, cerebral palsy, and bronchopulmonary dysplasia are well-known (Murphy and Kennea, 2007).

The rate of PB was high (9.3%) in Hungary (Bjerkedahl et al., 1983) and some other countries, e.g. USA (12–13%) (Goldenberg et al., 2008), therefore PB is the most common cause of infant mortality and morbidity (Saigal and Doyle, 2008). Vulvovaginal infections/diseases are believed to account for 25–40% of PBs (McGregor et al., 1990; Divers and Lilford, 1993; Chin and Lamon, 1997; Menon and Fortunate, 2007; Goldenberg et al., 2008).

Intrauterine infections have different origins and routes but the most frequent and serious access is ascending infection from the lower genital tract. Thus the infections and inflammatory diseases of the lower genital tract (cervix, vagina and vulva), i.e. *vulvovaginitis and bacterial vaginosis* (VV–VB) are the major causes of intrauterine infections. Intrauterine infections may have an onset in the decidua which later extends to the space between the amnion and chorion, finally reaching the amniotic cavity and the fetus. The preterm parturition syndrome due to intrauterine infections can be explained partly by the effect of certain microorganisms (e.g. endotoxins) and partly by the activation of the innate immune system (inflammatory chemokines and cytokines, like interleukin 8 and 1 beta, tumor necrosis factor, such as TNF alfa) (Goldenberg et al., 2000; Romero et al., 2006). Microbial endotoxins and proinflammatory cytokines stimulate the production of prostaglandins which increase uterine contractility. Other inflammatory mediators result in the degradation of extracellular matrix in the fetal membranes followed by their preterm premature rupture.

The association of some sexually transmitted diseases such as syphilis (Ingall and Norris, 1976; Grossman, 1977) or herpes genitalis (Brown et al., 1987; Baldwin and Whitley, 1989) with CAs were shown. However, to our best knowledge the possible association between VV–BV during pregnancy and CAs has not been analyzed in controlled epidemiological studies (Shepard and Lemire, 2004). On the other hand, the potential teratogenic effect of drugs used for the treatment of maternal VV–BV during pregnancy was frequently evaluated. For example the high dose of fluconazole (Pursley et al., 1995; Aleck and Bartley, 1997) was found to be teratogenic in the human.

Therefore there were four objectives of our study. The first objective was to evaluate pregnancy complications pregnant women affected with VV–BV. The second objective was to measure the risk for PB of the newborns of pregnant women with VV–BV with or without related treatment. Thirdly, we wanted to estimate the efficacy of the usual drug treatments in the prevention of VV–BV related PB. Finally, the fourth objective was to estimate the possible association between VV–BV during pregnancy and the risk of different CAs in their offspring.

16.2.1 Results of the Study (VI, VII)

The disease group of VV–BV included two main categories of acute infections/diseases of external genital organ in pregnant women:

Vulvovaginitis (i.e. vaginitis, vulvitis, inflammatory diseases of the vulva and/or the vagina frequently combined with cervicitis) as a clinical syndrome comprises not only discrete vulvar and vaginal lesions, but also abnormal vaginal secretions (Yarberry-Allen et al., 1986). Most cases of vulvovaginitis are due to specific microbiological agents.

Bacterial vaginosis is caused by bacteria or bacterial vaginosis-related organisms such as *Gardenella vaginalis, Mobiluncus, anaerobes, Mycoplasma hominis*.In Hungary the diagnosis of bacterial vaginosis is based on the presence of 3 of 4 Amsel's criteria (Amsell et al., 1983): (i) a homogeneous white adherent ("watery") vaginal discharge, (ii) vaginal fluid pH less than 4.5, (iii) release of a fishy odor on mixing 5–10% potassium hydroxide with vaginal secretion, i.e. amine test (Sonnex, 1995), and (iv) presence of vaginal epithelium cells covered with and the so-called clue cells, i.e. obscured by bacteria on fresh wet mount (Nugent et al., 1991).

Pregnant women with vulvovaginitis and bacterial vaginosis were included to the group of VV–BV in our data set, however, because on the basis of Gram stain it is difficult to differentiate normal and abnormal vaginal flora mixed together with the intermediate flora (Donders, 2002, 2007), only prospectively and medically recorded VV–BV in the prenatal maternity logbook of pregnant women were evaluated in the study.

VV–BV with pelvic inflammatory diseases, abscess of the Bartholin gland and the vulva, in addition to genital herpes were excluded from the study. Gonococcal and syphilitic infections were recorded in 4 case and 2 control mothers, respectively, but they were also excluded from this analysis.

Out of 22,843 cases, 2,027 (8.9%) had mothers with the diagnosis of VV–BV recorded in the prenatal maternity logbook and/or reported by mothers in the questionnaire, however we evaluated only 1,536 (6.7%) mothers who had prospectively and medically recorded diagnosis of VV–BV. Out of 1,536 case mothers, 215 (14.0%) were recorded as specified vulvovaginal candidiasis, 190 (12.4%) as trichomonal infections, 230 (15.0%) as bacterial vaginosis, while the rest of VV–BV was unspecified.

Out of 38,151 controls without CA, 3,326 (8.7%) had mothers with the diagnosis of VV–BV recorded in the prenatal maternity logbook and/or reported by mothers in the questionnaire, but only 2,698 (7.1%) pregnant women with medically recorded VV–BV were evaluated. The proportions of candidiasis, trichomoniasis, and bacterial vaginosis were the following in control mothers: 11.4% (n=307), 15.5% (n=418) and 16.6% (n=447), respectively.

There was no significant difference in the occurrence of VV–BV between case and control mothers (0.94, 0.88–1.01). The causes of bacterial vaginosis such as *Gardenella vaginalis, Mobiluncus*, anaerobes, *Mycoplasma hominis* were rarely mentioned in the prenatal maternity logbook. The distribution of different specified and unspecified etiological groups showed some differences between case and control mothers with VV–BV.

VV–BVs were recorded at the first visit in prenatal care clinics nearly in all pregnant women during II and/or III gestational month. Therefore, the onset of VV–BV likely occurred before the conception or very early in pregnancy. In general, the duration of VV–BV after diagnosis and treatment was shorter than one month.

The mean maternal age (25.0 vs. 25.5 year) was somewhat lower in pregnant women with VV–BV compared to pregnant women without VV–BV as reference. However, there was no difference in the mean birth order (1.7) between the two study groups. The distribution of their employment status was different due to the higher proportion of professionals (13.5% vs. 11.3%) and "others" including mainly students (7.4% vs. 5.9%), while semiskilled workers (13.5% vs. 15.3%) had a lower proportion among pregnant women with VV–BV. There was no difference in the use of folic acid between case (51.6% vs. 49.2%) and control mothers (55.0% vs. 54.4%) with or without VV–BV, however, case mothers used folic acid less frequently than control mothers with VV–BV (0.8, 0.7–0.9). The use of folic acid-containing multivitamins did not show difference among the study groups. The proportion of smokers was 22.1% in pregnant women with VV–VB among the mothers of children with CA visited at home, while 18.4% of pregnant women without VV–BV were smoker. The proportion of regular drinkers (more than one drink per week) was somewhat less than 1% in both subgroups of mothers visited at home.

Among other acute maternal diseases, only the infectious diseases of the urinary tract such as cystitis, pyelitis, pyelonephritis showed a higher incidence in pregnant women with VV–BV (8.2% vs. 6.0%, 1.4, 1.2–1.5). There was no difference in the prevalence of chronic maternal diseases such as diabetes mellitus or epilepsy among the study groups.

The evaluation of most frequently used drugs showed that the use of clotrimazole (58.7% vs. 3.9%) and metronidazole (33.0% vs. 1.7%) was much more frequent in pregnant women with VV–BV than in pregnant women without VV–BV. In addition, the treatment of ampicillin (9.8% vs. 6.8%), nitrofurantoin (4.5% vs. 2.9%), and sulphamethoxazole + trimethoprim (co-trimoxazole) (1.8% vs. 1.1%) was more frequent in mothers with VV–BV.

The first aim of the study was to evaluate pregnancy complications. Only anemia (18.8% vs. 16.5%, 1.2, 1.1–1.3) was more frequent in pregnant women with VV–BV compared to mothers without VV–BV.

Table 16.4 shows the distribution of gestational age at birth and weight groups, in addition to the rate of PB and LBW newborn of mothers with or without VV–BV.

The mean gestational age was 0.1 week longer, while mean birth weight was 28 g larger in babies born to mothers with VV–BV. This trend was in agreement with a lower rate of PB (7.5% vs. 9.3%) and LBW (4.8% vs. 5.8%).

In the next step the data of birth outcomes were stratified according to the most frequently used antimicrobial drugs for the treatment of VV–BV (Table 16.5).

Pregnant women with or without VV–BV and with or without *antimicrobial drug treatment* (ADT) were compared. Among ADT, four groups: clotrimazole, metronidazole, ampicillin, and others were differentiated. Clotrimazole was able to reduce

Table 16.4 Distribution of birth weight according to gestational age groups in newborn infants born to mothers with or without VV–BV

Gestational age (week)		36 or less		37–41		42 or more		Total				Gestational age[a]			
		With VV–BV	Without VV–BV	With VV–BV	Without VV–BV	With VV–BV	Without VV–BV	With VV–BV		Without VV–BV		With VV–BV		Without VV–BV	
Birth weight (g)		No.	No.	No.	No.	No.	No.	No.	%	No.	%	Mean	S.D.	Mean	S.D.
2,499 or less		70	1,213	58	775	1	50	129	4.8	2,038	5.8	35.8	3.4	35.6	3.2
2,500–4,499		133	2,080	2,162	27,575	246	3,473	2,541	94.2	33,128	93.4	39.6	1.6	39.6	1.7
4,500 or more		0	0	20	203	8	84	28	1.0	287	0.8	40.8	0.9	41.0	1.2
Total	No.	203	3,293	2,240	28,553	255	3,607	2,698	100.0	35,453	100.0	39.5	1.9	39.4	2.1
	%	7.5	9.3	83.0	80.5	9.5	10.2	100.0	–	100.0	–	–	–	–	–
Birth weight	Mean	2,500	2,483	3,335	3,323	3,647	3,613	3,302	–	3,274	–	–	–	–	–
	S.D.	465	435	440	429	507	484	511	–	511	–	–	–	–	–

Comparison of mean gestational age[a]: $t = 2.8$, $p = 0.005$ and mean birth weight[b]: $t = 2.7$, $p = 0.007$. Rate of PB[a]: OR = 0.8 (0.7–0.9) and LBW[b]: OR = 0.8 (0.7–0.9).

[a] Adjusted for maternal age, birth order, employment status, other maternal diseases, related drug treatments, folic acid supplementation.

[b] Adjusted for maternal age, birth order, employment status, other maternal diseases, related drug treatments, folic acid supplementation, and gestational age.

Table 16.5 Analysis of PB in the groups of pregnant women with both VV–BV and antimicrobial drug treatment (ADT) and pregnant women without VV–BV but with ADT compared to women without VV–BV and ADT as reference

	VV–BV = NO, ADT = NO			VV–BV = NO, ADT = YES			VV–BV = YES, ADT = YES		
Treatment	No.	%	OR (95% CI)	No.	%	OR (95% CI)	No.	%	OR (95% CI)
Clotrimazole	3,183	9.4	Reference	110	7.8	**0.8 (0.7–0.9)**	111	6.7	**0.7 (0.6–0.8)**
Ampicillin	3,124	9.4	Reference	169	7.2	**0.7 (0.6–0.9)**	17	6.5	0.7 (0.4–1.1)
Metronidazole	3,228	9.3	Reference	65	11.2	1.2 (0.9–1.6)	78	9.4	1.0 (0.8–1.3)
Others[a]	3,073	9.3	Reference	220	8.6	0.9 (0.8–1.1)	22	9.9	1.1 (0.7–1.6)

[a]Oxytetracycline, penamecillin, sulfamethoxazole + trimethoprim.

the rate of PB in pregnant women with VV–BV. However, out of 2,698 pregnant women with VV–BV, 307 were recorded with vulvovaginal candidiasis, but only 111 were treated by clotrimazole. Although the lowest rate of PB was found after ampicillin treatment in pregnant women with VV–BV, this association was not significant due to the limited number of subjects. However, the major finding is that the rate of PB in babies born to mothers with VV–BV diagnosed in early pregnancy followed by clotrimazole and ampicillin treatment was much lower (6.5–6.7%) than the PB rate of the Hungarian newborn population (9.3%). It is worth presenting that pregnant women without VV–BV but after clotrimazole and ampicillin treatment (likely due to other indications) also had a significantly lower PB rate (7.2–7.8%) than the national average PB rate (9.3%). Finally, 783 pregnant women with VV–BV but without ATD were recorded in the HCCSCA (these data are not shown in Table 16.5) and the number of newborns with PB was 60, thus its rate (7.7%) was also lower than the national average PB rate (9.3%). Out of these 60 pregnant women, 38 (63.3%) pregnant women were treated by boric acid or lactobacillus vaccine.

The fourth objective of our study was to evaluate the possible associations between VV–BV and different CAs. All case and control mothers affected by VV–BV at any time during pregnancy or in II and/or III months of pregnancy, i.e. the critical period of most major CAs, were compared. A higher prevalence of maternal VV–BV was not found in total CA (0.95, 0.89–1.02) or any CA group when calculating adjusted OR.

Finally, we evaluated the possible associations between maternal VV–BV with or without appropriate treatment and the risk of CAs in their offspring. Five drugs such as clotrimazole, metronidazole, ampicillin, nitrofurantoin, and co-trimoxazole (sulphamethoxazole + trimethoprim) used frequently for the treatment of VV–BV in pregnant women were evaluated separately and compared to the data of mothers with VV–BV but without treatment of these drugs. The risk for total CAs was significantly lower in the group of maternal VV–BV with appropriate treatment (0.85, 0.78–0.91) than in the group of maternal VV–BV without treatment (1.11, 0.90–1.32).

16.2.2 Interpretation of Results

We summarize our results according to the objectives of the study.

First, there is no higher risk for pregnancy complications in pregnant women with VV–BV, with the exception of anemia which had a somewhat higher incidence in pregnant women with VV–BV.

Second, we did not find an increase in the rate of PB in children of pregnant women with VV–BV.

Third, the previous unexpected finding can be explained by the effective medical intervention: when the diagnosis of VV–BV in early pregnancy was followed by clotrimazole and ampicillin treatment and these treatments resulted in a much lower (6.5–6.7%) rate of PB than the national average PB rate (9.3%). Thus these treatments were effective in the prevention of PB due to VV–BV. However, there is another important finding of the study. The rate of PB was lower in babies born to mothers without diagnosed and/or recorded VV–BV but had clotrimazole or ampicillin treatment for other reasons (7.2–7.8%).

Fourth, this first population-based case-control study epidemiological study did not show a higher risk for total CAs or any CA in the newborns of pregnant women with VV–BV. Therefore, localized infections and infectious diseases of the vagina with necessary treatment during early pregnancy do not disturb the organogenesis of the human embryo.

After the summary of results, it is necessary to better understand the causes of VV–BV.

Vaginal candidiasis (monilial vaginitis) caused mainly by *Candida albicans* and rarely *Candida glabrata*. Candida albicans as a saprophytic yeast which is part of the endogenous flora of the vagina and is present in the vagina of about 25% of sexually active females. However, candidas may become opportunistic pathogens when the defense mechanism of the host organism is compromised. Thus candidal VV is the second most frequent cause of VV following BV. Symptomatic candidal VV occurs in about 15% of pregnant women. The symptoms of candidal VV include pruritus and burning, dysuria, dyspareunia, excoriation with secondary infections, and thick, white, curd-like vaginal discharge. Microscopic examination of vaginal secretion using 10% potassium hydroxide is appropriate for the presumptive diagnosis of candidal VV, i.e. the identification of fungus. Sometimes the diagnosis needs cultures using selective media in pregnant women with negative potassium hydroxide smears.

Trichomonas vaginalis is another common cause of VV characterized by typical malodorous, yellow-green, frothy vaginal discharge, together with priritus and dysuria. The occurrence of trichomonal VV in pregnant women is between 10 and 50% depending on the number of sexual partners and socioeconomic status. The diagnosis of vaginal trichomoniasis is based on the microscopic examination of the vaginal discharge. Trichomonas vaginalis can be identified on the basis of their size (somewhat larger than leukocytes) and active flagella; however, the microscopic examination can reveal many leukocytes and bacteria as well.

The diagnostic criteria of BV were described previously; clinically the primary symptoms are vaginal discharge and odor. BV can be characterized by a major shift in vaginal flora from the normal predominance of lactobacilli to the predominance of anaerobes. The occurrence of these anaerobes increased 100-fold in BV compared to normal secretion. *Gardenella vaginalis* is also present in 95% pregnant women frequently associated with *Mycoplasma hominis*.

As our previous data showed, less than 50% of our pregnant women had specified diagnosis of BV, therefore it was better to evaluate them together. About 7% of pregnant women had medically recorded VV–BV and that is lower than expected (VIII). The explanation may be that only severe VV–BV were recorded in the prenatal care logbooks and/or some women with VV–BV were screened, diagnosed, and treated before the first visit in the prenatal care clinics.

Unfortunately, the PB preventive effect of some recently introduced drugs, e.g. clindamycin (Kurkinen et al., 2000; Rosenstein et al., 2000; Kekki et al., 2001; Ugwumadu et al., 2003; Ugwumadu, 2007) could not be evaluated in Hungary during the study period as these drugs were not used frequently at that time.

Our study confirmed the well-known association between VV–BV and infectious diseases of the urinary tract (cystitis, pyelitis, and pyelonephritis). Our study also underlined the importance of the treatment of common genital tract infection with effective antimicrobial drugs in pregnant women (McGregor et al., 1995).

Nearly all pregnant women with VV–BV were treated during pregnancy, thus an important finding of the study is that there was a significantly lower risk for the total group of CAs after the treatment of pregnant women with most frequently used drugs for VV–BV during the study pregnancy. This finding is an important argument against the teratogenic effect of metronidazole (41–43), clotrimazole (28), ampicillin (4), penamecillin (3), and nitrofurantoin (22). Additionally, these drugs can reduce the maternal VV–BV related PB in their babies; therefore their use is important during early pregnancy as well.

This recommendation is not in agreement with the results of the study performed by Cotch et al. (1998) because they did not find any association between candidal VV and higher risk for PB. However, a reduction in PB was also found after the treatment of pregnant women with commonly infected candidiasis in a prospective randomized controlled trial of Kiss et al. (2004). In addition, our studies indicated 30% reduction in the rate of PB in pregnant women treated with the antifungal clotrimazole (29, 30).

A possible explanation of this effect is the restoration of the abnormal colonization of the vagina due to infections and the less-known antibacterial and antiprotozoal – beyond its well-known antimycotic – effects of clotrimazole (Teichmann and Steigerwald, 1994; Engelmann, 1999).

Our study showed that ampicillin was able to reduce the risk for VV–BV-related preterm births; this finding confirmed the data of our previous study (5). Ampicillin was used for the prophylaxis in preterm premature ruptures of the membranes (Boyer and Gotoff, 1986; Ammon et al., 1988; Morales et al., 1989).

The PB preventive effect of metronidazole was published (Pfeifer et al., 1978; Malouf et al., 1982; Eschenbach et al., 1983; Morales et al., 1994; McDonald et al., 1997; Klebanoff et al., 2000) but our study did not confirm these findings. The explanation may be the different populations, time of treatment, study designs, or different microbial agents. In addition, other studies found a reduction of PB after metronidazole treatment only in women with heavy growth of G. vaginalis or BV who had a previous PB (Morales et al., 1994; McDonald et al., 1997).

The high rate of PB in the reference group (mothers without VV–BV and without antimicrobial treatment) may be related to their asymptomatic or undiagnosed VV–BV without appropriate treatment (Hay and Czeizel, 2007, Leitich and Kiss, 2007). Pregnant women without VV–BV but treated by clotrimazole or ampicillin for other indications or not recorded VV–BV had also a lower rate of PB. Thus other indications of antimicrobial treatment may have a beneficial "side" effect in pregnant women with asymptomatic Candida colonisation or undiagnosed VV–BV. Finally, a few of these pregnant women were treated with boric acid and/or lactobacillus vaccine treatment (Karkut, 1984; Lázár et al., 1988), their effect for the reduction of PB needs further studies.

Our data stress the importance of drug treatment of VV–BV although its efficacy was debated (Brucklehurst et al., 2000; Kenyon et al., 2001; Leitich et al., 2003). The differences might be explained by different genetic background of the given population (Romero et al., 2004; Genc and Schantz-Dunn, 2007), different agents of infections, the different time of treatment, and different drugs. The time of screening and treatment is a very crucial point because early spontaneous PB is more likely to have infectious etiology than PB just before term (Lamont, 2005). Thus the optimal time for the screening and treatment of abnormal vaginal flora including VV–BV is the prepregnancy-preconceptional period (VIII) or early pregnancy (29, 30) as this study also demonstrated. The longer the abnormal colonisation remains untreated, the greater the chance is for microorganisms to ascend through the cervix into the decidua initiating inflammatory process which eventually leads to labor. In several studies, the possible explanation for unsuccessful results was that antimicrobial drug treatment was initiated too late in pregnant women with genital infections.

We know the conclusion of ACOG (2001): "Currently there are insufficient data to suggest screening and treating women at either low or high risk will reduce the overall rate of preterm birth". Nevertheless, our Hungarian population-based data show the usefulness of treatment of pregnant women with VV–BV after their diagnosis due to screening or clinical symptoms. If we accept the Hungarian population figure regarding to the rate of PB, i.e. 9.3% and we suppose that screening is able to detect symptomatic and asymptomatic VV–BV, after appropriate antimicrobial treatment we have a chance to reduce it to 6.6%, thus about 30% of PBs are preventable (IX).

In conclusion, VV–BV associated with a lower rate of PB due to the effective drug treatment in the study. However, our study also showed the weaknesses of the usual clinical practice, i.e. high proportion of unspecified agents of VV–BV and the major part of VV–BV were not diagnosed or recorded. Furthermore, our population-based case-control study did not indicate a teratogenic risk of maternal VV–BV and related drug treatments during pregnancy for any CAs. Therefore, maternal VV–BV needs treatment during pregnancy as well because it helps to reduce the rate of PB without increasing the risk for CAs.

16.3 Erosion of the Cervix with or Without Cervicitis

When evaluating the diseases of the female genital organs an unexpected association was found between *erosion of cervix in pregnant women* (ECP) and a high risk of hypospadias and cardiovascular CAs in their offspring. To our best knowledge similar association has not been published before.

16.3.1 Results of the Study (X)

If pregnant women had acute pelvic inflammatory disease including oophoritis, salpingitis, parametritis, adnexitis, endometritis associated with cervicitis and vulvovaginitis, they were evaluated as acute pelvic inflammatory disease and the results of this study were shown in the first part of this chapter. Vulvovaginitis-bacterial vaginosis in our pregnant women frequently associated with cervicitis, but this pathological group was evaluated together in the part of this chapter. However, some pregnant women were recorded with the diagnosis of ECP with or without cervicitis or endocervicitis, but without pelvic inflammatory diseases or vulvovaginitis-bacterial vaginosis in the HCCSCA. Therefore, it seemed to be necessary to evaluate the pregnancy outcomes of women with ECP separately. Of course, pregnant women with other pathological conditions of the cervix such as incompetence, ectropion dysplasia, leukoplakia, laceration, stricture, stenosis, mucous polyp of the cervix were excluded from the study.

The medical term for cervical erosion is cervical ectopy because the cells at the os of the cervix changes from the squamous cells normally found at this region to columnar cells and this pathological condition gives a red and eroded appearance (Gabbe et al., 2001).

Two groups of ECP were differentiated: (i) previously known and documented erosion which existed in the study pregnancy, and (ii) erosion diagnosed at the time of the visit of pregnant women in the prenatal care clinic by obstetrician and confirmed by colposcopic examination. Thus ECP was medically recorded in the prenatal maternity logbook. If PAP smear showed atypical cells, cervical biopsy was performed and women with precancerous condition were also excluded from the study.

Out of 22,843 cases with CA, 40 (0.18%) had mothers with prospectively and medically recorded diagnosis of ECP in the prenatal maternity logbook, while out of 38,151 controls, 25 (0.07%) were born to pregnant women affected with medically recorded ECP.

ECP was recorded at the first visit, i.e. between the 6th and 10th gestational weeks in the prenatal maternity logbook in all pregnant women, thus the onset of ECP was considered to happen before conception or in early pregnancy. Out of 40 case mothers, 13 (32.5) had the diagnosis of ECP with cervicitis, while out of the 25 control mothers, 4 (16.0%) had combined diagnosis. In general, the end of ECP was not recorded therefore the usual duration of ECP could not be estimated.

Mean maternal age (25.8 vs. 25.5 year) and birth order (1.8 vs. 1.7) in mothers with ECP did not differ significantly from the figures of the reference sample. The proportion of unmarried women was somewhat higher in pregnant women with ECP (10.8% vs. 4.5%). Control pregnant women with ECP showed a higher socioeconomic status based on their employment status (16.0% vs. 10.0%) compared to case pregnant women with ECP. The use of folic acid during pregnancy was higher in control mothers particularly affected with ECP compared to case mothers (68.0% vs. 50.0%). A similar trend was seen in the use of multivitamins as well.

The incidence of acute diseases did not show significant differences between pregnant women with or without ECP. The evaluation of chronic maternal diseases showed that diabetes mellitus and epilepsy did not occur among pregnant women with ECP but the prevalence of hemorrhoids was higher both in case mothers (10.0% vs. 3.5%) and control mothers (12.0% vs. 4.3%) with ECP compared to pregnant women without ECP.

Two pregnancy complications showed a much higher incidence in pregnant women with ECP: threatened preterm deliveries (case mothers with ECP: 22.5% vs. 11.4%, control mother with ECP: 44.0% vs. 14.3%) and anemia (case mothers with ECP: 32.5% vs. 14.2%, control mothers with ECP: 28.0% vs. 16.7%).

The occurrences of ECP related drug treatments such as topical and oral antimycotic and antiparasitic drugs, mainly clotrimazole, metronidazole, or metronidazole+miconazole combination were much higher and they may indicate the suspicion of medical doctors that the causes of ECP were either candidiasis or trichomoniasis or both. Antibiotics (penamecillin and ampicillin) were used relatively rarely. Other drugs such as allylestrenol, diazepam, promethazine, and terbutaline are used for the treatment of threatened preterm delivery in Hungary. Nevertheless, the extremely high occurrence of allylestrenol in case mothers with ECP (22.5% vs. 15.2%) and particularly in control mothers with ECP (44.0% vs. 14.0%) is noteworthy.

The mean gestational age of newborns who had mothers with ECP was shorter (39.1 vs. 39.4 week; $p = 0.12$) but it did not associate with a higher rate of PB (8.0% vs. 9.2%; 0.9, 0.6–1.8). The mean birth weight was smaller by 39 g in newborns of mothers with ECP (3,237 vs. 3,276 g; $p = 0.49$) with a somewhat higher rate of LBW (8.0% vs. 5.7%; 1.2, 0.7–2.9) although the limited number of newborns does not allow drawing any conclusion.

The main objective of our study was the evaluation of possible associations of ECP with the risk of different CAs (Table 16.6). The different periods of gestation were not differentiated because ECP was diagnosed in early pregnancy thus this pathological condition may overlap with the critical time window of most CAs.

ECP demonstrated an increased risk for the total rate of CAs which is explained by the higher risks found in two particular CA groups. In the group of hypospadias, 9 cases resulted in a 4-fold higher risk, although, the minor anomaly manifestation of hypospadias (coronal type) was excluded. The distribution of cardiovascular CAs was the following: transposition of great vessels 1, tetralogy of Fallot 3, ventricular septal defect 3, congenital stenosis of aortic valve 1, persistent ductus arteriosus 1, unspecified.

16.3.2 Interpretation of Results

Thus our population-based case-control study showed a higher risk of hypospadias and cardiovascular CAs in the children of women with ECP. Transposition of great vessels, tetralogy of Fallot, and certain part of ventricle septal defects can be

Table 16.6 Estimation of possible associations of maternal ECP with different CAs in their offspring compared to the occurrence of ECP during the study pregnancy in case and control mothers

	Grand total	Pregnancy		
Study groups	N	No.	%	OR 95% CI
Controls	38,151	25	0.1	Reference
Isolated CAs				
Cardiovascular CAs	4,480	10	0.2	**3.4 1.6–7.1**
Undescended testis	2,052	3	0.1	2.2 0.7–7.4
Hypospadias	3,038	9	0.3	**4.5 2.1–9.7**
Clubfoot	2,424	3	0.1	1.9 0.6–6.3
Poly/syndactyly	1,744	3	0.2	2.6 0.8–8.7
Other isolated CAs	7,756	10[a]	0.1	1.5 0.6–3.7
Multiple CAs	1,349	2[b]	0.1	2.3 0.5–9.6
Total	22,843	40	0.2	**2.7 1.6–4.4**

[a]Spina bifida with hydrocephalus, cleft lip, cleft lip + palate, microtia, stenosis of the external auditory canal, tracheal stenosis, oesophageal atresia, anal atresia, cystic kidney, torticollis.
[b]Ventricular septal defect + cleft palate only + undescended testis; branchial cyst + rectal atresia + clubfoot.

combined in the group of conotruncal defects (Adams et al., 1989), and of 10 cases with cardiovascular CAs, 7 belonged to this group.

The crucial point of the study is the diagnostic validity of ECP. ECP is a symptom and not a clinical entity. The study design excluded secondary ECP due to microbial origin, however, the use of antimicrobial drugs questioned the diagnostic criteria of ECP in the study. In general data were not available regarding the possible electro- or cryocautery and diathermy in pregnant women with ECP.

Theoretically 3 causes are worth differentiating in the origin of ECP: (i) Trauma, however, it is not likely during early pregnancy. (ii) Topical chemicals (e.g. spermaticidal contraceptive creams) were not used by these pregnant women. (iii) The high level of estrogens in the body during pregnancy.

At the evaluation of the possible association between ECP and higher risk of hypospadias and conotruncal cardiovascular CAs, the effect of ECP itself, the causes of ECP, related drug treatments, other confounders and chance effect should be considered.

The direct effect of ECP for the organogenesis of embryo/fetus does not seem to be plausible.

The causes of ECP may have some association with higher risk of CAs. Our previous study showed an association of acute pelvic inflammatory diseases with 4.2-folds higher risk of atrial septal defect, type II, however, this type of cardiovascular CA did not occur in the study. Estrogens may have some teratogenic effect in particular circumstances. A higher risk of hypospadias was found in pregnant women exposed to an elevated estrogen intake from drugs or such dietary sources as milk or soy (Sharpe and Skakkeback, 1993). This hypothesis was supported by an experimental study in mice, showing that supraphysiological doses of synthetic estrogen during pregnancy induce hypospadias in 50% of the male fetuses (Kim et al., 2004). Some epidemiological studies indicated a causal association between sex hormones, particularly oral contraceptives and cardiovascular CAs (Janerich et al., 1977) but other studies did not confirm this association (Bracken, 1990). Obviously this possible association may occur only in women and/or fetuses with special genetic predisposition both for ECP and CAs triggered by these hormonal factors.

Thus our hypothesis is based on a special genetic predisposition in pregnant women with a much higher sensitivity for the high level of estrogens during pregnancy. This higher level of estrogens explains the common occurrence of ECP during pregnancy and may associate with a higher risk of hypospadias and conotruncal cardiovascular CAs in their offspring. Our population-based case-control study shows a higher risk for hypospadias in the children of women with ECP.

The secondary results of the study were the detection of a higher risk of threatened preterm delivery and shorter gestational age due to probably amnionitis in women with ECP. The higher rate of anemia can be explained partly by the higher rate of hemorrhoids but the higher rate of hemorrhoids would need further explanation in pregnant women with mean age of 25 years.

The drugs also might have a role in the origin of CAs. However, the teratogenic potential of antimicrobial drugs such as clotrimazole (29), metronidazole (41–43) metronidazole+miconazole (46), econazole (35), nystatin (32), natamycin (31), fluconazole (38), ampicillin (4), and penamecillin (3) used by pregnant women with ECP were checked in the HCCSCA and these drugs did not demonstrate any association with higher risk for hypospadias. The drugs used for the treatment of threatened preterm delivery such as diazepam (54) and promethazine (74) also did not show any association with increased risk for hypospadias. However, the allylestrenol (66) seemed to have some association with a higher risk of hypospadias; however, this hormone was used more frequently by control mothers compared to case mothers with ECP.

Finally, the effect of unknown confounders and the chance effect cannot be excluded.

In conclusion, our population-based case-control study showed an association between ECP in early pregnancy and a higher risk for hypospadias and conotruncal cardiovascular CAs. These findings are considered only as signals and further studies are needed to confirm or reject this association.

16.4 Cyst and/or Abscess of the Bartholin Gland

The infectious diseases of the Bartholin's gland occurred frequently in the past, recently their incidence has shown a decreasing trend, particularly in pregnant women.

16.4.1 Interpretation of Data in the HCCSCA

There were 5 cases and 8 controls. The distribution of CAs was the following: hypospadias 2, primary microcephaly, atresia of the bile duct, and exomphalos. Eight controls without CA were born between 37 and 42 gestational week with a mean birth weight of 3,100 g; however, two had intrauterine growth retardation with birth weight of 2,100 and 2,250 g born on the 37th and 38th gestational weeks, respectively.

16.5 Endometriosis

Endometriosis is a common disorder in women of reproductive age, with an estimated prevalence of approximately 10% (Wheeler, 1989). The rate of endometriosis is much higher among women with reduced fertility (about 30%) and among adolescents with severe dysmenorrhea or pelvic pain (about 50%). Endometriosis may be asymptomatic or it may cause a wide variety of symptoms. The diagnosis of endometriosis is based on the evaluation of symptoms but mainly on the histological analysis of biopsy specimens of the lesions. The direct cause of endometriosis is the transplantation of endometrial tissue from the uterus to ectopic locations (Olive, 2008)

16.5.1 Interpretation of Data in the HCCSCA

Out of 22,843 cases with CA, 16 (0.07%) had mothers with endometriosis, while out of 38,151 controls without CA, 26 (0.07%) were born to mothers with the diagnosis of endometriosis. Their mean maternal age (26.7 vs. 25.5 year) was somewhat higher but mean birth order (1.3 vs. 1.7) was lower. Among drugs, hydroxyprogesterone (9.5% vs. 1.2%) and particularly clomiphene (95.2% vs. 0.2%) were used more frequently in pregnant women with endometriosis. The mean gestational age of newborns without CA was longer (39.8 vs. 39.4 week) although the mean birth weight was similar (3,280 vs. 3,276 g) but PB and LBW newborns did not occur in the group of pregnant women with endometriosis. The risk of total CAs was not higher (1.0, 0.6–1.9) in cases born to mothers with endometriosis. Out of 16 cases with CA, 3 were affected with neural-tube defects (spina bifida aperta 2, encephalocele 1) (3.7, 1.1–12.1); however, this association disappeared after the consideration of clomiphene use in the adjusted OR. The distribution of other CAs was the following: ventricular septal defect 2, hypospadias 2, cleft lip + cleft palate, complex cardiovascular CA, cystic kidney, undescended testis, polydactyly, cong. limb deficiency, clubfoot, omphalocele, multiple CA 1–1.

In conclusion, endometriosis is a frequent cause of reduced fertility in women but if these patients achieve pregnancy, there is no higher risk for PB, LBW, or CAs.

16.6 Ovarian Cysts

Non-inflammatory disorders of the ovary include different manifestation of cysts such as follicular cyst, corpus luteum cyst, other or unspecified cysts, in addition to polycystic ovaries. In the data set of the HCCSCA, nearly all ovarian cysts were specified as follicular cyst; therefore, we were able to evaluate only pregnant women with *ovarian follicular cysts* (OFC). After the review of international literature it appeared that epidemiological studies on CAs in children of women affected with OFC have not yet been published. Therefore, this possible association was checked in the HCCSCA.

16.6.1 Results of the Study (XI)

The diagnosis of OFC was based on prospective medically recorded data in the prenatal maternity logbooks if the size of OFC exceeded 30 mm.

Out of 22,843 cases, 54 (0.24%), while out of 38,151 controls, 88 (0.23%) had mothers with preconceptional OFC. The mean maternal age (26.1 vs. 25.5 year) was higher, while mean birth order (1.4 vs. 1.8) was lower in pregnant women with OFC. The proportion of high socioeconomic status was larger (53.5% vs. 23.8%) among patients with OFC, while the use of folic acid (52.8% vs. 52.6%) and multivitamins (6.3% vs. 6.3%) was similar in pregnant women with or without OFC. However, there were no significant differences in these variables between case and control mothers with OFC.

The incidence of pregnancy complications and acute maternal diseases did not show significant difference between pregnant women with or without OFC. Among chronic diseases, infertility (35.5% vs. 2.2%) was recorded much more frequently in pregnant women with OFC.

Among drugs only clomiphene showed a higher rate in both case (*N*: 16, 29.4% vs. *N*: 67, 0.3%) and control (*N*: 25, 28.4% vs. *N*: 96, 0.3%) mothers with OFC than in mothers without OFC.

The birth outcomes of newborns without CA were characteristics: mean gestational age (39.7 vs. 39.3 week) was longer with similar mean birth weight (3,280 vs. 3,276 g), thus the rate of PB (5.7% vs. 9.2%) was lower without any difference in the rate of LBW newborns (5.7%).

The prevalences of different CAs occurring at least in 3 cases born to mothers with preconceptional OFC are shown in Table 16.7.

Out of 9 CA-groups, only *neural-tube defects* (NTD) associated with OFC. However, the adjusted OR including clomiphene treatment among confounders did not confirm this association because out of 7 cases with NTD, 3 were born to mothers who had OFC and were treated by clomiphene.

The possible association between clomiphene treatment and the risk for CAs was also checked (Table 16.7). Out of 22,843 cases, 67 (0.29%), while out of 38,151

Table 16.7 Estimation of the associations between the prevalence of ovarian follicular cyst (OFC) in mothers and different CAs in their offspring, in addition to a comparison between the occurrence of clomiphene treatment (CT) and different CAs

Study groups	Total No.	Mothers with OFC		Association: Crude		Association: Adjusted[a]		Mothers with CT		Association: Crude		Association: Adjusted[b]	
Isolated CAs		No.	%	OR	95% CI	OR	95% CI	No.	%	OR	95% CI	OR	95% CI
Neural-tube defects	1,202	7	0.58	**3.2**	**1.0–10.4**	1.7	0.4–6.9	7	0.58	**6.4**	**1.3–31.4**	4.5	0.7–6.7
Cleft lip ± palate	1,375	3	0.22	0.5	1.0–2.0	0.5	0.1–1.9	5	0.36	1.5	0.4–5.4	2.3	0.6–8.9
Hypospadias	3,038	10	0.33	0.9	0.4–2.0	0.8	0.3–1.9	10	0.33	1.4	0.6–3.1	1.7	0.7–4.2
Undescended testis	2,052	3	0.15	0.4	0.1–1.5	0.5	0.1–1.9	3	0.15	0.3	0.1–1.2	0.4	0.1–1.4
Cardiovascular CAs	4,480	12	0.27	1.3	0.6–2.9	1.3	0.6–2.8	14	0.31	1.3	0.6–2.5	1.3	0.6–2.8
Clubfoot	2,424	6	0.25	1.7	0.5–5.4	1.5	0.4–5.0	6	0.25	1.4	0.5–4.0	1.2	0.4–3.7
Poly/syndactyly	1,744	3	0.17	1.5	0.3–6.9	2.3	0.5–11.3	2	0.11	0.4	0.1–2.1	0.4	0.1–1.9
Other isolated CAs	5,179	7[c]	0.14	0.6	0.3–1.6	6.6	0.2–1.6	13[d]	0.25	1.1	0.5–2.2	1.3	0.6–2.6
Multiple CAs	1,349	3	0.22	5.8	0.6–57.4	4.7	0.4–50.4	7	0.52	3.9	0.9–15.2	3.1	0.8–12.6
Total	22,843	54	0.24	1.1	0.7–1.5	1.0	0.7–1.5	67	0.29	1.2	0.9–1.7	1.3	0.9–1.8
Controls without CA	38,151	88	0.23	Reference		Reference		96	0.25	Reference		Reference	

[a] Adjusted for maternal age, birth order, maternal marital, employment status, and the occurrence of CT.
[b] Adjusted for maternal age, birth order, maternal marital, employment status, and the occurrence of OFC.
[c] Obstructive CAs of the urinary tract 2, Robin sequence, oesophageal stenosis, limb deficiency in upper limb, exomphalos, gastroschisis 1–1.
[d] Renal a/dysgenesis 2, obstructive CAs of the urinary tract 2, limb deficiencies 2, cleft palate, oesophageal atresia, intestinal stenosis, rectal atresia, exomphalos, pectus excavatum, torticollis 1–1.

controls, 96 (0.25%) had mothers with medically recorded inadvertent clomiphene treatment in I and II gestational month. Again only NTD showed an association with clomiphene, however, adjusted OR including OFC among confounders did not confirm this association.

16.6.2 Interpretation of Results

A possible interaction between clomiphene treatment, OFC, and NTD was found in the study. The association between clomiphene treatment and OFC is well-known due to hyperstimulation (Asch and Greenblatt, 1976). The possible association between clomiphene treatment and NTD is debated (Nevin and Harley, 1976; Cuckle and Wald, 1989). Previously a weak association of clomiphene with NTD but not with other CAs was found in the data set of the HCCSCA (87).

In this study an association between maternal OFC and higher risk for NTD in their offspring was found, however, this association was lost after inclusion of clomiphene treatment among confounders. On the other hand, there was some association between clomiphene treatment in early pregnancy and a higher risk for NTD, but this association has also disappeared if OFC was included as a confounder. Thus the predisposition for OFC due to clomiphene may have some role in the origin of NTD. The higher rate of NTD in the offspring of mothers with clomiphene treatment cannot be explained only by the use of this drug, it needs maternal sensitivity for OFC as well.

Periconceptional folic acid-containing multivitamin supplementation (125, 131) and high doses of folic acid (99) were able to reduce the first occurrence of NTD in our previous trials/studies. If we considered folic acid/multivitamin use as confounder, the previously found association of OFC with NTD disappeared (2.0, 0.7–16.1).

This maternal sensitivity may be related to some pharmacogenetic susceptibility of certain females or the relaxed reproductive-selection due to medical intervention on infertile women (XII). These factors may explain the 3–4-fold higher risk for hypospadias (Wennerholm et al., 2000; Ericson and Kallen, 2001) and esophageal and rectal/anal atresia/stenosis (Ericson and Kallen, 2001; Reefhuis et al., 2008), the 3.5-fold higher risk for neural-tube defects (Ericson and Kallen, 2001), and a significant increase in the birth prevalence of retinoblastoma, Beckwith-Wiedemann, Angelman syndromes (Moll et al., 2003; Adamson and Bujjeni, 2003) in newborn infants born conceived by assisted reproductive technologies, such as in vitro fertilization (IVF) including intracytoplasmic sperm injection (ICSI). The results of an Australian study are worth showing (Table 16.8) because major CAs of singleton children conceived by IVF or ICSI evaluated at the end of their first year of age demonstrated a 2-fold higher frequency compared to naturally conceived infants (Hansen et al., 2002).

Table 16.9 summarizes the results of a comparative analysis of CAs in children born to mothers with natural conception, artificial homolog insemination (AIH), or IVF (van Voorhis et al., 2005) and the risk for CA in a meta-analysis based on 25

Table 16.8 The results of Australian study (Hansen et al., 2002)

CA	Reference (%)	IVF/ICSI (%)
Cardiovascular	0.6	1.3[a]
Urogenital	1.3	2.7
Musculo-skeletal	1.1	3.8[b]
Central nervous system	0.2	0.4
Chromosomal	0.8	0.7
Others	0.2	0.6
Total	4.2	9.5[a]

[a]<0.001.
[b]<0.05.

Table 16.9 The data of two important comparative analyses regarding to the association of AIH or IVF and CAs

Percentage figure of CAs in children according to the type of conception (Olson et al., 2005, USA)			Meta-analysis of children born to mothers with IVF/ICSI (Hansen et al., 2005)		
				CA risk	
Method	No.	CA (%)	Sample	OR	95% CI
Natural	8,422	4.4	All births	2.01	1.49–2.69
AIH	34.3	5.0	Singleton	1.35	1.20–1.51
IVF	1,462	4.4	Adjusted	1.40	1.28–1.53

studies including 28,638 children born to mothers with IVF/ICSI (Hansen et al., 2005). Thus about 40% higher risk for major CA should be expected after assisted reproductive technologies.

Thus the results of our study and the recent findings of assisted reproductive technologies show that women with infertility have a higher risk for some CAs. An important medical task is to reduce this risk as much as possible, e.g. by periconceptional folic acid/multivitamin supplementation.

In conclusion, there is an association between infertility, clomiphene treatment, OFC in women and a higher risk for neural-tube defect in their offspring. Therefore, if there are symptoms of hyperstimulation due to clomiphene treatment (like OFC), folic acid supplementation during the periconceptional period for the prevention of NTD is more important than in general. In addition, it is necessary to emphasize the early diagnosis of NTD by prenatal screening.

16.7 Polyp of the Cervix or Corpus Uteri

The location of this pathological condition may be both in the corpus uteri with endometrial origin or the cervix with mucous or adenomatous (i.e. benign tumor) origin.

16.7.1 Interpretation of Data in the HCCSCA

Out of 22,843 cases, 5 (0.02%) had mothers with recorded polyp, while out of 38,151 controls without CA, 12 (0.03%) were born to pregnant women with the diagnosis of "uterus polyp". Five CAs were different (spina bifida aperta, anal atresia, hypospadias, polydactyly in hand, multiple CA). Beyond one preterm baby (33 gestational week with 2,300 g), the other 11 newborns had mean birth weight of 3,356 g and their pregnancies ended between 38 and 42 gestational week.

16.8 Cervical Incompetence

The term *cervical incompetence/insufficiency in pregnant women* (CIP) means a resumed weakness of the cervix that might causes the loss of an otherwise healthy pregnancy, usually in the second trimester (Iams, 2004). The diagnosis of CIP has traditionally been made and is still most confidentially established by an obstetric history of recurrent passive and painless dilatation of the cervix in the second trimester. In the past this diagnosis was based on digital examination to assess cervical dilatation. However, this type of diagnosis was unreliable and subjective thus transvaginal imaging of the cervix by ultrasound examination resulted in a great progress in the diagnosis of CIP. As the study of Iams et al. (1995) showed the length of cervix corresponds to a normal bell curve distribution between 22 and 32 weeks of pregnancy, with the 50th percentile at about 35 mm and the 10th and 90th percentile at 25 and 45 mm, respectively.

The cervical changes during pregnancy can be summarized in three important steps (Iams, 2004) on the basis of the results of ultrasound examination: (i) Cervical effacement begins at the internal cervical os and proceeds caudal. (ii) This change is slow "chronic" process which occurs over a period of weeks rather than days. (iii) The risk of spontaneous preterm delivery increases as the cervical length decreases between the 16th and 32nd weeks.

The data set of the HCCSCA includes a very large number of pregnant women with the diagnosis of CIP, and the evaluation of case and control pregnant women with or without CIP helped us to define 5 objectives of the study.

The first objective of our study was to determine the prevalence of CIP in Hungary during the study period.

The second aim of the study was to check the incidence of pregnancy complications in pregnant women with CIP because beyond threatened preterm delivery and placental disorders we did not find such data in the international literature.

The third aim of the study was to measure the association between CIP and the risk for adverse birth outcomes, particularly the rate of PB, i.e. estimation of the risk for PB due to CIP. The rate of PB is extremely high (about 9%) in Hungary (Bjerkedahl et al., 1983) and preterm babies associated with about one-third of infant mortality in Hungary during the 2000s. In addition, a major part of mental retardation (XIV), visual (XV) and other handicaps (XVI) were related to PB. In other countries preterm births accounts for 75% of perinatal mortality and more than half of the long-term morbidity such as neurodevelopmental impairments, respiratory or gastrointestinal complications (McCormick, 1985). Thus it is an important public health task to reveal the possible causes of PB and to prevent them.

The fourth aim was to check the efficacy of available CIP treatment in the prevention of PB. At present time, two kinds of CIP treatment compete with each other in Hungary. One group of obstetricians prefers the prophylactic surgical intervention used previously the Shirodkar suture (1955), later therapeutic McDonald cerclage (1957). Another group of obstetricians gives preference to the conservative treatment based on lasting bed-rest alone because some previous studies were not able to show the advantage of therapeutic cerclage (Berghella et al., 1999). Thus we planned to evaluate the rate of PB as an indicator of efficacy after the above two medical treatments in women with CIP.

Finally the fifth objective of the study was to evaluate the possible association between CIP and different CAs in the offspring. We did not find any study regarding this potential risk in the international literature. The lack of these data is understandable because the "no association" hypothesis between CIP manifested in general during the second trimester of gestation and higher risk of different CAs with critical period mainly in II and III gestational months in their offspring is a biologically reasonable hypothesis.

16.8.1 Results of the Study (XIII)

In Hungary CIP was defined as a progressive dilatation of the uterine cervix and/or bulging membranes during the second trimester of pregnancy diagnosed by the manual examination of obstetrician in the prenatal maternity clinics in which circumstances preterm delivery seems inevitable without interference. The cervical length was measured rarely with the use of transvaginal ultrasonography and/or reported during the study period. According to our study design, CIP was accepted on the basis of medically recorded diagnosis in the prenatal maternity logbooks based on clinical examination or discharge summaries of hospitalized pregnant women due to therapeutic cerclage. CIP reported only by mothers in the questionnaire was excluded from the study.

In addition, women with previous history of cold knife conisation and uterine anomalies were also excluded from the study.

The preventive or therapeutical cervical cerclage was performed in Hungary according to the technique of McDonald (McDonald, 1957) when dilatation of the cervix and/or bulging membranes were present during the second trimester of pregnancy before the 27th gestational week. After therapeutic cerclage, according to the Hungarian practice, women needed a complete bed rest for 48 h. On the third day they were allowed to leave the bed to use the bathroom. On the fourth day they were allowed to mobilize 3 times for a quarter of an hour each time. Pregnant women were discharged from the hospital on the fifth day. At home they were allowed to mobilize 3 times for a quarter of an hour each time until the 32nd gestational week.

Cerclages were removed at the beginning of labor or electively in the 37th week of gestation.

Another group of women with CIP was only treated by bed rest alone until the 32nd gestational week.

Prophylactic transvaginal cervical cerclage before pregnancy or during the first trimester were excluded from the study to achieve the study sample as homogeneous as possible.

The case group consisted of 22,843 malformed newborns or fetuses ("informative offspring"), of whom 1,170 (5.12%) had mothers with CIP. Out of 38,151 controls, 2,795 (7.33%) were born to mothers with CIP.

Most CIP were recorded in V and VI gestational months in the prenatal maternity logbook. CIP was recorded only in 13.0 and 13.5% in case and control mothers before the 16th but after 12th gestational week, respectively.

The demographic characteristics of control mothers with or without CIP are shown in Table 16.10. (Case mothers did not show here because defects of their offspring may modify these data though there was no significant difference in the demographic characteristics of case and control mothers with CIP.)

The mean maternal age was somewhat higher in pregnant women with CIP compared to mothers without CIP although the distribution of age groups did not show significant differences between them. The mean birth order was also somewhat higher because the proportion of pregnant women with 2 or more pregnancies was larger in mothers with CIP. CIP was more frequent among professional and managerial women (44.6% vs. 37.5%).

Out of 2,640 case mothers visited at home and evaluated, 158 (6.0%) had medically recorded CIP and among them 32 (20.3%) were smoker during the study pregnancy while this figure was 24.0% among case mothers without CIP. The proportion of drinkers was 0.6 and 1.6% in case mothers with or without CIP. Out of 158 case mothers with CIP, 111 (70.3%) reported one or more previous induced abortions due to social reasons, while out of 2,482 case mothers without CIP, 672 (27.1%) mentioned previous induced abortions. Unfortunately the number of control mothers visited at home was too small for the evaluation of these lifestyle factors. The use of folic acid was higher in case mothers (72.8% vs. 64.1%) and particularly in control mothers (77.2% vs. 69.6%) with CIP than in case and control mothers without CIP. However, case mothers with CIP had lower rate of folic acid supplementation (0.8, 0.7–0.9). There was no difference in the use of multivitamins (about 6%) among the study groups.

The incidence of acute and the prevalence of chronic maternal diseases are shown in the study groups (Table 16.11).

The occurrence of acute infectious disease of the digestive system and hemorrhoids was higher in pregnant women with CIP. In addition, the frequency of influenza-common cold, acute diseases of the digestive system, and constipation was higher in case mothers with CIP than in control mothers with CIP.

The second aim of the study was to evaluate the incidence of other pregnancy complications (Table 16.12). Again only the data of control mothers are shown.

Table 16.10 Characteristics of women with cervical incompetence in pregnancy (CIP) or without CIP as reference, in addition to mothers with CIP treated by therapeutic cerclage or bed rest alone

Variables	Pregnant women with CIP (*N*=2,795)		Pregnant women without CIP (*N*=35,356)		Comparison	Pregnant women with CIP treated by therapeutic cerclage (*N*=1,112)		Comparison with pregnant women without CIP	Pregnant women with CIP and best rest alone (*N*=1,683)		Comparison with pregnant women without CIP
	No.	%	No.	%		No.	%		No.	%	
Maternal age (year)											
19 or less	226	8.1	3,051	8.6		90	8.1		133	7.9	
20–29	2,015	72.1	25,587	72.4	$p=0.40$	820	73.7	$p=0.59$	1,200	71.3	$p=0.14$
30 or more	554	19.8	6,718	19.0		202	18.2		350	20.8	
Mean, S.D.	25.6 ± 4.7		25.4 ± 4.9		**$p=0.03$**	25.4 ± 4.7		$p=0.97$	25.8 ± 4.8		**$p=0.006$**
Birth order											
1	1,132	40.5	17,077	48.3	**$p<0.0001$**	462	41.5	**$p<0.0001$**	674	40.0	**$p<0.0001$**
2 or more	1,663	59.5	18,279	51.7		650	58.5		1,009	60.0	
Mean, S.D.	1.8 ± 0.8		1.7 ± 0.9		**$p<0.0001$**	1.8 ± 0.9		$p=0.11$	1.8 ± 0.8		**$p<0.0001$**
Unmarried	96	3.4	1,375	3.9	$p=0.23$	49	4.4	$p=0.38$	48	2.8	**$p=0.03$**
Employment status											
Professional	370	13.2	3,983	11.3		139	12.5		234	13.9	
Managerial	876	31.3	9,258	26.2		385	34.6		492	29.2	
Skilled worker	786	28.1	10,904	30.8		292	26.3		495	29.4	
Semiskilled worker	430	15.4	5,353	15.1	**$p<0.0001$**	180	16.2	**$p<0.0001$**	252	15.0	**$p<0.0001$**
Unskilled worker	99	3.5	1,760	5.0		49	4.4		50	3.0	
Housewife	102	3.7	1,936	5.5		49	4.4		53	3.2	
Others	132	4.7	2,162	6.1		18	1.6		107	6.4	

Table 16.11 Maternal disorders during the study pregnancy

Maternal disorders	Case mothers				Control mothers				Comparison of case and control mothers with CIP
	With CIP (*N*=1,170)		Without CIP (*N*=21,673)		With CIP (*N*=2,795)		Without CIP (*N*=35,356)		
	No.	%	No.	%	No.	%	No.	%	OR (95% CI)
Acute disease groups									
Influenza – common cold	235	20.1	4,732	21.8	423	15.1	6,638	18.8	**1.4 (1.2–1.7)**
Respiratory system	120	10.3	1,998	9.2	240	8.6	3,215	9.1	1.2 (0.9–1.5)
Digestive system	62	5.3	687	3.2	88	3.2	851	2.4	**1.7 (1.2–2.4)**
Urinary tract	56	4.8	1,488	6.9	152	5.4	2,039	5.8	0.9 (0.6–1.2)
Genital organs	93	8.0	1,583	7.3	191	6.8	2,700	7.6	1.2 (0.9–1.5)
Chronic diseases									
Diabetes mellitus	0	0.0	56	0.3	4	0.1	48	0.1	–
Epilepsy	3	0.3	73	0.3	3	0.1	74	0.2	2.4 (0.5–11.9)
Constipation	31	2.7	534	2.5	43	1.5	670	1.9	**1.7 (1.1–2.8)**
Varicosity	11	1.0	321	1.5	30	1.1	536	1.5	0.9 (0.4–1.8)
Hemorrhoids	44	3.8	525	2.4	131	4.7	1,137	3.2	0.8 (0.6–1.1)
Others	131	11.2	2,091	9.7	325	11.6	4,111	11.6	1.0 (0.8–1.2)

Table 16.12 Incidence of pregnancy complications of control mothers with or without CIP

Pregnancy complications	Mothers with CIP (N=2,795)		Pregnant women without CIP (N=35,356)		Comparison	Pregnant women with CIP treated by therapeutic cerclage (N=1,112)		Comparison with pregnant women without CIP	Pregnant women with CIP and bed rest alone (N=1,683)		Comparison with pregnant women without CIP
	No.	%	No.	%	OR (95% CI)	No.	%	OR (95% CI)	No.	%	OR (95% CI)
Nausea-vomiting, severe	1,491	53.4	18,477	52.3	1.0 (0.9–1.1)	602	54.1	1.1 (0.9–1.2)	893	53.18	1.0 (0.9–1.1)
Threatened abortion	654	23.4	5,858	16.6	**1.5 (1.4–1.7)**	283	25.5	**1.7 (1.5–2.0)**	371	22.0	**1.4 (1.3–1.6)**
Preeclampsia-eclampsia	203	7.3	3,018	8.5	**0.8 (0.7–0.9)**	88	7.9	0.9 (0.7–1.1)	115	6.8	0.8 (0.6–1.0)
Placental disorders[a]	74	2.7	518	1.5	**1.8 (1.4–2.3)**	39	3.5	**2.4 (1.8–3.4)**	35	2.1	**1.4 (1.0–2.0)**
Poly/oligohydramnios	23	0.8	182	0.5	**1.6 (1.0–2.5)**	7	0.6	1.2 (0.6–2.6)	16	1.0	**1.8 (1.1–3.1)**
Gestational diabetes	25	0.9	245	0.7	1.3 (0.9–1.9)	9	0.8	1.2 (0.6–2.3)	17	1.0	1.5 (0.9–2.4)
Anemia	592	21.2	5,764	16.3	**1.4 (1.3–1.5)**	141	12.7	**0.7 (0.6–0.9)**	453	26.9	**1.9 (1.7–2.1)**

[a]Placenta previa, premature separation of the placenta, antepartum hemorrhage.

Threatened preterm delivery was not evaluated because it was equivalent with CIP. The occurrence of threatened abortions, placental disorders, particularly premature separation of the placenta (abruptio placentae), and anemia was higher in mothers with CIP compared to mothers without CIP. Poly/oligohydramnios showed marginally higher risk, while the incidence of preeclampsia-eclampsia was lower in women with CIP.

There was a higher frequency of drugs used for the treatment of threatened abortion and preterm delivery in Hungary such as promethazine (34.2% vs. 14.7%), terbutaline (33.5% vs. 8.8%), allylestrenol (29.5% vs.13.4%), diazepam (27.4% vs. 10.1%),) magnesiums (24.5% vs. 13.3%), drotaverine (16.6% vs. 8.6%), and aminophylline (13.1% vs. 5.5%) in pregnant women with CIP compared to pregnant women without CIP. In addition, the use of antifungal clotrimazole (10.0% vs. 7.6%) and laxative senna (4.3% vs. 2.0%) was also higher by pregnant women with CIP. However, only diazepam (1.2, 1.1–1.5) were used somewhat more frequently by case mothers with CIP than by control mothers with CIP. Terbutaline was used for tocolytic treatment completed with aminophylline, in addition, the sedative diazepam and promethazine, the spasmodic drotaverine, the progestogen allylestrenol, and magnesium for the treatment of threatened abortion/preterm delivery. The higher occurrence of senna can be explained by more frequent constipation in women with CIP, while clotrimazole was used more frequently for the treatment of CIP associated vulvovaginal infections.

The third and main objective of the study was the evaluation of birth outcomes to estimate the risk for PB of babies born to mothers with CIP (Table 16.13).

There was no difference in sex ratio between the two study groups. Among pregnancy outcomes, stillbirths and elective terminations of pregnancy after the prenatal diagnosis of fetal defects could not be occurred in control newborns due to the criteria of selection.

The evaluation of live-births showed a somewhat higher rate of twins among babies born to case and control mothers with CIP. The gestational age and birth weight were evaluated mainly in control newborns because the CA in cases may have a more drastic effect for these variables than CIP. The mean gestational age was shorter by 0.4 week and mean birth weight was smaller by 82 g. The rate of PB was 11.2% in controls born to mothers with CIP (and 19.7% in cases) compared to 9.0% of control mothers without CIP. The rate of LBW newborns was also higher (7.8%) in control newborns. However, the lower mean birth weight and higher rate of LBW newborns can partly be explained by the shorter gestational age. The rates (e.g. PB) and means of birth outcomes (e.g. birth weight) in newborn infants born to mothers without CIP corresponded well to the Hungarian newborn population in the study period.

This analysis was repeated including only primiparous pregnant women, but the birth outcomes of their babies did not deviate from the associations shown in Table 16.13.

The fourth objective of the study was to estimate the efficacy of two main types of CIP treatments based on birth outcomes namely the rate of PB.

Control pregnant women with CIP were differentiated into two subgroups: (i) CIP treated by therapeutic cerclage and bed rest (*N*: 1,112, i.e. 2.9%). Later this

Table 16.13 Pregnancy outcomes of mothers with or without CIP and birth outcomes of their newborn infants

	Case group				Control group			
	With CIP (*N*=1,170)		Without CIP (*N*=21,673)		With CIP (*N*=2,795)		Without CIP (*N*=35,356)	
Variables	No.	%	No.	%	No.	%	No.	%
Pregnancy outcomes								
Livebirth	1,157	98.9	21,201	97.8	2,795	100.0	35,356	100.0
Stillbirth (late fetal death)	5	0.4	376	1.7	0	0.0	0	0.0
Elective termination after the diagnosis of fetal defect	0	0.0	104	0.5	0	0.0	0	0.0
Birth outcomes liveborn babies								
Quantitative	Mean	S.D.	Mean	S.D.	Mean	S.D.	Mean	S.D.
Gestational age (week)	38.3	2.9	38.8	2.8	39.0	2.2	39.4	2.0
Birth weight (g)	2,950	688	3,005	673	3,200	527	3,282	509
Categorical								
Twin	38	3.3	370	1.7	63	2.3	347	1.0
PB	230	19.7	3,143	14.5	314	11.2	3,185	9.0
LBW	243	20.8	3,960	18.3	218	7.8	1,949	5.5

Comparison of control newborns in the groups of mothers with or without CIP.
Gestational age: $p > 0.0001$.
Birth weight: $p > 0.0001$.
PB: 1.3, 1.1–1.4; LBW: 1.5, 1.3–1.7.

subgroup will be referred as therapeutic cerclage. (ii) CIP treated by bed rest alone (*N*: 1,683, i.e. 4.4%).

Therapeutic cerclage was performed before the 27th gestational week. As we mentioned previously, all CIP were medically recorded in prenatal maternity logbooks, however, it is worth mentioning that CIP was reported in the questionnaire by 99% and 72% of mothers with CIP with or without cerclage (i.e. bed rest alone) as well, respectively.

There was some demographic difference in pregnant women with CIP according to the type of treatment (Table 16.10). The mean maternal age was somewhat elder in the group of bed rest alone (25.8 year) compared to the groups of cerclage (25.4 year). Mean birth order (1.8) was similar in these two subgroups. The proportion of unmarried pregnant women was lower in women with bed rest alone (2.8% vs. 4.4%). Maternal employment status did not show obvious differences between these two subgroups.

When evaluating pregnancy complications (Table 16.12), threatened abortion (25.5% vs. 22.0%), preeclampsia-eclampsia (7.9% vs. 6.8%), and placental disorders (3.5% vs. 2.1%) were more frequent in the subgroup of cerclage, while the rate of anemia (12.7% vs. 26.9%) was lower in the cerclage group.

Among the frequently used drugs, allylestrenol (23.0% vs. 32.8%) was used less frequently, while aminophylline use (16.3% vs. 10.8%) was more frequent by mothers with cerclage. The frequency of other drug uses was similar.

The use of folic acid was more frequent by pregnant women with CIP treated by cerclage (64.2%) compared to pregnant women with CIP and bed rest alone (60.6%), although both figures exceeded the reference value of women without CIP.

After identifying these confounding factors, it worth evaluating the birth outcomes of newborns of mother with CIP according to the two types of treatments (Table 16.14).

There was no significant difference in sex ratio (i.e. in the proportion of boys) of newborns and the rate of twins between the groups of therapeutic cerclage and bed rest alone. As previously we showed, the mean gestational age at delivery was shorter in newborns who had mothers with CIP compared to mothers without CIP; however, this difference was 0.2 week in the subgroup of mothers with CIP treated by cerclage while 0.5 week in the subgroup of mothers treated by bed rest alone. This difference was reflected in the rate of PB, it did not differ significantly in the subgroup of pregnant women with CIP treated by cerclage from the figure of the reference sample. However, the rate of PB was 12.7% in the subgroup of mothers with CIP and bed rest alone and this figure was significantly higher than in the reference sample, and significantly higher than the rate of PB in babies born to mothers with CIP treated by cerclage (p=0.04). The mean birth weight was significantly lower in both subgroups of mothers with CIP, but was somewhat larger (15 g) in babies born to mothers with CIP and bed rest alone than in the newborns of mothers with CIP treated by cerclage. Nevertheless, the rate of LBW newborns did not have significant difference between subgroups of CIP treated by cerclage and bed rest alone. These differences were not changed after the excluding 27 and 36 twin births from the study groups.

Table 16.14 Birth outcomes of newborns infants born to pregnant women with CIP and without CIP treated by therapeutic cerclage or bed rest alone

Variables	Pregnant women with CIP (N=2,795)		Pregnant women without CIP (N=35,356)		Comparison		Pregnant women with CIP treated by therapeutic cerclage (N=1,112)		Comparison with pregnant women without CIP		Pregnant women with CIP and best rest alone (N=1,683)		Comparison with pregnant women without CIP	
Quantitative	Mean	S.D.	Mean	S.D.	t	P	Mean	S.D.	t	p	Mean	S.D.	t	p
Gestational age (week)[a]	39.0	2.2	39.4	2.0	**8.3**	**<0.0001**	39.2	2.0	**3.0**	**0.003**	38.9	2.3	**9.6**	**<0.0001**
Birth weight (g)[b]	3,200	527	3,282	509	7.9	**<0.0001**	3,192	501	**7.0**	**<0.0001**	3,207	544	**4.1**	**<0.0001**
Categorical	No.	%	No.	%	OR (95% CI)		No.	%	OR (95% CI)		No.	%	OR (95% CI)	
PB[a]	314	11.2	3,185	9.0	**1.3 (1.1–1.4)**		101	9.1	1.0 (0.8–1.3)		213	12.7	**1.5 (1.3–1.7)**	
LBW[b]	218	7.8	1,949	5.5	**1.5 (1.3–1.7)**		80	7.2	**1.4 (1.1–1.9)**		138	8.2	**1.2 (1.0–1.4)**	
Postterm birth[a]	201	7.2	3,661	10.4	**0.7 (0.6–0.8)**		87	7.8	**0.7 (0.6–0.9)**		114	6.8	**0.6 (0.5–0.8)**	
Large birthweight[b]	11	0.4	304	0.9	**0.5 (0.2–0.8)**		5	0.5	0.6 (0.2–1.4)		6	0.4	0.5 (0.2–1.1)	

[a] Adjusted for maternal age, birth order, and maternal employment status.
[b] Adjusted for maternal age, birth order, maternal employment status, and gestational age.

The proportion of postterm births was lower in both subgroups of mothers with CIP compared to the figure of mothers without CIP, while the occurrence of large birth weight newborns did not show significant difference explained partly by the limited number of subjects. The rate of postterm births and large birthweight newborns did not show significant difference between the two types of treatment.

Finally, the fifth aim of the study was the comparison of cases with different CAs and their *all matched controls* (Table 16.15).

Only three CAs: diaphragmatic CAs, intestinal and rectal/anal atresia/stenosis had OR higher than 1.0 but these associations were not significant. However, isolated congenital hydrocephaly, neural-tube defects, poly/syndactyly, cleft lip $\pm$ palate and multiple CAs had an obviously lower (0.6 or less OR), while undescended testis, cardiovascular CAs, and clubfoot had a marginally lower adjusted OR. The exclusion of stillborn and electively terminated cases, in addition to twins and finally recurrent/familial CAs from this analysis did not change the OR values significantly (Table 16.15).

The general pattern was similar in the two subgroups of CIP with different treatment, although this association was found only in cases with cleft lip $\pm$ palate, hypospadias, undescended testis, cardiovascular CAs, and clubfoot born to mothers treated by cerclage. Cleft palate alone and congenital pyloric stenosis showed an association with CIP treated by bed rest.

16.8.2 Interpretation

The evaluation of the results will follow the five objectives stated above.

(1) The prevalence of CIP was 7.33% in control mothers who later delivered babies without CAs. This CIP prevalence is much higher than the about 1% prevalence of CIP in other countries (Rust et al., 2000; Althuisius et al., 2001). Theoretically there are two possible explanations for this significant difference: (i) Different diagnostic criteria. In general, the length of cervical canal was not measured by transvaginal ultrasonography in Hungary during the study period. The diagnosis of CIP, therefore, was based on digital assessment by different obstetricians, and this is not comparable with recent data of international studies. This also might result in an overdiagnosis which could not be excluded in the lack of appropriate standard diagnostic criteria. However, both in case and control mothers with CIP in the study had the same diagnostic criteria and methods; therefore, within the study the groups are comparable. (ii) Different origin of CIP in Hungary. It is worth differentiating natural (congenital) and induced (by surgery or trauma) CIP. Congenital CIP is a developmental anomaly characterized by short cervix of the uterus, while induced CIP is associated with the insufficiency of cervical musculature due to mechanical insult.

We suppose that most CIP were caused by D+C method of induced abortions in Hungary, although, unfortunately we had no information regarding to the number of previous induced abortion in the total data set. The data of prenatal

Table 16.15 Estimation of risk for CAs in the comparison of cases and their matched controls born to pregnant women with CIP

	Grand total	Mothers with CIP			Mothers with CIP treated by cerclage			Mothers with CIP treated by bed rest alone		
Study groups	No.	No.	%	Adjusted OR[a]	No.	%	OR (95% CI)[a]	No.	%	OR (95% CI)[a]
Isolated CAs										
Neural-tube defects	1,202	46	3.8	**0.5 (0.3–0.7)**	20	1.7	**0.5 (0.3–0.8)**	26	2.2	**0.5 (0.3–0.7)**
Cleft lip ± palate	1,375	64	4.7	**0.6 (0.4–0.8)**	21	1.5	**0.4 (0.2–0.7)**	43	3.1	0.7 (0.5–1.1)
Cleft palate only	601	29	4.8	0.7 (0.4–1.1)	12	2.1	1.0 (0.5–2.3)	17	2.9	**0.5 (0.3–0.9)**
Oesophageal atresia/stenosis	217	7	3.2	0.6 (0.3–1.6)	1	0.5	0.2 (0.0–2.1)	6	2.8	0.9 (0.3–2.5)
Congenital pyloric stenosis	241	11	4.6	0.6 (0.3–1.1)	6	2.5	1.1 (0.4–3.2)	5	2.1	**0.3 (0.1–0.9)**
Intestinal atresia/stenosis	158	9	5.7	1.1 (0.4–2.9)	5	3.3	1.0 (0.2–4.5)	4	2.6	1.1 (0.3–4.4)
Rectal/anal atresia/stenosis	231	12	5.2	1.1 (0.5–2.3)	3	1.4	0.7 (0.2–3.0)	9	4.1	1.2 (0.5–3.0)
Obstructive urinary CAs	343	21	6.2	0.5 (0.2–1.0)	10	2.9	1.0 (0.7–1.3)	11	3.21	0.6 (0.3–1.2)
Hypospadias	3,038	168	5.5	0.8 (0.7–1.0)	44	1.5	**0.6 (0.4–0.8)**	124	4.1	1.0 (0.8–1.2)
Undescended testis	2,052	102	5.0	**0.7 (0.5–0.9)**	32	1.6	**0.6 (0.4–0.9)**	70	3.4	0.7 (0.6–1.0)
Exomphalos/ gastroschisis	255	6	2.4	0.6 (0.2–1.7)	2	0.8	0.7 (0.1–4.0)	4	1.7	0.6 (0.2–2.1)
Microcephaly, primary	111	5	4.5	0.6 (0.2–2.1)	1	0.9	0.4 (0.0–6.9)	4	3.7	0.8 (0.2–2.9)
Congenital hydrocephaly	314	9	2.9	**0.3 (0.1–0.6)**	3	1.0	**0.2 (0.1–0.6)**	6	1.9	**0.4 (0.1–0.9)**
Ear CAs	354	20	5.7	0.7 (0.4–1.4)	7	2.0	1.0 (0.3–3.3)	13	3.7	0.7 (0.3–1.4)

Table 16.15 (continued)

	Grand total	Mothers with CIP			Mothers with CIP treated by cerclage			Mothers with CIP treated by bed rest alone		
Study groups	No.	No.	%	Adjusted OR[a]	No.	%	OR (95% CI)[a]	No.	%	OR (95% CI)[a]
Cardiovascular CAs	4,480	241	5.4	**0.8 (0.6–0.9)**	71	1.6	**0.6 (0.4–0.8)**	170	3.8	0.9 (0.7–1.1)
Clubfoot	2,424	129	5.3	**0.8 (0.6–0.9)**	35	1.4	**0.6 (0.4–0.9)**	94	3.9	0.9 (0.7–1.2)
Limb deficiencies	548	30	5.5	0.8 (0.5–1.3)	9	1.6	0.7 (0.3–1.5)	21	3.8	0.9 (0.5–1.5)
Poly/syndactyly	1,744	76	4.4	**0.5 (0.4–0.7)**	26	1.5	**0.4 (0.3–0.7)**	50	2.9	**0.6 (0.4–0.8)**
CAs of the musculoskeletal system	585	36	6.2	0.7 (0.4–1.3)	19	3.3	0.8 (0.3–1.9)	17	2.9	0.5 (0.2–1.4)
Diaphragmatic CAs		12	4.9	1.2 (0.6–2.7)	3	1.2	0.5 (0.1–2.0)	9	3.7	2.2 (0.8–6.5)
Other isolated CAs	976	79	7.4	1.0 (0.7–1.2)	40	4.1	1.3 (0.9–1.9)	39	4.09	0.9 (0.6–1.4)
Multiple CAs	1,349	58	4.3	**0.5 (0.4–0.7)**	21	1.6	**0.4 (0.3–0.7)**	37	2.7	**0.6 (0.4–0.9)**
Total cases	22,843	1,170	5.1	**0.7 (0.6–0.8)**	391	1.7	**0.6 (0.5–0.7)**	779	3.4	**0.8 (0.7–0.8)**
Total controls	38,151	2,803	7.4	–	1,112	2.9	–	1,691	4.4	–

[a]Matched OR adjusted for maternal age, birth order, employment status, influenza-common cold, drugs for CIP (i.e. threatened abortion and preterm delivery), and folic acid use in conditional logistic regression model.

maternity logbooks regarding to the previous induced abortions are not reliable and our questionnaire did not include question about previous induced abortions due to social reasons. However, our subsample based on the personal interview of mothers at the home visit of regional nurses and several Hungarian studies also confirmed this association. Thus the high rate of CIP could be explained by previous induced abortions in Hungary and it is necessary to consider these differences at the evaluation of high prevalence of CIP in Hungary.

The explanation of this high Hungarian rate of CIP may be on one hand the extremely high number of previous induced abortions due to social reason (XVII) because it was the main method of birth control in Hungary during last decades. After the introduction of the Hungarian Abortion Law in 1956, induced abortion due to social reason has become free. The ratio of livebirths and induced abortions due to mainly social reasons was 1.00:1.19 (2,499,248 vs. 2,971,250) between 1957 and 1973. The Abortion Law was restricted in 1973, after this but before the period of this study; this ratio was 1.00:0.51 (1,072,031 vs. 546,362) between 1974 and 1979. The ratio of livebirths and induced abortion was 1.00:0.65 (2,146,574 vs. 1,397,188) during the study period (i.e. 1980–1996) of this project. On the other hand, the method of induced abortion was the mechanical dilatation of cervical canal by Hegar devices followed by the evacuation/curettage (D+C) of the uterus. (The use of laminaria for the dilatation of cervical canal in primiparae was introduced only in the 1990s.)

Therefore, the incidence of CIP in Hungarian pregnant women is an appropriate way to estimate the harm of this old-fashion medical interruption of pregnancy. The late adverse effect of induced abortions caused a 1.1–2.9 higher risk for PB due to CIP in consecutive pregnancies (Hulka and Higgins, 1961; Henshaw and Host, 1996; Thorp et al., 2003; Moreau et al., 2006) with an increasing risk with the number of previous induced abortions. These associations were found by Hungarian experts as well (Barsy and Sárkány, 1963; Lampé et al., 1980). Unfortunately the use of abortion pills was not introduced in Hungary in order to prevent CIP until now, although this method does not associate with CIP (Chen et al. 2004). Thus CIP can be considered one of the most frequent causes of PB in Hungary.

(2) The threatened preterm delivery is an obligatory criterion of CIP, thus CIP was included to this group of pregnancy complications in the data set of the HCCSCA. Among other pregnancy complications, threatened abortions, placental disorders particularly premature separation of the placenta (abruption of the placenta), and anemia occurred more frequently in mothers without CIP. The higher incidence of threatened abortions may be related to CIP itself or doctors being aware of existing CIP may lower their subjective diagnostic threshold. The association between CIP and higher risk for placental disorders is biologically plausible considering the more frequently abnormal position of the placenta in a uterus with CIP. This finding of the study was in agreement with the finding of other studies as well (Rust et al., 2000). The higher prevalence of anemia may be related – at least partly – to a higher occurrence of hemorrhoids.

(3) There was an about 30% higher risk for PB in newborns of pregnant women with CIP. This risk is high but in fact lower than expected due to the theoretically 100% risk for preterm delivery in pregnant women with CIP. On the other hand, this figure is in agreement with the results of other studies (Page, 1958; Iams et al., 1996; Goldenberg et al., 2008) and can be explained by the early diagnosis of CIP followed by appropriate treatment.

The occurrence of PB in previous pregnancies was unknown because gestational ages at delivery of previous pregnancies were not mentioned. This part of previous pregnancy history would be important because women with prior preterm delivery had a 2.5-fold increased risk for PB in their next pregnancies (Mercer et al., 1999). However, about 40% of our pregnant women with CIP were primiparae and the evaluation of primiparous women with or without CIP resulted in similar findings as in the total data set. Finally, we were unable to differentiate the three categories of PB: induced delivery or caesarean section of delivery due to maternal or fetal indications (30–35%), spontaneous preterm labor with intact membrane (40–45%), and preterm premature rupture of membranes, irrespective of whether delivery is vaginal or by caesarean section (20–25%) (Goldenberg et al., 2008). However, we know that the proportion of caesarean section was about 7% in the data set of the HCCSCA. We also need to emphasize that twins may have some association with CIP and a higher risk for PB due to CIP.

(4) When evaluating the two kinds of medical management of CIP, i.e. cerclage and bed rest alone, the data indicated that cerclage was more effective in reducing the rate of PB. However, the PB preventive effect of cerclage also was associated with a mild intrauterine growth retardation of the fetus.

We assumed a similar bias and compliance with medical orders in the two subgroups of pregnant women with CIP treated by cerclage or bed rest alone. In addition our data were not appropriate to evaluate the causes for the choice of cerclage or bed rest alone treatment. Therefore, we did not know whether more severe CIPs were selected for therapeutic cerclage or the selection only depended on the attitude of obstetricians in the given medical institutions. Also, we were unable to compare pregnant women without CIP as reference and treated CIP, because we had no data on CIP without treatment.

As far as we know, previously three observational studies evaluated the effect of cerclage compared to no cerclage treatment after detection of short cervical length. Two studies indicated the benefit of cerclage based on longer gestational age and lower rate of PB (Heath et al., 1998; Hibbard et al., 2000), while there was no significant difference in these variables between cerclage and bed rest alone groups in the third study (Berghella et al., 1999). The results of two randomized controlled trials showed controversial findings. Rust et al. (2000) randomly allocated 61 pregnant women with a cervical length of <25 mm or prolapse of the fetal membranes into the endocervical canal for more than 25% of the original cervical length, measured between 16 and 24 weeks of gestation to receive a therapeutic McDonald cerclage with bed rest or bed rest alone.

There was no statistically significant difference in mean gestational age at delivery (33.5 vs. 34.7 week) and in the prevalence of PB. However, Althuisius et al. (1999) reported that therapeutic McDonald cerclage resulted in a longer cervical length (measured by transvaginal ultrasonography) in women with CIP. The final results of the Cervical Incompetence Prevention Randomized Cerclage Trial (CIPRACT) (Althuisius et al., 2001) based on 35 women showed that therapeutic cerclage with bed rest reduced PB (before the 34th weeks of gestation) in women with risk factors and/or symptoms of CIP and cervical length of <25 mm before the 27th weeks of gestation. In addition, the comparison of McDonald cerclage and bed rest versus bed rest alone indicated that PB was more frequent with a higher admission to the neonatal intensive care unit (as indicator of neonatal morbidity) or neonatal death in the group of women with CIP and bed rest alone.

Our findings showed the higher efficacy of therapeutic McDonald cerclage in the reduction of PB in women with CIP compared to bed rest alone in Hungary. However, it is necessary to consider the very high prevalence of CIP in Hungarian pregnant women due to the extreme frequent induced abortions due to social reason and old-fashion clinical diagnosis of CIP.

The possible intrauterine growth retardation of fetus after the surgical intervention of CIP by cerclage would need further studies because a lower birth weight was found in the CIPRACT (Althuisius et al., 2001) as well. However, the CIPPART included antimicrobial (amoxicillin, clavulanic acid, and metronidazole) treatment in women with CIP and indomethacin suppository to inhibit possible contractions caused by cerclage. The Hungarian protocol of therapeutic cerclage did not contain these complementary treatments, although several pregnant women were also treated by antimicrobial drugs. On the other hand, the rate of LBW newborns was not higher and the proportion of large birthweight newborns was not smaller in babies born to mothers with CIP treated by cerclage than in women with CIP and bed rest alone and these findings are against intrauterine fetal growth retardation.

(5) The most unexpected result of the study is the possible association found between CIP and the lower risk for different CAs in their offspring. We did not expect any association, but our data showed an inverse association (i.e. seemingly preventive effect) of CIP for some CAs, particularly for congenital hydrocephaly, neural-tube defects, poly/syndactyly, cleft lip $\pm$ palate, and multiple CAs.

Of course, the first thought was a systemic error related to some methodological problems, positive/negative biases, or uncontrolled confounders. The major causes of this seemingly absurd association may be the unclear diagnostic criteria of CIP in Hungary and other weaknesses of this data set:

(i) Our analysis was based on the medically recorded CIP, however, we were not able to check whether Hungarian obstetricians followed the recommended diagnostic criteria of CIP or not. As Iams (2004) stated: "Few subjects in obstetrics generate as much controversy as does abnormal cervical competence, or cervical incompetence..." This controversy is explained mainly by the different definition and/or diagnostic criteria of CIP in different countries and institutions based on only digital or ultrasound examination, in addition to the confusion between the diagnosis of CIP as categorical (yes or no) or continuous (based on the measurement of cervical length) variable (Leitich et al., 1999). Both length and diameter-dilation of the cervical canal is a continuum (Iams et al., 1995), thus the diagnosis of CIP is not easy.

(ii) Unfortunately the data of cervical length were not available in our study; therefore it was not possible to differentiate short cervix and CIP (Goldenberg et al., 2008). At the beginning of labor, the cervix shortens, softens, and dilates. Premature shortening of the cervix is a risk factor for preterm delivery. In pregnant women at 24th week of gestation, a cervical length of less than 25 mm is associated with an increased risk for PB (Copper et al., 1990, Iams et al., 1996, Andrews et al., 2000). In Hungary the diagnosis of CIP was based on a digital assessment of obstetricians and the severity of CIP was not known. However, these weaknesses were similar in the groups of case and controls mothers.

(iii) We had no information regarding to the origin of CIP. Our questionnaire requested information on the outcomes of previous pregnancies, but induced abortions due to social reasons were omitted from this list. However, regional nurses obtained data regarding to prior induced abortions from mothers visited at home based on the personal interview and a 2.8-fold higher rate of previous induced abortions was found in case mothers with CIP than in case mothers without CIP.

(iv) Our data set includes the history of previous pregnancy outcomes and CAs of the parents, thus recurrent and/or familial CAs are known, although, the completeness of these data were not checked. However, about 40% of our pregnant women with CIP had no previous birth and the evaluation of primiparae with or without CIP resulted in similar findings than the total data set.

(v) The frequency of maternal smoking and drinking during the study pregnancy as confounder were not known in the total data set. These data were collected only in a minor part of the data set of the HCCSCA based on the cross interview of women and their family members at the home visit. The proportion of smokers was 20.3% vs. 24.0% in case mothers with or without CIP in this subsample, respectively. Mothers of cases with common isolated CAs were evaluated separately in our previous studies and the proportion of smokers during the study pregnancy of mothers with or without CIP was 16 and 23% (XVIII). The figure of smoker control mothers (19.0%) in the study corresponded well to the rate of smoking among Hungarian pregnant women (XIX). However, this small subsample was not appropriate for the estimation of proportion of smokers in control mothers with or without CIP. The proportion of regular drinkers during the study pregnancy was about 1% in our samples.

The second thought to explain this unexpected association was related to other biases. However, selection bias is limited in our population-based material; in addition, recall bias was excluded by the use of only medically recorded CIP and CAs.

The third hypothesis suspects confounders behind the non-specific "preventive effect" of CIP on CAs. Our data indicated a higher socioeconomic status and/or a better medical care (including folic acid supplementation) and healthier lifestyle (e.g. smoking) in mothers with CIP, but there was a lower use of folic acid in case mothers than in control mothers with CIP. The periconceptional folic acid-containing multivitamin or folic acid supplementation reduces the first occurrence of neural-tube defects (125–127, 131, Berry et al., 1999), in addition, folic acid containing multivitamins can reduce the risk for some other CAs as well (126–129, 131, Botto and Olney, 2004). Thus the decrease of CAs should be rather addressed as coincidental finding in pregnant women with CIP as this group was offered more advanced and detailed prenatal care. However, maternal employment status as indicator of socioeconomic status and folic acid supplementation with other possible confounders (such as fever related influenza) were considered at the calculation of adjusted OR and there was no difference in the use of multivitamins among the study groups. However, we also need to consider other unevaluated confounders.

The fourth possibility is chance effect because we can expect a false association explained by the chance in every 20th analysis. However, 8 out of 22 CAs showed this association which is against this theory.

A further important criterion for the proof of human teratogenicity or for the justification of "antiteratogenic effect" is that the association needs to make scientific sense. It is not an easy task in this situation but we need to attempt the generation of a biologically plausible hypothesis for these findings. The proportion of malformed stillborn fetuses was 0.4% vs. 1.7% in case mothers with or without CIP, respectively. There was a higher rate of threatened abortions and placental disorders in mothers with CIP compared to pregnant women without CIP, therefore a more intensive very early selection of malformed fetuses could not be excluded. In addition, CIP poses a higher risk for spontaneous abortion (Page, 1958; Madsen et al., 1979). Unfortunately we were unable to measure the rate of clinically recognized miscarriages or unrecognized very early embryonic loss. The fact is that about 50% of all conceptions end as early loss (Wilcox et al., 1988). In addition, we found an extreme high rate of early loss in pregnant women who attempted suicide with large doses of drugs in early pregnancy (XX). Thus our hypothesis is based on the speculation that CIP may be a marker for certain structural and/or functional defects of the cervical canal and endometrium of the uterus as a late effect of induced abortions or other factors which more intensively expel the abnormal embryos in the early pregnancy.

Obviously we need further studies to confirm or refuse these unexpected, seemingly illogical finding in other datasets. These findings seemed to be too illogical to publish them in international periodicals.

In conclusion, our study showed that CIP is very frequent in Hungary probably due to the extremely high number of induced abortion with D+C method. Our findings also confirmed the higher risk for PB in pregnant women with CIP even though their CIP was treated. The available data suggested that PB can be prevented more effectively by therapeutic cerclage than by bed rest alone; however, this concept is against the accepted view of Hungarian obstetricians. Finally, our study showed that CIP associated with a lower risk for some CAs, particularly for congenital hydrocephalus, neural-tube defects, poly/syndactyly, cleft lip ± palate, and multiple CAs. However, it is necessary to consider the old-fashion unreliable diagnostic criteria of CIP and the very high rate of CIP in Hungary. Thus this unexpected association needs confirmation or rejection in other populations.

16.9 Non-inflammatory Disorders of Vagina and Vulva

Finally, some pregnant women were affected with different disorders of the vagina or the vulva; therefore we summarize their data here.

16.9.1 Interpretation of Data in the HCCSCA

Out of 22,843 cases, 11 (0.05%) had mothers with this group of disorders including leukoplakia of the vagina 2, stricture of the vagina 2, vaginal or vulvar laceration 5, leukoplakia of the vulva 2. Out of 38,151 controls without CA, 25 (0.07%) were born to pregnant women with this group of disorders comprising leukoplakia of the vagina 8, vaginal and vulvar laceration 7, leukoplakia of the vulva 8, atrophia of the vulva 2. The mean age of these pregnant women was higher (27.6 vs. 25.5 year) with somewhat higher mean birth order (1.9 vs. 1.8) compared to national average. Unexpectedly the mean gestational age (40.0 vs. 39.4 week) was longer and birth weight (3,318 vs. 3,276 g) was higher in the newborns of pregnant women with these vaginal and/or vulvar disorders. The distribution of CAs in 11 cases was cardiovascular CAs 3, clubfoot 3, undescended testis 2, hypospadias 1, microtia 1, absence of the gallbladder 1. There was no association of these maternal disorders with any CA group.

16.10 Cystic Mastopathy of the Breast

There were 4 controls and 1 case who had mothers with benign mammary dysplasia. It is worth mentioning that all the 5 children were boy, the case was affected with undescended testis, while controls were born on 39–40th gestational week with a mean birth weight of 3,850 g.

16.11 Conclusions

The infectious diseases of the lower genital organs in pregnant women cause the most frequent complains during pregnancy. Most of these diseases are not severe but they have a strong association with the higher risk for PB. At present time PB is the most decisive factor in infant mortality and in the origin of different handicaps in Hungary. The results of our studies showed that this increased risk is preventable by appropriate treatment. Therefore, an early and effective treatment of pregnant women with infectious diseases of the genital organs is an outstandingly important task for obstetricians during prenatal care.

References

ACOG: American College of Obstetricians and Gynecologists. Assessment of risk factors for preterm birth. ACOG Pract Bull 2001; 31.

Adams FH, Emmanouilideas GC, Riemenschneider TA (eds.). Heart Disease in Infants, Children, and Adolescents. Williams and Wilkins, Baltimore, 1989.

Adamson GD, Bujjeni V. Birth defects and assisted reproductive technologies (ART): a reproductive endocrinologist's review and perspective. Birth Defects Res 2003; 67: 332.

Aleck XA, Bartley DL. Multiple malformation syndrome following fluconazole use in pregnancy. Am J Med Genet 1997; 72: 253–256.

Althuisius SM, Dekker GA, van Geijn HP, Himmel P. The effect of therapeutic McDonald cerclage on cervical length as assessed by transvaginal ultrasonography. Am J Obstet Gynecol 1999; 180: 366–369.

Althuisius SM, Dekker GA, Hummel P et al. Final results of the Cervical Incompetence Prevention Randomized Cerclage Trial (CIPRACT): therapeutic cerclage with bed rest versus bed rest alone. Am J Obstet Gynecol 2001; 185: 1106–1112.

Ammon E, Lewis SV, Sibai BM et al. Ampicillin prophylaxis in preterm premature rupture of the membranes: a prospective randomised study. Am J sObstet Gynecol 1988; 159: 539–543.

Amsell R, Totten PA, Spiegel CA et al. Nonspecific vaginitis. Diagnostic criteria and microbial and epidemiological associations. Am J Med 1983; 74: 14–22.

Andrews WW, Copper RL, Hauth JC et al. Second-trimester cervical ultrasound: associations with increased risk for recurrent early, spontaneous delivery. Obstet Gynecol 2000; 95: 222–226.

Asch RH, Greenblatt RB. Update on the safety and efficacy of clomiphene citrate as a therapeutic agent. J Reprod Med 1976; 17: 175–180.

Baldwin S, Whitley RJ. Intrauterine herpes simplex virus infection. Teratology 1989; 39: 1–10.

Barsy G, Sárkány J. Impact of induced abortion on the birth (Hungarian with English abstract). Demográfia 1963; 6: 427–450.

Berghella V, Daly SF, Tolosa JE et al. Prediction of preterm delivery with transvaginal ultrasonography of the cervix in patients with high-risk pregnancies: does cerclage prevent prematurity? Am J Obstet Gynecol 1999; 181: 809–815.

Berry RJ, Li Z, Erickson JD, Moore CA et al. Prevention of neural-tube defects with folic acid in China. China-US Collaborative Project for Neural Tube Defects Prevention. N Engl J Med 1999; 341: 1485–1490.

Bjerkedahl T, Czeizel AE, Hosmer DW. Birth weight of single livebirths and weight specific early neonatal mortality in Hungary and Norway. Paediat Perinat Epidemiol 1983; 3: 29–40.

Botto LD, Lynberg MC, Erickson JD. Congenital heart defect, maternal febrile diseases and multivitamin use: a population-based study. Epidemiology 2001; 12: 485–490.

Botto LD, Olney RS. Vitamin supplements for risk of congenital anomalies other than neural-tube defects. Am J Med Genet 2004; 1256: 12–21.

Boyer KM, Gotoff SP. Prevention of early-onset neonatal group B streptococcal diseases with selective intrapartum chemoprophylaxis. N Engl J Med 1986; 314: 1665–1669.

Bracken MB. Oral contraception and congenital malformations in offspring: a review and meta-analysis of the prospective studies. Obstet Gynecol 1990; 736: 552–557.

Brown ZA, Vontrer LA, Benedetti J et al. Effects on infants of a first episode of genital herpes during pregnancy. N Engl J Med 1987; 317: 1246–1250.

Brucklchurst P, Hannah M, McDonald H. Interventions for treating bacterial vaginosis in pregnancy. Cochrane Database Syst Rev 2000; 2: CD000262.

Chen A, Yuan W, Meirik L et al. Mifepristone-induced early abortion and outcome of subsequent wanted pregnancy. Am J Epidemiol 2004; 160: 110–117.

Chin BM, Lamon RF. The microbiology of preterm labor and delivery. Contemp Rev Obstet Gynaecol 1997; 9: 285–296.

Cibley LJ. Cytolytic vaginosis. Am J Obstet Gynecol 1991; 165: 1245–1249.

Copper RL, Goldenberg RL, Davis RQ et al. Warning symptoms, uterine contractions, and cervical examination findings in women at risk of preterm delivery. Am J Obstet Gynecol 1990; 62: 748–754.

Cotch MF, Hillier SL, Gibbs RS et al. Epidemiology and outcomes associated with moderate to heavy Candida colonization during pregnancy. Am J Obstet Gynecol 1998; 178: 374–380.

Cuckle H, Wald N. Ovulation induction and neural tube defects. Lancet 1989; 2: 1281.

Divers MJ, Lilford RJ. Infection and preterm labour: a meta-analysis. Contemp Rev Obstet Gynaecol 1993; 5: 71–84.

Donders GGG. Definition and classification of abnormal vaginal flora. Best Pract Res Clin Obstet Gynaecol 2007; 21: 355–373.

Donders GGG, Vereecken A, Bosmanic E et al. Definition of a type of abnormal vaginal flora that is distinct from bacterial vaginosis: aerobic vaginitis. Br J Obstet Gynaecol 2002; 109: 1–10.

Ericson A, Kallen B. Congenital malformations in infants born after IVF: a population-based study. Hum Reprod 2001; 16: 504–509.

Engelmann E: Sporspilze. In: Hahn H, Falke D, Kaufmann SHE, Ullmann U (eds.) Medizinische Mikrobiologie und Infektologie. Springer, Berlin, 1999. p. 693.

Eschenbach DA, Critchlow CW, Watkins M et al. A dose-duration study of metronidazole for the treatment of nonspecific vaginosis. Scand J Infect Dis 1983; 40: 73–80.

Ferencz C, Loffredo C, Correa-Villasenor A. Genetic and environmental factors of major cardiovascular malformations: the Baltimore-Washington Infant study 1981–1989. Futura Publishing Co. Inc., Armonk, NY, 1997.

Gabbe SG, Niebyl JR, Simpson JL (eds.). Obstetrics: Normal and Problem Pregnancies. 4th ed. Churchill Livingstone, New York, 2001.

Genc MR, Schantz-Dunn J. The role of gene-environment interaction in predicting adverse pregnancy outcome. Best Pract Res Clin Obstet Gynaecol 2007; 21: 491–504.

Gjonaess H. Pelvic inflammatory diseases: etiologic studies with emphasis on chlamidial infection. Obstet Gynecol 1982; 59: 550–554.

Goldenberg RL, Culhane JF, Iams JD, Romero R. Epidemiology and causes of preterm birth. Lancet 2008; 271: 75–84.

Goldenberg RL, Hauth JC, Andrews WW. Intrauterine infection and preterm birth. N Engl J Med 2000; 342: 1500–1507.

Grossman J. Congenital syphilis. Teratology 1977; 16: 217–224.

Hansen M, Kurinczuk J, Bower C, Webb S. The risk of major birth defects after intracytoplasmic sperm injection and in vitro fertilization. N Engl J Med 2002; 346: 725–730.

Hansen M, Bower C, Milne E et al. Assisted reproductive technologies and the risk of birth defects – a systematic review. Hum Reprod 2005; 20: 328–338.

Hay Ph, Czeizel AE. Asymptomatic trichomonas and candida colonization and pregnancy outcome. Best Pract Res Clin Obstet Gynaecol 2007; 21: 403–409.

Heath VC, Sonka AP, Erasmus I et al. Cervical length at 23 weeks of gestation: the value of Shirodkar suture for the short cervix. Ultrasound Obstet Gynecol 1998; 12: 318–322.

Henshaw SK, Kost K. Abortion patients in 1994–1995: characteristics and contraceptive use. Fam Plann Perspect 1996; 28: 140–147, 158.

Hernandez-Diaz S, Werler MM, Walker AM, Mitchell AA. Folic acid antagonists during: pregnancy and the risk of birth defects. N Engl J Med 2000; 343: 1608–1914.

Hulka JF, Higgins G. Trauma to the internal cervical os during dilatation for diagnostic curettage. Am J Obstet Gynecol 1961; 82: 913–917.

Hibbard JU, Snow J, Moawad AH. Short cervical length by ultrasound and cerclage. J Perinatol 2000; 20: 161–165.

Iams JD. Abnormal cervical competence. In: Creasy RK, Resnik R (eds.) Maternal-Fetal Medicine. 5th ed. Saunders, Philadelphia, 2004. pp. 603–622.

Iams JD, Goldenberger RL, Meis PJ et al. The length of cervix and the risk of spontaneous premature delivery. N Engl J Med 1996; 334: 567–572.

Iams JD, Johnson FF, Sonek J et al. Cervical competence as a continuum: a study of ultrasonographic cervical length and obstetric performance. Am J Obstet Gynecol 1995; 172: 1097–1103.

Ingall D, Norris L. Syphilis, infectious diseases of the fetus and newborn infant. Chapter 9. In: Demington JS, Klein JO (eds.) Saunders Col, Philadelphia, 1976. pp. 414–463.

Janerich DT, Dugan JM, Standfast SJ, Strite L. Congenital heart disease and prenatal exposure to exogenous sex hormones. Br J Med 1977; i: 1058–1060.

Kallen BAJ, Olausson PO. Maternal drug use in early pregnancy and infant cardiovascular defect. Reprod Toxicol 2003; 17: 255–261.

Karkut G. Wirkung einer Lactobazillus-Immuntherapie auf die Genitalinfektion der Frau (Solcotrichovac/Gynatren) Geburtsch Frauenheilk 1984; 44: 311–314.

Kekki J, Kurki T, Pelkonen J et al. Vaginal clindamycin in preventing preterm birth and perinatal infections in asymptomatic women with bacterial vaginosis. A randomized, controlled trial. Obstet Gynecol 2001; 97: 643–648.

Kenyon SL, Taylor DJ, Tarnow-Mordi W. Broad spectrum antibiotics for spontaneous preterm labour: the ORACLE II. Randomized trial. ORACLE Collaborative Group. Lancet 2001; 357: 989–994.

Kim KS, Torres CR Jr, Yucel S et al. Induction of hypospadias in a murine model by maternal exposure to synthetic estrogens. Environ Res 2004; 94: 267–275.

Kiss H, Petricevic L, Husslein P. Prospective randomised controlled trial of an infection screening programme to reduce the rate of preterm delivery. Br Med J 2004; 329: 371–374.

Klebanoff MA, Hauth JC, Hiller SL, Thom EA, Ernest JM et al. Metronidazole to prevent delivery in pregnant women with asymptomatic bacterial vaginosis. N Engl J Med 2000; 343: 534–540.

Kurkinen R, Vuopala S, Koskela M et al. A randomised controlled trial of vaginal clindamycin for early pregnancy bacterial vaginosis. Br J Obstet Gynaecol 2000; 107: 1427–1432.

Lamont RF. Can antibiotics prevent preterm birth – the pro and con debate. Br J Obstet Gynecol 2005; 112(Suppl. 1): 67–73.

Lampé L, Bernard RP, Batár I. Outcome of current birth by previous induced abortion. interaction with smoking and prenatal care. J Foetal Med 1980; 43: 1–3.

Lázár E, Varga Gy, Institoris L, Ujhelyi K. Examination of factors affecting premature delivery in Kazincbarcika, with special regard to lactobacillus vaccination (Hungarian with English abstract). Magyar Nőorvosok Lapja 1988; 51: 353–356.

Leitich H, Kiss H. Asymptomatic bacterial vaginosis and intermediate flora as risk factors for adverse pregnancy outcome. Best Pract Res Clin Obstet Gynaecol 2007; 21: 375–390.

Leitich H, Brunhauer M, Bodner-Adler B et al. Antibiotic treatment of bacterial vaginosis in pregnancy: a meta-analysis. Am J Obstet Gynecol 2003; 188: 752–758.

Leitich H, Brumbauer M, Kaider A et al. Cervical length and dilatation of the internal as detected by vaginal ultrasonography as marker for preterm delivery: a systematic review. Am J Obstet Gynecol 1999; 181: 1465–1472.

Madsen M, Obel E, Ostergaard E. Gestation birth weight and spontaneous abortion in pregnancy after induced abortion. Lancet 1979; i: 142–145.

Malouf M, Fortier J, Morin F, Dube JL. Treatment of Hemophilus vaginalis vaginitis. Obstet Gynecol 1982; 57: 711–714.

McCormick MC. The contribution of low birth weight to infant mortality and childhood morbidity. N Eng J Med 1985; 312: 82–90.

McDonald IA. Suture of cervix for inevitable miscarriage. J Obstet Gynecol Emp 1957; 146: 346–350.

McDonald HM, O'Loughlin JA, Vigneswaran R et al. Impact of metronidazole therapy on preterm birth in women with bacterial vaginosis flora (Gardnerella vaginalis): a randomised, placebo controlled trial. Br J Obstet Gynaecol 1997; 104: 1391–1393.

McGregor JA, French JI, Richter R et al. Antenatal microbiological maternal risk factors associated with prematurity. Am J Obstet Gynecol 1990; 163: 1465–1473.

McGregor JA, French JL, Parker R et al. Prevention of premature birth by screening and treatment for common genital tract infection: results of a prospective controlled evaluation. Am J Obstet Gynecol 1995; 173: 157–167.

Mercer BM, Goldenberg RL, Moawad AH et al. The preterm prediction study: effect of gestational age and cause of preterm birth on subsequent obstetric outcome. Am J Obstet Gynecol 1999; 181: 1216–1221.

Menon R, Fortunate SJ. Infection and the role of inflammation in preterm premature rupture of the membrane. Best Pract Res Clin Obstet Gynaecol 2007; 21: 467–478.

Miettinen OS, Reiner ML, Nadas AS. Seasonal incidence of coarctation of the aorta. Br Heart J 1970; 32: 103–107.

Moll AC, Inhof SM, Crysberg RM et al. Incidence of retinoblastoma in children born after in-vitro fertilization. Lancet 2003; 361: 309–310.

Monga M, Sanborn BM. Biology and physiology of the reproductive tract and control of myometrial contraction. In: Creasy RK, Resnik R (eds.) Maternal-Fetal Medicine. 5th ed. Saunders, Philadelphia, 2004. pp. 69–78.

Morales WJ, Angel JL, O'Brien WF, Knuppel RA. Use of ampicillin and corticosteroids in premature rupture of the membranes: a randomised study. Obstet Gynecol 1989; 73: 721–726.

Morales WJ, Schorr S, Albritton J. Effect of metronidazole in patients with preterm birth in preceding pregnancy and bacterial vaginosis: a placebo-controlled, double-blind study. Am J Obstet Gynecol 1994; 171: 345–347.

Moreau C, Kaminsky M, Ancel PY et al. Previous induced abortions and the risk of very preterm delivery: results of the EPIPAGE study. Br J Obstet Gynecol 2006; 112: 430–437.

Murphy V, Kennea NL. Antenatal infection/inflammation and fetal tissue injury. Best Pract Res Clin Obstet Gynaecol 2007; 21: 479–489.

Nevin NC, Harley JMG. Clomiphene and neural tube defects. Ulster Med J 1976; 45: 59–64.

Nugent RP, Krohn MA, Hillier SL. Reliability of diagnosing bacterial vaginosis is improved by a standard method of Gram stain interpretation. J Clin Microbiol 1991; 29: 297–301.

Olive DL. Gonadotropoin-releasing hormone agonist for endometriosis. N Engl J Med 2008; 359: 1136–1142.

Olson CK, Keppler-Noreuil KM, Romitti PA et al. In vitro fertilization is associated with an increase in major birth defects. Fertil Steril 2005; 84: 1380–1315.

Page EW. Incompetent internal os of the cervix causing late abortion and premature labour. Technique for surgical repair. Obstet Gynecol 1958; 12: 509–515.

Pfeifer TA, Forsyth PS, Durfee MA et al. Nonspecific vaginitis: role of Hemophilus vaginalis and treatment with metronidazole. N Engl J Med 1978; 298: 1429–1434.

Pursley TJ, Blomquist IK, Abraham J et al. Fluconazole-induced congenital anomalies in three infants. Clin Infect Dis 1995; 22: 336–340.

Reefhius J. Honein MA, Schieve LA et al. Assisted reproductive technology and major structural birth defects in the United States. Hum Reprod 2008; doi:10.1093/humrep/den387

Romero R, Chaiworaponga T, Kuivaniemi H, Tromp G. Bacterial vaginosis, the inflammatory response and the risk of preterm birth: a role for genetic epidemiology in the prevention of preterm birth. Am J Obstet Gynecol 2004; 190: 1509–1519.

Romero R, Espinoza J, Kusanovic JP et al. The preterm parturition syndrome. Br J Obstet Gynaecol 2006; 113: 17–42.

Rosenstein IJ, Morgan DJ, Sheelan Dore CJ, Lamont RT, Taylor-Robinson D. Effect of vaginally applied clindamycin on the outcome of pregnancy and on vaginal microbial flora in women. Infect Dis Obstet Gynecol 2000; 8: 158–165.

Rust OA, Atlas RO. Jones KJ et al. A randomized trial of cerclage versus no cerclage among parents with ultrasonographically detected second-trimester preterm dilatation of the internal os. Am J Obstet Gynecol 2000; 183: 830–835.

Saigal S, Doyle LW. An overview of mortality and sequelae of preterm birth from infancy to adulthood. Lancet 2008; 271: 261–269.

Sharpe RM, Skakkeback NE. Are estrogens involved in falling sperm counts and disorders of the male reproductive tracts? Lancet 1993; 341: 1392–1395.

Shepard TH, Lemire RJ. Catalog of teratogenic agents. 11th ed. Johns Hopkins University Press, Baltimore, 2004.

Shirodkar VN. A new method of operative treatment for habitual abortion in the second trimester of pregnancy. Antiseptic 1955; 52: 299–300.

Sonnex C. The amine test: a simple, rapid, inexpensive method for diagnosing bacterial vaginosis. Br J Obstet Gynaecol 1995; 102: 160–161.

Stacey CM, Munday PM, Taylor-Robinson D et al. A longitudinal study of pelvic inflammatory disease. Br J Obstet Gynaecol 1992; 99: 994–999.

Teichmann AT, Steigerwald U. Infektionen in Gynekologie und Geburtshilfe. Wissenschaftliche Verlagsgeselschaft, Stuttgart, 1994.

Thorp JM, Hartmann KE, Shadigan E. Long-term physical and psychological health consequences of induced abortion: review of the evidence. Obstet Gynecol Surv 2003; 58: 67–79.

Tikkanen J, Heinonen OP. Maternal hyperthermia during pregnancy and cardiovascular malformations in the offspring. Eur J Epidemiol 1991; 7: 628–359.

Tikkanen J, Heinonen OP. Risk factors for hypoplastic left heart syndrome. Teratology 1994; 50: 112–117.

Torfs CP, Velie EM, Oechsli FW et al. A population-based study of gastroschisis: demographic, pregnancy and lifestyle risk factors. Teratology 1994; 50: 44–53.

Ugwumadu A, Manyonda I, Reid F, Hay P. Effect of early oral clindamycin on late miscarriage and preterm delivery in asymptomatic women with abnormal vaginal flora and bacterial vaginosis: a randomised controlled trial. Lancet 2003; 361: 983–988.

Ugwumadu A. Role of antibiotic therapy for bacterial vaginosis and intermediate flora in pregnancy. Best Pract Res Clin Obstet Gynaecol 2007; 21: 391–402.

Werler MM, Mitchell AA, Shapiro S. Demographic reproductive, medical and environmental factors in relation to gastroschisis. Teratology 1992; 45: 353–360.

Wennerholm U-B, BerghC, Hamberger K et al. Incidence of congenital malformations in children born after ICSI. Hum Reprod 2000; 15: 944–948.

Westron L. Incidence, prevalence and trends of acute pelvic inflammatory disease and its consequences in industrialized countries. Am J Obstet Gynecol 1980; 138: 880–886.

Wheeler JM. Epidemiology of endometriosis-associated infertility. J Reprod Med 1989; 34: 41–46.

Wilcox AJ, Weinbeg CR, O'Connor JF et al. Incidence of early loss of pregnancy. N Engl J Med 1988; 319: 189–194.

Yarberry-Allen P, Ledger WJ, Milstein SJ. Infections of the female genital tract. In: Roberts RB (ed.) Infectious Diseases: Pathogenesis, Diagnosis and Therapy. Year Book Medical Publ., Chicago, 1986.

Own Publications

I. Ács F, Bánhidy F, Puho HE, Czeizel AE. Possible association between acute pelvic inflammatory disease in pregnant women and congenital abnormalities in their offspring. A population-based case-control study. Birth Defects Res A 2008; 82: 563–570.

II. Ács N, Bánhidy F, Puho HE, Czeizel AE. Maternal influenza during pregnancy and risk of congenital abnormalities in the offspring. Birth Defects Res A 2005; 73: 989–996.

III. Czeizel AE, Ács N, Bánhidy F et al. Primary prevention of congenital abnormalities due to high fever related maternal diseases by antifever therapy and folic acid supplementation. Curr Women's Health Rev 2007; 3: 1–17.

IV. Ács N, Bánhidy F, Puhó E, Czeizel AE. Population-based case-control study of the common cold and congenital abnormalities. Eur J Epidemiol 2006; 21: 61–75.

V. Czeizel AE, Ács N, Bánhidy F, Vogt G. Possible association between maternal diseases and congenital abnormalities. In: Engel JV (ed.) Birth Defects New Research. NOVA Scientific Publ. New York, 2006. pp. 55–70.

VI. Ács F, Bánhidy F, Puho HE, Czeizel AE. No association between vulvovaginitis-bacterial vaginosis and related drug treatments of pregnant women and congenital abnormalities in their offspring. A population-based case-control study. Cent Eur J Med 2008; 3: 332–340.

VII. Bánhidy F, Ács F, Puho HE, Czeizel AE. Rate of preterm births in pregnant women with common lower genital tract infection: a population-based study based on clinical practice. J Mat-Fetal Neonat Ned 2009; XX: 1–9.

VIII. Czeizel AE. Ten years' experience in periconception care. Eur J Obstet Gynecol Reprod Biol 1999; 84: 43–49.

IX. Czeizel AE, Puhó E, Kazy Z. The use of data set of the Hungarian Case-Control Surveillance of Congenital Abnormalities for the evaluation of birth outcomes beyond congenital abnormalities. Cent Eur J Publ Health 2007; 15: 147–153.

X. Ács F, Bánhidy F, Puho HE, Czeizel AE. Possible association between cervical erosion in pregnant women and congenital abnormalities in their offspring – population-based case-control study. Health, 2010 (in press).

XI. Bánhidy F, Ács N, Czeizel AE. Ovarian cysts, clomiphene therapy, and the risk of neural tube defects. Int J Gynecol Obstet 2008; 100: 86–88.

XII. Czeizel AE, Rothman KJ. Does relaxed reproductive selection explain the decline in male reproductive health? A new hypothesis. Epidemiology 2002; 13: 113–114.

XIII. Bánhidy F, Ács N, Puhó HE, Czeizel AE. Association of very high Hungarian rate of preterm birth with cervical incompetence in pregnant women. Cent J Publ Health 2010; 18: 8–15.

XIV. Czeizel AE, Lányi-Engelmayer Á, Klujber L et al. Etiological study of mental retardation in Budapest, Hungary. Am J Ment Def 1980; 85: 120–128.

XV. Czeizel AE, Törzs E, Diaz LG et al. An aetiological study on 6 to 14 years-old children with severe visual handicap in Hungary. Acta Paediatr Hung 1991; 31: 365–377.

XVI. Czeizel AE, Skripeczky K, Mester E, Sankararanarayan K. The load of genetic and partially genetic disease in man. IV. Severe visual handicaps and profound childhood deafness in Hungarian school-age children. Mutat Res 1992; 270: 103–114.

XVII. Czeizel AE. Mortality and morbidity of legal induce abortion. Lancet 1971; ii: 209.

XVIII. Czeizel AE, Tusnady G. Aetiological Studies of Isolated Common Congenital Abnormalities in Hungary. Akadémai Kiadó, Budapest, 1984.

XIX. Czeizel AE, Kodaj I, Lenz WC. Smoking during pregnancy and congenital limb deficiency. Br Med J 1994; 308: 1473–1476.

Chapter 17
Pregnancy, Childbirth, and the Pueperium

First our analyses focused on cases with CA but case-control studies also needed matched controls without CA. The control group of HCCSCA also helped us to evaluate PB and LBW. The third aspect of our analysis was the evaluation of pregnancy complications as possible co-morbidities of maternal diseases. In these studies we only used medically recorded information from the prenatal maternity logbook because in our validation studies the retrospective maternal information proved to be inaccurate regarding to the diagnoses of maternal illnesses and were significantly distorted by recall bias.

Another topic which needs further discussion is the list of pregnancy complications published in our papers and different chapters of this monograph. We followed the strategy of recent handbooks (Creasy et al., 2004) and presented the data of *preeclampsia-eclampsia* and *gestational hypertension* in Chapter 10 of the diseases of the circulatory system because it helps to better understand the different aspects of the same symptom, i.e. hypertension. However, *secondary hypertension due to renal disease* was discussed among the diseases of the urinary tract in Chapter 15. *Gestational diabetes* is presented together with the other form of diabetes mellitus in Chapter 5. The ICD (WHO) classifies *cervical incompetence* among the pathological conditions of the female genital organs thus we followed this concept. Finally, *nausea and vomiting in pregnancy* was included in the Chapter 12, i.e. among the diseases of the digestive system.

The rest of pregnancy complications are presented here. In general, we focus on the data of control pregnant women because pregnancy complications in case mothers may be modified by the effect of fetal defects. In addition, we follow the structure of our previous way of presentation while summarizing the data in tables.

Table 17.1 shows maternal age and birth order, in addition to the use of folic acid and multivitamins as the indicator of the quality of periconceptional and prenatal care. We also need to consider these measures when evaluating CAs due to the preventive attributes of folic acid and multivitamins on CAs.

Table 17.2 summarizes the possible co-morbidities of maternal disease, and pregnancy complications with significant associations with other pregnancy complications.

Birth outcomes compared to the rate of PB and LBW, in addition to mean gestational age and birth weight are presented in Table 17.3.

N. Ács et al., *Congenital Abnormalities and Preterm Birth Related to Maternal Illnesses During Pregnancy*, DOI 10.1007/978-90-481-8620-4_17,

Table 17.1 Characteristics of control mothers with (+) or without (–) pregnancy complications

Pregnancy complications	Maternal age		Birth order		Folic acid	Multivitamin
	Mean	S.D.	Mean	S.D.	+/–(%)	+/–(%)
Threatened abortion	25.7	4.8	1.7	0.9	59.4/55.4	9.3/7.30
Placental disorders	26.7	5.0	1.8	0.9	66.1/54.3	11.0/6.5
Polyhydramnios	25.4	5.4	1.8	0.9	64.9/54.4	11.5/6.6
Oligohydramnios	27.7	6.1	2.1	1.0	78.6/54.4	–
Oedema/excessive weight gain	25.2	4.9	1.6	0.8	52.7/54.5	–
Threatened preterm delivery	25.5	4.9	1.8	0.9	62.1/53.4	7.0/6.6
Reference	25.4	5.0	1.7	1.0	59.6/52.6	8.5/5.8

Table 17.2 Occurrence of acute and chronic diseases and pregnancy complications in control mothers with (+) or without (–) pregnancy complications

Pregnancy complications	Acute disease groups (%)*	Chronic diseases (%)*	Other pregnancy complications (%)*
Threatened abortion	–	EH 9.2/6.6	TPD 22.2/12.7 PD 3.0/1.2
Placental disorders	–	EH 11.6/7.0	TA 33.4/16.8 TPD 23.9/14.1
Polyhydramnios	–	EH 9.9/7.0	TA 25.1/17.0 TPD 22.0/14.2
Oligohydramnios	RS 28.6/9.0	RH 28.6/4.2	TA 42.9/17.1 TPD 23.9/14.1
Oedema/excessive weight gain	–	EH 12.3/6.9	PE 8.7/2.9 TPD 26.6/14..4
Threatened preterm delivery	–	EH 14.9/5.9	TA 27.0/15.7

RS = respiratory system; EH = essential hypertension; TA = threatened abortion; RH = recorded haemorrhoid; TPD = threatened preterm delivery; PD = placental disorders; PE = preeclampsia-eclampsia.

*with or without pregnancy complication studies

Finally, the possible direct and indirect associations of pregnancy complications with different CAs are shown in Table 17.4.

17.1 Threatened Abortion

In general, the preliminary symptoms of early fetal loss, i.e. spontaneous abortion (miscarriage) are uterine spasm and/or uterine-vaginal bleeding. These preliminary symptoms without fetal loss are defined as threatened abortion.

Out of 22,843 cases, 3,497 (15.3%) had mothers with the diagnosis of threatened abortion. However, these women were all able to continue with their pregnancy as informative offspring in the HCCSCA includes only liveborn infants, stillborn

Table 17.3 Birth outcomes of newborn infants born to control pregnant women with pregnancy complications

Pregnancy complications	No. of controls	Gestational age (week)		Birth weight (g)		PB		LBW	
		Mean	S.D.	Mean	S.D.	No.	%	No.	%
Threatened abortion	6,510	39.2	2.2	3,239	535	700	10.8	461	7.1
Placental disorders	593	39.1	2.4	3,179	607	67	11.3	65	11.0
Polyhydramnios	191	39.4	2.5	3,288	645	22	11.5	19	9.9
Oligohydramnios	14	38.1	3.0	2,930	580	3	21.4	2	14.3
Oedema/excessive weight gain	912	39.4	2.0	3,381	495	80	8.8	31	3.4
Threatened preterm delivery	396	39.1	2.2	3,191	542	45	11.4	34	8.6
Reference	27,813	39.4	2.0	3,286	501	2,503	9.0	1,502	5.4

Table 17.4 Estimated risk of CAs in cases born to mothers with pregnancy complications

Pregnancy complications	No. of cases	Total CA		Isolated CA		Multiple CA	
		OR	95% CI	OR	95% CI	OR	95% CI
Threatened abortion	3,497	0.9	0.8–0.9	AA	1.3, 1.0–1.8	1.1	1.0–1.3
Placental disorders	296	0.8	0.7–1.0	HY	1.9, 1.0–3.6	1.1	0.7–1.6
Polyhydramnios	211	**1.9**	**1.5–2.3**	**OA**	**27.4, 15.6–48.0**	**8.1**	**6.0–11.1**
Oligohydramnios	33	**3.9**	**2.1–7.4**	**RA**	**42.6, 5.6–296.1**	**14.2**	**5.7–35.3**
				OU	**32.0, 7.2–146.6**		
Oedema/excessive weight gain	428	0.8	0.7–0.9	–		0.6	0.4–1.0
Threatened preterm delivery	518	0.8	0.8–0.9	SK	1.3, 1.1–1.7	0.8	0.6–0.9

AA = anal/rectal atresia/stenosis; DI = diaphragmatic CA; HY = hydrocephalus, congenital; OA = oesophageal atresia/stenosis; OU = obstructive CA of the urinary tract; RA = renal a/dysgenesis; SK = CAs of the musculo-skeletal system's.

fetuses and electively terminated malformed fetuses after prenatal diagnosis. The ratio of vaginal bleeding and uterine spasm was 85.8% and 14.2%, together 33.3%.

Out of 38,151 controls, 6,510 (17.1%) were born to mothers with threatened abortion. The proportion of vaginal bleeding and uterine spasm was 58.0% and 15.0%, together 41.7%.

Thus the rate of uterine bleeding was less frequent in case mothers with a plausible biological explanation that fetal loss followed these symptoms occurred more frequently in pregnant women who had malformed fetuses.

The mean maternal age was somewhat higher while birth order did not deviate from the reference value, i.e. the Hungarian population figures. There was no significant difference in the rate of folic acid and multivitamin supplementation during the study pregnancy between women with or without threatened abortion (Table 17.1)

There was no association of threatened abortion with acute disease groups; however, essential hypertension occurred more frequently in pregnant women with threatened abortion. The incidence of two other pregnancy complications: placental disorders and threatened preterm delivery was higher in pregnant women with threatened abortions. These associations may reflect placental disorders as the common cause behind certain part of threatened abortion and preterm delivery (Table 17.2).

Birth outcomes of newborns born to mothers with previous threatened abortion may show somewhat increased risk for PB because mean gestational age was somewhat (0.2 week) PB and birth weight (47 g) was lower, and this trend was reflected in the higher rate of PB and LPW newborns (Table 17.3).

On the other hand, threatened abortion did not associate a higher risk for total CA (Table 17.4) and among 24 CA-groups only anal/rectal atresia/stenosis showed a marginal association with prior threatened abortion. The risk of multiple CAs was somewhat higher but the analysis of component CAs of these multimalformed cases did not reveal any characteristic pattern. Therefore, these crude OR values does not indicate any real risk of higher prevalence of CAs in pregnant women with prior threatened abortion.

In conclusion, there is no higher risk for CAs after the symptoms of threatened abortion. Probably, seriously affected fetuses were selected out by spontaneous abortion while the "surviving" fetuses had no defects but implantation failure or other maternal problems may explain the symptoms of threatened abortion.

17.2 Placental Disorders

Three manifestations of placental disorders have been differentiated in the data set of the HCCSCA.

Placenta previa means a low-lying placenta in the uterus, i.e. the lower margin of placenta covers the internal cervical os (Clark, 2004). In the past, partial (placenta partially covers the os) and complete (placenta completely covers the os) placenta previa were differentiated. Recently, due to the progress of ultrasonography a new classification has been introduced: placenta previa, when the placenta covers the internal os in the third trimester and marginal placenta previa, when the placenta lies within 2–3 cm of the internal os but does not cover it.

The incidence of placenta previa is estimated about 0.5% of pregnancies by the time of birth, and is getting more and more frequent with advanced age, multiparity, previous cesarean section, induced abortion, and cigarette smoking.

Premature separation of placenta (abruptio placentae) means the separation of a normally implanted placenta before the birth of the fetus. The diagnosis is most commonly made in the third trimester and is presented by bleeding into the decidua basalis. Abruption of the placenta is a very dangerous condition for both the mother and the fetus.

The incidence of premature separation of placenta is 0.8% in pregnant women during the third trimester. There is no generally accepted theory of etiology behind this pregnancy complication.

The third group of placental disorders is the so called *antepartum hemorrhage*, which is a symptom and not a pathological condition. It is used when physicians cannot differentiate one of the above two placental disorders.

Out of 22,843 cases, 239 (1.1%), 37 (0.2%) and 20 (0.1%) had mothers with placenta previa, premature separation of placenta, and antepartum hemorrhage, respectively. Together the number of these three placental disorders was 296, i.e. 1.30%.

Out of 38,151 controls, 471 (1.2%), 86 (0.2%) and 36 (0.1) were born to mothers with placenta previa, abruption placentae, and antepartum hemorrhage, respectively. These figures with the total percentage of 1.55% were somewhat higher compared to case mothers.

The maternal characteristics of pregnant women with placental disorders may indicate the history of some unsuccessful previous pregnancies: the mean maternal age and birth order was somewhat higher and their folic/multivitamin uses were more frequent (Table 17.1). On the other hand, these variables may only reflect the effect of a more advanced maternal age.

There was no association between any acute maternal disease group and the above mentioned placental disorders. However, there was a higher prevalence of essential hypertension in pregnant women with placental disorders. Both threatened abortion and preterm delivery occurred more frequently in the pregnancy of women with placental disorders (Table 17.2). It is worth mentioning that the incidence of preeclampsia-eclampsia was not significantly higher in control pregnant women with placental disorders (4.2% vs. 3.0%) but this association was strong in case pregnant women (7.8% vs. 2.9%).

Birth outcomes of babies born to mothers with placental disorders showed the pathological importance of this pregnancy complication (Table 17.3). The mean gestational age was shorter by 0.3 week and it associated with a higher rate of PB. However, the lower mean birth weight of 107 g was associated with a very significant increase in the rate of LBW newborns. These variables might indicate intrauterine growth retardation of the fetuses in the pregnancies with placental disorders.

Fortunately placental disorders of pregnant women did not associate with a higher risk of total CA and multiple CA in their offsprings. Among 25 CA-groups studied, only congenital hydrocephalus showed a marginally higher risk.

17.3 Pathological Forms of Amnion Fluid

The quantity of the amniotic fluid increases progressively throughout pregnancy. The volume of amniotic fluid is 10 mL at 10th, 190 mL at 16th, and 780 mL at 32–35th weeks of gestation. After the 35th week there is a decrease to the average volume of 700 mL at term. Fetal urine first enters the amniotic space between the 8th and 11th week of pregnancy and fetal urine becomes the major source of amniotic fluid in the second half of pregnancy. The human fetus begins swallowing the amniotic fluid from the 10th gestational week and this volume increases to 210–760 mL/day during the last months. The third factor which influences the amniotic fluid is intramenbranous absorption (Brace, 2004).

Polyhydramnios means an access of amniotic fluid of 1.5–2 L between 32nd and 36th gestational weeks. Polyhydramnios has a relatively wide range of volume and if it occurs during the second trimester, polyhydramnios, spontaneously resolves in 40–50% of pregnancies with a good pregnancy outcome.

Oligohydramnios means a very low volume of amniotic fluid (in general less than 0.5 L in mid-pregnancy) and it associated with poor pregnancy outcome.

Out of 22,843 cases, 211 (0.92%) had mothers with the diagnosis of polyhydramnios, while among 38,151 controls, 191 (0.50%) pregnant women were affected with this pregnancy complications. The incidence of oligohydramnios is much lower, 33 (0.14%) case mothers and 14 (0.04%) mothers had this pregnancy complication.

The mean maternal age and birth order of pregnant women with *polyhydramnios* did not differ significantly from the reference values. These pregnant women used folic acid and multivitamins more frequently than pregnant women without these pregnancy supplements (Table 17.1).

Among maternal diseases, only essential hypertension showed a weak association with polyhydramnios. However, polyhydramnios associated with a higher risk of threatened abortion and preterm delivery (Table 17.2).

Birth outcomes of newborns in this group of pregnancy complications showed controversial pattern (Table 17.3). On one hand, the mean gestational age and birth weight did not differ significantly from the reference values. On the other hand, the rate of PB and LBW newborns was higher.

The data of Table 17.4 shows the obvious association of polyhydramnios with certain CAs therefore there is a higher risk in both total CA-group and in multiple CAs. The higher risk of total CA-group is explained mainly by the much higher occurrence of oesophageal atresia but the evaluation of other CA showed a higher risk of congenital hydrocephalus (3.9, 1.7–8.8) and CAs of the diaphragm

(8.5, 4.4–16.2). There was a predominance of these CAs and intestinal/rectal/anal atresias among the component CA in 53 multimalformed cases.

In conclusion, polyhydramnios associates with a much higher risk of certain CAs which can be explained by the amniotic fluid dynamics.

Oligohydramnios shows a more severe pathological condition, but fortunately occurred rarely. The higher mean maternal age and birth order shows the importance of advanced maternal age and multiparity. Surprisingly, folic acid usage was the highest in mothers affected by oligohydramnios among all pregnancy complications (Table 17.1).

Oligohydramnios in pregnant women associated with a high incidence of acute disease of the respiratory system. Among chronic diseases, nearly 30% of pregnant women with oligohydramnios were affected with severe hemorrhoid. Oligohydramnios also associated with a higher risk of threatened abortion and preterm delivery. However, it is worth emphasizing the extremely high number (43%) of threatened abortion in this group of pregnancy complications (Table 17.2).

Oligohydramnios associated with the shortest mean gestational age and lowest mean birth weight. These pathological variables explain the very high rate of PB and LBW in newborns (Table 17.3).

Oligohydramnios resulted in the highest risk both in the total CA-group and in multimalformed cases. These high risks are explained by the extreme high rate of renal a/dysgenesis and obstructive CAs of the urinary tract among isolated CAs but these CAs dominated among the component CAs of 7 cases with multiple CA. Of course, the high risk of these CAs is in agreement with our knowledge regarding to the amniotic fluid dynamics.

In conclusion, oligohydramnios can be considered one of the most dangerous pregnancy complications that is associated with very poor pregnancy outcomes.

17.4 Oedema and Excessive Weight Gain Without Hypertension

According to the recommendation of expert committees, three groups of weight gain during pregnancy in women are differentiated on the basis of their prepregnancy weight or their body mass index (BMI):

Underweight women (BMI less than 19.8)	12.5–18 kg weight gain
Normal weight (BMI: 19.8–26.0)	11.5–16 kg weight gain
Overweight (BMI over 26.0–29.0)	<11.5 kg weight gain

The first task of medical doctors to find the factors in the origin of edema and excessive weight gain because, in general, they might be the symptom of different diseases (Abrams, 1993). The treatment and/or reduction of the severity of these underlying causes are much more effective than general advices on symptomatic treatment.

Out of 22,843 cases, 428 (1.9%), while out of 38,151 controls, 912 (2.4%) had mothers with these pregnancy complications.

As Table 17.1 shows, pregnant women with this pregnancy complication was somewhat younger with lower birth order and with a lower quality of periconceptional and prenatal care (the use of folic acid was the lowest in this group).

Oedema and excessive weight gain occurred more frequently in pregnant women with essential hypertension and was associated with a higher risk of preeclampsia-eclampsia and threatened preterm delivery (Table 17.2).

Birth outcomes of newborns in these pregnant women showed a characteristic pattern. Mean gestational age and rate of BP corresponded to the values of the reference sample, but the mean birth weigh was much higher and the rate of LBW newborns was lower (Table 17.3).

There was no higher risk of CA in this group of pregnancy complications (Table 17.4).

17.5 Threatened Preterm Delivery

Beyond CA, PB is the "protagonist" of this monograph and we present the Hungarian data regarding to the possible associations of different maternal diseases with preterm delivery and PB. There are three steps in the prevention of PB. The first step is optimal preconceptional planning and prenatal care. The second step is the treatment of threatened preterm delivery and postponing labor. The third step includes direct attempts to avoid preterm labor by the most modern tocolytic and other methods.

There are two main groups of pregnant women with threatened preterm delivery in the data set of the HCCSCA. The first group includes pregnant women with cervical incompetence and this topic was discussed in detail in previous chapters. The rest of pregnant women in the second group had different etiologies.

Out of 22,843 cases, 1,688 (7.4%) had mothers with the diagnosis of threatened preterm delivery and among them 1,170 were affected by cervical incompetence (which is equivalent with threatened preterm delivery) and 518 pregnant women had symptoms of threatened preterm delivery due to other causes. Out of 38,151 controls, 3,191 (8.4%) were born to mothers who had previous diagnosis of threatened preterm delivery. Among them, 2,795 belonged to the group of cervical incompetence and 396 to the rest. Here only pregnant women with threatened preterm delivery without cervical incompetence are evaluated.

The maternal characteristics do not show any special in pregnant women with threatened preterm delivery (Table 17.1), their mean age and birth order fit the value of reference sample.

Only essential hypertension occurred more frequently in pregnant women with threatened preterm deliver and among other pregnancy complications, threatened abortion had a higher incidence (Table 17.2).

Threatened preterm delivery associated with a higher risk of PB and LBW newborns partly explained by the shorter gestational age (0.3 week) and lower mean weight (95 g) (Table 17.3).

Fortunately, threatened preterm birth did not associate with a higher risk of total CA-group and multiple CAs. In fact, these OR values show a somewhat lower risk (the upper limit of CI is less than 1). Among 24 isolated CA-groups, only CAs of the musculo-skeletal system had a somewhat higher risk. In the analysis of different subgroups of mild CAs, torticollis showed a higher prevalence at birth. This CA is generally more common in preterm babies.

In conclusion, threatened preterm delivery is associated with a higher risk for PB, which shows that the available medical management is not totally effective. However, fortunately this pregnancy complication was not associated with increased risk for any CAs.

17.6 Others

The data of prolonged pregnancy, isoimmunisation, etc were not appropriate for scientific based analyses.

17.7 Conclusions

Only two pregnancy complications: polyhydramnios and oligohydramnios have casual association with CA. The other pregnancy complications are important when evaluating birth outcomes, although in general they have no direct causal relationship.

References

Abrams B. Preventing low birth weight: Does WIC work? A review of evaluation of the Special Supplemented Food Program for Women, Infants and Children. Ann N Y Acad Sci 1993; 678: 306–344.

Brace RA. Amniotic fluid dynamics. In: Creasy RK, Resnik R, Iams JD (eds.) Maternal-Fetal Medicine. 5th ed. Saunders, Philadelphia, 2004. pp. 45–53.

Clark SL. Placenta previa and abruptio placentae. In: Creasy RK, Resnik R, Iams JD (eds.) Maternal-Fetal Medicine. 5th ed. Saunders, Philadelphia, 2004. pp. 707–722.

Creasy RK, Resnik R, Iams JD (eds.). Maternal-Fetal Medicine. 5th ed. Saunders, Philadelphia, 2004.

Chapter 18
Congenital Malformations, Deformations, and Chromosomal Abnormalities

CAs also might occur in pregnant women, i.e. mothers of cases and controls as well. In this chapter the offspring of mothers who are affected by congenital malformations, deformations, or chromosomal abnormalities will be analyzed. Three CA-groups had more than 10 case mothers in the data set of the HCCSCA

18.1 Cardiovascular CAs

The group of cardiovascular CAs shows the highest total prevalence among CAs in general. The prevalence of cardiovascular CAs in Hungary is about 1% (I–III). However, cardiovascular CAs comprise of very heterogeneous manifestations of CAs with different origin, and most common groups (e.g. ventricular septal defect) usually have multifactorial etiology (IV, V).

18.1.1 Interpretation of Data in the HSCCSCA

Out of 22,843 cases, 32 (0.14%), while out of 38,151 controls, 41 (0.11%) had mothers affected with cardiovascular CA. All of them were medically recorded in the prenatal care logbook. Unfortunately, the type of medical interventions (e.g. cardiac surgery) was not mentioned in most pregnant women.

The mean maternal age (26.2 vs. 25.5 year) and birth order (2.0 vs. 1.8) was somewhat higher without obvious difference in the socioeconomic status of pregnant women with or without cardiovascular CAs. The use of folic acid was much higher both in case mothers (62.5% vs. 49.4%) and in control mothers (61.0% vs. 54.4%), while the folic acid containing multivitamin supplementations did not show difference among the study groups.

Among pregnancy complications, the lower incidence of severe nausea and vomiting in pregnancy (5.5% vs. 9.2%) and the higher occurrence of anemia (21.9% vs. 15.7%) in pregnant women with cardiovascular CA are worth mentioning. The evaluation of maternal diseases showed a higher incidence of acute infectious respiratory diseases (15.1% vs. 9.1%) and much higher prevalence of hypertension

N. Ács et al., *Congenital Abnormalities and Preterm Birth Related to Maternal Illnesses During Pregnancy*, DOI 10.1007/978-90-481-8620-4_18,

(35.6% vs. 7.1%). The latter pathological condition also explained the higher use of hypertension related drugs in pregnant women with cardiovascular CAs.

The mean gestational age was somewhat shorter (39.2 vs. 39.4 week) with much lower mean birth weight (3,057 vs. 3,276 g) which was associated with an increased rate of LBW newborns (9.8% vs. 5.7%). The rate of PB was similar (9.8% vs. 9.2%).

The risk of total CAs was not higher (1.3, 0.8–2.1). However, out of 32 cases, 12 had cardiovascular CA (2.4, 1.1–5.6), while other specified CA-groups did not show a higher risk in the offspring of pregnant women with cardiovascular CAs. The distribution of cardiovascular CAs in the 12 cases was the following: ventricular septal defect 4, atrial septal defect 2, transposition of the great vessels, tetralogy of Fallot, congenital stenosis of the pulmonary valve, congenital mitral insufficiency, and persistent ductus arteriosus 1–1.

In conclusion, pregnant women with cardiovascular CAs had a higher risk of acute infectious respiratory diseases and hypertension, while their fetuses had intrauterine fetal growth delay and higher risk for recurrence of cardiovascular CA confirming the results of our previous studies (IV, VI).

18.2 CA of the Uterus

This group of CA includes aplasia/agenesis/absence of uterus that excludes fertility. The hypoplasia is common but pregnancies help uterus to develop further. The major group of uterus CAs comprises the atavistic developmental disturbance of the Müllerian (paramesonephric) ducts which normally fuse caudally at the 8th postconceptional week of human embryos forming the uterus, the cervix, and the upper part of the vagina. However, a single defect of this developmental process avoids the caudal fusion of these ducts resulting in an incomplete atretic proximal vagina and rudimentary bicornuate uterus, or uterus unicornis, a uterus with only one functioning horn, the so-called Rokitansky sequence. In addition, doubling of the uterus, the cervix or even the vagina or in milder cases septum in the uterus may occur. The major manifestation of these CAs needs surgical corrections. The affected women have a very high (25–50%) risk for PB (Raga et al., 1997).

18.2.1 Results of the Study

Out of 22,843 cases, 57 (0.25%) were born to pregnant women with CA of their uterus. Among 38,151 controls without CA, 67 (0.18%) had mothers with this CA. All CAs of the uterus were prospectively and medically recorded in the prenatal maternity logbook but unfortunately the exact description/diagnosis of the CA was not mentioned in one-third of pregnant women, Uterus bicornis was recorded in 27 case mothers and 32 control mothers, in addition uterus unicornis and septus in 4 and 7 case mothers and in 6 case and 6 control mothers, respectively. The type of medical interventions (e.g. surgery) was not mentioned in most pregnant women.

The mean maternal age (26.5 vs. 25.5 year) was higher, while the mean birth order (1.6 vs. 1.8) was lower possibly indicating some previous pregnancy losses. The proportion of professional and managerial women was much higher among pregnant women who had CA of the uterus (65.7% vs. 38.5%) and had higher folic acid consumption (61.2% vs. 54.4%).

Among pregnancy complications, the incidence of threatened abortion (35.8% vs. 17.0%) was much higher, while the recorded incidence of threatened preterm delivery was only somewhat higher (22.4% vs. 14.3%). The incidence of influenza-common cold during the study pregnancy was also higher (37.3% vs. 18.3%) and the CA of the uterus was also associated with increased prevalence of acute infectious diseases of the urinary tract (10.4% vs. 6.0%). Among chronic diseases, the prevalence of hypertension (12.9% vs. 7.0%) and hemorrhoids (10.5% vs. 4.0%) was higher in pregnant women with uterus CA.

There was a lower proportion of boys by 10% among newborn infants without CA. In addition, the mean gestational age was much shorter (35.9 vs. 39.4 week) which associated with a much lower mean birth weight (2,365 vs. 3,276 g). Therefore, the rate of PB was 67.2% compared to the 9.2% in pregnant women without uterus CA as reference. The rate of LBW newborns was also much higher (44.8% vs. 5.7%).

The rate of total CAs showed a higher risk in the offspring of pregnant women with uterus CA explained mainly by the higher rate of multiple CAs, limb deficiencies and cardiovascular CAs (Table 18.1).

Of these 10 multimalformed cases, 7 had typical postural deformity association: congenital dislocation of hip + clubfoot 2, clubfoot + torticollis 2, depression in

Table 18.1 Estimation of risk for total and different CAs in the offspring of pregnant women with uterus CAs and in their matched controls

		Crude			
Study groups	Grand total *N*	No.	Percent	OR 95% CI	Adjusted[a] OR 95% CI
Controls	38,151	67	0.2	Reference	Reference
Isolated CAs					
Neural-tube defects	1,202	3	0.2	1.4 0.4–4.5	1.4 0.4–4.6
Hypospadias	3,038	6	0.2	1.1 0.5–2.6	1.2 0.5–2.8
Undescended testis	2,052	4	0.2	1.1 0.4–3.0	1.2 0.4–3.4
Cardiovascular CAs	4,480	13	0.3	1.7 0.9–3.0	*1.9 1.0–3.4*
Clubfoot	2,425	7	0.3	1.6 0.8–3.6	1.7 0.8–3.8
Limb deficiencies	548	3	0.6	3.1 0.9–10.0	*3.3 1.0–10.5*
Other isolated CAs	7,749	11[b]	0.1	0.8 0.4–1.5	0.9 0.5–1.7
Multiple CAs	1,349	10	0.7	3.8 1.9–7.7	*4.7 2.4–9.1*
Total	22,843	57	0.2	1.4 1.0–2.0	*1.5 1.1–2.2*

[a]OR adjusted for maternal age and employment status, birth order and folic use during the study pregnancy.

[b]Cleft palate 2, cleft lip 1, cleft lip + cleft palate 1, oesophageal atresia/stenosis 2, torticollis 2, cong. pyloric stenosis 1, rectal atresia 1, polydactyly 1.

skull + congenital dislocation of hip + clubfoot + torticollis 1, congenital dislocation of hip + clubfoot + torticollis 1, clubfoot + deformation of neck (torticollis?) + undescended testis 1. Of these 7 cases, 5 were preterm baby born on 26–37 gestational weeks with 800, 1,450, 1,800, 2,150 and 2,270 g birth weight. The other 3 multiple CAs included ventricular septal defect + clubfoot, microtia + cleft palate, cystic kidney + clubfoot. Thus, out of these 3 multimalformed children, 2 were affected with clubfoot.

There was a marginally higher risk of isolated limb deficiencies, unfortunately without specification of different types. One case had unimelic, two were affected with multimelic limb deficiencies.

There was also a marginally higher risk for isolated cardiovascular CAs explained by the unusual distribution of different types. Of these 13 cases, 6 were affected with persistent ductus arteriosus.

18.2.2 Interpretation of Results

Our population-based case-control study confirmed the well-known higher risk of PB in pregnant women with uterus CAs. However, the major finding of the study is the higher risk of multiple CAs particularly the so-called *postural deformity association* (VII) in the children of pregnant women with uterus CAs.

Deformation is a special manifestation of CAs due to mechanical causes and this group of CAs includes the major part of clubfoot, dislocation of the hip, torticollis, deformation of vertebral column, skull, face as the most typical manifestations of deformations. This study showed an association of uterus CAs in pregnant women with a higher risk of postural deformity association which is biologically plausible due to the anatomic configuration of these uterus CAs, i.e. the so-called Rokitansky sequence (1928). This sequence later was called as Rokitansky-Kuster-Hauser syndrome as well and sometimes associated with defects of other derivatives of the mesonephric ridge, such as renal agenesis, and vertebral and/or rib abnormalities (Jarcho, 1943; Anger et al., 1966; Winter 1968; Buttram and Gibbons, 1979; Buttram 1983; Ancien, 1993).

This anatomic defect associating with serious shape restriction of uterus explains the much higher rate of spontaneous abortions (Probst and Hill, 2000) and PB. The latter was confirmed in our study, while the higher rate of spontaneous abortion was shown indirectly by the lower proportion of males among newborns (i.e. a possible higher prenatal selection among them) and lower mean birth order (parity) of pregnant women with uterus CAs though they were elder. In addition these data were confirmed by the higher mean pregnancy order (2.1, including miscarriages beyond births) of case and control mothers with uterus CAs. The higher use of vitamin E is also an argument for the previous unsuccessful pregnancy outcomes.

The anatomic defect of uterus associates with the higher risk of both isolated deformation-type CAs and their associations well. Among isolated CAs, there were 7 cases with clubfoot and 2 cases with torticollis. Three cases with limb deficiencies were not specified but the so-called amniogenic type may associate with uterus CAs

(VIII). In addition it is necessary to remind that one of the most common deformation type CAs, congenital dysplasia/dislocation of the hip was excluded from the study due to the criteria of case selection in the HCCSCA. Among cardiovascular CAs the rate of persistent ductus arterious was 46.2% though the expected figure was 12.0%. However, persistent ductus arteriosus is more frequent in preterm babies but the diagnosis of this CA was accepted only after the third postnatal week in general and after the third postnatal month in preterm infants in the HCAR.

There is an unusual ratio of isolated and multiple CAs: 82.5%:17.5% in the study instead of the usual 94%:6%, because deformations prefer to associate with each other as postural deformity association. In addition a higher rate of isolated deformation-type CAs also occurred. There were 3 other multiple CAs and 2 had postural deformities (clubfoot) as component CA. One of these cases may be the Potter or oligohydramnios sequence due to the severe kidney disease. The second multimalformed case is a typical example for the previously introduced term "additive congenital abnormality pattern" (IX) when one isolated CA such as ventricular septal defect associated with clubfoot due to uterus CA.

Thus it is reasonable to suppose that there is an overlapping between postural deformity association in preterm babies and uterus CA in their mothers. The prevention/reduction of PB therefore may associate with the reduction of this postural deformity association entity as well.

The secondary results of the study were the detection of a higher risk of constipation and hemorrhoid in pregnant women with uterus CAs.

In conclusion there is an association between uterus CAs, mainly uni- or bicornuate uterus in pregnant women and a higher risk for postural deformities, mainly postural deformity association in their children.

18.3 Congenital Dislocation of the Hip

Congenital dislocation of the hip (CDH) was the most common CA in Hungary; about 1% of girls were affected with this CA (X, XI). However, due to the introduction of neonatal orthopedic screening based on the detection of Ortolani click in Hungary in 1973, most of these CAs were treated early. The origin of CHD can be explained by the multifactorial etiology (XII, XIII).

18.3.1 Interpretation of Data in the HCCSA

Out of 22,843 cases, 18 (0.08%), while out of 38,151 controls without CA, 30 (0.08%) had mothers with CDH. Only one-third of these pregnant women were recorded in the prenatal maternity logbook, thus most were reported by mothers in the questionnaire.

The mean maternal age (26.0 vs. 25.5 year) and birth order (1.6 vs. 1.7) was somewhat lower with a higher proportion of professional and managerial women (56.7% vs. 38.5%) and folic acid use (66.7% vs. 54.4%).

There was no difference in the occurrence of pregnancy complications, acute and chronic maternal diseases between pregnant women with or without CHD.

The mean gestational age was the same (39.4 week) and the mean birth weight (3,219 vs. 3,276 g) was similar in cases and controls. Thus the rate of PB (10.0% vs. 9.2%) and LBW newborns (6.7% vs. 5.7%) did also not show significant differences.

The risk for total CAs (0.7, 0.3–1.6) or any specific CA groups was not increased. The distribution of 18 CAs was the following: hypospadias 5 (2.1, 0.8–5.4), cardiovascular CAs 4, clubfoot 3, spina bifida cystica, cleft palate, atresia of the bile duct, renal agenesis, undescended testis, limb deficiency. However, it is a biased pattern because CDH with multifactorial origin associates with a high recurrence risk (XII) but cases with CDH were excluded from the data set of the HCCSCA.

In conclusion, CDH does not pose any risk for adverse birth outcomes.

18.4 Others

Spina bifida aperta/cystica is the most common manifestation of neural-tube defect in Hungary (of 2.78/1,000 informative offspring, 1.55) (XIV). There were only 2 controls in the HCCSCA; these two boys were born on the 36th and 40th gestational week with 2,630 and 3,750 g.

Congenital cerebral cyst was recorded in one pregnant women and her fetus was affected by occipital encephalocele.

CAs of the eye had heterogeneous manifestations and origin in pregnant women without recurrence. Seven cases were affected with different CAs (transposition of the great vessels, ventricular septal defect, cleft lip with cleft palate, oesophageal atresia, hypospadias, clubfoot, and exomphalos). Four controls were born in term (between the 39th and 41st gestational weeks) with birth weight of 2,790, 2,900, 3,350 and 3,550 g. These cases and controls were evaluated in details (XV).

CAs of the kidney occurred in 4 controls and they were born between the 37th and 41st gestational weeks with 3,735 g mean birth weight.

Scoliosis is also a group of heterogeneous entities, some of these CAs are caused by teratogenic agent or inherited, but most are called as adolescent idiopathic scoliosis with multifactorial origin and manifested mainly in teenage girls (XVI, XVII). There are 2 controls with intrauterine retardation (the boy was born on 42nd gestational week with 2,650 g, while the girl was born on the 40th gestational week with 2,750 g) and one case with hypospadias in the data set of the HCCSCA.

18.5 Conclusions

There is drastic improvement in the treatment and care of cases with CA thus their survival rate has increased significantly. Many of these affected females reach the reproductive age with a hope of babies, thus it is necessary to estimate their recurrence and other risks to help them to deliver healthy newborn infants.

References

Acien P. Reproductive performance of women with uterine malformations. Hum Reprod 1993; 8: 122–129.

Anger D, Hemet J, Ensel J. Forme familiale du syndrome de Rokitansky-Kuster-Hauser. Bull Fed Soc Gynecol Obstet Lang Fr 1966; 18: 229–236.

Buttram VC, Jr. Müllerian anomalies and their management, Fertil Steril 1983; 40: 159–166.

Buttram VC, Jr, Gibbons WE. Mullerian anomalies: a proposed classification (an analysis of 144 cases). Fertil Steril 1979; 32: 40–49.

Jarcho J. Malformations of the uterus. Review of the subjects, including embryology, comparative anatomy, diagnosis and report of cases. Am J Surg 1946; 71: 106–111.

Probst AM, Hill JA. Anatomic factors associated with recurrent pregnancy loss. Semin Reprod Med 2000; 18: 341–349.

Raga E, Bauset C, Remohi J et al. Reproductive impact of congenital Müllerian anomalies. Hum Reprod 1997; 12: 2277–2281.

Rokitansky K. Über sog. Verdoppeling des Uterus. Med Jahrb des Österreich Staates 1928; 26: 39–77.

Winter JSD. A familial syndrome of renal, genital, and middle ear anomalies. J Pediatr 1968; 72: 88–93.

Own Publications

I. Czeizel AE, Kamarás J, Balogh Ö, Szentpéteri J. Incidence of congenital heart defects in Budapest. Acta Paediatr Acad Sci Hung 1972; 13: 191–202.

II. Mészáros M, Nagy A, Czeizel AE. Incidence of congenital heart disease in Hungary. Hum Hered 1975; 25: 513–519.

III. Mészáros M, Czeizel AE. Point prevalence at birth of ventricular septal defect in Hungary. Acta Paediatr Acad Sci Hung 1978; 19: 51–54.

IV. Czeizel AE, Mészáros M. Two family studies of children with ventricular septal defectz. Eur J Paediatr 1981; 136: 81–85.

V. Mészáros M, Czeizel AE. ECG-conduction disturbance in the first-degree relatives of children with ventricular septal defect. Clin Genet 1981; 19: 298–301.

VI. Czeizel AE, Pornoi A, Péterffy E, Tarczal E. Study of children of parents operated on for congenital cardiovascular malformation. Br Heart J 1982; 47: 290–293.

VII. Pazonyi I, Kun A, Czeizel AE. Congenital postural deformity association. Acta Paediat Acad Sci Hung 1982; 23: 431–445.

VIII. Czeizel AE, Evans JA, Kodaj I, Lenz W. Congenital Limb Deficiencies in Hungary. Akadémiai Kiadó, Budapest, 1994.

IX. Czeizel AE. Additive congenital anomaly pattern. Am J Med Genet 1988; 29: 727–738.

X. Czeizel AE, Vizkelety T, Szentpéteri J. Congenital dislocation of the hip in Budapest, Hungary. Br J Prev Soc Med 1972; 26: 15–22.

XI. Czeizel AE, Szentpéteri J, Kellermann M. Incidence of congenital dislocation of the hip in Hungary. Br J Prev Soc Med 1974; 28: 265–267.

XII. Czeizel AE, Szentpéteri J, Tusnády G, Vizkelety T. Two family studies on congenital dislocation of the hip after early orthopedic screening in Hungary. J Med Genet 1975; 12: 125–130.

XIII. Czeizel AE, Tusnády G, Vaczó G. Vizkelety T. The mechanism of genetic predisposition in congenital dislocation of the hip. J Med Genet 1975; 12: 121–124.

XIV. Czeizel AE, Révész C. Major malformations of the central nervous system in Hungary. Br J Prev Soc Med 1970; 24: 205–222.

XV. Vogt G, Szunyogh M, Czeizel AE. Birth characteristics of different ocular congenital abnormalities. In Hungary. Ophthal Epidemiol 2006; 13: 159–166.
XVI. Bellyei Á, Czeizel AE, Barta O et al. Prevalence of adolescent idiopathic scoliosis in Hungary. Acta Orthop Scand 1977; 18: 177–180.
XVII. Czeizel AE, Bellyei Á, Barta O et al. Genetics of adolescent idiopathic scoliosis. J Med Genet 1978; 15: 424–442.

Part III
Summary of Results and Recommendations

Andrew E. Czeizel, Nándor Ács, and Ferenc G. Bánhidy

Chapter 19
Association of Maternal Diseases During Pregnancy with Higher Risk of Congenital Abnormalities (CAs) in Their Children

The systematic analysis of possible associations between maternal diseases and CAs revealed several known and some new findings. The objective of this chapter is to summarize them, to draw conclusions, and to define recommendations for the medical society.

19.1 High Fever Related Maternal Diseases During Pregnancy and CAs in Their Offspring

Out of 8 maternal infectious diseases or groups, 7 showed an increased risk for total CAs. However, this increase was explained by a higher risk of some specific CAs, and acute pelvic inflammatory disease associated only with a higher risk of cardiovascular CAs (Table 19.1). The common route of this maternal teratogenic effect may be the high fever. One of the main symptoms of these maternal diseases is high fever. There are three main arguments of the maternal-teratogenic effect of these high fever related maternal diseases: (i) these maternal diseases associated with some specific CAs; therefore one of the main rules of human teratology is that teratogens induce specific CA, was proved, (ii) the teratogenic effect of these fever related maternal disease was shown only in the critical period of these specific CAs, and (iii) the teratogenic effect of these high fever related maternal diseases was preventable by antipyretic drugs.

The human evidence for the teratogenicity of high fever is continuing to accumulate, although hyperthermia-induced CAs were detected first in animal investigations. Brinsmade and Rubsaamen (1957) produced fever by injecting milk on the 7th and 8th gestational days in pregnant rabbits, and found microcephaly or encephalocele in 3 of 65 embryos, this 4.6% rate was higher than in the offspring of untreated pregnant animals. Skreb and Frank (1963) immersed one uterine horn in water of 40 to 41°C for 40–60 min on the 8th to 16th gestational days of pregnant rats and produced neural-tube defects, cleft palate, CAs of eye and limbs. In addition, severe histological alterations of the central nervous system and high resorption rate were found in offspring. Hofmann and Dietzel (1966) also produced CAs of the central nervous system in rat fetuses by diathermy in their pregnant mothers.

N. Ács et al., *Congenital Abnormalities and Preterm Birth Related to Maternal Illnesses During Pregnancy*, DOI 10.1007/978-90-481-8620-4_19,

Table 19.1 Incidence of high fever related maternal diseases in II and/or III gestational month in case and control mothers and the risk for total CA-group (OR with 95% CI) and specified CAs

High fever related maternal diseases	Case mothers ($N = 22,843$) No.	%	Control mothers ($N = 38,151$) No.	%	Total OR	(95% CI)	Specified CAs with higher risk
Infectious diarrhea	82	0.36	70	0.18	3.1	(1.8–5.2)	CL ± CP, CLD, MCA
Orofacial herpes, recurrent	429	1.88	572	1.50	1.6	(1.3–1.9)	NTD, CL ± CP, CCM, CLD, MCA
Unspecified virus infections	80	0.35	49	0.13	3.7	(2.0–7.0)	NTD, CL ± CP
Common cold with secondary complications	3,827	16.75	3,455	9.06	1.4	(1.3–1.6)	CT, CL ± CP
Influenza	1,328	5.81	1,838	4.82	1.5	(1.3–1.7)	NTD, CT, CL ± CP, CP, CCM
Tonsillitis	674	2.95	1,165	3.05	1.2	(1.0–2.8)	NTD, CT, CL ± CP, MCA
Cholecystitis, complicated	109	0.48	145	0.38			NTD
Acute pelvic inflammatory diseases	87	0.38	15.8	0.41	1.0	(0.7–1.3)	CCM
Total	6,616	28.96	7,452	19.53		1.5 (1.2–2.2)	

CCM = cardiovascular malformation, CL ± CP = cleft lip ± cleft palate, CP = cleft palate, CLD = congenital limb deficiency, CT = congenital cataract, MCA = multiple CA, NTD = neural-tube defect.

The major contributor of this topic was M. J. *Edwards* (1967, 1969a, b, 1971, 1986; Edwards et al., 1995) who studied the teratogenic effect of 1 h daily exposure of guinea pigs to 43°C external temperature. Fetal deaths including resorption were common due to this treatment before the 18th day of gestation while 86% of the fetuses had multiple CAs including microcephaly, limb deficiencies, exomphalos, and renal agenesis. The major target of hyperthermia was the brain. Its maldevelopment caused a wide spectrum of functional and structural defects from prenatal growth retardation to CAs such as neural-tube defect. In addition, the secondary consequences of brain damage may be neurogenic contractures, i.e. arthrogryposis multiplex congenita. Webster and Edwards (1984) produced exencephaly by hyperthermia in mice. Harding and Edwards (1991) found a higher rate of microcephaly in rats exposed twice to 44°C for 10 min on days 13 and 14 of pregnancy.

In addition, Hartley et al. (1974) increased the body temperature to 40–41°C for 9 h daily in pregnant ewes and a high incidence of brain cavitation and microcephaly was found in their lambs. Kilham and Fern (1976) produced exencephaly by hyperthermia in hamster, while Sasaki et al. (1995) had rats swim in water at a temperature of 40.5°C for 3 min on 9 gestational day which resulted in the rectal temperature of these animals about 42°C and encephalocele, CAs of the eye, maxillary hypoplasia and gastroschisis were found in 69% of the offspring. Several experimental animal investigations showed an association between high body temperature in pregnant animals and a higher risk for behavioral and learning impairments of their offspring (Jonson et al., 1976; Shiota and Kayamura, 1989), but this topic is not presented here. However, it is necessary to mention that some animal investigations did not show an association between CAs and high temperatures (e.g. Buckiova and Brown, 1999).

Among human studies the teratogenic effect of hot tub and sauna bathing related hyperthermia (Chambers, 2006) are not shown here, only the possible association of high fever related maternal diseases with CAs mentioned in Table 19.1 is discussed here, although the teratogenic effect of hyperthermia was proved to have a role in the origin of other CAs as well such as microphthalmia (Fraser and Skelton, 1978), facial defects like micrognathia, midfacial hypoplasia, external ear CA, micropenis (due to LH deficiency), and neurogenic contractures (Smith et al., 1978; Jones, 2004). However, we know a limited number of human studies which were unable to find an association between hyperthermia and CAs (Kleinbrecht et al., 1979; Chambers et al., 1998).

19.1.1 Neural-Tube Defects (NTD)

Chance and Smith (1978) evaluated the pregnancy history of 43 women who gave birth to infants with meningomyelocele (i.e. spina bifida cystica) and 3 had fever over 38.9°C between the 25th and 28th day of gestation. Halperin and Wilroy (1978), in addition to Miller et al. (1978) found an association between high maternal temperature and higher risk for NTD. Clarren et al. (1979) showed a wide spectrum of CAs associated with hyperthermia depending on the time of febrile illness, if it occurred between 21st and 28th postconceptional days, NTD was found in approximately 10% of offspring. Layde et al. (1980) studied the possible association between maternal fever and NTD and found a significant increase in fever among mothers who delivered infants with spina bifida cystica. Fisher and Smith (1981) analyzed the pregnancy history based on personal interview in the mothers of 30 infants with major CAs of the central nervous system and 4 had high fever (1.5°C above normal) between the 20th and 28th gestational days. Shiota (1982) evaluated a collection of 113 embryos with NTD. Out of 50 embryos with anecephaly, 9 (18%), while in matched controls without CA only 4.9% had mothers with high fever. The difference was significant. Out of 63 embryos with myeloschisis (spina bifida cystica), 7 (11.1%) had mother with fever during pregnancy. Hunter (1984) studied 264 mothers who delivered infants with NTD, 229 women did not recall fever, 3 were unsure and 32 reported fever. Of these 32 women, 13 had fever during the first 4 weeks and 9 had newborns with anencephaly. The evaluation of large human materials later also confirmed the etiologic role of high fever related maternal disease in the origin of NTD (Milunsky et al., 1992; Lynberg et al., 1994). Shaw et al. (1998) found a higher risk for NTD (1.91, 1.35–2.72) in the offspring of pregnant women with febrile illnesses during the first trimester in a case-control population-based study.

Our previous studies also showed a strong association between high fever related maternal diseases and NTD in their offspring (Table 19.1). Out of these 8 infectious maternal diseases, 5 associated with a higher risk for NTD.

19.1.2 Microcephaly

Previous animal experiments studies indicated that microcephaly is one of the most sensitive outcomes in offspring of pregnant animals with high fever. Some human studies confirmed it, e.g. Smith et al. (1978) evaluated 13 infants born to mothers with hyperthermia during the first trimester in a retrospective study and all infants had some alteration in the development of central nervous system including 3 cases with microcephaly.This association was not so obvious in the data set of the HCCSCA due to the limited number of cases with primary microcephaly. However, we have found an association between fever related complications of acute appendicitis due to the delay of surgical intervention and higher risk for primary microcephaly.

19.1.3 Congenital Cataract

Smith et al. (1996) reported a high rate of cataract in the lens of guinea pig offspring exposed to temperatures of 2.5–3.5°C above normal core temperature for 60 min of varying times during pregnancy.

Vogt et al. (LXII in Chapter 1) showed a much higher risk for congenital cataract in the children of pregnant women with high fever related influenza-common cold with secondary complications and tonsillitis in the HCCSCA. However, the higher risk for congenital cataract was found not only in the critical period of this CA (i.e. the development of lens in II and III gestational months) but after this time window. Therefore, congenital cataract may be the result of high fever attack in the second and third trimesters of pregnancy as well.

19.1.4 Orofacial Clefts

There are two main manifestations of orofacial clefts: cleft lip with or without cleft palate (CL ± CP) and cleft palate only (CPO, this abbreviation is used if Robin sequence is excluded from this CA-group); however, it is necessary to differentiate isolated CL ± CP and CPO and multiple CL ± CP and CP when these CAs are the component of MCA-syndromes or unclassified multiple CAs. Here we discuss cases only with isolated orofacial clefts. As the data of Table 19.1 show there was a higher risk of CPO and particularly CL ± CP in the children of mothers with high fever related diseases during pregnancy. This association was presented first by Métneki et al. (XL in Chapter 1) in the population-based data set of the HCCSCA. A higher risk for CL ± CP was found in the children of pregnant women with influenza, common cold with secondary complications, tonsillitis, recurrent orofacial herpes (due to provoking high fever in the recurrence of this herpes disease), and infectious diarrhea.

19.1.5 Cardiovascular Malformations

The group of cardiovascular malformations is the most common major CA including several subgroups and types with heterogeneous origin. Miettinen et al. (1970) found a secular trend in the birth prevalence of coarctation of the aorta explained by seasonal changes of virus infections. Tikkanen and Heinonen (1994) reported an association between upper respiratory tract infection during the first trimester of pregnancy and hypoplastic left heart syndrome. Ferencz et al. (1997) found an association between maternal urinary tract infections and some types of cardiovascular CA, such as heterotaxies, transposition of the great vessels, and atrial septal defects in The Baltimore Washington Infant Study. Finally some studies indicated an association between cardiovascular CA and high fever during the critical period of these CAs (Tikkanen and Heinonen, 1991; Botto et al., 2001). Our hypothesis is that the cause of the possible association between recurrent orofacial herpes, influenza and acute pelvic inflammatory disease in early pregnancy and the higher risk for cardiovascular CAs, particularly atrial septal defect type II, may be the high fever which is characteristic for these maternal diseases (Table 19.1).

19.1.6 Congenital Limb Deficiencies

Congenital limb deficiencies (CLD) comprise several groups and types of deficiencies such as terminal (transverse and amniogenic), longitudinal (radial-tibial, ulnar-fibular, split hand ± foot), intercalary (phocomelia and femoral aplasia), in addition, it is worth differentiating uni- and multimelic CLD and, of course, isolated and multiple CLD. The previous Hungarian studies (LXXIII in Chapter 1) showed a higher risk of terminal transverse type CLD in the children of pregnant women with high fever related acute diseases of the respiratory system. The present analysis revealed an association of fever related infectious diarrhea with CLD as well (Table 19.1).

19.1.7 Multiple Congenital Abnormalities (MCAs)

To our best knowledge the higher risk for MCA in the offspring of pregnant women with high fever related diseases was shown first in the population-based data set of the HCCSCA (I), therefore, this topic is discussed here in detail.

The definition of MCA is a concurrence of two or more CAs in the same person affecting at least two different organ systems. Cases with CA were selected for the HCCSCA from the Hungarian Congenital Abnormality Registry (HCAR). MCAs had a special evaluation procedure in the HCAR as the most sensitive indicators of environmental (teratogenic and mutagenic) agents, and three groups of MCA cases were differentiated:

(1) Cases with notified *MCA-syndromes* caused by gene mutations, chromosomal aberrations, and teratogenic factors were excluded from this study.
(2) *MCA-associations* such as VACTERL, MURCS, CHARGE, Schisis, Postural deformity, GAM (*g*enital *a*nomalies of *m*ales) CA-associations with well-defined component CAs were also excluded from the study.
(3) *MCA cases with specified component CAs* but without the identification of MCA-syndromes and MCA-associations. These cases were evaluated critically according to the number (2, 3, 4, 5 or more) of component CAs (see Chapter 1). Minor anomalies were also evaluated in MCA cases, however, in the calculations of number of component CAs they were not considered.

The data set of the HCCSCA included 1,349 cases with MCA, 2,405 matched controls without CA and 21,494 malformed controls with isolated CA. Table 19.2 shows the birth characteristics of cases with MCA, controls, and malformed controls.

Stillbirths and elective abortions did not occur in the group of controls due to the selection criterion; therefore, ORs were not calculated. The proportion of stillbirths was larger in the group of cases with MCA compared to the group of malformed controls with isolated CA. The proportion of prenatally diagnosed and terminated malformed fetuses was low and similar in the case and malformed control groups because, as we mentioned previously, chromosomal aberrations were excluded from this analysis during the study period.

There was a male excess among the cases with MCA and their matched controls compared to the sex ratio of the Hungarian newborn population (about 51% of

Table 19.2 Pregnancy outcomes and birth characteristics of cases with MCA, controls, and malformed controls

	Cases with MCA (N = 1,349)		Controls (N = 2,405)			Malformed controls (N = 21,494)		
Variables	No.	%	No.	%	OR (95% CI)	No.	%	OR (95% CI)
Pregnancy outcomes								
Livebirth	1,288	95.5	2,405	100.0	–	21,054	97.9	0.4 (0.3–0.5)
Stillbirth[a]	55	**4.1**	0	0.0	–	342	1.6	**2.6 (2.0–3.5)**
Elective termination	6	0.4	0	0.0	–	98	0.5	1.0 (0.4–2.2)
Sex ratio, males	803	**59.5**	1,437	59.7	1.0 (0.9–1.1)	14,126	65.7	**0.8 (0.7–0.9)**
Birth outcomes								
Categorical[b]								
Preterm birth	394	**30.6**	252	10.5	**3.5 (3.0–4.2)**	3,216	15.3	**2.3 (2.1–2.6)**
Low birthweight	606	**47.1**	126	5.2	**14.9 (12.1–18.3)**	3,841	18.2	**3.7 (3.3–4.1)**
Quantitative[b]	Mean	S.D.	Mean	S.D.	Student t-test	Mean	S.D.	Student t-test
Gestational age (week)	**37.4**	4.6	39.3	2.0	$t = 14.6$, $\boldsymbol{p < 0.0001}$	38.7	3.4	$t = 10.4$, $p <$ **0.0001**
Birth weight (g)	**2,494**	797	3,279	504	$t = 32.6$, $\boldsymbol{p < 0.0001}$	3,005	699	$t = 22.9$, $p <$ **0.0001**

[a]Fetal death after the 28th gestational week, but this definition was changed to 24th gestational week in 1988.
[b]Without stillborn babies and electively terminated malformed fetuses.

males, it is not shown in Table 19.2). However, the proportion of males was significantly larger also in the group of malformed controls due to the high rates of CAs in male genital organs such as hypospadias and undescended testis.

The mean gestational age was the shortest in the case and the longest in the control group. These findings were in agreement with the rate of PB which was 2.0- and 2.9-fold higher in the case group than in the malformed and control groups, respectively. The mean birth weight was also much smaller in MCA cases compared to malformed controls and particularly controls. The proportion of LBW newborns in the case group was 2.6- and 9.1-fold larger than in the malformed and control groups, respectively. The data of controls corresponded well to the Hungarian newborn population.

The birth characteristics of cases with MCA confirmed the well-known experiences that MCA represent the most severe category of CAs with increased rate of stillbirths, PB, and LBW newborns.

The incidence of acute infectious diseases of mothers during pregnancy particularly during II and III gestational months were evaluated in the group of cases with MCA, controls, and malformed controls (Table 19.3).

Influenza and common cold with secondary complications, in addition to tonsillitis and recurrent orofacial herpes occurred more frequently during II and III month of pregnancy in case mothers than in control mothers. This association was seen only in common cold and tonsillitis at the comparison of case and malformed control mothers. High fever (38.5°C or more) was defined on the basis of the results of our previous studies. About 92% of pregnant women with influenza reported high fever, while 57% of pregnant women who had common cold with secondary complications informed us about high fever. The proportion of high fever was 47% in mothers with tonsillitis. Most recurrent orofacial herpes diseases were manifested after fever. The rate of rubella-virus infection was low and these 2 cases corresponded to the well-known rubella MCA-syndrome including eye CAs (cataract and microphthalmia) and cardiovascular CAs (patent ductus arteriosus and ventricular septal defect).

When evaluating only medically recorded acute diseases, the previously found association was confirmed in influenza, common cold, and tonsillitis but not in recurrent orofacial herpes in the comparison of case and control group.

Among chronic maternal diseases, the prevalence of diabetes mellitus and migraine was higher in case mothers than in control and malformed control mothers (Table 19.3). Of course, these associations are not connected with high fever.

The major finding of our study is that high fever related diseases such as influenza, common cold with secondary complications, tonsillitis, and recurrent orofacial herpes are associated with a higher risk for MCA. These fever related illnesses during II and/or III gestational months increased the risk for MCA by 2.3-fold (I).

Previous studies showed the association between high fever-related diseases and isolated CAs. Only two studies indicated an association between high fever and a specified MCA-syndrome. Graham et al. (1988) reported 3 infants with Moebius syndrome born to mothers with hyperthermia in the late first or early second trimester of pregnancy. Lipson et al. (1989) also evaluated cases with Moebius syndrome (or sequence, although recently the name oromandibular-limb hypogenesis

Table 19.3 Occurrence of maternal diseases in the study groups

Maternal diseases	Cases with MCA ($N = 1{,}349$)				Controls ($N = 2{,}405$)				Comparison of entire pregnancy	Malformed controls ($N = 21{,}494$)				Comparison of entire pregnancy
	II–III months		Total		II–III months		Total			II–III months		Total		
Acute	No.	%	No.	%	No.	%	No.	%	OR[a] (95% CI)	No.	%	No.	%	OR[b] (95% CI)
Influenza	29	2.2	78	5.8	27	1.1	121	5.0	**2.1 (1.2–3.8)**	425	2.0	1,250	5.8	1.1 (0.8–1.6)
Common cold	108	8.0	281	20.8	100	4.2	336	14.0	**2.2 (1.6–2.9)**	1,228	5.7	3,546	16.5	**1.5 (1.2–1.8)**
Respiratory system														
Sinusitis	5	0.4	12	0.9	6	0.3	16	0.7	1.6 (0.5–5.5)	54	0.3	129	0.6	1.5 (0.6–3.8)
Tonsillitis	29	2.2	51	3.8	23	1.0	67	2.8	**2.2 (1.3–3.9)**	216	1.0	623	2.9	**2.2 (1.5–3.3)**
Pharyngitis	12	0.9	34	2.5	10	0.4	55	2.3	2.1 (0.8–5.3)	199	0.9	607	2.8	1.0 (0.5–1.7)
Laryngitis–tracheitis	8	0.6	25	1.9	18	0.8	54	2.3	0.8 (0.3–1.9)	139	0.7	379	1.8	0.9 (0.5–1.9)
Bronchitis–bronchiolitis	10	0.7	32	2.4	7	0.3	26	1.1	2.4 (0.9–6.7)	104	0.5	307	1.4	1.5 (0.8–3.0)
Pneumonia	3	0.2	12	0.9	5	0.2	12	0.5	1.3 (0.3–5.7)	34	0.2	104	0.5	1.4 (0.4–4.5)
Digestive system														
Infectious diarrhea	3	0.2	6	0.4	3	0.1	7	0.3	2.3 (0.4–12.1)	29	0.1	76	0.4	1.7 (0.1–5.6)
Urinary tract	21	1.6	102	7.6	34	1.4	156	6.5	1.3 (0.7–2.3)	336	1.6	1,487	6.9	1.0 (0.6–1.5)
Genital organs	34	2.5	106	7.9	54	2.3	178	7.4	1.1 (0.7–1.8)	439	2.0	1,570	7.3	1.3 (0.9–1.8)
Orofacial herpes	15	1.1	36	2.7	11	0.5	36	1.5	**2.9 (1.3–6.4)**	148	0.7	393	1.8	1.7 (0.9–2.8)
Rubella	2	0.2	4	0.3	1	0.0	3	0.1	3.2 (0.7–14.7)	7	0.0	28	0.1	2.4 (0.8–6.7)
Chickenpox	2	0.2	3	0.2	0	0.0	4	0.2	1.4 (0.3–6.7)	7	0.0	28	0.1	1.7 (0.5–5.7)

Table 19.3 (continued)

Maternal diseases	Cases with MCA ($N = 1{,}349$) II–III months		Total		Controls ($N = 2{,}405$) II–III months		Total		Comparison of entire pregnancy	Malformed controls ($N = 21{,}494$) II–III months		Total		Comparison of entire pregnancy
Chronic														
Diabetes mellitus	8	0.6	9	0.7	1	0.0	3	0.1	**4.5 (1.1–17.8)**	53	0.3	70	0.3	**2.1 (1.0–4.1)**
Epilepsy	4	0.3	5	0.4	5	0.2	5	0.2	1.4 (0.4–4.8)	62	0.3	71	0.3	1.1 (0.4–2.8)
Migraine	29	2.2	47	3.5	30	1.3	50	2.1	**1.6 (1.1–2.4)**	386	1.8	518	2.4	**1.5 (1.1–2.0)**
Hypertension	7	0.5	35	2.6	18	0.8	71	3.0	0.9 (0.6–1.4)	139	0.7	542	2.5	1.0 (0.7–1.4)
Varicose veins of lower extremities	7	0.5	26	1.9	10	0.4	48	2.0	0.9 (0.5–1.4)	80	0.4	306	1.4	1.4 (0.9–2.0)
Hemorrhoids	9	0.7	28	2.1	20	0.8	82	3.4	0.6 (0.4–0.9)	124	0.6	541	2.5	0.8 (0.6–1.2)

[a]OR = odds ratios adjusted for maternal age, birth order, maternal employment, and marital status in conditional logistic regression model.
[b]OR = odds ratios adjusted for maternal age, birth order, maternal employment, and marital status in unconditional logistic regression model.

spectrum was suggested for this CA-entity). Out of 15 cases, 2 mothers had high fever in the 7–8th gestational weeks. The third case-control study showed that 14% of cases with Schisis-association had mothers with high fever during pregnancy and this figure was only 6% in their matched controls in Hungary (IV in Chapter 1).

However, as far as we know, the possible association between high fever and MCA has not been published. Previously the *hyperthermia-induced spectrum of CAs* (HISCA) included isolated CAs such as NTD, microcephaly, microphthalmia, facial CAs such as micrognathia and midfacial hypoplasia, CP, CAs of the external ears, neurogenic contractures, and micropenis were described. However, as Jones (2004) stated "much more investigation is required".

Therefore, the spectrum of the HISCA was checked in the data set of the HCCSCA and the delineation of the maternal high fever related MCA-syndrome based on the specific pattern of the component CAs was attempted (II).

Our data set included 1,349 cases with MCA, among them 181 cases were born to mothers with one of four high fever-related diseases such as influenza, common cold with secondary complications, tonsillitis, and recurrent orofacial herpes during II and/or III months of gestation. These 181 MCA cases had 498 component CAs.

In the first step the *observed number* of component CAs of MCA cases was compared with their *expected number* based on the data set of the HCCSCA. The observed number was significantly higher (showed a "cluster") in 4 component CAs: *microphthalmia* (MPH), *indeterminate sex or pseudohermaphroditism* (ISP), *arthrogryposis-neurogenic contractures* (ANC) and CL $\pm$ CP.

In the second step, the so-called *pairwise analysis of component CA pairs in MCA cases* (VIII in Chapter 1) showed a possible association between high fever-related maternal diseases during II and/or III gestational months and two schisis-type CAs: NTD (including anencephaly, spina bifida aperta, encephalocele, and craniorachischisis) and orofacial clefts (including CL $\pm$ CP and CP) (Table 19.4).

The proportion of cases with Schisis MCA-association was 0.5% in MCA cases of the HCCSCA; however, their proportion was 6.6% among 181 MCA cases born

Table 19.4 Number of MCA cases with the combination of two schisis-type CAs (NTD and CL $\pm$ CP or CP = OFC) and other high fever-related CAs of the so-called hyperthermia-induced spectrum CA (HISCA)

	Cases		
Component CA	No.	%	Abbreviation and number of HISCA
NTD + OFC	12	46.2	–
NTD + HISCA	3	7.7	MPH 1, ISP 1, ANC 1
OFC + HISCA	9	34.6	MPH 1, ISP 1, ANC 7
NTD + OFC + HISCA	3	11.5	ISP, ANC 2
Total	26	100.0	

NTD = neural-tube defect; MPH = microphthalmia; OFC = orofacial cleft; ANC = arthrogryposis-neurogenic contracture; HISCA = high fever-related spectrum CAs ISP = indeterminate sex and pseudohermaphroditism.

to mothers with high fever-related disorders during II and/or III gestational months. The combination of two schisis-type CAs such as NTD and CL ± CP or CP as cardinal symptoms of HISCA associated with MPH, ANC, ISP in 15 cases. Therefore, these 26 MCA cases represented 14.4% of 181 MCA cases studied.

Furthermore CAs of the external ear, face (micrognathia, midfacial hypoplasia), and microcephaly, i.e. component CAs of HISCA were combined with the previously mentioned CAs of HISCA in further 8 cases. Thus, the delineation of the so-called "*HI-MCA syndrome*" (II) was based on the combination of two schisis-type CAs and six other CAs (ANC, ISP, MPH, microcephaly, CAs of the external ear and face) (Fig. 19.1) and this HI-MCA syndrome was identified in 34 (18.8%) cases, i.e. about one fifth of 181 MCA cases.

In conclusion, HI-MCA syndrome showed a strong association with high fever maternal diseases ($p < 0.0001$) and these 34 cases represented 2.5% of 1,349 MCA cases in the HCCSCA.

The major part of MCAs is not delineated as MCA-syndromes or MCA-associations and the origin of these MCA cases are mostly unknown. Only about 25% of MCAs can be explained by random combination of component CAs (LXXVII in Chapter 1). The rest is still undelineated, therefore, we have to do our best to delineate as many MCA-syndromes as possible and identify their origin to effectively prevent these abnormalities CAs. HI-MCA syndromes may be responsible for about 2.5% of all MCAs.

After the recognition of the high fever induced isolated CAs and HI-MCA syndrome, we have a chance for their prevention by antipyretic therapy (III). On the other hand, the knowledge of high fever induced CAs may help us to suggest specific ultrasound scanning at the 20th gestational week in pregnant women affected by high fever-related diseases in their early pregnancy.

In conclusion, maternal fever-related illnesses during the critical period of some CAs may induce specific isolated CAs and a specific pattern of HI-MCA syndrome (Fig. 19.1).

Animal investigations produced important data regarding to the mechanism of teratogenic effect of hyperthermia. Edwards (1967, 1969a, b) showed that maternal hyperthermia of 1.5°C above normal tended to stop the growth of neuronal mitotic cells in the ependymal layer of the developing brain, and elevation of 3.0°C or more tended to kill these cells. Cockroft and New (1978) found that the temperature of 40°C reduced both the size and protein content of the brain of rat embryos. Mirkes (1985) studied the association between the duration and degree of temperature and cell necrosis in the central nervous system of rat embryos. Necrosis was found after 60 min at 42°C and after 2–4 h at 41°C. German et al. (1985) showed that an elevation of temperature for 1 h at 2.5°C was the threshold of teratogenesis in rats immersed in water. Shiota (1988) found a brief period of decreased mitoses followed by a burst of activity in the central nervous system of mouse embryos exposed to high temperature by immersing their mothers into hot water. With a 42°C at 10 min, no increase in CAs was found, but at 15 min, 31% of embryos had CAs. Rao et al. (1990) reported that in the nerve tissue culture from rat embryos exposed to hyperthermia had a significantly lower level of acetylcholine. Mirkes (1997) described the molecular/cellular biology of the heat stress response and its role in agent-induced

CAs (structural birth defects)

	Brain	Eye	Face
Cardinal schisis type CA:	NTD		CL±CP or PCO
	Microcephaly	Microphthalmia	Other facial CAs,
	Neurogenic contractures	Cataract	(micrognathia, Moebius syndrome,
	CAs of the male genital organs due to luteal hormone (LH) deficiency		midfacial hypoplasia)
			External CAs of the ear

Functional deficits:

Mental deficiency

Hypotonia – hypotonic diplegia

Seizures

NTD = neural-tube defects

CL±CP = cleft lip with or without cleft palate

CPO = cleft palate only

Fig. 19.1 The spectrum of high fever related CAs and the delineation of high fever related multiple congenital abnormality (HI-MCA) syndrome

teratogenesis. Umpierre et al. (2001) investigated mouse embryos exposed to hyperthermia and found that the increased number of cells undergoing apoptosis localized caspase-3 and demonstrated extensive DNA fragmentation. Little and Mirkes (2003) studied the induction of heat shock apoptosis in whole rat embryo culture and found that one or more of the pro-apototic proteins regulate the cytochrome C efflux (NOXA, PUMA, and DP5).

Finally, one animal study indicated the importance of genetic predisposition in the teratogenic effect of hyperthermia. Lundberg et al. (2003) crossed and backcrossed different mice strains and they showed that the highest exencephaly rate was found after maternal exposure to hyperthermia (bath water at 43°C for 10 min) on E8.5 SWV/Fnn (SWV) × SWV mice. These findings help us to understand why only a small proportion of offspring is affected with specific CA in mothers with high fever related diseases during pregnancy.

19.1.8 Conclusions

Both animal investigations and human studies indicated the role of high fever related maternal diseases in the origin of some specific CAs; however, the timing and duration, in addition to the severity of maternal hyperthermia are also important.

1. There is no doubt that temperature over 40°C has teratogenic effect; however, the teratogenic effect threshold is very likely to be at 38.5°C.
2. Based on human experiences one or more days seem to be the critical duration of hyperthermia.

3. The timing of hyperthermia determines the risk for specific CAs. If the neuronal cell population cannot recover from the antimitotic insult and heat stress response of hyperthermia, mainly the development of the brain is affected. If it occurs during the time of neural tube closure (i.e. between 21st and 28th postconceptional days, i.e. third postconceptional week), there is a higher risk for NTD. Severe hyperthermia between 4th and 6th gestational week can associate with a higher risk for CL ± CP, microphthalmia, cardiovascular CA, congenital limb deficiencies, and HI-MCA syndrome. Hyperthermia between the 7th and 14th gestational weeks can disturb the fusion of palate (i.e. CP), in addition, it may induce other facial or ear CAs and spinal cord morphogenesis with neurogenic contractures (e.g. arthrogryposis) related functional defects such as hypotonia. Finally, higher risk for congenital cataract may associate with high fever related maternal diseases during any time of pregnancy.
4. High fever can induce both isolated CAs and HI-MCA syndrome, probably the spectrum of high fever induced spectrum of component CAs in this HI-MCA syndrome depends on the severity and time of fever. It is possible that the spectrum of isolated CAs and component CAs of this HI-MCA syndrome will be expanded in the future. However, here it is worth stressing that high fever can induce both isolated and multiple CAs.
5. Last but not least high fever related CAs are preventable by specific (e.g. influenza vaccination) and general (antipyretic drugs) medical interventions (III).

19.2 Confirmed Associations of Maternal Diseases with CA

Our studies confirmed some previously found associations between maternal diseases and CA.

19.2.1 Diabetes Mellitus, Type 1

The risk of CAs in the offspring of pregnant women with overt *diabetes mellitus* (DM) prior to conception was estimated 4- to 8-fold higher based on a meta-analysis of several studies. This high risk was explained by the teratogenic effect of hyperglycemia in the first trimester because there is no higher risk of CA in the children of diabetic fathers, normoglycemic pregnant women and women with gestational diabetes if its onset was after the first trimester. Another important argument for the teratogenic effect of DM is that this maternal disease associated with a specific spectrum of CAs such as neural-tube defects, cardiovascular CAs (particularly transposition of the great vessels, double outlet right ventricle, and common truncus), kidney CA (renal a/dysgenesis), CAs of the urinary tract, congenital limb deficiency (mainly the aplasia of femoral head), and CAs of the skeletal system (CAs of the spines). In addition, *caudal dysplasia sequence* may occur in the offspring of pregnant women. Caudal dysplasia sequence includes cardinal primary CA of the caudal region, i.e. the incomplete development of the sacrum which is often associated with the CA of the lumbar vertebrae (sometimes with typical spina bifida aperta) and CA (a/hypoplasia) of the femoral head, renal a/dysgenesis, and imperforate anus with the secondary consequences of the primary CAs like clubfoot, flexion or abduction deformity of the hips, popliteal webs, in addition to incontinence of urine and feces due to neurologic impairment of the distal spinal cord.

DM type 1 (DM-I) with insulin treatment, *DM type 2* (DM-II) in general without insulin treatment and *gestational diabetes* (GDM) with the onset during the study pregnancy were differentiated in the data set of the HCCSCA. There was no higher risk for CA in the children of pregnant women with DM-II and GDM. The total (birth + fetal) prevalence of different CAs was 1.5-fold higher in the group of DM-I explained by a higher risk of some specific types/groups of CAs in their offspring. Three isolated CA groups (renal a/dysgenesis, obstructive CA of the urinary tract, and cardiovascular CA) and multiple CA occurred more frequently. Out of 9 multiple CAs, 4 (44.4%) were diagnosed as caudal dysplasia sequence.

Our study showed a relatively lower risk for specific CAs (1.5-fold instead of the previous 4- to 8-fold) suggesting that appropriate antidiabetic medical management including insulin and oral antidiabetics of diabetic pregnant women can reduce the risk in their offspring (see later). Another argument for the recent progress in specific medical care of diabetic pregnant women is that 71.4% of cases with diabetes related CAs was born in the 1980s. Finally, our study first showed that recent periconceptional high dose (in general 6 mg) folic acid or folic acid-containing multivitamin supplementation may contribute to the reduction or prevention of some specific diabetes related CAs. Our hope is that the reduction of previously found increased risk for neural-tube defects, spine CAs, and congenital limb deficiencies is explained mainly by folic acid supplementation.

In conclusion, the maternal teratogenic effect of DM-I can reduce by appropriate periconceptional and prenatal care.

19.2.2 Epilepsy

About 45% of epileptic pregnant women have a higher seizure frequency explained partly by the decreasing serum levels of antiepileptic drugs during pregnancy. Most epileptic pregnant women therefore need treatment during pregnancy as well, sometimes with an increase in dosage to maintain the effective plasma level of antiepileptic drugs. When selecting antiepileptic drugs the type of epilepsy is the most important factor, however, the teratogenic effect of the antiepileptic drugs should also be considered.

Previous studies showed about 3-fold higher risk of CA in the offspring of epileptic pregnant women and this increased risk for CAs was related to the teratogenic potential of the applied antiepileptic drugs. However, the cluster of seizures in pregnant women without appropriate treatment induces an even higher risk for CAs. Different type of antiepileptic drugs have different risks and spectrums of CAs but the most important fact is that monotherapy associates with lower risk (2.8) than polytherapy (4.2). Certain specific CAs such as CL ± CP, CP, cardiovascular CA, and NTD have a higher risk, and higher dose of antiepileptic drugs associates with a higher risk for specific CAs.

Our data confirmed the higher risk of NTD, CL ± CP, CP, and cardiovascular CA after the use of antiepileptic drugs, but a higher risk for oesophageal atresia/stenosis was also found in the offspring of epileptic pregnant women. Polytherapy always showed a higher risk than monotherapy. Our data indicated the teratogenic effect of trimethadione, primidone, sultiame, valproate, phenytoin, mephenytoin but could not confirm phenobarbital and diazepam as teratogenic agents.

The main result of our studies was that association between antiepileptic drugs and CAs tended to be lower among pregnant women who took folic acid supplement in early pregnancy compared to mothers who did not receive this supplementation (see Subchapter 19.4).

In conclusion, epileptic pregnant women have a higher risk for some CAs. Nevertheless, at present, pregnancy of epileptic women does not need to be discouraged if they wish to have babies; however, specific and high standard care is necessary.

19.2.3 Infectious Teratogenic and Fetopathogenic Agents

Rubella-virus is important from both historical and medical aspect in human teratology because this virus was the first proved infectious teratogenic agent in 1941 and the introduction of rubella vaccination was the first and good example of primary prevention of a specific CA-entity, i.e. rubella MCA-syndrome.

In Hungary 10.6% of females were seronegative before the first pregnancy, thus only 32 cases with different CA were evaluated in the HCCSCA and only one part of these CAs had association with maternal rubella infection/disease during the study pregnancy (however, deafness could not be diagnosed immediately after birth in Hungary during the study period). Out of 4 multiple CAs, three had typical *rubella CA-syndrome* (microphthalmia-congenital cataract + patent ductus arteriosus-ventricular septal defect with or without microcephaly) in newborns of pregnant women with rubella infection in their II and/or III gestational months. Among 28 cases with isolated CAs, microcephaly occurred in 4, patent ductus arteriosus in 4, ventricular septal defect in 3, and complex cardiovascular CAs (ventricular + atrial septal defects and ventricular septal defect + patent ductus arteriosus) in 2 cases and these CAs may associate with rubella infection due to the time of exposure. All cases were born before the introduction of rubella vaccination in Hungary in 1989.

In conclusion, rubella virus is a good example demonstrating that teratogens induce specific CAs and particularly MCA-syndrome, and it is important to know that this severe CA-entity is preventable.

The *varicella zoster virus* infection of pregnant women may associate with a low risk (about 1%) of congenital anomaly in their fetuses. Maternal antibodies due to previous infection or vaccination usually protect the fetus. The affection of the fetus is not a MCA-syndrome; therefore, we use the term *fetal varicella disease*. The latter is explained by the critical period of fetal varicella disease, which is between 10th and 21st gestational (i.e. 8th and 19th postconceptional) weeks. The symptoms of fetal varicella disease are the consequence of fetal varicella skin lesions which consist of cuteneous scars and secondary limb hypoplasia (caused by the massive scars of skin on the flexible, developing bones) and anomalies of auricles (e.g. microtia).

The data of the HCCSCA showed an increasing trend of fetal varicella disease during the study period. Out of 31 cases, 28 were isolated and 3 had multiple CAs. Of these 28 isolated CAs, 3, while of the 3 multiple CAs, two were considered as fetal varicella disease due to the symptoms of infants and the time of maternal infection during the study pregnancy.

The risk of fetal varicella disease is low; however, this low fetal risk causes serious anxiety in pregnant women. Thus it is very important to stress that fetal varicella disease is preventable by vaccination which is available as attenuated virus vaccine.

In conclusion, an important task is to clarify previous varicella disease in the history of every woman in the preconceptional period because the administration of varicella vaccine is recommended in prospective pregnant women with seronegativity or unsure history of varicella.

Cytomegalovirus (CMV) is very large therefore its transplacental transmission in general does not attack the embryo before the 12th gestational week. Fetuses could be infected during the last two trimesters but the highest risk for the so-called *fetal cytomegalovirus disease* (FCD) is expected after the primary infection of CMV between IV and VI gestational months. The most obvious symptoms of FCD are microcephaly and intrauterine growth retardation at birth, completed by chorioretinitis, optic atrophy (blindness), hepatosplenomegalia with hyperbilirubinemia, i.e. jaundice after birth.

There were 16 (0.07%) cases born to mothers with CMV infection in the data set of the HCCSCA, 6 were affected with cardiovascular CAs, all other CAs occurred only once. Among them one case with microcephaly and one case with multiple CA including microcephaly and unspecified eye CA that are worth mentioning because they may fit into the diagnostic criteria of FCD.

In conclusion, the ascertainment of cases with FCD due to the lack of specific symptoms of maternal infection/disease and unspecific anomalies in newborn infants is difficult; therefore, its diagnosis occurred rarely in the HCCSCA.

Syphilis is caused by the spirochete *Treponema pallidum*. After the introduction of penicillin in the 1940s, syphilis has become treatable and *fetal syphilis disease* is preventable in the offspring of infected pregnant women. In Hungary all pregnant women are screened for syphilis at the first visit in the prenatal care clinics, and positive cases are treated. Thus typical fetal syphilis disease was not recorded in the data set of HCCSCA. Only 3 cases with coincidental isolated microcephaly, ventricular septal defect, and renal dysgenesis, respectively, were born to pregnant women with syphilis in the data set of the HCCSCA.

In conclusion, fetal syphilis disease is extremely rare in Hungary.

Toxoplasmosis is caused by a parasite: *Toxoplasma gondii*, the host of this parasite is the cat. The sexual cycle of *T. gondii* happens in the intestinal tract of cats; therefore, the main source of infection is coccidian oocysts in the feces of cats.

Fetal toxoplasmosis (i.e. a fetal disease) may occur after the primary infection of pregnant women after the first trimester. The large parasites cannot cross the placenta before the 14th gestational week and fetal immunocompetence develops after this period when the fetal immune system can react with inflammatory disease of this infection. After the primary infection of pregnant women about 40% of fetuses get infected. However, the classical tetrad of fetal toxoplasmosis as symptoms of fetal meningoencephalitis: (i) chorioretinitis, (ii) periventricular calcification, (iii) secondary microcephaly or hydrocephaly (ventriculomegaly), and (iv) seizures, paresis, mental retardation can be diagnosed only in a minor part of these infants after birth.

There were 35 cases in the data set of the HCCSCA who had mothers with suspected toxoplasma infection during the study pregnancy. However, the distribution of CAs did not show characteristic pattern, only 2 cases with hydrocephalus and out of 3 cases with multiple CA, two may have some association with fetal toxoplasmosis.

In conclusion, suspected toxoplasmosis in pregnant women is associated with a higher risk for fetal toxoplasmosis; however, identification of these cases is difficult in clinical practice.

19.2.4 Cardiovascular CAs in Pregnant Women

Among different major CAs, cardiovascular CAs represent the most common CA-group with about 1% prevalence at birth in Hungary. Recently the life-expectancy of these patients has increased significantly due to cardio-surgical interventions; therefore the number of pregnant women with cardiovascular CAs is increasing (Tennant et al., 2010). Most cardiovascular CAs have multifactorial (polygenic predisposition with triggering environmental factors) origin therefore a recurrence risk is expected.

In the HCCSCA 32 (0.14%) pregnant women with different cardiovascular CAs were recorded and 12 had children with cardiovascular CA (2.4, 1.1–5.6) while other CA-groups did not show increased risk in the offspring of pregnant women with cardiovascular CAs.

In conclusion, the higher risk for recurrence of cardiovascular CAs in the children of affected mothers was confirmed.

19.2.5 Conclusions

The population-based HCCSCA was appropriate to confirm the teratogenic/fetopathogenic effect of some previously known maternal diseases, to check the efficacy and progress of their medical management. In addition, these data helped us to better understand the difficulties in the diagnosis of some infectious agents during pregnancy.

Three groups of unexpected associations between maternal diseases during pregnancy and higher risk of CAs in their offspring are differentiated: (i) associations with reasonable etiological hypothesis, (ii) strong associations without plausible explanation, and (iii) weak associations with or without plausible hypothesis.

19.3 Unexpected Association of Maternal Disease During Pregnancy With Higher Risk of CAs in Their Children But With Reasonable Etiological Hypothesis

19.3.1 Migraine

The primary event of migraine attack is the release of neuroinflammatory peptides such as serotonin 5-hydroxytriptamine in response to stressors both in peripheral and central portions of the trigeminal nerve. The release of these peptides causes vasoconstriction and later, after the drop of their levels, vasodilatation which induces pain around the temples and eyes.

Migraine is among the most frequent chronic diseases and it is more common among females than males. The typical onset of migraine is between 10 and 30 years of age, therefore migraine occurs frequently in pregnant women as well. The possible teratogenic/fetotoxic effects of antimigraine drugs during pregnancy have been evaluated frequently but the possible hazard of underlying maternal disease, e.g. migraine was studied only in one clinical study but higher rate of CAs was not found.

In the data set of the HCCSCA 565 (2.5%) pregnant women with migraine during the study pregnancy had children with CA (1.3, 1.2–1.5). The risk of congenital limb deficiencies in children born to mothers with medically recorded maternal migraine during II and/or III gestational months of the study pregnancy was higher (2.7, 1.1–6.5). Most cases of this CA group had terminal transverse type limb deficiencies and this association cannot be explained by related drug treatments or other confounders.

The critical period of unimelic terminal transverse type congenital limb deficiencies is between the 4th and 9th gestational week and it is caused by vascular disruption. The pathogenesis of migraine attacks also involves vascular effects, thus the higher risk of unimelic terminal transverse limb deficiency in children born to pregnant women with severe migraine attacks during II and/or III months of gestation can be explained by available scientific findings.

In conclusion, a higher occurrence of congenital limb deficiencies was found in infants born to mothers with severe migraine during II and/or III gestational month.

19.3.2 Paroxysmal Supraventricular Tachycardia

Among cardiac dysrhythmias, paroxysmal supraventricular tachycardia occurred most frequently. Of 45 cases with different CAs born to mothers affected with paroxysmal supraventricular tachycardia, 25 (55.5%) had cardiovascular CAs (2.1,

1.2–3.7). However, the distribution of these cardiovascular CAs was very interesting, because 12 cases (48.0%) had ventricular septal defect and 8 (32.2%) were affected with atrial septal defect, type II, i.e. cardiac septal defect. When these cases were compared with their matched controls, a strong association was found in cases with ventricular septal defect (2.8, 1.4–4.4) and particularly in cases with atrial septal defect, type II (5.6, 2.8–14.4) with maternal paroxysmal supraventricular tachycardia. The critical period of ventricular septal defect and atrial septal defect, type II is in II and/or III gestational months, and 8 and 7 mothers of cases with ventricular septal defect and atrial septal defect, type II, respectively, had mothers with paroxysmal supraventricular tachycardia during this time window.

Thus intraventricular conduction disturbance may be a subthreshold sign of septal defect in mothers which may be manifested as septal CA in their children.

19.3.3 Ovarian Follicular Cysts

Ovary may have different cysts; ovarian follicular cysts were evaluated in the study.

In the data set of the HCCSCA 54 (0.24%) case pregnant women were reported with medically recorded preconceptional ovarian follicular cysts. Among drugs only clomiphene showed a higher usage (29.4%) in these pregnant women.

Only neural-tube defects (NTD) were associated with ovarian follicular cysts (3.2, 1.0–10.4). However, of these 7 cases with NTD, 3 were born to mothers with ovarian follicular cysts and clomiphene treatment together. In the HCCSCA 67 (0.29%) case pregnant women had medically recorded inadvertent clomiphene treatment in I and II gestational month. Again only NTD showed an association with clomiphene (6.4, 1.3–31.4).

However, the detailed analysis of these pregnant women showed an obvious interaction among clomiphene treatment, ovarian follicular cysts, and NTD. The association between clomiphene treatment and ovarian follicular cysts is well-known due to hyperstimulation. The possible association between clomiphene treatment and NTD was shown in some papers but debated in others. Our data show that the predisposition for ovarian follicular cysts due to clomiphene may have some role in the origin of NTD. The higher rate of NTD in the offspring of mothers with clomiphene treatment cannot be explained only by the use of this drug, it needs maternal sensitivity for ovarian follicular cysts as well. Thus the predisposition for ovarian follicular cysts in women and NTD in the offspring may be related to pharmacogenetic susceptibility to clomiphene.

In conclusion, women with infertility have a higher risk for some CAs and this study showed an association between infertility, clomiphene treatment, ovarian follicular cysts in women, and a higher risk of NTD in their offspring.

19.3.4 CAs of the Uterus

The developmental defect of caudal fusion of the Müllerian (paramesonephric) ducts results in an incomplete atretic proximal vagina and rudimentary bicornuate uterus, or uterus unicornis, or uterus with only one functioning horn, the so-called Rokitansky sequence.

In the HCCSCA 57 (0.25%) pregnant women were affected with CAs of uterus, mainly by bicornuate uterus and the total rate of CAs in their children showed a higher risk (1.5, 1.1–2.2). However, the distribution of CAs showed an unusual very characteristic pattern. On the one hand, specific deformation-type CAs dominated among isolated CAs: clubfoot 7, unspecified limb deficiencies 3, torticollis 2. (In addition we have to remind the reader that cases with isolated congenital dislocation of the hip were excluded from the data set of the HSSCA.). Thirteen cases had isolated cardiovascular CAs, but among them 6 were affected with persistent ductus arteriosus. On the other hand, out of these 57 cases, 10 had multiple CA (4.7, 2.4–9.1) and out of 10 multimalformed children, 7 were affected with typical postural deformity MCA-association, i.e. combination of clubfoot, congenital dislocation of the hip, torticollis. Finally, out of these 7 cases with postural deformity MCA-association, 5 were preterm baby and 4 were affected with persistent ductus arteriosus. Thus, there is an obvious adverse birth outcome pattern in children of pregnant women with bicornuate uterus including PB, deformity types of CAs, and postural deformity MCA-association. The anatomic defect associating with serious shape restriction of uterus may explain the higher risk of mechanical oriented deformity types CA in the children of pregnant women with these CAs of uterus.

In conclusion, a higher risk for specific isolated CAs, i.e. deformities and multiple MCA-association, i.e. postural deformity MCA-association is noteworthy in the preterm newborns of pregnant women with bicornuate uterus due to the pathological structure of their uterus.

19.4 Unexpected Strong Association of Maternal Disease During Pregnancy With Higher Risk of CAs in Their Children But Without Reasonable Etiological Hypothesis

19.4.1 Panic Disorder

Most pregnant women with anxiety disorders were diagnosed as *panic disorder* (PD) in Hungary; therefore, the study was focused on pregnant women with PD.

In the data set of the HCCSCA 210 (0.9%) pregnant women had PD and their diagnosis was medically recorded in the prenatal maternity logbooks in 93.8% of these pregnant women. Most pregnant women with PD were treated by benzodiazepines: diazepam (34.2%), chlordiazepoxide (20.9%), tofisopam (5.4%), nitrazepam (2.7%), medazepam (1.6%), and alprazolam (1.1%).

Fifteen CA-groups were evaluated and isolated cleft lip ± palate occurred more frequently in children of pregnant women with PD (5.4, 1.5–19.4). This association cannot be explained by related drug treatments (the details of this analysis are shown in Section 19.7).

In conclusion, our study showed a higher occurrence of cleft lip ± palate in children of pregnant women with PD.

19.4.2 Coronary Artery Disease

The incidence of *coronary artery disease* (CAD) is low in pregnant women due to the dominance of CAD in males and in the advanced aged population. Angina pectoris is the most common manifestation of CAD which frequently precede acute myocardial infarction

In the HCCSCA 22 case pregnant women were affected with angina pectoris and all of them were treated with recommended anti-ischemic nitrates.

Out of 22 pregnant women with angina pectoris, 6 had children with isolated cleft lip ± cleft palate (13.3, 4.9–35.9) while 2 children were affected with cleft palate (10.5, 2.3–47.6). This association cannot be explained by related drug treatments or other known confounders.

In conclusion, a very high risk for isolated cleft lip ± cleft palate and cleft palate was found in the children of pregnant women with CAD.

19.4.3 Periodontal Infectious Diseases

Periodontal infectious diseases include gingivitis, periodontitis, stomatitis, glossitis, etc., and in general this group of diseases was neglected in pregnant women. However, recent studies showed association of periodontal infectious diseases with a higher risk for PB.

In the HCCSCA 21 (0.09%) children with CA had mothers with periodontal disease in pregnancy. Of these 21 cases, 6 (28.6%) were affected with cleft lip ± palate (9.8, 3.9–25.0) and 2 with cleft palate (7.5, 1.7–32.5). This strong association cannot be explained by related drug treatment but smoking seemed to show an important interaction both with periodontal infection and isolated orofacial clefts.

In conclusion, there is an unexpected very strong association between maternal periodontal infectious diseases in pregnant women and isolated orofacial clefts in their children.

19.5 Unexpected Weak Association of Maternal Disease During Pregnancy With Higher Risk of CAs in Their Children With or Without Plausible Hypothesis

25 CA-groups were evaluated in the data set of the HCCSCA; however, if a significant association was found between any CA-group and a maternal disease, we attempted to split the different manifestations of the given CA-group to find the specific CA which associated with the maternal disease. For example, the very frequently evaluated NTD includes anencephaly, spina bifida aperta/cystica with or without hydrocephalus, spinal dysraphism, anencephaly + spina bifida, i.e. craniorachischisis and encephalocele (although recently the inclusion of the latter CA into the group of NTD has been debated). It is necessary to stress this important

methodological aspect because multiple comparisons may produce non-causal association in every 20th calculation due to chance if the level of significance is 0.05. However, the Bonferroni correction or setting the significance level to 0.01 may help to limit the chance of type I error. On the other hand, if a significant weak association is found on the basis adjusted risk figures in controlled epidemiological studies, it is worth publishing this finding as signal because only other studies based on different populations can confirm or reject this association. If the association is confirmed it helps us to better understand the etiology of the given CA which is the most important step towards the prevention of CAs and optimal medical management.

19.5.1 Hyperthyroidism

The prevalence of hyperthyroidism is 0.2–0.5% in pregnant women, 90–95% of hyperthyroid females have Graves disease. The teratogenic potential of methimazole used for the treatment of hyperthyroidism was shown.

In the data set of the HCCSCA 71 (0.31%) pregnant women had medically recorded diagnosis of hyperthyroidism in their prenatal maternity logbooks. There was no higher risk in the group of total CAs (1.0, 0.8–1.4), but the maternal hyperthyroidism associated with a higher risk of obstructive CA of the urinary tract (4.9, 2.0–11.9), oesophageal atresia/stenosis (4.6 1.4–14.6), and congenital pyloric stenosis (4.1 1.3–13.1) in their children. These associations cannot be explained by the drugs used for the treatment of hyperthyroidism. In fact the lack of appropriate treatment of these pregnant women seems to be the major problem. The risk of antithyroid medication in pregnant women affected with hyperthyroidism is much lower than the risk of untreated hyperthyroidism regarding to pregnancy complications and adverse birth outcomes including CAs.

In conclusion, a higher risk of some specific CAs was found in the children of mothers with hyperthyroidism in the study.

19.5.2 Otitis Media

In general otitis media occurs in children but sometimes pregnant women are also affected by this inflammatory disease of the ear.

In the data set of the HCCSCA 58 (0.25%) cases had mother with medically recorded diagnosis of otitis media.

The incidence of otitis media in II and/or III gestational months was associated with a higher risk of total CAs (2.8, 1.4–5.6) explained mainly by the higher rate of ear CAs (0.85% vs. 0.04%; 16.0, 3.6–71.3); however, based only on 3 cases.

In conclusion, a higher risk of ear CAs in the children of pregnant women with otitis media raises the possibility that the anatomic configuration of middle ear and auditory canal may associate with a higher risk for the developmental error of the ears and later otitis media.

19.5.3 Essential Hypertension

Primary or *essential hypertension* (EH) occurs about 95% of hypertensive patients caused by the interaction of polygenic liability and hazardous environmental factors. Hypertension can be present before and during pregnancy in 1–5% of women. In our study pregnant women with secondary hypertension, preeclampsia-eclampsia, preeclampsia superimposed upon chronic hypertension, and gestational hypertension were excluded

In the data set of the HCCSCA 1,030 (4.5%) case pregnant women had medically recorded diagnosis of EH in the prenatal maternity logbook. Of these 1,030 case mothers, only 37 (3.6%) were not treated; therefore, we calculate that most pregnant women with EH had Stage II hypertension.

The total rate of CAs (1.1, 1.0–1.2) was somewhat higher in the offspring of pregnant women with EH explained by two CA-groups, namely oesophageal atresia/stenosis (3.1, 1.4–6.8) and multiple CAs (1.6, 1.1–2.2). However, the higher rate of multimalformed children disappeared after the exclusion of 2 cases with the teratogenic effect of captopril while the higher rate of oesophageal atresia/stenosis with or without tracheal fistula was not related to drug treatments or other confounders.

In conclusion, a higher risk for oesophageal atresia/stenosis was found in children of pregnant women with treated EH. The muscular layer of arteries is a target tissue of EH. In addition, the maldevelopment of musculature may also be an important factor in the origin of oesophageal atresia/stenosis; therefore, these two pathological conditions may have some common genetic predisposition.

19.5.4 Varicose Veins of the Lower Extremities

Primary varicosities tend to be familial; however, pregnancy induces dilatation and proliferation of blood vessels, therefore *varicose veins of the lower extremities* (VVLE) are common in pregnant women.

In the data set of the HCCSCA 332 (1.45%) case mothers had medically recorded and treated VVLE during the study pregnancy. The total rate of cases with CA (1.0, 0.9–1.1) and any specified CA-group did not show a higher risk in the children of pregnant women with VVLE in the first trimester. However, the evaluation of the subgroups of musculo-skeletal system's CAs showed a higher risk for pectus excavatum in children of mothers with VVLE ($p = 0.002$; after Bonferroni correction 0.03) and this association cannot be explained by related drug treatment or other confounders.

In conclusion, a higher risk for pectus excavatum was found in children born to mothers with VVLE. Both VVLE and pectus excavatum are related to mesodermal connective tissue, therefore they also may have common genetic origin.

19.5.5 Hemorrhoids

Hemorrhoids are common pathological conditions, more frequent in females, particularly in pregnant women.

Only prospectively and medical recorded hemorrhoids were evaluated in the study with related drug treatments. In the data set of the HCCSCA 795 (3.5%) case mothers had hemorrhoids and about one-third was affected with hemorrhoid before conception. The rest of pregnant women had new-onset hemorrhoids with a peak between VII and VIII gestational months.

The possible risk of hemorrhoid for CAs was estimated using the data of mothers who had hemorrhoids in II and/or III gestational months of their pregnancies. There was no higher risk for the total group of CAs (0.8, 0.7–0.9) or any CA group in the offspring of mothers with hemorrhoid. However, the detailed evaluation of the cases in the group of other isolated CAs showed that 8 cases had malposition/malrotation of the digestive organs resulting in a significant association with maternal hemorrhoid. ($p= 0.002$; after Bonferroni correction 0.01).

In conclusion, a higher risk for malposition-malrotation of the digestive organs was found in the offspring of pregnant women with hemorrhoid.

19.5.6 Dyspepsia and Gastro-Oesophageal Reflux Disease

Dyspepsia is a complex of symptoms originating in the upper gastrointestinal tract including gastro-oesophageal reflux disease. Dyspepsia is particularly common in the second part of gestation. The aim of our study was to check the possible association of different CAs and adverse birth outcomes with maternal dyspepsia and related drug treatments.

In the data set of the HCCSCA 175 (0.77%) case mothers had medically recorded dyspepsia in the prenatal maternity logbook. We evaluated 148 (0.65%) case mothers with *severe chronic dyspepsia* (SCD), all women were treated by medications.

There was no higher risk for total CA (1.2, 0.9–1.4) but the evaluation of cases with different CAs showed that cases with isolated rectal/anal atresia/stenosis had mothers with significantly higher rate of SCD (4.3, 1.7–10.5) based on 5 cases. After the so-called Bonferroni correction, the p value was 0.0015. This association cannot be explained by related drug treatment or other confounders.

In conclusion, 4-fold higher risk for isolated rectal/anal atresia/stenosis was found in children of pregnant women with SCD.

19.5.7 Ulcerative Colitis

Ulcerative colitis (UC) occurs in women of childbearing age and therefore during pregnancy as well.

In the data set of the HCCSCA 71 (0.3%) case mothers were affected by UC, and 60 (84.5%) were medically recorded in their prenatal maternity logbook. All pregnant women had the onset of UC before conception, and most of them were treated by sulfasalazine and promethazine.

The risk of total CAs in the children of mother with UC was not higher (1.3, 0.9–1.8). However, a higher risk for congenital limb deficiencies (6.2, 2.9–13.1) was found. The evaluation of 8 cases with congenital limb deficiencies showed that only one limb was affected in all cases, 6 occurred on the upper limbs and 2 on the lower limbs. Their estimated diagnosis was terminal transverse type which is caused by vascular disruption of the limb buds. This association cannot be explained by related drug treatment or other confounders.

In conclusion, our study indicated a higher risk of limb deficiencies in the children of pregnant women with UC.

19.5.8 Glomerulonephritis

In general the term *glomerulonephritis* (GN) encompasses a range of immune-mediated disorders that cause inflammation within the glomerules and other compartments of the kidney.

In the data set of the HCCSCA 309 (1.35%) cases with different CAs had mothers with the diagnosis of medically recorded GN during pregnancy. Only pregnant women with the onset of GN 3 or more months before the study pregnancy were evaluated. The persistent proteinuria was the principal marker of kidney damage in this group of kidney diseases.

A higher risk for isolated intestinal atresia/stenosis (6.8, 1.3–37.4) was found in the children of pregnant women with GN based on 5 cases.

In conclusion, there is an association between maternal GN during the study pregnancy and higher risk for isolated intestinal atresia/stenosis in their children.

19.5.9 Erosion of Cervix

Three major groups of pregnant women with inflammatory diseases of the genital organs were evaluated: (i) acute pelvic inflammatory disease (including oophoritis, salpingitis, parametritis, adnexitis, endometritis associated with or without cervicitis or vulvovaginitis), (ii) vulvovaginitis-bacterial vaginosis, frequently associated with cervicitis, but this pathological group was evaluated together, and (iii) genital herpes. However, some pregnant women were recorded with the diagnosis of *erosion of the cervix in pregnant women* (ECP) with or without cervicitis and endocervicitis, but without pelvic inflammatory disease and vulvovaginitis-bacterial vaginosis in the HCCSCA. Thus, it seemed to be necessary to evaluate the pregnancy outcomes of women with ECP separately.

In the data of the HCCSCA 40 (0.18%) case mothers had medically recorded diagnosis of ECP. ECP was recorded at the first visit in the prenatal care clinic, i.e. between the 6th and 10th gestational weeks in all pregnant women; therefore the onset of ECP probably occurred before conception.

The total rate of CAs (2.7, 1.6–4.4) showed a higher risk and it was explained mainly by the higher rate of hypospadias (4.4, 2.1–9.7) and cardiovascular CAs (3.4, 1.6–7.1) in children born to mothers with ECP.

At the evaluation of 9 cases with hypospadias, the minor manifestation of this CA (coronal type) was excluded. Of 10 cases with cardiovascular CAs, 7 belonged to the so-called conotruncal CAs. The related drug treatments cannot explain this association, although previously allylestrenol used for the treatment of threatened abortion and other high risk pregnancies seemed to show some association with the elevated risk for hypospadias; however, this hormone was not used more frequently by case mothers compared to control mothers with ECP in the data set of the HCCSCA.

In conclusion, an association was found between ECP in early pregnancy and a higher risk for hypospadias and conotruncal cardiovascular CAs.

19.6 Conclusions

The evaluation of the large population-based HCCSCA revealed some new and unexpected associations between maternal diseases and specific CAs in their children. In general, only medical recorded maternal diseases in the prenatal maternity logbooks were evaluated. In addition, the validity of CAs is good because cases were reported by medical doctors and diagnoses were checked by experts and were updated later based on recent medical examinations. Therefore, these findings are published here as signals. We encourage all clinical researchers to study these findings in other populations to confirm or reject the associations found in the Hungarian database.

19.7 The Teratogenic Potential of Related Drug Treatments

During pregnancy the possible teratogenic effect of a drug is an important factor in estimating the total benefit of applying the given medicine. However, as we previously mentioned, according to our opinion, the underlying diseases, i.e. the indications of drug treatments were frequently neglected when evaluating the teratogenic effect of drugs. We tried to avoid the same mistake; therefore, when analyzing the teratogenic potential of maternal diseases related drug treatments were also evaluated as the most important confounders. Here the main experiences about drug teratogenicity are summarized.

In the data set of the HCCSCA the possible teratogenic potential of drugs used for treatment of maternal diseases studied was also evaluated as confounder. Here only those related drug treatments are discussed which showed some special character of drugs.

19.7.1 Antiepileptic Drugs

Previously about 3-fold higher risk for CAs in the offspring of epileptic pregnant women was detected mainly explained by the teratogenic effect of antiepileptic drugs. The risk of CA is lower with monotherapy than with polytherapy. In addition, different antiepileptic drugs have different teratogenic risks for different specific CAs.

In Hungary the spectrum of antiepileptic drugs (phenobarbital, phenytoin, trimethadione, phenacemid, sultiame, ethosuximide, morsuximide, mephenytoin, primidone, clomethiazol, diazepam, clonazepam, carbamazepine, and valproate) was different than in Western countries during the study period, therefore it provides an opportunity for the evaluation of teratogenic potential of some less-known drugs.

Our data confirmed the higher risk of NTD, CL ± CP, CP, and cardiovascular CA after the use of antiepileptic drugs, but a higher risk for oesophageal atresia/stenosis was also found. There was also a higher risk after polytherapy than after monotherapy. The Hungarian data indicated the teratogenic effect of *trimethadione, primidone, sultiame, valproate, phenytoin, mephenytoin* but phenobarbital and diazepam did not show increased teratogenic effect.

The main result of our study was to show that periconceptional folic acid supplementation was able to reduce the teratogenic risk of some antiepileptic drugs.

Finally, it is worth summarizing the major recommendations for epileptic women at the preparation of their pregnancies.

The first task is to educate epileptic women about the importance of planning their pregnancies.

The second task is in the preconceptional care to check their antiepileptic drugs and to attempt to change teratogenic drugs (e.g. valproate) to a less (e.g. carbamazepine) or non-teratogenic (lamotrigine) drugs under the supervision of a specialist. In general drug selection is determined by the type of seizure and clinical status. If a teratogenic drug is necessary (because the loss of seizure control during pregnancy is more dangerous than the teratogenic epileptic drugs), monotherapy is preferred. In addition, it is recommended to use the lowest effective dose of the given drug because there is a dose-effect relation in teratogenic potential of antiepileptic drugs such as valproate. Regular blood test is also necessary to check the levels of seizure medications because frequently there is a decreasing trend in the blood concentration of drugs during pregnancy partly due to dilution effect of increasing plasma volume.

The third task is to strongly recommend periconceptional folic acid supplementation for epileptic pregnant women. Unfortunately the optimal dose of folic acid is not known yet.

The fourth task is the monitoring of the fetal development with high resolution ultrasound because the cardinal CAs associated with different teratogenic antiepileptic drugs are detectable at about the 20th gestational week. Fortunately these defects are diagnosed rarely, but if it is happened, pregnant women have the right to decide to keep or terminate their pregnancies.

The final fifth task is related to the preparation of delivery. Sometimes clinical or subclinical coagulopathy may occur in newborn infants born to epileptic mothers with some antiepileptic treatment caused by vitamin K deficiency. Maternal ingestion of vitamin K1 (10 mg/day) during the last month of pregnancy may prevent this complication.

In conclusion, epileptic pregnant women have a higher risk for some CAs. Nevertheless, at present pregnancy in epileptic women does not need to be discouraged but supported with specific and high standard care is necessary.

19.7.2 Ergotamine

The main objective of our study was to evaluate the birth outcomes of children born to mothers affected by migraine attacks during pregnancy. Of course, beyond the effect of migraine, the related drugs treatments were also analyzed. The preliminary analysis of risk of different CAs showed a somewhat higher risk for NTD in the offspring of pregnant women with migraine. The detailed analysis of these mother-offspring pairs revealed that the major part of these pregnant women was treated with high dose of *ergotamine*. Therefore, we decided to evaluate the teratogenic potential of this drug in the data set of the HCCSCA and its teratogenic effect was proven. However, teratogenic effect of low dose ergotamine or other antimigraine drugs was not found.

In conclusion, migraine improves during pregnancy therefore several women do not need medication. However, some pregnant women have severe migraine attacks sometimes with symptoms of severe nausea and vomiting resulting in dehydration. These women need drug treatments. In pregnant women with serious symptoms it is necessary to simultaneously consider the improvement of migraine, the teratogenic/fetotoxic effects of drugs and migraine itself. Triptans are appropriate for this purpose sometimes with other analgesic and preventive drugs. Although special caution is always necessary when we recommend drug treatment for pregnant women, at present the possible teratogenic effects of antimigraine drugs are surely exaggerated. Beyond high doses of ergotamine, our study did not show any teratogenic effect of other antimigraine drugs.

19.7.3 Certain Antihypertensive Drugs

Hypertension is one of the most common chronic diseases. Nevertheless, hypertension is frequently neglected because blood pressure is a continuous variable and therefore there is no obvious natural threshold between normal and pathological blood pressure. In addition, there are no symptoms in the early phase of the disease. According to the classification of hypertension, Stage 1 (140–159/90–99 mmHg) and Stage 2 (160/100 or over mmHg) can be differentiated and hypertension with Stage 2 always needs treatment.

In the data set of the HCCSCA nearly all pregnant women with hypertension were treated. The frequency order of drugs used was terbutaline, verapamil, metoprolol, nifedipin, fenoterol, and methyldopa in pregnant women with essential hypertension, while this order was methyldopa, clopamide, dihydralazine, nifedipin, metoprolol in pregnant women with gestational hypertension.

The first aim of the study was to check the efficacy of antihypertensive treatment of pregnant women with hypertension and the Hungarian data showed that antihypertensive treatment was not able to neutralize the harmful effect of hypertension for some pregnancy complications particularly intrauterine growth retardation. In general, monotherapy is preferred instead of polytherapy in pregnant women. However, the polytherapy seems to be more effective in patients with hypertension therefore it would be necessary to introduce a more effective drug combination in the treatment of pregnant women with severe hypertension.

Only *captopril*, an ACE (angiotensin converting enzyme) inhibitor was associated with increased risk for CAs. No other drugs used for the treatment of hypertension indicated elevated risk. ACE inhibitors and angiotensin-II-receptor antagonists are contraindicated in pregnant women due to their fetotoxic effect. Nevertheless, 10 pregnant women with essential hypertension were treated with captopril in the data set of the HCCSCA and 2 had malformed offspring. The pattern of their CAs corresponded to the expected oligohydramnios sequence.

In conclusion, there is a wide spectrum of antihypertensive drugs for the treatment of pregnant women, however, ACE (angiotensin converting enzyme) inhibitors and angiotensin-II-receptor antagonists are contraindicated. In addition, it is necessary to introduce a more effective treatment protocol.

19.7.4 "Warfarin"

The diseases of the veins, such as superficial thrombophlebitis and deep vein thrombophlebitis with or without thrombosis of the lower extremities, in addition to pulmonary embolism in pregnant women are severe complications. Anticoagulation therapy is the mainstay of therapy for these diseases; however, their administration needs special expertise during pregnancy due to the teratogenic potential of coumadin derivatives such as warfarin.

Our study showed that Hungarian pregnant women with venous diseases of the lower extremities generally were treated by heparin and/or *acenocoumarol* (Syncumar®), a coumadin derivative. In our data set 8 pregnant women were treated orally with Syncumar® in early pregnancy without demonstrating any increased risk for CAs. The characteristic pattern of "warfarin syndrome" was not observed in the 3 cases with CA, while the other 5 pregnant women delivered healthy babies. Both unfractionated and low-molecular-weight heparin was available for parenteral treatment frequently complemented with the oral treatment of tribenoside and local treatment with phenylbutazone. Heparin is safe during pregnancy because it cannot cross the placenta.

A higher risk for total CAs or any CA was not found in children of pregnant women with superficial thrombophlebitis and deep vein thrombophlebitis treated with Syncumar®. However, human teratogenic effect of coumadin derivates is widely accepted, our study seemingly not confirmed it probably due to the limited number of pregnant women. In addition, 3 pregnant women were treated with Syncumar® only in I gestational month.

In conclusion there was no higher risk for CAs in the offspring of pregnant women with thrombophlebitis and treated by "warfarin", this finding is explained by the limited number of pregnant women and the weak teratogenic potential of this drug.

19.7.5 Methimazole

Most hyperthyroid pregnant women had Graves disease which is an autoimmune disease. Its symptoms frequently ameliorated during pregnancy. The optimal onset of treatment of pregnant women with hyperthyroidism is prior to pregnancy; however, treatment is frequently continued during pregnancy as well.

An antithyroid drug, *methimazole* was shown to have teratogenic potential inducing a specific pattern of CAs with the cardinal symptom of scalp defect.

Out of 71 case mothers with hyperthyroidism, only 4 (methimazole 3, propylthiouracyl 1), while out of 116 control mothers with this disease, 8 (methimazole 7, propylthiouracyl 1) were treated with antithyroid drugs in the data set of the HCCSCA. Previously most of them were treated by these drugs, but their physicians suggested stopping these drugs because of their teratogenic potential.

As we showed previously a higher risk for obstructive CA of the urinary tract, oesophageal atresia/stenosis, and congenital pyloric stenosis was found in the children of mothers with hyperthyroidism. However, the teratogenic potential of methimazole or propylthiouracyl treatment was not seen because mothers of children with the above CAs were not treated with these drugs.

In conclusion hyperthyroidism associates with a high risk for pregnant women. On the one hand, maternal hyperthyroidism associates with a higher incidence of pregnancy complications like preeclampsia-eclampsia. On the other hand, a higher risk for some specific CAs was found in the study and this association cannot be explained by drugs used for the treatment of hyperthyroidism. In fact the lack of appropriate treatment of these pregnant women seems to be the major problem because the risk of antithyroid medication in pregnant women affected with hyperthyroidism is much lower than the risk of untreated hyperthyroidism regarding to pregnancy complications and adverse birth outcomes including CAs.

19.7.6 Phenolphthalein

Constipation is one of the most frequent pathological conditions which affect 11–38% of pregnant women. Some clinical reports even stated that over half of the pregnant women had complaints of constipation during pregnancy. Sometimes the usual management of constipation by diet is not enough therefore medications are necessary and possible teratogenic and/or fetotoxic effect of related drug treatments may cause a dilemma in clinical practice. Severe constipation during pregnancy associates frequently with anemia due to hemorrhoids but no higher risk for unsuccessful birth outcomes could be detected.

In Hungary the oral treatment of senna and phenolphthalein was used most frequently for severe constipation. The use of *phenolphthalein* showed a significantly higher frequency in case mothers compared to control mothers with severe constipation (4.0, 2.4–18.2). After using phenolphthalein in II and III gestational months, there was a higher risk for Hirschsprung's disease ($p = 0.01$). On the other hand, the teratogenic potential of senna was also studied without showing any teratogenic effect.

In conclusion, if severe constipation needs medication senna is recommended, because the old fashion phenolphthalein was found to have a weak teratogenic potential.

19.8 The So-called "Antiteratogenic" Drugs

This term is not used in the international literature, although it would be worth introducing this term for some drugs, when related drug treatment of maternal diseases in pregnant women has some protective effect on CAs.

19.8.1 Antipyretic Drugs

Our studies showed the obvious teratogenic effect of hyperthermia. However, the major findings of our studies were that this teratogenic effect could be prevented or reduced by the parallel use of antipyretic drugs. The triggering factor of the recurrence of orofacial herpes is generally the high fever. If this fever had been treated with antipyretic drugs, the possible teratogenic effect of recurrent orofacial herpes was not seen.

As far as we know first we showed the *multiple CA* (MCA) inducing effect of high fever (see Section 19.1). Our studies demonstrated the antiteratogenic effect of antipyretic drugs in this severe and common group of CAs and the major findings are shown here in Table 19.5.

Thus, the effect of antipyretic drugs (acetylsalicylic acid, paracetamol, aminophenazone, and dipyrone) was checked for the risk of MCA associated with the above four fever related diseases during II and/or III months of gestation. Table 19.5 shows the data regarding to the critical period of most major CAs, i.e. II and/or III gestational months. Antipyretic drugs were able to reduce the MCA inducing effect of these diseases both in the comparison of case and control groups or case and malformed control groups. Common cold with secondary complications

Table 19.5 Risk (adjusted OR) for MCA in cases, controls, and malformed controls born to mothers without high fever related maternal disorders and antipyretic drug treatment during the study pregnancy as reference, in addition to 4 high fever related maternal disorders together with or without treatment of antipyretic drugs

Study groups	Comparison MCA cases vs. controls OR	95% CI	Comparison MCA cases vs. malformed controls OR	95% CI
Pregnant women without high fever related disorders and without antipyretic drug treatment	Reference (1.0)		Reference (1.0)	
Pregnant women with high fever related disorders and without antipyretic drug treatment	**2.2**	**1.7–2.9**	**1.4**	**1.2–1.7**
Pregnant women with high fever related disorders and with antipyretic drug treatment	1.6	0.9–2.9	1.3	0.9–2.2

was the most sensitive while tonsillitis was the less sensitive for the MCA reducing effect of antipyretic drugs.

Of course, the teratogenic potential of antipyretic drugs used in Hungary was evaluated in the data set of the HCCSCA without showing increased risk for total CAs or any CA groups. These drugs therefore have no contraindication during pregnancy.

In conclusion, data of the HCCSCA showed that the major part of high fever related CAs – beyond the previously known NTD, orofacial clefts, congenital limb deficiencies, and cardiovascular CA as well – can be reduced by the parallel use of antipyretic drugs. In addition, our study first found an association between higher risk for MCAs and high fever related maternal diseases such as influenza, common cold with secondary complications, tonsillitis and recurrent orofacial herpes. The major new finding of our study is that high fever related maternal diseases induced CA also could be prevented by antipyretic drug therapy.

19.8.2 Insulin

Diabetes mellitus (DM) is a common disease and at the first level of classification 3 types of DM can be differentiated. The onset of *Type 1 (DM-I)* is predominantly under 30 years with a peak of 9 years and needs insulin treatment for life. The characteristics of this type of DM explain its other terms: juvenile or insulin dependent DM. *Type 2* (DM-II) is characterized by variable insulin level and generally with slow appearance of symptoms. Patients need diet control and/or oral hypoglycemic drugs. The onset of DM-II is predominantly over 30 years (explaining its previous term: adult-onset or non-insulin dependent DM, although the past 12–20 years have seen a dramatic increase in the prevalence of DM-II in younger persons). Insulin treatment may also be required later to control hyperglycemia in these patients. *Gestational DM* (GDM) is defined as glucose intolerance of any degree that begins or is first recognized during pregnancy. Pregnant women with GDM need medical nutritional therapy and insulin when necessary.

The risk of specific CAs in the offspring of pregnant women with overt DM prior to conception was 4- to 8-fold higher. These specific CAs and a MCA-syndrome with specific component CAs ("diabetic embryopathy") were shown in our studies of pregnant women with DM-I as well, but the risk was relatively lower (1.5-fold instead of the previous 4- to 8-fold) reflecting the recent progress in the specific medical care of diabetic pregnant women. If we consider the annual distribution of cases with DM-I related CAs, out of 42 cases, 30 (71.4%) were born in the 1980s. Therefore we can speculate that special periconceptional and prenatal care of diabetic pregnant women with appropriate insulin treatment was able to prevent the teratogenic effect of maternal DM.

In conclusion, the teratogenic effect of maternal DM is preventable by high standard periconceptional and prenatal care including appropriate insulin therapy if necessary. Thus, an important message is that insulin and other antidiabetic drugs can reduce the teratogenic risk of DM related hyperglycemia during the critical period of CAs in diabetic pregnant women.

19.8.3 Antipanic Drugs

As we showed previously isolated *cleft lip±palate* (CL ± CP) occurred more frequently in children of pregnant women with panic disorder (5.4, 1.5–19.4). The question was whether this association could be explained by related drug treatments, maternal disease itself, lifestyle factors, or by other confounders. Thus, we attempted to differentiate the effect of panic disorder and their related drug treatments (alprazolam, chlordiazepoxide, diazepam, medazepam, meprobamate, nitrazepam, phenobarbital, tofisopam) for CL ± CP and the data are presented here.

The reference sample included pregnant women without panic disorder and without antipanic drug treatments, their value is 1.0. Panic disorder had the onset before conception and continued during pregnancy; therefore II and/or III gestational months were not evaluated separately. Antipanic drugs were evaluated only in II gestational month of pregnancy, i.e. the critical period of CL ± CP. The total risk of CL ± CP in the children of pregnant women with panic disease was 2.1, 1.2–3.5. There were three other study groups: pregnant women with panic disorder and without antipanic drug treatment (3.1, 1.4–6.9), pregnant women without panic disorder and with antipanic drug treatment obviously due to other indications (1.8, 0.8–2.8) and pregnant women with panic disorder and antipanic drug treatment (1.5, 0.7–3.2). The highest risk was found in pregnant women with panic disease and without antipanic treatment, the lowest risk occurred in pregnant women with panic disease and antipanic drugs. Therefore drugs used for the treatment of this disease seemed to be protective for CL ± CP.

These findings suggest that Cl ± CP in the children of pregnant women with panic disorder is not caused by antipanic drugs (mainly benzodiazepines) but by the psychiatric disorder and related lifestyle. Consequently panic disorder and its related lifestyle or their interaction seems to be important risk factors in the origin of CL ± CP. Among direct effects of panic disorder, different quantity and/or pathogenic effect of neurotransmitters or other brain chemicals of the disease itself can be considered particularly without appropriate drug treatment. If pregnant women are affected by pathological conditions (e.g. influencing by released neurotransmitters from the brain), it may have adverse effect on the fetus as well. In addition among panic disorder related lifestyle factors like higher occurrence of substance use/abuse behaviors, alcohol drinking was not found in the study, additionally CL ± CP does not fit into the characteristics of fetal alcohol syndrome. However, the proportion of smokers was larger in pregnant women with panic disorder. Recent studies showed a higher risk for CL ± CP in children of smoker women with some genetic predisposition.

In conclusion, a higher risk for CL ± CP was found in children born to pregnant women with panic disorder; however, after the differentiation of these pregnant women according to antipanic treatment (mainly benzodiazepines) this higher risk was only found in children of mothers with panic disorder and without antipanic drug treatment. Therefore, antipanic treatment seemed to be protective for CL ± CP in pregnant women with panic disorder.

19.9 Conclusions

Among several thousand drugs used at present, less than 50 have been proved as human teratogen. Of course, an important task is to avoid the use of teratogenic medications during pregnancy if possible (e.g. accutane-isotretinoin due to acne) or we need to attempt to change to a less teratogenic drugs if treatment is necessary (e.g. in epileptic pregnant women). However, at present the major problem in Hungary is that the necessary drug treatments are frequently neglected due to presumed teratogenic potential of drugs (e.g. in high fever related maternal diseases). Thus it would be incredibly important for all doctors to understand that most drugs have no teratogenic potential and some drugs like antipyretic drugs or insulin even have antiteratogenic effect.

19.10 Maternal Diseases with Preventive Effect on CAs

We are aware of the fact again that the title of this section is unusual, but our studies demonstrated that two pathological conditions of pregnant women associated with a lower risk for CAs in their children.

19.10.1 Nausea and Vomiting in Pregnancy

Nausea and vomiting in pregnancy (NVP) is a collection of symptoms of nausea alone, or nausea in combination with vomiting that begins in early pregnancy but always before the 20th gestational week. It is not associated with primary maternal diseases such as gastrointestinal infections.

Several studies showed that women with NVP had a lower risk for miscarriage than women who did not experience NVP. In addition, our study showed some protective effect of NVP for some CAs as well.

Three categories of NVP were differentiated in the data set of the HCCSCA:

(i) mild NVP based on retrospective maternal information. They were rarely treated by antiemetics (only 7.0% of case and 8.2% of control mothers),
(ii) severe NVP based on medical records in the prenatal maternity logbook. All pregnant women were treated by antiemetics,
(iii) very severe NVP with significant weight loss. These women needed hospitalization and intensive treatment including infusion. This group is also called as hyperemesis gravidarum and happened in 0.1% of case and 0.2% of control mothers.

There was a severity dependent prevention association between NVP and total CA group. In addition, mild and severe NVP associated with a lower risk for 3 and 10 CA-groups, respectively. The number of cases with different CAs was too small for evaluation in the very severe NVP group.

Finally, pregnant women with mild NVP (because the maternal retrospective maternal information regarding NVP was too subjective) and very severe NVP (due the too small number of patients) were excluded from the analysis, and only medically recorded and treated severe NVP were evaluated in detail.

Out of 25 CA-groups, 5 CA groups (cleft lip ± cleft palate, cleft palate, renal a/dysgenesis, obstructive CAs of the urinary tract, and cardiovascular CAs) showed a lower risk.

NVP is the most common pregnancy complication and our study showed an inverse association between severe NVP and risk of some CAs. Severe NVP was associated with a 26% protective effect against the occurrence of total CAs.

The possible causal association between severe NVP and the reduction of some CAs needs explanation. The possible CA-protective effect of antiemetic drugs is also worth attention. Vitamin B6 showed a protective effect for cardiovascular CAs (0.9, 0.7–0.9) in our study (73) and vitamin B6 (i.e. pyridoxine) was used very frequently (60%) in pregnant women with NVP. The teratogenic potential of dimenhydrinate treatment was also evaluated (71) and there was no higher risk for total CAs (0.9, 0.8–1.0) or any CA-group. In fact, there was a lower risk for obstructive CA of the urinary tract (0.3, 0.1–0.9). The study of thiethylperazine treatment did not show increased risk for total CA group (72); however, there was a marginally higher risk for cleft lip ± cleft palate (2.0, 1.0–4.0). The effect of these antiemetics was considered as confounder in the calculation of adjusted OR regarding to the effect of NVP.

Our favorite hypothesis for the explanation of this beneficial effect on NVP for CAs is based on higher blood level of human chorionic gonadotropin and estrogens from the larger placenta in pregnant women with NVP. An important argument is that the peak of NVP occurs during gestational weeks 5–10 which just correspond to the organ-forming period when embryonic susceptibility to teratogens is most obvious and when the level of human chorionic gonadotropin is the highest. Thus this hormonal milieu may have a protective effect for some CAs and the higher estrogen concentration induces a hyperacuity of the olfactory system to odors which may be the primary stimulus for NVP.

In conclusion, there is a significant reduction in the total prevalence of some CAs and total CAs in pregnant women with severe NVP.

19.10.2 Cervical Incompetence

The term *cervical incompetence/insufficiency in pregnant women* (CIP) means a resumed weakness of cervix that causes the loss of an otherwise healthy pregnancy usually in the second trimester. The diagnosis of CIP has traditionally been made and is still most confidentially established by an obstetric history of recurrent passive and painless dilatation of the cervix in the second trimester. In the past this diagnosis was based on digital examination to assess cervical dilatation. However, this type of diagnosis was unreliable and subjective therefore transvaginal imaging of the cervix by ultrasound examination resulted in a great progress in the diagnosis of CIP.

The data set of the HCSCA included a very large number of pregnant women with the diagnosis of CIP. One of the objectives of our study was to evaluate the possible association between CIP and different CAs in the offspring. In the international literature we did not find any study regarding to potential risk of CIP for CAs. CIP generally manifested during the second trimester of gestation and the critical period of most major CAs is in II and/or III gestational months. We, therefore, could not create a biologically plausible hypothesis explaining this association.

In Hungary CIP was defined as a progressive dilatation of the uterine cervix and/or bulging membranes during the second trimester of pregnancy diagnosed by manual examination of an obstetrician in the prenatal maternity clinics in which circumstances preterm delivery seemed inevitable without interference. According to our study design, CIP was accepted based on medically recorded diagnosis in the prenatal maternity logbooks or discharge summaries of hospitalized pregnant women after therapeutic cerclage.

In the data set of the HCCSCA 1,170 (5.12%) case mothers and 2,795 (7.33%) control mothers had medically recorded CIP, and most CIP were diagnosed in V and VI gestational months. The total rate of CAs (0.7, 0.6–0.8) was lower in the offspring of pregnant women with CIP explained mainly by the lower risk of isolated congenital hydrocephaly, neural-tube defects, poly/syndactyly, cleft lip ± palate, and multiple CAs (0.6 or less OR).

The proportion of malformed stillborn fetuses was 0.4 and 1.7% in case mothers with and without CIP, respectively. There was a higher rate of threatened abortions and placental disorders in mothers with CIP than in pregnant women without CIP, thus a more intensive very early selection of malformed fetuses cannot be excluded. In addition, CIP poses a higher risk for spontaneous abortion and in general about 50% of all conceptions end as early loss. Thus our hypothesis was based on the speculation that CIP might be a marker of certain structural and/or functional defects of the cervical canal and endometrium in uterus due to the late effect of induced abortions or other factors which expulsed more intensively the abnormal embryos in the early pregnancy.

In conclusion, our study showed that CIP is very frequent in Hungary probably due to the extremely high number of induced abortions with D+C method and CIP associated with a lower risk for some CAs, particularly for congenital hydrocephalus, neural-tube defects, poly/syndactyly, cleft lip ± palate and multiple CAs. This unexpected association needs more data from other populations to confirm or to reject these findings.

19.10.3 Conclusions

An important rule of epidemiology is that "unexpected is expected". Nevertheless, the systematic evaluation of all maternal diseases in our population-based data set resulted in too many unexpected findings; among them the above described "CA protective" maternal diseases. Our hope is that these associations will be checked in other populations as well to decide whether they were Hungarian specialties or they might have general importance.

19.11 Primary Prevention of CAs

CAs represent a defect condition, therefore complete recovery from a CA, although that is the most desirable outcome, is difficult to achieve. For this reason prevention is the best, almost the only feasible option in the medical care of CAs.

Here three possibilities for the prevention of CAs are discussed.

19.11.1 Vaccination

The introduction of population-based vaccination has resulted in a great success in the prevention of CAs associated with *rubella-virus* infection of pregnant women in Hungary. Vaccine is available for the prevention of fetal *varicella* disease, but this facultative vaccination is used rarely before conception in pregnant women with negative history of varicella in Hungary. In addition, the *influenza* vaccine prevents or diminishes the fetal consequence of high fever related influenza in pregnant women beyond the lower maternal mortality.

19.11.2 Avoidance of Teratogens

The prevention of teratogenic lifestyle factors such as alcohol drinking, smoking, illicit drug uses seems to be the most important task but unfortunately has only limited success.

An important medical mission is to select the non-teratogenic (e.g. heparin vs. warfarin) or less teratogenic (among antiepileptics) drugs for the necessary medical treatment of pregnant women with specific diseases.

In addition, it is worth mentioning the previously shown so-called "antiteratogenic" drugs, e.g. antipyretics and insulin which can neutralize the teratogenic effect of maternal diseases (e.g. high fever and diabetes mellitus).

Finally, our opinion is that the human teratogenic risk of drugs is exaggerated. There are several explanations for the unbalanced risk/benefit estimation of drug treatments during pregnancy:

(i) positive findings of animal investigations are frequently extrapolated for the human fetus in spite of the differences between species;
(ii) previous human teratological studies had methodological weaknesses, e.g. drug exposures were based on retrospective maternal information during the first trimester of pregnancy with strong recall bias, though most teratogens did not induce CA in I gestational month;
(iii) editors prefer publish positive findings;
(iv) self-defensive attitude of medical doctors, pharmaceutical factories, and regulatory agencies;
(v) the wish of prospective parents to have "100%" healthy babies.

In fact, there are about 50 human teratogenic drugs – most of them with a risk less than 10% – among the several thousand medicinal products. The exaggeration of teratogenic risk of drugs causes serious hazards:

(i) Several pregnancies are terminated due to anxiety and fear created by the motion that nearly all drugs cause CAs.
(ii) Many pregnant women with chronic (e.g. panic disorder or migraine) and acute (e.g. high fever related) diseases do not get the necessary drug treatment and it associates with serious consequences both for the mothers (e.g. pandemic influenza associates with a higher mortality) and the fetuses (high fever related influenza can induce neural-tube defects or congenital cataract, although these CAs are preventable by antipyretic drugs). Nevertheless, most pregnant women with influenza are not treated.
(iii) Pregnant women using necessary drug treatment may suffer permanent psychological stress due to the rumor of teratogenic risk of drugs till the end of pregnancy.

Obviously it is necessary to estimate the risk and benefit of the necessary drug treatment during pregnancy and generally we should not recommend drugs with teratogenic effect. Also, if a drug has teratogenic effect it should, if possible, be avoided in the preparation period for conception or during pregnancy. However, if pregnant women used necessary teratogenic drugs during the pregnancy, there is no reason to suggest pregnancy termination. All true human teratogenic drugs induce specific CAs, generally MCA-syndromes, and at present these CAs are recognizable by 4D ultrasound examination on the 20th week of gestation; therefore, it is possible to identify malformed cases. The Hungarian law allows terminating the pregnancy after the diagnosis of severe fetal defects until the 24th week of gestation. The life of many healthy fetuses could be protected by utilizing this strategy.

19.11.3 Folic Acid or Folic Acid-Containing Multivitamin Supplementation in General

Periconceptional multivitamin/folic acid supplementation resulted in a breakthrough of primary preventive of CA. As some of our studies in Part II showed folic acid/multivitamin supplementation is appropriate and effective method for the prevention/reduction of maternal disease related CAs as well. Here the main messages of these studies will be summarized but first the history of this new preventive method is presented shortly.

19.11.3.1 Historical Background

First Smithells et al. (1980, 1989) reported the possible prevention of the recurrence of *neural-tube defects* (NTD) by periconceptional administration of a multivitamin (Pregnavite forte F®) supplement containing folic acid (0.36 mg) based on their non-randomized intervention study. Their final results in Yorkshire showed a *91% reduction in recurrent NTD* while the other part of the study in Northern Ireland resulted in 83% reduction (Nevin and Seller, 1990).

The *Hungarian Periconceptional Service* (HPS) was launched in 1984 embracing all the methods for the prevention of CAs and PB known at that time (121–124). (The term "periconceptional" is preferred rather than "preconceptional" because prenatal care usually begins between the 8th and 12th weeks of pregnancy, thus the most sensitive and vulnerable early period of fetal development, from the 5th to the 10th gestational week calculated from the first day of the last menstrual period, i.e. from the 3rd week post-conception until the 8th week, is not covered by the standard medical health service, leaving embryos uncared for and in general unprotected.) The new primary preventive method of NTD was incorporated into the protocol of HPS (Table 19.6) using a multivitamin (Elevit prenatal®) containing 12 vitamins including folic acid (0.8 mg), vitamin B12 (4.0 μg), B6 (2.6 mg), B2 (1.8 mg), thus it was possible to test its efficacy for the prevention of a first affected child with an NTD in the family, i.e. the first occurrence or primary case of NTD in a *randomized controlled trial* (RCT). The Hungarian RCT, based on HPS participants, was designed to answer two major questions. The first of these was: "Does folic acid-containing multivitamin supplementation reduce the risk of *first* occurrence of

Table 19.6 The three stages of the Hungarian Periconceptional Service, and activities undertaken at each stage

(1) *Reproductive health check-up*
- (a) Family history of prospective mother and father, and obstetric history of females
- (b) Case history and available medical records of females, e.g., epilepsy, diabetes
- (c) Vaginal and cervical smear screening for sexually transmitted infections/disorders
- (d) Sperm analysis to detect subfertility and pyosperm (i.e. pus cells in the semen as indicators of sexually transmitted infections)
- (e) Psychosexual assessment
- (f) Blood screening of women to detect rubella seronegativity, or lack of previous exposure to varicella (vaccination will be offered), or HIV positivity. In addition, carrier screening for cystic fibrosis and, more recently, predictive genetic diagnostic tests are carried out at this stage

(2) *The 3-month preparation for conception period*
- (a) Protection of germ cells: avoidance of tobacco, alcohol or narcotic consumption, and unnecessary drugs
- (b) Discontinuation of oral contraception, and removal of IUDs (condoms are provided)
- (c) Occupational history of females
- (d) Menstrual history; measurement of basal body temperature for detection of hormonal dysfunction (and commencement of further investigation and treatment, if necessary)
- (e) Start of preconceptional multivitamin supplementation
- (f) Recommendation that dental status should be checked
- (h) Guidelines for physical exercise
- (i) Guidelines for healthy diet

(3) *Better protection of early pregnancy*
- (a) Undertaking of all additional investigations/treatments necessitated by conditions and disorders detected at the preconception check-up
- (b) Appropriate investigation and treatment of women demonstrating hormonal dysfunction
- (c) Optimal timing of conception in relation to ovulation
- (d) Early pregnancy confirmation using pregnancy tests and ultrasound scanning
- (e) Postconceptional multivitamin supplementation
- (f) Avoidance of teratogenic and other risks
- (g) Referral of pregnant women to prenatal care clinics

NTD?" About 95% of women delivering infants with NTD do not have a previous NTD pregnancy, so the prevention of primary NTD would be a real public health success. The second question concerned dosage. We wished to test the efficacy of a folic acid dose of less than 1 mg.

The Hungarian RCT was carried out at the HPS co-coordinating centre in Budapest between 1984 and 1991 (125–130), all participants were supplied with one of two types of apparently identical capsules according to a randomization scheme and asked to intake one capsule per day for at least 1 month prior to conception and at least 2 months following conception.

19.11.3.2 Results of the Hungarian RCT

The final data of the Hungarian RCT included 5,502 women whose pregnancies were confirmed and NTD cases were not found amongst the informative offspring

Table 19.7 First occurrence of neural tube defects (NTD) in informative offspring of "supplemented" women (those taking periconceptional folic acid-containing multivitamin-micronutrient supplementation) and "unsupplemented" women in the two Hungarian intervention studies

Intervention trials	Supplement	No supplement
Randomized controlled trial		
Number of offspring	2,471	2,391
Expected/observed number of NTD	6.9/0	6.7/6[a]
RR (with 95% CI)	0.07 (0.04–0.13)	
Cohort controlled trial		
Number of offspring	3,056	3,056
Expected/observed number of NTD	8.5/1[b]	8.5/9[c]
OR (with 95% CI)	0.11 (0.01–0.91)	
Pooled data		
Number of offspring	5,527	5,447
Expected/observed number of NTD	15.4/1	15.2/15
OR (with 95% CI)	0.08 (0.01–0.47)	

[a] 2 anencephaly, 2 anencephaly + spina bifida (1 lumbar, 1 thoracolumbar), 2 spina bifida (1 thoracolumbar, 1 lumbosacral).
[b] 1 anencephaly.
[c] 1 anencephaly, 8 spina bifida (1 thoracolumbar, 4 lumbar, 3 lumbosacral).

in the "multivitamin" group, but 6 NTD cases among the informative offspring of the "placebo-like" group ($p = 0.01$) (Table 19.7). Thus, the Hungarian RCT demonstrated that a multivitamin containing 0.8 mg of folic acid prevented *about 90% of primary NTD.*

The Hungarian RCT was performed in parallel with the MRC Vitamin Study (MRC, 1991) which also commenced in 1984 and Hungary was one of seven countries that collaborated in this RCT and contributed 43% of the participants. The MRC Vitamin Study found that a *pharmacological dose (4 mg) of folic acid supplementation alone reduced NTD recurrence by 71%.* In 1992, on the basis of these results, the US Public Health authorities recommended periconceptional folic acid (0.4 mg) supplementation for all women seeking to become pregnant (CDC, 1992). However, at that time there was no scientific evidence to support the recommended dose (in the Smithells study, 0.36 mg folic acid was a component of the multivitamin preparation used, and had not been individually tested). Subsequently the efficacy of this amount of folic acid in preventing primary NTD was evaluated in a Chinese intervention study (Berry et al., 1999). These workers found that folic acid (0.4 mg) daily was sufficient to reduce the risk of NTD in areas with a *high rate of NTD (6.5 per 1,000) by about 79%, while in areas with low rates of NTD (0.8 per 1,000) cases with NTD were reduced by 41%.*

Furthermore the Hungarian RCT also generated an unexpected finding. Periconceptional multivitamin supplementation was also associated with a significant reduction in *the total rate of informative offspring with major CA*: 20.6 per 1,000 in the "multivitamin" group and 40.6 per 1,000 in the "placebo-like" group (0.53, 0.35–0.70). When 6 NTD cases were excluded, this difference in the rates of major CA between the two study groups remained very highly significant ($p < 0.0001$). Thus, periconceptional multivitamin supplementation reduced not only the occurrence of NTD but also the rate of other major CAs. The detailed analysis of the final data set from the Hungarian RCT, which was based on personal medical examination of all children born to participants in the RCT, indicated a significant reduction in two further groups of *CA: the urinary tract and the cardiovascular system* (Table 19.8). The reduction was most marked in the case of obstructive CAs of the urinary tract and conotruncal cardiovascular CAs including ventricular septal defects (3 vs. 10; 0.09–0.97). There was also some reduction in the prevalence at birth of congenital limb deficiencies, congenital pyloric stenosis, and Down syndrome in the "multivitamin" group but this difference between the two groups in the RCT was not significant. There was no difference between the rates of cases with two frequent types of orofacial cleft: cleft palate and cleft lip ± palate, in addition to unclassified multiple CAs in the multivitamin and placebo-like groups.

19.11.3.3 Results of the Hungarian Cohort Controlled Trial

For ethical reasons, it was not possible to continue the Hungarian RCT. Therefore a *cohort controlled trial* (CCT) was designed to collect further data in order to confirm or reject the efficacy of periconceptional folic acid-containing multivitamin supplementation in preventing CAs other than NTD. Supplemented women were recruited via the HPS co-coordinating centre in Budapest and the 31 HPS subsidiary centers between 1993 and 1996. All participants were supplemented with the same folic acid (0.8 mg)-containing multivitamin (Elevit prenatal®) during the periconceptional period. Women in the supplemented cohort were followed until the 14th week of gestation, while a cohort of unsupplemented women was recruited from the Regional Prenatal Care Clinics at the 14th week of pregnancy. None of these women had received supplementation with folic acid, folic acid-containing multivitamins, or any multivitamins either before conception or in the first trimester of pregnancy. Women in the unsupplemented cohort were matched to each pregnant woman in the supplemented cohort based on age, socio-economic status, and place of residence. As in the RCT, the pediatric examinations (which included a cardiological assessment) were similar in the two CCT study groups.

The final data set of 3,056 supplemented and unsupplemented matched pairs showed that the cohort of supplemented pregnant women recruited via the HPS appeared to have a higher rate of morbidity (e.g. diabetes mellitus and epilepsy), and of previous unsuccessful pregnancy outcomes (miscarriages and CA, including NTD), compared to the cohort of unsupplemented pregnant women recruited through the Regional Prenatal Care clinics. This may have been due to the good reputation of the HPS in establishing optimal conditions for conception and providing care in early pregnancy which might have attracted women who had previously experienced problems in pregnancy. Thus the majority of supplemented women were at high risk for adverse pregnancy outcome, while most unsupplemented

Table 19.8 The efficacy of periconceptional folic acid-containing multivitamin (micronutrient) supplementation in the primary prevention of some major groups of CAs

	Hungarian intervention trials				Pooled data	
	RCT		CCT			
CA groups	No supplement ($n = 2{,}391$)	Supplement ($n = 2{,}471$)	No supplement ($n = 3{,}056$)	Supplement ($n = 3{,}056$)	No supplement ($n = 5{,}447$)	Supplement ($n = 5{,}527$)
Urinary tract CAs						
Renal a/dysgenesis	3	0	0	2	3	2
Cystic kidney	1	1	0	2	1	3
Obstructive CAs						
Pelvicoureteric junction	4	0	13	2	17	2
Other locations	1	1	6	8	7	9
Total	9	2	19	14	28	16
OR (95% CI)	**0.21 (0.05–0.95)**		0.71 (0.33–1.50)		0.56 (0.30–1.04)	
Cardiovascular CAs						
Conotruncal						
Ventricular septal defect	8	2	19	5	27	7
Others	2	1	1	3	3	4
Subtotal	10	3	20	8	30	11
Others	10	7	30	23	40	30
Total	20	10	50	31	70	41
OR (95% CI)	**0.42 (0.19–0.98)**		**0.60 (0.38–0.96)**		**0.57 (0.39–0.85)**	
Congenital limb deficiencies						
Terminal transverse	2	1	3	1	5	2
Others	3	0	0	0	3	0
Total	5	1	3	1	8	2
OR (95% CI)	0.19 (0.03–1.18)		0.33 (0.01–3.71)		0.25 (0.05–1.16)	
Congenital pyloric stenosis	8	2	2	0	10	2
OR (95% CI)	0.24 (0.05–1.14)		0.00 (0.00–26.8)		**0.20 (0.04–0.90)**	

Table 19.8 (continued)

CA groups	Hungarian intervention trials: RCT No supplement ($n = 2,391$)	RCT Supplement ($n = 2,471$)	CCT No supplement ($n = 3,056$)	CCT Supplement ($n = 3,056$)	Pooled data No supplement ($n = 5,447$)	Pooled data Supplement ($n = 5,527$)
Anal/rectal atresia/stenosis	1	0	4	1	5	1
OR (95% CI)	–		0.31 (0.02–2.52)		0.20 (0.02–1.69)	
Orofacial clefts						
Cleft lip ± palate	3	4	2	3	5	7
Cleft palate	2	0	1	1	3	1
Total	5	4	3	4	8	8
OR (95% CI)	0.77 (0.22–2.69)		1.63 (0.31–2.88)		0.99 (0.37–2.63)	
Down syndrome	5	2	8	8	13	10
OR (95% CI)	0.39 (0.07–1.99)		1.00 (0.33–1.73)		0.76 (0.33–1.73)	
Unclassified multiple CAs	5	6	15	12	20	18
OR (95% CI)	1.16 (0.35–3.81)		0.79 (0.40–1.48)		0.89 (0.47–1.68)	

women could be considered to be at low risk. The presence of these important confounding factors was undesirable from the scientific point of view, but since both the CCT and the RCT were performed under the umbrella of the HPS, with its role in the provision of primary health care for women seeking to become pregnant, it was felt that we had no right to exclude "high-risk" couples. In addition, when the study design for the CCT was being prepared, this unexpected bias was not taken into account because our previous experience came from the RCT which had mainly involved women in their first pregnancy.

The CCT confirmed the protective effect of folic acid-containing multivitamin supplementation, and its role in reducing the total prevalence of NTD: we found one NTD among the informative offspring in the supplemented group and nine NTDs among informative offspring in the unsupplemented cohort (Table 19.7). However, 34 informative offspring in the supplemented cohort had 36 previous sibs with NTD (two had two NTD siblings). In addition, six mothers and two fathers had NTD themselves (including 3 mothers and 2 fathers who had the mild form of NTD, the so-called spinal dysraphism). There was no recurrent NTD in our supplemented cohort. In the unsupplemented cohort, three women with previous NTD offspring had informative offspring, and one of these had a recurrence of NTD.

Table 19.8 shows the occurrence of other CAs in the supplemented and unsupplemented groups. Cardiovascular CAs are heterogeneous in their origin and manifestation, and have different critical periods, but their total occurrence (31 vs. 50) was again significantly reduced in the supplemented cohort. This can be explained mainly by the reduction in the number of *ventricular septal defects* (5 vs. 19) (0.26, 0.09–0.72) in the supplemented cohort. Urinary tract CAs are also very heterogeneous in their origin and manifestation, but there was no significant difference in their occurrence between the supplemented and unsupplemented cohorts (14 vs. 19 cases). However, within the subgroup of obstructive CAs (10 vs. 19), *stenosis of the pelvicoureteric junction* (2 vs. 13) showed a significant reduction in the supplemented cohort (0.19; 0.04–0.86). The causes and manifestation of limb deficiencies are many and heterogeneous, and there was again a trend towards reduction in incidence in the supplemented cohort (1 vs. 3): it is perhaps worth mentioning that all children in the unsupplemented cohort had unimelic terminal transverse type defects. *Congenital pyloric stenosis* was diagnosed in two infants in the unsupplemented cohort but was not found in the supplemented cohort. There was no reduction in the incidence of cleft lip $\pm$ palate or cleft palate in the supplemented group.

Finally, two "syndromic" groups with multiple CAs were evaluated. There was no difference in the rate of *Down syndrome* between the supplemented and unsupplemented cohorts. We did not detect any change in the rate of unclassified *multiple CAs* following periconceptional supplementation.

The results of the Hungarian CCT were thus in agreement with the findings of the previous RCT showing that periconceptional multivitamin supplementation protects against some CAs of the cardiovascular system (principally ventricular septal defects) and obstructive CAs of the urinary tract, particularly stenosis of the pelvicoureteric junction. These preventive effects were clearly evident despite the fact that the supplemented pregnant women represented a cohort at high risk due to a higher rate of maternal morbidity and a greater number of unsuccessful previous pregnancies.

The efficacy of folic acid-containing multivitamin supplementation in preventing cardiovascular CAs (mainly conotruncal defects e.g. common truncus, transposition of the great vessels and tetralogy of Fallot, and certain types of ventricular septal defects) was also demonstrated in two US studies (Botto et al., 1996; Botto et al., 2000b). Their results, together with our results from the RCT and CCT trials, suggest that periconceptional multivitamin supplementation was associated with an approximately 40% reduction in risk for cardiovascular CAs. The effect of early postconceptional supplementation with a pharmacological dose (6 mg) of folic acid alone in protecting against cardiovascular CAs was also discernible in the data set of the HCCSCA (99). Recently, two groups reported raised plasma homocysteine levels and methylenetetrahydrofolate reductase (MTHFR) gene polymorphisms in association with cardiovascular CA (Kapusta et al., 1999; van Beynum et al., 2006). However, three other US studies (Shaw et al., 1995; Werler et al., 1999; Scanlon et al., 1998) failed to demonstrate a significant protective effect of periconceptional multivitamin supplementation for cardiovascular outflow tract defects, although the reduction was close to significance (0.7, 0.5–1.1) in the study of Shaw et al. (1995). Incidentally, cardiovascular CAs were induced by pteroylglutamic acid deficiency during gestation in rat fetuses (Baird et al., 1954; Monie and Nelson, 1963).

In both the Hungarian RCT and CCT the incidence of obstructive CAs of the urinary tract (more precisely stenosis of the pelvicoureteric junction) was reduced in infants born to mothers who had received multivitamin supplementation (see Table 19.8). In the 1950s Monie et al. (1954, 1957) had been able to produce CAs of the urinary tract in folic acid-deficient rat embryos, while Li et al. (1995) and Werler et al. (1999) also observed a significant reduction in the rate of human urinary tract CAs following multivitamin supplementation in the first trimester of pregnancy.

One US study showed a significant reduction in congenital limb deficiencies following multivitamin supplementation (Yang et al., 1997). Two other studies (Shaw et al., 1995; Werler et al., 1999) also found reductions in incidence (RR: 0.50 and 0.64), but these differences were not significant, as the confidence intervals were too wide. In human embryos the teratogenic effects of folate deficiency due to folic acid antagonists were associated with, amongst other CAs, limb deficiencies (Warkany et al., 1959; Hernandez-Diaz et al., 2000).

The combined incidence of pyloric stenosis in the Hungarian RCT and CCT showed a significant reduction after periconceptional multivitamin supplementation. However, this finding was not confirmed in a US study (Werler et al., 1999).

In the China/US Collaborative Project for Neural Tube Defect Prevention (Berry et al., 1999), a somewhat lower occurrence of rectal atresia/stenosis was found following periconceptional folic acid supplementation (Myers et al., 2001). The Hungarian RCT and CCT showed a similar trend (1 vs. 5) (see Table 19.8).

In 1982, Tolarova reported that periconceptional supplementation with a multivitamin and very high dose folic acid (10 mg) formulation was effective in reducing the recurrence rate of cleft lip. However, the Hungarian RCT and CCT failed to show a reduction in the birth prevalence of cleft lip ± palate and cleft palate following supplementation with a multivitamin preparation containing a low dose (0.8 mg) of folic acid (see Table 19.8). On the other hand, a significant reduction was observed in the data set from the HCCSCA following a high dose (usually 6 mg) of folic acid alone (100). Thus a dose-dependent preventive role for folic acid in the prevention of orofacial clefting cannot be excluded. Other studies yielded controversial results, varying according to dosage, population genetic background, and the socioeconomic status and lifestyle, particularly the diet, of the women studied (Botto et al., 2004).

Botto et al. (2002c) found a lower rate of omphalocele in newborn infants born to mothers following periconceptional multivitamin supplementation (0.4, 0.2–1.0). The supplemented and unsupplemented groups of the Hungarian RCT and CCT contained 1:1 and 3:1 infants with omphalocele, respectively.

Recent publications had suggested an association between polymorphisms in genes involved in folate metabolism and maternal risk of Down syndrome (James et al., 1999; Hobbs et al., 2000; Barkai et al., 2003; Gueant et al., 2003).We therefore sought to explore this putative association in the HCCSCA, which indicated that supplementation with a high dose (usually 6 mg) of folic acid and iron had some impact in preventing Down syndrome (104).

We did not find any difference in the incidence of cases with *unclassified multiple CA* in the RCT and CCT following multivitamin supplementation during the periconceptional period (132) (see Table 19.8). However, the birth defect registries of Shaw et al. (2000) and Yuskin et al. (2005) reported a higher occurrence of multiple CAs following periconceptional multivitamin supplementation. We therefore sought to evaluate this in the data set of the HCCSCA. However, while our data showed that periconceptional folic acid/multivitamin supplementation did not reduce the incidence of multiple unclassified CAs; neither did it cause an increase in the number of cases (103).

The total reduction in CAs was just 20.0/1,000 (40.6–20.6/1,000) in the Hungarian RCT. The rate of NTD was 2.5/1,000 in the "trace element" group and this figure was near the previously determined prevalence at birth of NTD (2.8/1,000) in Hungary. Thus the total reduction of CAs without NTD was 17.5/1,000 in the multivitamin group, which is approximately 6.3–7.0 times greater that the incidence of NTD in Hungary, indicating the importance of folic acid-containing multivitamins in the reduction of risk for CAs other than NTD. This reduction is principally due to a reduction of cardiovascular CAs, because the birth prevalence of cardiovascular CAs was 10.2/1,000 in Hungary which is 3.6 times greater than the total (birth + fetal) prevalence of NTD. Thus, the role of this new primary preventive measure in preventing other CAs is at least as important, from a public health point of view, as its role in preventing NTD. In the light of this finding, it is strange that, while the value of folic acid/multivitamin supplementation for prevention of NTD was accepted with enthusiasm by the international scientific community in the early 1990s, and prompted fresh recommendations for practical implementation, these novel data have been received with reservations and have failed to stimulate any further recommendations for exploiting their protective effect against other CAs. On one hand, these reservations are understandable because different CAs have different origins making it difficult to believe that an intervention as simple as multivitamin supplementation can reduce the incidence of CAs of distinctly different origins. On the other hand, several studies (Botto et al., 2004) have confirmed its role in preventing or reducing the incidence of CAs other than NTD. It is clearly necessary, therefore, to identify and clarify the mechanism by which periconceptional folic acid/folic acid-containing multivitamin supplementation acts to reduce the incidence of specific CAs.

At present 20–25% of infant mortality in industrialized countries can be attributed to CAs, and CAs are among the leading causes of loss of life.

In conclusion, folic acid or folic acid-containing multivitamin supplementation offers a breakthrough in the primary prevention of NTD and some other CAs, because of its ability to reduce the incidence of CAs by about one third (Tarusco, 2004). It constitutes a better alternative than so-called secondary prevention (that is, termination of a pregnancy following diagnosis of severe fetal defect).

19.11.4 Folic Acid or Multivitamin in Reduction of Maternal Disease Related CAs

At present there are three important topics in this field.

19.11.4.1 High Fever Related Maternal Diseases

As previously presented there is an important association between high fever related maternal disease and some specific CAs. Antipyretic drugs can reduce this risk, however, as the findings of Botto et al. (2001, 2002a) showed first, folic acid-containing multivitamins can also reduce high fever related CA risk. Later Shaw et al. (1998) reported a 7.4 fold increased risk for NTD in mothers with fever who did not take folic acid-containing multivitamins. The HCCSCA data set showed that folic acid/multivitamin supplementation can reduce and/or protect against the teratogenic effects of high fever in some (NTD and CL $\pm$ CP), but not all CAs. For example, periconceptional multivitamin/folic acid supplementation cannot reduce the high fever related risk for MCA.

In conclusion, the teratogenic effect of high fever related maternal diseases can be reduced by antipyretic drugs; however, folic acid/multivitamin supplementation should also be administered to further reduce the risk for CAs.

19.11.4.2 Maternal Epilepsy

Our study based on the data set of the HCCSCA confirmed the higher risk of NTD, CL $\pm$ CP, CP, and cardiovascular CA after the use of antiepileptic drugs. Our data indicated the teratogenic effect of trimethadione, primidone, sultiame, valproate, phenytoin, mephenytoin. However, phenobarbital and diazepam did not increase the risk for CAs.

The effect of high dose of folic acid (3–9 mg, the estimated mean about 5.6 mg) supplementation during the time of organogenesis was evaluated. We investigated whether this primary preventive method can reduce the prevalence of total or specific CAs among children exposed to these antiepileptic drugs. The risk of CL ± CP and NTD in offspring of mothers treated with antiepileptic drugs without folic acid was higher than in the offspring of pregnant women treated with antiepileptics and folic acid together. Thus the risk of 1.5 (1.1–1.5) in the total CA group was reduced to 1.3 (0.8–1.9). In addition, it is worth mentioning that this risk reduction was after monotherapy from 1.4 (1.1–1.8) to 1.2 (0.8–1.8) and mainly after polytherapy from 5.2 (1.4–19.3) to 2.4 (0.5–10.8). However, there was an unexpected finding: the risk of multiple CA increased after the concomitant use of antiepileptic drugs and high dose of folic acid.

Folic acid CA-reducing effect was also evaluated in different antiepileptic drugs. The risk of all CA after carbamazepine treatment without folic acid was 3.3 (1.5–7.5) but with concomitant folic acid supplementation only 1.3 (0.4–4.0). A similar risk reduction was found in pregnant women with primidone treatment and folic acid use together from 5.2 (1.7–16.3) to 2.5 (0.8–7.5). There was a risk reduction after the parallel use of phenytoin and folic acid as well, but this reduction did not reach the level of significance. The teratogenicity reducing effect of valproate was not found with the parallel use of folic acid.

In conclusion, the evaluation of concomitant use of high dose folic acid demonstrated risk reducing effect in women taking antiepileptic drugs, particularly with specific drugs such as carbamazepine or primidone.

19.11.4.3 Maternal Diabetes Mellitus

Our study confirmed the higher risk of some specific CAs in the offspring of pregnant women with DM-I. However, as far we know our study was the first showing that high dose folic acid supplementation was able to reduce some DM-I related CAs in the offspring of diabetic pregnant women. Folic acid or folic acid-containing multivitamin supplementation during early pregnancy changed the spectrum of DM related CAs. There was a significant reduction in neural-tube defect, CAs of the spine, and congenital limb deficiencies.

In conclusion, there was a significant improvement in the preconceptional and prenatal care of diabetic pregnant women during the last decades which resulted in a decrease in the frequency of DM related CAs. However, the implementation of folic acid or folic acid-containing multivitamin supplementation into the protocol of diabetic pregnant women's care may further improve the efficacy of this preventive effort.

19.12 General Conclusions

Folic acid or folic acid containing multivitamin supplementation in early pregnancy was shown to be an effective method in preventing NTD and some other CAs in general. However, recent studies indicated that folic acid or folic acid-containing multivitamin supplementation was appropriate for the prevention of CAs related to specific causes such as high fever, antiepileptic drugs, or diabetes mellitus in pregnant women.

References

Baird CD, Nelson MM, Monie IW, Evans HM. Congenital cardiovascular anomalies induced by pteroylglutamic acid deficiency during gestation in the rat. Circ Rev 1954; 2: 544–548.

Barkai G, Arbuzova S, Berkenstadt M et al. Frequency of Down's syndrome and neural-tube defects in the same family. Lancet 2003; 361: 1331–1335.

Berry RJ, Li Z, Erickson JD, Li S et al. Prevention of neural-tube defects with folic acid in China. China-US Collaborative Project for Neural Tube Defect Prevention. N Engl J Med 1999; 341: 1485–1490.

Botto LD, Erickson JD, Mulinare J et al. Maternal fever, multivitamin use and selected birth defects: evidence or interaction. Epidemiology 2002a; 13: 620–621.

Botto LD, Khoury MJ, Mulinare J, Erickson JD. Periconceptional multivitamin use and the occurrence of conotruncal heart defects. Results from a population-based case-control study. Pediatrics 1996; 98: 911–917.

Botto LD, Lynberg MC, Erickson JD. Congenital heart defects, maternal febrile illness, and multivitamin use: a population-based study. Epidemiology 2001; 12: 485–490.

Botto LD, Mulinare J, Erickson JD. Occurrence of congenital heart defects in relation to maternal multivitamin use. Am J Epidemiol 2000b; 151: 878–884.

Botto LD, Mulinare J, Erickson JD. Occurrence of omphalocele in relation to maternal multivitamin use: a population-based study. Pediatrics 2002c; 109: 904–908.

Botto LD, Olney RS, Erickson JD. Vitamin supplements and the risk for congenital anomalies other than neural tube defects Am J Med Genet C 2004; 125C: 12–21.

Brinsmade AB, Rubsaamen H. Zur Teratogenetischen Wirkung von Unspezifischem Fieber auf den sich Entwickelnden Kaninchenembryo. Beitr Pathol Anat 1957; 117: 154–164.

Buckiova D, Brown NA. Mechanism of hyperthermia effects on CNS development: rostral gene expression domains remain, despite severe head truncation, and the hindbrain/octocyst relationship is altered. Teratology 1999; 59: 139–147.

CDC: Centers for Disease Control. Recommendations for the use of folic acid to reduce the number of cases of spina bifida and other neural tube defects. MMWR 1992; 41: 1233–1238.

Chambers CD. Risk of hyperthermia associated with hot tub or spa use by pregnant women. Birth Defects Res A 2006; 76: 569–573.

Chambers CD. Johnson KA, Di LM et al. Maternal fever and birth outcome: a prospective study. Teratology 1998; 58: 251–237.

Chance PF, Smith DW. Hyperthermia and meningomyelocele and anencephaly. Lancet 1978; 1: 769–770.

Clarren SK, Smith DW, Harvey MAS et al. Hyperthermia: a prospective evaluation of a possible teratogenic agent in man. J Pediatr 1979; 95: 81–83.

Cockroft DL, New DAT. Abnormalities induced in rat embryos by hyperthermia. Teratology 1978; 17: 277–284.

Edwards MJ. Congenital defects in guinea pigs following induced hyperthermia during gestation. Arch Pathol 1967; 84: 42–47.

Edwards MJ. Congenital defects in guinea pigs: prenatal retardation of brain growth of guinea pigs following hyperthermia during gestation. Teratology 1969a; 2: 239–245.

Edwards MJ. Congenital defects in guinea pigs: fetal resorptions, abortions and malformations following induced hyperthermia during early gestation. Teratology 1969b; 2: 313–328.

Edwards MJ. The experimental production of arthrogryposis multiplex congenita in guinea pigs by maternal hyperthermia during gestation. J Pathol 1971; 104: 221–228.
Edwards MJ. Hyperthermia as a teratogen: a review of experimental studies and their clinical significance. Terat Carcinog Mutag 1986; 6: 563–582.
Edwards MJ, Shiota K, Walsh DA, Smith MS. Hyperthermia and birth defects. Reprod Toxicol 1995; 9: 411–425.
Ferencz C, Loffredo C, Correa-Villasenor A. Genetic and environmental factors of major cardiovascular malformations: the Baltimore-Washington Infant study 1981–1989. Futura Publishing Co. Inc., Armonk, NY, 1997.
Fisher NL, Smith DW. Occipital encephalocele and early gestational hyperthermia. Pediatrics 1981; 68: 480–483.
Fraser FC, Skelton J. Possible teratogenicity of maternal fever. Lancet 1978; 2: 634. (only)
German MA, Webster WS, Edwards MJ. Hyperthermia as a teratogen: parameters determining hyperthermia-induced head defects in the rat. Teratology 1985; 31: 265–272.
Graham JM, Edwards MJ, Lipson AH, Webster WS. Gestational hyperthermia as a cause for Moebius syndrome. Teratology 1988; 37: 461–462.
Gueant JL, Gueant-Rodriguez RM, Anello G et al. Genetic determination of folate and vitamin B12 metabolism: a common pathway in neural tube defects and Down syndrome? Clin Chem Lab Med 2003; 41: 1473–1477.
Halperin LR, Wilroy RS Jr. Maternal hyperthermia and neural-tube defects. Lancet 1978; 2: 212–213.
Harding AJ, Edwards MJ. As a results of prenatal hyperthermia three week old rats display microcephaly absent in the newborn. Teratology 1991; 44: 477–478.
Hartley WJ, Alexander G, Marshall MJ. Brain cavitation and microcephaly in lambs exposed to prenatal hyperthermia. Teratology 1974; 9: 299–304.
Hernandez-Diaz S, Werler MM, Walker AM, Mitchell AA. Folic acid antagonists during pregnancy and risk of birth defects. N Engl J Med 2000; 343: 1608–1614.
Hobbs CA, Sherman SL, Yi P, Hopkins SE et al. Polymorphisms in genes involved in folate metabolism as maternal risk factors for Down syndrome. Am J Hum Genet 2000; 67: 623–630.
Hofmann D, Dietzel F. Abort und Missbildungen nach Kurzwellemdurchflutung in der Schwangerschaft. Geburts Frauenheilk 1966; 26: 378–390.
Hunter AGW. Neural tube defects in eastern Ontario and western Quebec: demography and family data. Am J Med Genet 1984; 19: 45–63.
James SJ, Pogribna M, Pogribny IP et al. Abnormal folate metabolism and mutation in the methylenetetrahydrofolate-reductase gene may be maternal risk factors for Down syndrome. Am J Clin Nutr 1999; 70: 495–501.
Jones KL. Hyperthermia-induced spectrum of defects. In: Jones KL (ed.) Smith's Recognizable Patterns of Human Malformation. 4th ed. WB Saunders Co., Philadelphia, 2004. pp. 516–519.
Jonson KM, Lyle JG, Edwards MJ, Penny RHC. Effect of prenatal heat stress on brain growth and serial discrimination reversal learning in the guinea pig. Brain Res Bull 1976; 1: 133–150.
Kapusta L, Haagmans MLM, Steegers EAP et al. Congenital heart defects and derangement of homocysteine metabolism. J Pediat 1999; 135: 773–774.
Kilham L, Fern VH. Exencephaly in fetal hamsters exposed to hyperthermia. Teratology 1976; 14: 323–326.
Kleinbrecht J, Michaelis H, Michaelis J, Koller S. Fever in pregnancy and congenital defects. Lancet 1979; 1: 1403.
Layde PM, Edmonds LD, Erickson JD. Maternal fever and neural tube defects. Teratology 1980; 21: 105–108.
Li DK, Daling JR, Mueller BA, Hickock DE et al. Periconceptional multivitamin use in relation to the risk of congenital urinary tract anomalies. Epidemiology 1995; 6: 212–218.
Lipson AH, Webster WS, Brown-Woodman PDC, Osborn RA. Moebius syndrome: animal model – human correlations and evidence for a brainstem vascular etiology. Teratology 1989; 40: 339–350.

Little SA, Mirkes PE. Increased levels of 3 pro-apoptotic Bcl-2 genes, NOXA, PUMA and DP5, in day 9 mouse embryos exposed to hyperthermia (HS) or 4-hydroperoxycyclophosphamide (4-CP) (Abstract). Birth Defects Res A 2003; 67: 323.

Lundberg YW, Wing MJ, Xiong W et al. Genetic dissection of hyperthermia-induced neural tube defects in mice. Birth Defects Res A 2003; 67: 409–413.

Lynberg MC, Khoury MJ, Lu X, Cocian T. Maternal flu, fever and the risk of neural-tube defects: a population-based case-control study. Am J Epidemiol 1994; 140: 244–255.

Miettinen OS, Reiner ML, Nadas AS. Seasonal incidence of coarctation of the aorta. Br Heart J 1970; 32: 103–107.

Miller P, Smith DW, Shepard TH. Hyperthermia as one possible etiology of anencephaly. Lancet 1978; 1: 519–521.

Milunsky A, Ulcickas M, Rothman KJ et al. Maternal heat exposure and neural-tube defects. J Am Med Assoc 1992; 268: 882–885.

Mirkes PE. Effects of acute exposures to elevated temperatures on rat embryo growth and development in vitro. Teratology 1985; 32: 259–266.

Mirkes PE. Molecular/cellular biology of the heat stress response and its role in agent-induced teratogenesis. Mut Res 1997; 396: 163–173.

Monie IW, Nelson MM. Abnormalities of pulmonary and other vessels in rat fetuses from maternal pteroylglutamic acid deficiency. Anat Rec 1963; 147: 397–401.

Monie IW, Nelson MM, Evans HM. Abnormalities of the urinary system of rat embryos resulting from maternal pteroylglutamic acid deficiency. Anat Rec 1954; 120: 119–136.

Monie IW, Nelson MM, Evans HM. Abnormalities of the urinary system of rat embryos resulting from transitory deficiency of pteroylglutamic acid during gestation in the rat. Anat Rec 1957; 127: 711–724.

MRC Vitamin Study Research Group. Prevention of neural tube defects: results of the Medical Research Council Vitamin study. Lancet 1991; 338: 131–137.

Myers MF, Li S, Correa-Villasenor A, Li Z et al. Folic acid supplementation and risk for imperforate anus in China. Am J Epidemiol 2001; 154: 1051–1056.

Nevin NC, Seller MJ. Prevention of neural tube defect recurrences. Lancet 1990. 1: 178–179.

Rao GS, Abraham V, Fink BA et al. Biochemical changes in the developing rat central nervous system due to hyperthermia. Teratology 1990; 41: 327–332.

Sasaki J, Yamaguchi A, Nabeshima Y et al. Exercise at high temperature causes maternal hyperthermia and fetal anomalies in rats. Teratology 1995; 51: 233–236.

Scanlon KS, Ferencz C, Loffredo CA et al. Preconceptional folate intake and malformations of the cardiac outflow tract. Baltimore-Washington Infant Study Group. Epidemiology 1998; 9: 95–98.

Shaw GW, O'Malley CD, Wasserman CR, Tolarova MM. Maternal periconceptional use of multivitamin and reduced risk for conotruncal heart defects and limb deficiencies among offspring. Am J Med Genet 1995; 59: 536–545.

Shaw GM, Croen LA, Todoroff K, Tolarova MM. Periconceptional intake of vitamin supplements and risk of multiple congenital anomalies. Am J Med Genet 2000; 93: 188–193.

Shaw GM, Todoroff K, Velie EM, Lammer EJ Maternal illness, including fever, and medication use as risk factors of neural-tube defects. Teratology 1998; 57: 1–7.

Shiota K. Neural-tube defects and maternal hyperthermia in early pregnancy. Epidemiology in a human embryo population. Am J Med Genet 1982; 12: 281–288.

Shiota K. Induction of neural tube defects and skeletal malformations in mice following brief hyperthermia in utero. Biol Neonat 1988; 53: 86–97.

Shiota JK, Kayamura T. Effects of prenatal heat stress on postnatal growth, behaviour and learning capacity in mice. Biol Neonat 1989; 56: 6–14.

Skreb N, Frank Z. Developmental abnormalities in the rat induced by heat shock. J Embryol Exp Morphol 1963; 11: 445–457.

Smith DW, Clarren SK, Harrey MA. Hyperthermia as a possible teratogenic agent. J Pediatr 1978; 92: 878–883.

Smith M, Edwards MJ, Waugh P. Maternal hyperthermia and the formation of cataract in the lens of the embryonic and fetal guinea pig. Cong Anom (Kyoto) 1996; 36: 7–19.

Smithells RW, Sheppard S, Schorah CJ et al. Possible prevention of neural tube defects by periconceptional vitamin supplementation. Lancet 1980; 1: 339–340.

Smithells RW, Sheppard S, Wild J, Schorah CJ. Prevention of neural tube defect recurrences in Yorkshire: final report. Lancet 1989; 2: 498–499.

Tarusco D, editor. Folic Acid: From Research to Public Health Practice. Rapporti ISTISAN 04/26, Rome, 2004.

Tennant PWG, Pearce MS, Bythell M, Rankin J. 20-year survival of children born with congenital anomalies: a population-based study. Lancet 2010; 375: 649–656.

Tikkanen J, Heinonen OP. Maternal hyperthermia during pregnancy and cardiovascular malformations in the offspring. Eur J Epidemiol 1991; 7: 628–635.

Tikkanen J, Heinonen OP. Risk factors for hypoplastic left heart syndrome. Teratology 1994; 50: 112–117.

Tolarova M. Periconceptional supplementation with vitamins and folic acid to prevent recurrence of cleft lip. Lancet 1982; 2: 217.

Umpierre CC, Little SA, Mirkes PE. Co-localization of active caspase-3 and DNA fragmentationn (TUNEL) in normal and hyperthermia-induced abnormal mouse development. Teratology 2001; 63: 134–145.

Van Beynum IM, Kapusta L, den Heijer M et al. Maternal MTHFR 677C>T is a risk factors for congenital heart defects: effect modification by periconceptional folate supplementation. Eur Heart J 2006; 27: 981–987.

Warkany J, Beaudry PH, Hornstein S. Attempted abortion with 4-aminopteroylglutamic acid (aminopterin): malformations of the child. Am J Dis Child 1959; 97: 274–281.

Webster WS, Edwards MJ. Hyperthgermia and the induction of neural tube defects in mice. Teratology 1984; 29: 417–425.

Werler MM, Hayes C, Louik C. Multivitamin use and risk of birth defects. Am J Epidemiol 1999; 150: 675–682.

Yang Q, Khoury MJ, Olney RS, Mulinare J. Does periconceptional multivitamin use reduce the risk for limb deficiency in offspring? Epidemiology 1997; 8: 157–161.

Yuskin N, Honein MA, Moore CA. Reported multivitamin supplementation and the occurrence of multiple congenital anomalies. Am J Med Genet A 2005; 136A: 1–7.

Own Publications

I. Czeizel AE, Puho HE, Ács N, Bánhidy F. High fever-related maternal diseases as possible cause of multiple congenital abnormalities: A population-based case-control study. Birth Defects Res A 2007; 79: 544–551.

II. Czeizel AE, Puho HE, Ács N, Bánhidy F. Delineation of multiple congenital abnormality syndrome in the offspring of pregnant women affected with high fever-related maternal disorders. A population-based study. Cong Anom (Kyoto) 2008; 48: 126–136.

III. Czeizel AE, Ács N, Puho HE, Bánhidy F. Primary prevention of congenital abnormalities due to high fever-related maternal diseases by antifever therapy and folic acid supplementation. Curr Woman's Health Rev 2007; 3: 1–12.

Chapter 20
Associations of Maternal Diseases with Higher Risk for Pretem Birth (PB) and Low Birth Weight (LBW) Newborns

The rate of PB is extremely high (about 9%) in Hungary and PB associated with about one-third of infant mortality during the 2000s. In addition, a major part of mental retardation, visual and other handicaps of children was related to PB. LBW as indicator of intrauterine fetal growth retardation was also associated with short- and long-term complications of newborns infants.

The data of PB and LBW newborns were evaluated using data only from the control pregnancies without CA because CAs may have a more drastic effect for these adverse birth outcomes than the maternal diseases themselves. First, some local and infectious maternal diseases will be presented in Sections 20.1 and 20.2 followed by the general evaluation of all maternal diseases and pregnancy complications in Sections 20.3 and 20.4. Finally, possible specific and general preventive methods of PB will be summarized in Sections 20.6 and 20.7.

20.1 Local Causes

20.1.1 CA of the Uterus

The developmental defect of the caudal fusion of the Müllerian (paramesonephric) ducts causes incomplete atretic proximal vagina and rudimentary bicornuate uterus, uterus unicornis or the so-called *Rokitansky sequence*.

In the data set of the HCCSCSA 67 (0.18%) mothers were affected with bicornuate uterus.

Mean gestational age of their newborns was much shorter (35.9 vs. 39.4 week) which also associated with a much lower mean birth weight (2,365 vs. 3,276 g). Thus the rate of PB was 67.2% compared to the 9.2% in pregnant women without uterus CA as reference. CA of the uterus therefore associated with 7.3 fold higher risk for PB. The rate of LBW newborns (44.8% vs. 5.7%) was also 7.9 times higher.

In conclusion, uterus CA, mainly bicornuate uterus, is associated with a high risk for PB and LBW.

N. Ács et al., *Congenital Abnormalities and Preterm Birth Related to Maternal Illnesses During Pregnancy*, DOI 10.1007/978-90-481-8620-4_20,

20.1.2 Cervical Incompetence

In the data set of the HCCSCA 2,795 (7.33%) mothers had medically recorded diagnosis of CIP in the prenatal maternity logbook. Most CIP were recorded in V and VI gestational months based on progressive dilatation of the uterine cervix and/or bulging membranes during the second trimester of pregnancy diagnosed by the manual examination of obstetrician in the prenatal care clinics which circumstances preterm delivery seemed inevitable without interference. All pregnant women with CIP recorded in the HCCSCA were treated due to this pathological condition.

One of the two types of treatment was used in all women with CIP. The preventive or therapeutical cervical cerclage was performed in certain part of Hungarian pregnant women according to the technique of McDonald. The treatment was complete bed rest in another part of women with CIP.

The mean gestational age was shorter by 0.4 week and mean birth weight was smaller by 82 g in pregnant women with CIP. The rate of PB was 11.2% compared to 9.0% of newborns of mothers without CIP. The rate of LBW newborns was also higher (7.8% vs. 5.5%). However, the lower mean birth weight and higher rate of LBW newborns can be explained by the shorter gestational age. The rates (e.g. PB) and means of birth outcomes (e.g. birth weight) in newborn infants born to mothers without CIP corresponded well to the Hungarian newborn population in the study period.

There was a higher rate of PB in the newborns of women with CIP, this rate is about 30% higher than the Hungarian population figure. However, it is necessary to consider that all pregnant women with CIP were treated due to CIP.

In conclusion there was an about 30% higher risk for PB in newborns of pregnant women with treated CIP, thus CIP was one of the most frequent causes of PB in Hungary.

20.2 Microbial Causes

Table 20.1 summaries the birth outcomes of newborns without CA born to mothers with acute infectious diseases during the study pregnancy if the given disease occurred in 20 or more pregnant women.

20.2.1 Acute Maternal Infectious Diseases During the Study Pregnancy

An unexpected finding of this summary (Table 20.1) is that nearly all acute maternal infectious diseases from salmonellosis to unspecified virus infection, in addition to influenza was associated with somewhat longer gestational age. The explanation may be that the duration of these diseases e.g. influenza was short and frequently

Table 20.1 Birth outcomes of newborn without CA of women with acute infectious diseases during the study pregnancy

Acute diseases	No.	Gestational age (week)	Birth weight (g)	Rate (%) Preterm birth	Low birthweight
Reference	38,151	39.4	3,279	9.3	5.7
Salmonellosis	23	39.9	3,395	0.0	0.0
Infectious diarrhea	70	40.0	3,298	1.4	4.3
Chickenpox	56	39.7	3,235	5.4	5.4
Viral genital warts	25	38.0	2,980	28.0	12.0
Rubella	38	39.7	3,386	7.9	5.3
Mumps	49	39.5	3,260	12.2	6.1
Unspecified virus infections	49	39.8	3,327	6.1	6.1
Toxoplasmosis	27	39.1	3,300	11.1	3.7
Otitis media	56	39.6	3,370	7.3	3.6
Common cold	5,475	39.3	3,305	9.8	4.2
Influenza	1,838	39.5	3,311	8.0	4.7
Sinusitis	250	39.6	3,348	5.6	5.2
Pharyngitis	1,048	39.6	3,364	5.8	3.4
Tonsillitis	1,165	39.7	3,340	5.4	4.8
Laryngitis-tracheitis	804	39.8	3,349	4.0	4.9
Bronchitis-bronchiolitis	398	39.1	3,271	12.3	6.5
Pneumonia	182	38.9	3,271	15.4	8.8
Gastritis-duodenitis	78	39.5	3,317	6.4	5.1
Appendicitis	25	39.5	3,302	8.0	4.0
Cholecystitis	145	39.1	3,293	11.0	9.0
Glomerulonephritis, acute	479	39.1	3,252	14.8	6.0
Bacteriuria	1,767	39.3	3,250	10.8	6.5
Cystitis, acute	178	39.4	3,302	7.9	6.2
Pyelonephritis, acute	243	39.2	3,200	10.3	8.6
Pelvic inflammatory disease, acute	28	39.1	3,207	14.1	8.6
Vulvovaginitis-bacterial vaginosis[a]	2,698	39.5	3,302	7.5	4.8
Erosion of the cervix	25	39.1	3,237	8.0	8.0

occurred in early pregnancy without any effect on the last trimester of pregnancy. Another important observation of this project is that these pregnant women were treated with antimicrobial drugs due to this infectious disease. However, these drugs might have some beneficial effect for the undiagnosed and/or asymptomatic urogenital infections. The latter plays an important role in the origin of PB thus the treatment of acute maternal infectious diseases may provide some protective effect against PB.

There were two exceptions from the above mentioned trend. Viral genital warts were associated with a very high rate of PB and therefore it will be discussed separately among the acute infections of the genital organs. While shorter gestational age in pregnant women with toxoplasmosis may be related to intrauterine infection of the fetus.

Of course, in general longer gestational age was associated with lower rate of PB; however, there was one exception from this rule: mumps. The newborns of mothers with mumps had somewhat longer gestational age while they had a higher rate of PB suggesting a not normal distribution of gestational age in this group.

Among acute infectious diseases of the respiratory and digestive system, only bronchitis-bronchiolitis, pneumonia, and cholecystitis (severe diseases with longer duration) were associated with higher risk for PB. In general, other diseases of these organs had somewhat longer mean gestational age and somewhat lower rate of PB, and these unexpected findings may have similar explanation which was mentioned previously regarding to acute infectious disease.

Urinary tract infections will be discussed in the next section; here only acute glomerulonephritis needs to be commented because this severe and relative long condition was associated with shorter gestational age and higher rate of PB. However, this disease had no real effect for mean birth weight and rate of LBW newborns.

The mean birth weight was determined mainly by the gestational age, the gestational age specific birth weight rarely showed deviation from this rule. Thus intrauterine fetal growth retardation is not characteristic for the pregnancy of mothers with acute diseases. Only the cholecystitis seems to be exceptional, however, as it was shown in Part B, most of these pregnant women were affected with complicated cholecystitis.

In conclusion, acute maternal diseases – except infectious diseases of the urogenital system – generally were not associated with higher risk for PB or LBW newborns.

20.2.2 Urinary Tract Infections

The urinary tract represents one of the most common sites of bacterial infections, particularly in women; 10–15% of the adult female population is affected by *urinary tract infection* (UTI) at some time in their lives. UTI is one of the most frequently seen complications in pregnant women because pregnancy is a risk factor for UTI due to the changes of the urinary tract during pregnancy. Bacteria, mainly Escherichia coli, in addition to Enterobacter, Klebsiella, Pseudomonas, and Proteus can ascend from the bladder to the upper part of the urinary tract.

The main objective of our study was to check the association of UTI in pregnant women with adverse birth outcomes of their newborns. Three diagnoses of UTI were differentiated for evaluation: (i) significant or true bacteriuria, (ii) acute cystitis, or lower UTI, and (iii) acute pyelonephritis, or upper UTI.

In the data set of the HCCSCA 2,188 (5.74%) mothers were affected with UTI, 90.0% had medically recorded diagnosis of UTI in the prenatal maternity logbooks. The distribution of different manifestations of UTI was the following: true bacteriuria with symptoms of genital infections in 1,767 (80.8%), acute cystitis in 178 (8.1%), and acute pyelonephritis in 243 (11.1%) pregnant women. Most pregnant women with UTI were treated with antibacterial or antiseptic drugs

The mean gestational age was somewhat shorter in newborn infants born to mothers with UTI (Table 20.1) compared to pregnant women without UTI. The mean birth weight was slightly smaller in the babies of mothers with UTI. However, these statistical significant differences were caused only by 0.1 week and 27 g which are clinically not important. The proportion of PB was larger in the group of mothers with UTI but the similar trend in the proportion of LBW newborns did not reach the level of significance (Table 20.1).

However, there was a severity-effect relation in the rate of PB and LBW newborns. The acute pyelonephritis associated with a higher rate of PB while the rate of PB was lower in the newborns of pregnant women with acute cystitis compared to the reference value. However, it is necessary to stress that most pregnant women with UTI were treated with antimicrobial drugs. The exception was true bacteriuria with the highest rate of PB which was related to parallel genital infections of pregnant women. Therefore, PB inducing effect of true bacteriuria was associated with the infections of lower genital organs in our study.

Another important message of this study is that up to 30% of mothers developed acute pyelonephritis if true bacteriuria was left untreated, while antibiotic treatment is effective in reducing the risk of pyelonephritis in pregnancy and related PB.

In conclusion, this study confirmed that maternal UTI increases the rate of PB.

20.2.3 Infections of the Genital Organs

20.2.3.1 Diseases of the Upper Genital Organs

Pelvic inflammatory diseases are clinical diagnosis of acute or chronic infections/diseases in the upper genital tract. *Acute pelvic inflammatory disease* (APID) was evaluated in the study based on the medically recorded diagnosis of acute oophoritis, salpingitis, adnexitis and endometritis in the prenatal maternity logbook or discharge summaries during pregnancy. APID is frequently associated with cervicitis and/or vulvovaginitis; therefore, pregnant women with these conditions were also included into the group of APID.

In the data set of the HCCSCA 158 (0.41%) pregnant women were recorded with APID. However, finally only 128 (0.34%) mothers with medically recorded APID and antimicrobial treatment were evaluated. In most women the onset of APID occurred in early pregnancy.

Mean gestational age was 0.3 week shorter and mean birth weight was 72 g smaller in newborns of mothers with APID compared to babies born to mothers without APID. The rate of PB was 14.1% while the rate of LBW newborns was 8.6%, higher than in the reference sample (9.1 and 5.7%).

In conclusion, there was a somewhat higher rate of PB in the newborns of pregnant women with APID in early pregnancy despite of antimicrobial treatment.

20.2.3.2 Infections/Diseases of the Lower Genital Organs

Lower genital tract infections such as vulvovaginal infections are among the most frequent diseases during pregnancy and the association between antenatal infection/inflammation of the lower genital tract and higher risk of preterm premature rupture of membranes, i.e. PB is well-known. Thus, the infections and inflammatory diseases of the lower genital tract (cervix, vagina, and vulva), i.e. *vulvovaginitis and bacterial vaginosis* (VV–VB) are believed to account for 25–40% of PB.

In the data set of the HCCSCA 3,326 (8.7%) pregnant women had the diagnosis of VV–BV recorded in the prenatal maternity logbook and/or reported by mothers in the questionnaire. However, only 2,698 (7.1%) pregnant women with medically recorded VV–BV in the prenatal maternity logbooks were evaluated. Candidiasis was diagnosed in 11.4% of these pregnant women while trichomoniasis was identified in 15.5% of pregnant women. The diagnosis was bacterial vaginosis in 16.6% of these pregnant women. The rest of women had unspecified VV–BV.

VV–BVs were recorded in nearly all pregnant women at the first visit in gestational months II and/or III. Therefore, the onset of VV–BV was likely before the conception or in early pregnancy. In general, the duration of VV–BV was less than 1 month.

Only about 7% of pregnant women had medically recorded VV–BV which is lower than expected. The explanation may be that only severe VV–BV were recorded in the prenatal maternity logbooks and/or some women with VV–BV were screened, diagnosed and treated before the first visit in the prenatal clinics.

The mean gestational age was 0.1 week longer, while mean birth weight was 23 g larger in babies born to mothers with VV–BV. This trend was in agreement with a lower rate of PB (7.5% vs. 9.3%; 0.8, 0.7–0.9) and of LBW newborns (4.8% vs. 5.8%; 0.8, 0.7–0.9).

In conclusion, our study resulted in unexpected findings showing lower rate of PB in children of pregnant women with VV–BV. This finding might be explained by the applied antimicrobial treatment for all evaluated women in our study which, additional to the treatment of VV–BV, may have resulted in some protective effect for amnionitis and PB.

20.2.3.3 Genital Herpes

Genital herpes caused by *Herpes simplex virus* (HSV) infection of the genital tract is one of the most common sexually transmitted viral infections, caused mainly by HSV-2.

In the data set of the HCCSCA 228 (0.60%) babies had mothers with reported and/or recorded genital herpes during the study pregnancy. Of these 228 mothers,

88 (38.6%) had medically recorded genital herpes in the prenatal maternity logbook and only 2 had primary genital herpes. Finally, 86 (0.23%) mothers with medically recorded *recurrent genital herpes* (RGH) were evaluated in our study. These women were treated by different drugs but effective antiviral treatment was not available during the study period.

Mean gestational age was 0.5 week shorter and the rate of PB was 14.0%, which is higher than the reference value (9.3%). The shorter gestational age was reflected in 113 g lower mean birth weight and in a higher rate of LBW newborns of pregnant women with RGH (10.5% vs. 5.7%). We evaluated these birth outcomes according to different trimesters and there was an obvious trend reflecting an increasing severity of consequences. Mean gestational age was 39.5, 39.2 and 38.7 weeks, mean birth weight was 3,348, 3,147, and 3,112 g, PB rate was 6.7%, 15.4%, and 23.5% and LBW rate was 3.3, 12.8, and 17.7% in the first, second, and third trimesters, respectively. The shortest gestational age and the highest rate of PB were found in the third trimester.

In conclusion, an association was found between maternal RGH in the third trimester and higher rate of PB.

20.2.3.4 Viral Genital Warts

Viral genital warts (VGW) (previously in general called as condyloma accuminatum) are pedunculated masses developing from the skin of the vulva with very wide range of size. VGW are caused by certain types of *human papillomaviruses* (HPV). Up to date, more than 100 types of HPV have been identified; however, VGW are most frequently caused by low risk HPV types like 6 and 11, rarely 42, 43, 44, and 54. Only serotype 54 belongs to the high oncogenic risk category.

In the data set of the HCCSCA 25 (0.07%) pregnant women were recorded with VGW in the prenatal maternity logbook during pregnancy. The evaluation of birth outcomes showed an obvious reduction of gestational age (38.0 week) and a much higher rate of PB (28.0%). The latter was 3 fold higher compared to reference sample. The mean birth weight was also smaller and it was associated with a 2.1 fold increase in the rate of LBW newborns. Therefore we can conclude that VGW drastically shortens fetal life and is associated with a very high rate of PB.

In conclusion, this strikingly high rate of PB in pregnant women with VGW was an unexpected finding which requires further studies.

The erosion of cervix is part of infectious diseases of genital organs and had an association with shorter gestational age; however, the rate of PB was not higher in affected women.

20.3 Chronic Maternal Diseases During Pregnancy

Table 20.2 summarizes the birth outcomes of newborns without CA born to mothers with chronic diseases during pregnancy if the given disease occurred in 20 or more pregnant women. Of course, the previously discussed uterus CAs such as

Table 20.2 Birth outcomes of newborns without CA of women with chronic diseases during pregnancy

		Mean		Rate of	
Chronic diseases	No.	Gestational age (week)	Birth weight (g)	Preterm birth (%)	Low birth weight newborns (%)
Reference	38,151	39.4	3,279	9.3	5.7
Tuberculosis	26	39.8	3,492	7.7	0.0
Orofacial herpes, recurrent	572	39.7	3,309	3.5	4.2
Genital herpes, recurrent	86	38.9	3,163	14.0	10.5
Dermatomycosis	71	39.1	3,271	12.7	2.8
Anemia	6,358	39.4	3,278	9.1	5.0
Leiomyoma	71	39.6	3,370	12.7	5.6
Hypothyroidism	31	39.6	3,264	3.2	3.2
Hyperthyroidism	116	39.3	3,210	10.3	6.9
Diabetes mellitus, type I	88	38.9	3,324	12.5	12.5
Diabetes mellitus, type II	141	39.7	3,273	4.3	2.8
Obesity	29	39.9	3,566	10.8	5.9
Maniac-depression	22	39.3	3,268	10.8	5.9
Panic disorder	187	39.0	3,209	17.1	8.6
Epilepsy	90	39.7	3,255	8.9	8.9
Migraine	713	39.3	3,266	9.8	6.6
Other headaches	1,268	39.4	3,280	8.7	4.9
Essential hypertension, treated	1,522	38.9	3,143	12.9	12.0
Paroxysmal supraventricular tachycardia	149	39.1	3,272	11.4	4.7
Superficial thrombophlebitis	778	39.5	3,417	6.8	3.6
Deep vein thrombophlebitis with or without thrombosis	192	39.3	3,322	8.3	5.2
Varicose veins of the lower extremities	566	39.4	3,349	7.1	3.5
Hemorrhoids	1,617	39.4	3,340	8.5	4.8
Hypotension	1,268	39.4	3,288	8.6	4.2
Allergic rhinitis	148	39.8	3,344	3.9	4.2
Bronchial asthma	757	38.8	3,102	14.1	9.0
Dyspepsia	270	39.7	3,317	4.2	4.7
Peptic ulcer disease	104	39.5	3,309	3.5	5.2

Table 20.2 (continued)

		Mean		Rate of	
Chronic diseases	No.	Gestational age (week)	Birth weight (g)	Preterm birth (%)	Low birth weight newborns (%)
Ulcerative colitis	95	38.7	3,249	18.9	4.2
Constipation, severe	144	39.8	3,275	4.2	4.2
Cholelithiasis	119	39.4	3,298	6.7	3.4
Atopic dermatitis	91	38.0	3,234	13.2	9.9
Psoriasis	40	39.7	3,368	2.5	0.0
Pruritus	25	39.3	3,273	16.0	4.0
Allergic urticaria	187	39.4	3,294	7.0	5.3
Rheumatoid arthritis	68	39.5	3,409	4.4	5.9
Lumbago	80	40.0	3,438	3.8	1.3
Kidney stones	147	39.5	3,387	5.4	6.1
Renal diseases related secondary hypertension	49	39.3	3,268	13.0	6.7
Endometriosis	26	39.8	3,280	0.0	0.0
Ovarian follicular cyst	88	39.7	3,280	5.7	5.7
Cervical incompetence	2,795	39.0	3,200	11.2	7.8
Cardiovascular CA	41	39.2	3,057	9.8	9.8
CA of the uterus	67	35.9	2,365	67.2	44.8
Congenital dislocation of the hip	30	39.4	3,219	10.0	6.7

Rokitansky sequence and cervical incompetence, in addition to recurrent genital herpes are omitted from this section.

Seven different groups are worth differentiating:

1. Chronic maternal diseases without effect on these birth outcomes such as anemia (nearly all anemic pregnant women were treated with iron products), migraine and other headaches (the short attacks of these pathological conditions did not modify the fetal development), deep vein thrombophlebitis, hypotension, cholelithiasis, allergic urticaria, and congenital dislocation of the hip.
2. Chronic maternal disease with seemingly beneficial effect on these birth outcomes. The longer gestational age associated with a lower rate of PB in the newborns of pregnant women with lumbago (intervertebral disc disorder) and tuberculosis likely explained by the physical limitation of motion and bed rest,

in addition to recurrent orofacial herpes and allergic rhinitis, perhaps due to immunosuppressive status of pregnant women. Dyspepsia, peptic ulcer disease, and severe constipation likely due to better diet. Finally, ovarian follicular cyst, rheumatoid arthritis, and kidney stone also belong to this group with longer gestational age and lower rate of PB, although the rate of LBW was not lower.

3. Chronic maternal disease with beneficial effect for fetal growth. The mean gestational age of these newborns did not deviate significantly from the reference figure but the mean birth weight was larger and in general it associated with a lower rate of LBW newborns. Varicose veins of the lower extremities, superficial vein thrombophlebitis, hemorrhoids, psoriasis, and endometriosis can be inserted into this group obviously with different hypothetic explanation, e.g. more bed rest or specific treatments.
4. Chronic maternal disease of pregnant women with higher rate of PB without significant change in the mean birth weight of their babies. The typical examples for this group are hyperthyroidism, maniac-depression, paroxysmal supraventricular tachycardia, dermatomycosis, pruritus, renal disease related hypertension with more-or-less usual gestational age and higher rate of PB. Newborns of pregnant women with leiomyoma had longer gestational age but higher rate of PB.
5. Chronic maternal diseases with both shorter gestational age and a lower mean birth weight, thus a higher rate of PB and LBW newborns. Typical examples for this group are bronchial asthma, recurrent genital herpes, atopic dermatitis, panic disorder, and severe essential hypertension.
6. Chronic maternal diseases with higher rate of LBW newborns but usual or longer gestational age might indicate slower intrauterine fetal growth. Epilepsy and cardiovascular CAs belong to this group. Pregnant women with hypothyroidism had longer gestational age with somewhat lower mean birth weight and these data also indicate some slower intrauterine growth, though the rate of LBW newborns was not higher.
7. Diabetes mellitus type 1 represents a special group inducing both large babies and intrauterine fetal growth retardation. The mean gestational age was significantly shorter while the mean birth weight was larger thus these data indicate a faster intrauterine growth in agreement with so many prior publications. The newborns of pregnant women with diabetes mellitus type 2 had a longer gestational age with the usual mean birth weight indicating moderate intrauterine fetal growth delay, though a higher rate of LBW newborns was not found. Maternal obesity was associated with longer gestational age and larger mean birth weight but the rate of PB was higher without the change in the rate of LBW newborns.

In conclusion, chronic maternal diseases generally have a strong effect for fetal development therefore they play an important role in the origin of PB and LBW newborns.

20.4 Pregnancy Complications During the Study Pregnancy

Table 20.3 summaries the birth outcomes of children without CA born to mothers with different pregnancy complications during the study pregnancy if the given complications occurred in 20 or more pregnant women.

Table 20.3 Birth outcomes of newborns without CA of women with pregnancy complications during pregnancy

		Mean		Rate of	
Pregnancy complications	No.	Gestational age (week)	Birth weight (g)	Preterm birth (%)	Low birth weight newborns (%)
Reference	38,151	39.4	3,279	9.3	5.7
Nausea-vomiting, severe	3,777	39.7	3,291	6.4	5.0
Threatened abortion	6,510	39.2	3,239	10.8	7.1
Gestational diabetes	229	39.4	3,390	7.0	5.7
Gestational hypertension	1,098	39.2	3,280	9.7	10.5
Preeclampsia	972	39.3	3,316	10.4	7.6
Preeclampsia superimposed upon chronic hypertension	250	39.2	3,170	11.2	14.0
Eclampsia	45	39.4	3,264	6.7	13.3
Eclampsia superimposed upon chronic hypertension	19	38.6	3,114	10.5	15.8
Placental disorders	593	39.1	3,179	11.3	11.0
Polyhydramnios	191	39.4	3,288	11.5	9.9
Threatened preterm delivery	396	39.1	3,191	11.4	8.6
Oedema/excessive gain	912	39.4	3,381	8.8	3.4

The evaluation of *severe nausea and vomiting* in pregnant women resulted in some unexpected findings. The mean gestational age was longer and it associated with a significantly lower rate of PB.

Unexpectedly *threatened abortion* and *preterm delivery* associated with only 0.2 and 0.3 day shorter gestational age, respectively, and with a moderate increase in the rate of PB in newborns of pregnant women with threatened preterm delivery but a lower rate of PB was found in pregnant women with threatened abortion. The mean birth weight corresponded to the mean gestational age and a significantly higher rate of LBW newborns was found only in the group of pregnant women with threatened preterm delivery.

The newborns of pregnant women with *gestational diabetes* and reference pregnant women had the same mean gestational age, but the mean birth weight was higher in the group of gestational diabetic pregnant women.

The effect of *gestational hypertension* was seen in the higher rate of LBW newborns, which indicated intrauterine fetal growth delay.

The different manifestations of *placental disorders* associated with shorter mean gestational age and lower mean birth weight, but these changes caused mainly a higher rate of LBW newborns indicating again intrauterine fetal growth delay.

Unexpectedly the effect of *polyhydramnios* did not cause a shorter mean gestational age and lower mean birth weight, but the rate of PB and mainly LBW newborns was higher. In these cases the distribution of the data is skewed which indicates multiple etiology behind the symptom of polyhydramnion. Some of those result in increased rate of PB and LBW, like genetic disorders, while others like esophagus atresia does not effect the rate of PB and LBW.

The effect of *oedema/excessive weight gain in pregnant women* could be detected only on the larger mean birth weight of their newborns.

In conclusion, the pregnancy complications associated frequently with adverse birth outcomes but both may have a common origin therefore the role of pregnancy complications as confounders are debated.

20.5 General Discussion

Obviously the study of associations between exposure (e.g. maternal diseases) and effect: outcome (e.g. preterm birth) needs precise and specific definition and analysis. In the above sections we attempted to demonstrate the evaluation of different maternal diseases in a population-based large material mainly based on prospective and medically recorded diagnoses of these diseases. However, these diagnoses reflected the medical standard in Hungary with some weaknesses (e.g. at the diagnostic criteria of cervical incompetence) and the lack of some important diseases such as parvovirus, chlamydia, SLE. Pregnancy outcomes such as PB and LBW were classified according to the international recommendations of the WHO. In addition, we followed the recent first level classification of PB, i.e. spontaneous and induced, i.e. cesarean section PB, but we were not able to use the second level classification of PB as spontaneous preterm labor with intact membrane and preterm premature rupture of membranes.

Finally, the associations studied can be biased and/or modified by confounders. In general, in the analysis of these associations we considered maternal demographic variables, other disorders, and related drug treatments. The role of drugs is very important in the origin of CAs but less important in the etiology of PB. However, our studies showed the effect of some drugs for PB and LBW, e.g. paracetamol associated with a lower risk of PB due to longer gestational age (78), furosemide seemed to be a fetal growth promoter with the usual mean gestational age but 123 g larger birth weight and 1.7 fold lower LBW newborns (79) while ergotamine particularly in the third trimester associated with a higher risk of LBW newborns (86).

In conclusion, to our best knowledge this is the first attempt to evaluate the association of *all recorded maternal diseases* with PB and LBW in a population-based large material; however, we are aware of the weaknesses of our approach and we hope that our results will be further studied and confirmed or rejected in other studies based on different populations.

Adverse birth outcomes such as PB and LBW frequently cause early death or long-term handicaps. Additionally, they often predestinate for other acquired disorders; therefore, their prevention is considered to be the best option in medical management. Thus, in the last sections we demonstrate some preventive efforts to avoid these adverse birth outcomes.

20.6 Specific Prevention of PB and LBW

Two main approaches are worth differentiating in the preventive strategies of PB and LBW. The first is based on specific methods according to the type of PB and/or LBW while the second approach attempts to provide a general preventive effect for PB and LBW.

20.6.1 The Medical Management of Cervical Incompetence in Pregnant Women

At present two kinds of treatment compete with each other in Hungary to prevent or reduce PB in the newborns of females with *cervical incompetence/insufficiency in pregnancy* (CIP). One group of obstetricians prefers prophylactic surgical interventions like Shirodkar suture or the more modern therapeutic McDonald cerclage. Another group of obstetricians gives preference to conservative treatment based on lasting bed-rest alone based on some previous studies which were unable to demonstrate the advantage of therapeutic cerclage.

The data set of the HCCSCA was appropriate to evaluate the rate of PB. The rate of PB can be used as the indicator of the efficacy of the above mentioned two medical managements in women with CIP.

The rate of PB in the newborns of pregnant women with CIP treated by therapeutic cerclage was 9.1% and this rate was not significantly higher than the rate of PB (9.0%) in the newborns of pregnant women without CIP (1.0, 0.8–1.3). Compared to untreated CIP group (PB rate: 11.2%) therapeutic cerclage showed a significantly lower PB rate. However, in the newborns of pregnant women with CIP treated by bed rest alone the rate of PB was 12.7% (1.5, 1.3–1.7).

Thus the available data suggested that PB can be reduced more effectively by therapeutic cerclage than by the bed rest alone.

In conclusion, the evaluation of the two kinds of medical management of CIP (cerclage vs. bed rest alone), showed that cerclage was more effective in reducing the risk of PB.

20.6.2 Prevention of Urinary Tract Infections

The PB preventive effect of different drugs was evaluated in mothers with *urinary tract infections*(UTI). Two groups of drugs were differentiated. Antimicrobial drugs included ampicillin, cefalexin, and cotrimoxazole, while the so-called urinary tract antiseptics such as nitrofurantoin and nalidixic acid were sorted into the other group.

Antimicrobial drugs were effective in the prevention of PB. The rate of PB was reduced from 10.4 to 7.4% in mothers with UTI. However, antiseptic drugs did not show any preventive effect. In addition, it is worth mentioning that pregnant women with UTI together with appropriate antimicrobial treatment had a lower rate of PB (7.4%) than the PB rate of the Hungarian pregnant population (9.1%) during the study period.

In conclusion, the important message of this study is that the major part of PB in pregnant women with UTI are preventable by antimicrobial drugs such as ampicillin, cefalexin, and cotrimoxazole and their beneficial effect can explain the low rate of PB in mothers with UTI; therefore, early treatment of UTI in pregnancy is strongly recommended.

20.6.3 Prevention of Vulvovaginitis-Bacterial Vaginosis

Most pregnant women with *vulvovaginitis–bacterial vaginosis* (VV–BV) were treated by clotrimazole (58.7%) and metronidazole (33.0%), in addition, ampicillin (9.8%), nitrofurantoin (4.5%), and sulphamethoxazole + trimethoprim (co-trimoxazole) (1.8%) was also used for their treatment.

The evaluation of PB rate according to the use of antimicrobial drugs resulted in important findings. Pregnant women without VV–BV and without *antimicrobial drug treatment* (ADT), as reference, were compared to two groups: (i) ADT without VV–BV, and (ii) ADT with VV–BV. The reference rate of PB was 9.3%. Among ADT, clotrimazole, metronidazole, and ampicillin were differentiated. Clotrimazole was able to reduce the rate of PB in the newborns of women with VV–BV to 6.7% (0.7, 0.6–0.8) though only a minor part of these women had recorded vulvovaginal candidiasis. Ampicillin treatment also seemed effective resulting in a PB rate of 6.5% (0.7, 0.4–1.1) however; this association was not significant due to the limited number of subjects. The rate of PB was 9.4% after the treatment of metronidazole (1.0, 0.8–1.3); therefore, this drug was ineffective.

However, the major finding of this study was that the rate of PB in babies born to mothers with VV–BV diagnosed in early pregnancy followed by clotrimazole and ampicillin treatment was much lower (6.5–6.7%) compared to the PB rate of the Hungarian newborn population (9.3%). This finding was confirmed by the data of the group having ADT without VV–BV because there was a significantly lower rate of PB (7.2–7.8%) after clotrimazole and ampicillin treatment compared to the Hungarian reference figure of 9.3%.

Nearly all pregnant women with VV–BV were treated during pregnancy, thus an important finding of the study was a significantly lower risk for PB after the treatment of pregnant women with clotrimazole or ampicillin during the study pregnancy. However, the major and unexpected finding of our study was the high rate of PB in the reference group (mothers without VV–BV and without antimicrobial treatment). Major part of these pregnant women likely had asymptomatic or undiagnosed VV–BV without appropriate treatment. This view is supported by the data of pregnant women without VV–BV but treated by clotrimazole or ampicillin due to other indications or unrecorded VV–BV because they also had a lower rate of PB. Thus the other indication of antimicrobial treatment may have some beneficial "side" effect in pregnant women with asymptomatic candida colonisation or undiagnosed VV–BV.

If we accept that population PB rate is 9.3% and we assume that screening is able to detect symptomatic and asymptomatic VV–BV, with appropriate antimicrobial treatment we have a chance to reduce the rate of PB to 6.6%; therefore, about 30% of PB is preventable.

The time of screening and treatment is a very crucial point because early spontaneous PB is more likely to be of infectious origin than PB just before term. Thus, the optimal time for screening and treatment is the prepregnancy-preconceptional period or early pregnancy as this study has also shown. The longer the abnormal colonisation remains untreated, the greater the chance is for microorganisms to ascend into the uterus initiating inflammatory process which may lead to early labor. The explanation of unsuccessful results in several studies was that antimicrobial drug treatment was administered too late in genital infections.

In conclusion, VV–BV associated with a lower rate of PB compared to Hungarian population rate of PB probably due to effective drug treatment. Our study showed the weaknesses of general clinical practice. High proportion of unspecified agents of VV–BV and a major part of VV–BV were not diagnosed or recorded. We must emphasize the importance accurate diagnosis and treatment of VV–BV, because it helps to reduce the rate of PB without increasing the risk for CAs.

20.6.4 Prevention of Bronchial Asthma Related PB

Bronchial asthma is one of the most common disorders during pregnancy. As our study showed there was a significantly shorter mean gestational age in pregnant women with asthma and it associated with a much higher rate of PB (14.1%). In addition, the rate of LBW newborns was also higher: 9.0% compared to the population-based figure of 5.7%. However, another important observation of our study was that two-third of pregnant women were treated with appropriate antiasthmatic drugs while the rest one-third went untreated due to the anxiety of possible teratogenic potential of drugs. Therefore, it was possible to compare the rate of PB and LPW in pregnant women with and without treatment. The results teach us a very important lesson: the rate of LBW was not significantly higher in babies of asthmatic pregnant women with appropriate treatment (6.6% vs. 5.6%); however, this figure increased by 2.5 fold in newborns of pregnant women without treatment (13.7% vs. 5.6%). A similar trend was seen in the rate of PB at the comparison of treated (10.8% vs. 9.1%) and untreated (20.7% vs. 9.1%) pregnant women with asthma. Obviously asthma attacks during pregnancy result in a risk for fetal development proportional with the number of attacks while a much more undisturbed development is provided for the fetuses of asthmatic pregnant women with appropriate treatment.

In conclusion, the hazard of fetuses associated with asthmatic attack of pregnant women is preventable by appropriate treatment.

20.6.5 Prevention of Iron Deficient Anemia Related PB

Anemia is common among pregnant women. In Hungary it is caused by iron deficiency in almost all anemic pregnant women. Our study showed the beneficial effect of iron supplementation in these pregnant women.

Out of 6,358 anemic pregnant women, only 214 had no iron treatment. The mean gestational age of their newborns was 38.9 week compared with 39.4 week in the newborns of iron supplemented pregnant women. These figures were in agreement with the increased rate of PB (15.0%) in the untreated group compared to the rate of PB (9.4%) in the treated group.

In conclusion, the higher rate of PB in newborns of anemic pregnant women is preventable by iron treatment.

20.7 General Prevention of PB

Periconceptional folic acid or folic-acid-containing multivitamin supplementation has been shown to have a clear preventive effect on the recurrence and first occurrence of neural-tube defects and some other CAs; therefore, this primary preventive method is recommended for all prospective pregnant women.

In Hungary most pregnant women use high doses of folic acid during pregnancy mainly after the first visit in the prenatal care clinics. However, the question is frequently raised whether it is worth continuing this supplement after the first trimester of pregnancy or not. Meta-analyses of supplementation studies recommended further researches to measure the effect of dietary folate or folic acid intake during pregnancy on reducing the rate of PB and LBW newborns as an "urgent priority" (Mohammed, 1993, Haider and Bhutta, 2006). On the other hand, recently the fetal weight promoting effect of folic acid and/or multivitamins has been stated by some medical doctors as an argument against this preventive method because large birth weight may associate with increased risk for birth complications of newborns.

The population-based dataset of the HCCSCA was appropriate to test the hypothesis regarding to the possible fetal growth promoting and/or PB reducing effect of folic acid and/or folic acid containing multivitamin supplementation during pregnancy, particularly in the third trimester, i.e. during the time of the most intensive fetal growth.

20.7.1 Results of the Study (I)

The objective of the study was to compare the length of gestation at delivery and birth weight, in addition to the rate of PB and LBW newborns as main outcome measures in pregnant women. Women with prospectively and medically recorded folic acid or folic acid-containing multivitamin use in the prenatal maternity logbook were compared to pregnant women who did not take these supplements during their pregnancy. Multiple pregnancies and the history (e.g. PB or CA) in previous pregnancies may have effects for these birth outcomes therefore only singletons without CA in primiparae were evaluated.

Five study groups were differentiated:

(1) *Folic acid (FA)* alone. Only one type of 3 mg FA tablet was available in Hungary during the study period. Women used 1–3 tablets per day. The intake was 2 tablets in 69% of pregnant women, thus the estimated daily dose was 5.6 mg.
(2) FA containing micronutrient combinations, the so-called *multivitamins* (MV). The three most frequently used micronutrient combinations were Elevit prenatal® (55.3%; containing 0.8 mg FA), Materna® (39.0%, containing 1.0 mg FA) and Polyvitaplex-10® (2.9%; containing 0.1 mg FA) during the study period. Most pregnant women (about 98%) used one tablet; the estimated daily dose of FA was 0.85 mg.
(3) Micronutrient combinations without FA with very heterogeneous products used mainly for body building and other purposes were excluded.
(4) MV + FA together. The proportion of Elevit prenatal®, Materna®, and Polyvitaplex-10® use was 42.6%, 31.9%, and 24.3% in this group, respectively. Nearly all women consumed one tablet from each of MV and FA; however, the proportion of different MV was different than in the MV group, therefore the estimated daily intake of FA was 3.7 mg.
(5) The reference group included pregnant women without any FA or MV supplementation prior to conception (at least 3 months) and during the study pregnancy.

The study sample included 38,151 newborns, therefore represented 1.8% of all Hungarian births, however, twins, newborn infants born to mothers supplemented with micronutrient combinations without FA, without medically recorded FA and/or MV use and mothers with previous birth were excluded from the study.

The main objective of the study was the evaluation of pregnancy/birth outcomes in different study groups (Table 20.4). (The sex ratio of newborns did not show difference among the study groups.)

The mean gestational age was 0.3 and 0.6 week longer after FA alone and MV + FA supplements during pregnancy than in the reference sample, respectively. The mean birth weight exceeded the reference figure by 74 g in the groups of MV. The rate of PB was significantly lower after FA alone (–3.5%), MV (–4.7%), and MV + FA (–6.6%) supplements compared to reference value. The rate of LBW newborns was also lower in FA alone (–0.7%), MV (–0.7%) and MV + FA (–1.1%) supplemented groups than in the reference sample, but these differences did not reach the level of significance.

Table 20.5 summarizes the data of FA alone supplementation according to the trimesters of the study pregnancy. 92.9% of pregnant women belonged to this study group.

The longest gestational age and lowest rate of PB was found after FA alone supplementation during the entire pregnancy, i.e. I–III trimesters (39.8 week and 4.9%) and the II–III trimesters (39.9 week and 3.8%), followed by the III trimester alone (39.5 week and 7.6%). This trend resulted in 39.8 week of mean gestational age and 4.8% rate of PB in the group of III trimester together (III + II–III + I–III trimesters). Our data suggest that the third trimester is the key time window of FA supplementation for the reduction of PB.

In addition, it is worth mentioning that mean gestational age was shorter and rate of PB was higher if pregnant women were supplemented with FA alone only during the first trimester and particularly only during the third trimester.

Pregnant women with the III trimester supplementation (III, II–III, I–III trimesters together) of MV and MV + FA showed larger mean birth weight by 75 and 89 g than in the reference group, while the mean gestational age did not change significantly in these two supplement groups (data not shown). The rate of PB changed from 6.4 to 6.9% in the group of MV and from 4.5 to 4.3% in the group of MV+FA. There was no difference in the rate of LBW after supplementation in the III trimester compared to the figures of the entire pregnancy.

Thus, trimester-dependent PB rate reduction effect was found only after FA alone supplementation.

20.7.2 Interpretation of the Study

Our findings showed that fetal growth promoting effect of vitamin supplements was limited (32–79 g during pregnancy, and 43–89 g in the third trimester), which does not seem to be important from clinical aspect. In addition, this minor increase in the birth weight can be explained partly by the longer gestational age and general effect (i.e. not third trimester specific) of MV. On the other hand, we found an obvious PB

Table 20.4 Birth outcomes of newborns of pregnant women using folic acid (FA) alone, multivitamins (MV), and MV+FA, in addition to reference pregnant women without FA and MV use

		Gestational age (week)		Birth weight (g)		Preterm birth		Low birth weight newborns	
Study groups	No.	Mean	S.D.	Mean	S.D.	No.	%	No.	%
Reference sample (without FA and MV)	16,177	39.2	2.1	3,262	509	1,792	11.1	933	5.8
FA alone	19,102	**39.5**	2.0	3,294	501	1,461	**7.6**	968	5.1
p/OR =		<0.0001		0.82		0.68, 0.63–0.73		0.88, 0.62–1.14	
MV	685	39.4	1.8	**3,336**	534	44	**6.4**	35	5.1
p/OR =		0.28		0.001		0.63, 0.46–0.86		0.87, 0.44–1.51	
MV+FA	1,410	**39.8**	1.8	3,341	511	64	**4.5**	66	4.7
p/OR =		<0.0001		0.28		0.40, 0.31–0.51		0.81, 0.43–1.38	

Table 20.5 Birth outcomes of singletons born to primiparae with prospectively and medically recorded use folic acid supplement alone by trimesters of use

		Gestational age (week)[a]		Birth weight (g)[b]		Preterm birth[a]		Low birth-weight[b]	
Trimester of use	No.	Mean	S.D.	Mean	S.D.	No.	%	No.	%
Reference[c]	7,319	39.2	2.1	3,216	486	864	11.8	416	5.7
I	1,118	39.1	2.1	3,229	478	133	11.9	54	4.8
p/OR		0.50		0.19		1.00 (0.82–1.21)		0.81 (0.58–1.13)	
II	896	**38.8**	2.3	3,218	505	136	**15.2**	49	5.5
p/OR		<0.001		0.49		1.31 (1.04–1.85)		0.96 (0.76–1.22)	
III	514	**39.5**	1.8	3,278	481	39	**7.6**	26	5.1
p/OR		<0.001		0.14		0.62 (0.45–0.87)		0.89 (0.40–1.66)	
I-II	88	39.4	2.1	3,241	480	9	10.2	7	8.0
p/OR		0.26		0.77		0.86 (0.43–1.72)		1.40 (0.31–4.11)	
II-III	1,622	**39.9**	1.7	**3,257**	455	61	**3.8**	68	4.2
p/OR		<0.0001		0.004		0.29 (0.23–0.38)		0.74 (0.34–1.27)	
I-III	2,055	**39.8**	1.8	3,270	494	101	**4.9**	115	5.6
p/OR		<0.0001		0.30		0.39 (0.32–0.49)		0.98 (0.51–1.58)	
Total	6,293	**39.5**	1.9	3,253	482	479	**7.6**	319	5.1
p/OR		<0.0001		0.86		0.62 (0.55–0.70)		0.89 (0.68–1.13)	
III together	4,191	**39.8**	1.8	3,266	478	201	**4.8**	209	5.0
(I-III, II-III, III)		<0.0001		0.08		0.38 (0.33–0.45)		0.88 (0.56–1.27)	

[a]Adjusted for maternal age and socioeconomic status.
[b]Adjusted for maternal age and socioeconomic status, in addition to gestational age.

rate reducing effect of these vitamin supplements particularly high dose FA alone in the III trimester.

Three intervention trials have shown some increase in birth weight after the use of prenatal FA containing MV while three others have failed to show an effect (Spencer, 2003). Other studies found some association between the low maternal folate intake or blood level and intrauterine growth retardation (Ek, 1982, Goldenberg et al., 1992, Neggers et al. 1997, Scholl et al., 1997, Shaw et al., 1997, Scholl and Johnson, 2000; Relton et al., 2005).

Mothers who delivered prematurely generally have lower dietary folate intake and/or FA supplement during pregnancy (Scholl et al., 1996, Siega-Riz et al., 2000). Folate demand is increased in pregnancy (McPartlin et al., 1993) and without adequate dietary intake of folate or FA supplementation, concentrations of folate in maternal plasma and red blood cells decrease from gestational month V onwards (Cikot et al., 2001) and parallel with these changes higher blood homocysteine levels were found (Vollset et al., 2000, Ronnenberg et al., 2002).

Periconceptional multivitamin supplementation was associated with the reduction of PB and the rate of small-for-gestational-age birth (Catov et al., 2007). The association of short interpregnancy intervals with higher rate of PB was also explained by the role of folate depletion during pregnancy and postpartum period (Smiths and Essed, 2001). A recent US study showed in 34,480 women with low-risk singleton pregnancies that preconceptional FA supplementation for 1 year or longer associated with a 70% decrease in the risk of spontaneous PB between 20 and 28 and a 50% reduction in PB of 28–32 weeks. After 32 weeks, no significant effect of preconceptional FA supplementation on PB was found (Bukowski et al., 2009).

After the review of international literature we attempt to interpret the results of our study. The first hypothesis for the explanation of 36–59% PB rate reduction due to FA alone supplementation during the III trimester was based on the well-known fact that pregnant women who used vitamin supplements may be associated with a better preconceptional and/or prenatal care and/or a generally better lifestyle. This hypothesis was supported by somewhat lower socioeconomic status and a somewhat higher rate of smokers in the group of unsupplemented pregnant women. However, we considered socioeconomic status in the calculations of adjusted OR and known confounders cannot explain the trimester dependent trend of FA supplementation. In addition, there is some dose-effect relation in the PB rate reducing effect of FA during the III trimester: the rate of PB was 6.9% after the use of MV containing low dose (0.1–1.0 mg) of FA, 4.9% in the FA group with an estimated dose of 5.6 mg, and 4.3% in the MV+FA group with an estimated 3.7 mg dose of FA. Finally, there is an obvious trimester dependent PB rate reduction effect of FA alone.

Our present hypothesis is that the reduced maternal folate status may be associated with elevated homocysteine related placental vasculopathy (van der Molen et al., 2000, Ferguson et al., 2001, Eskes, 2002) which can be neutralized by high dose of FA supplementation during pregnancy particularly in the III trimester. Johnson et al. (2005) showed an interaction between a pregnant woman's dietary folate intake and the presence or absence of a deletion allele in a folate-metabolizing gene.

Out of 136 million total births per year worldwide, more than 4 million newborns die within the first days or weeks of life. The major causes of their death are PB, birth asphyxia, and infections (WHO, 2005). Thus, the reduction of PB by FA supplementation would be an outstanding public health success.

In conclusion, the high dose of FA supplementation during pregnancy particularly in the III trimester reduces the risk of PB.

20.8 General Conclusions

The rate of PB is very high in Hungary, and as our studies showed there are many heterogeneous factors in the origin of PB. However it is worth emphasizing three main chances for the reduction of this high PB rate. (i) There is very high rate of cervical incompetence in Hungarian pregnant women explained by the extreme high number of previous induced abortions by D + C method. There are two urgent tasks to reduce this important cause of PB: the education of our people to use the modern effective contraceptive method instead of induced abortion with medical and moral problems. On the other hand it would be necessary to use abortion pills instead of the old fashion and risky surgical interruption of pregnancy if women insisting on this dangerous method of birth control. (ii) Our data showed that urogenital infections of pregnant women had not appropriate medical care in Hungary, i.e. early screening and effective treatment. Thus vulvovaginitis-bacterial vaginosis are frequently not diagnosed, and if diagnosed most of these pregnant women are not treated because of the anxiety of potential teratogenic effect of drugs. These two etiological factor groups may explain about 30 and 25% of PB, respectively, in Hungary, thus their appropriate medical management would result in a drastic drop in the very high Hungarian rate of PB. (iii) Finally we recommend using the potential preventive effect of folic acid during the third trimester of pregnancy for PB. Of course, all possible causes of PB need restriction, but these three factors seem to be the most important and their use can protect the life and health of several hundred newborn infants.

20.9 Final Conclusion

Preventive approaches are often classified as primary (due to the avoidance of causes), secondary (early detection and medical treatment; previously elective abortion was also classified as secondary prevention, but now we do not use the term of prevention for the termination of pregnancy in malformed fetuses) and tertiary (early surgical or other correction of CAs) prevention. Obviously primary prevention is the easiest and most effective way of prevention. At present many CAs can be prevented, therefore, CAs should not be considered as an unchangeable component of perinatal mortality and handicaps. However, as CAs vary so greatly, there is no single strategy for their prevention, still, periconceptional folic acid/multivitamin supplementation can prevent a wide spectrum of CAs.

References

Bukowski R, Malone FD, Porter FT et al. Preconceptional folate supplementation and the risk of spontaneous preterm birth: a cohort study. PLoS Med 2009; 6: e10000061.
Catov JM, Bodnar LM, Ness RB et al. Association of periconceptional multivitamin and risk of preterm or small-for-gestational-age births. Am J Epidemiol 2007; 166: 296–303.
Cikot RJLM, Steegers-Theunissen RPM, Thomas CMG et al. Longitudinal vitamin and homocysteine levels in normal pregnancy. Br J Nutr 2001; 85: 49–58.
Ek J. Plasma and red cell folate in mothers and infants in normal pregnancies. Relation to birth weight. Acta Obstet Gynecol Scand 1982; 61: 17–20.
Eskes TKAB. Vascular disease in women. Folate and homocysteine. In: Massaro EJ, Rogers JM (eds.) Folate and Human Development. Humana Press, Totowa, NJ, 2002. pp. 299–328.
Ferguson SE, Smith GN, Walker MC. Maternal plasma homocysteine levels in women with preterm premature rupture of membranes. Med Hypotheses 2001; 56: 85–90.
Goldenberg RL, Tamura T, Cliver SP et al. Serum folate and fetal growth retardation: a matter of compliance? Obstet Gynecol 1992; 79: 719–722.
Haider BA, Bhutta ZA. Multiple-micronutrients supplementation for women during pregnancy. Cochrane Database Syst Rev 2006; 18(4): CD004905.
Johnson WG, Scholl TO, Spychala JR et al. Common dihydrofolate reductase 19-base deletion allele: a novel risk factors for preterm delivery. Am J Clin Nutr 2005; 81: 664–668.
McPartlin J, Halligan A, Scott JM, Darling M, Weir DG. Accelerated folate breakdown in pregnancy. Lancet 1993; 341: 148–149.
Mohammed K. Routine folate supplementation in pregnancy. In: Enkin MW, Keirse MJCN, Renfreq MJ, Nielson JP (eds.) Pregnancy and Childbirth Module. Cochrane Database of Systematic Reviews, No. 03158, April 1993.
Neggers YH, Goldenberg RL, Tamura T et al. The relationship between maternal dietary intake and infant birth weight. Acta Obstet Gynecol Scand 1997; 165(Suppl.): 71–75.
Relton CL, Pearce MS, Parker L. The influence of erythrocyte folate and serum vitamin B12 status on birth weight. Br J Nutr 2005; 93: 593–599.
Ronnenberg AG, Goldman MB, Chen D et al. Preconception homocysteine and B vitamin status and birth outcomes in Chinese women. Am J Clin Nutr 2002; 76: 1385–1391.
Scholl TO, Hediger ML, Schall JI et al. Dietary and serum folate: their influence on the outcome of pregnancy. Am J Clin Nutr 1996; 63: 520–525.
Scholl TO, Hediger ML, Bendich A et al. Use of multivitamin/mineral prenatal supplements: influence on the outcome of pregnancy. Am J Epidemiol 1997; 146: 134–141.
Scholl TO, Johnson WG. Folic acid influence on the outcome of pregnancy. Am J Clin Nutr 2000; 71: 1285S–1303S.
Shaw GM, Liberman RF, Todoroff K, Wasserman CR. Low birth weight, preterm delivery, and periconceptional vitamin use. J Pediatr 1997; 130: 1013–1014.
Siega-Riz AM, Savitz SA, Zeisel SH et al. Second trimester folate status and preterm birth. Am J Obstet Gynecol 2000; 191: 851–857.
Smiths LJM, Essed GGM. Short pregnancy intervals and unfavorable pregnancy outcomes: role of folate depletion. Lancet 2001; 358: 2074–2077.
Spencer N. Social and environmental determinants of birth weight. In: Weighing the Evidence. How is Birthweight Determined? Radcliffe Medical Press, Oxford, 2003. pp. 87–121.

van der Molen EF, Verbruggen B, Nokalova I et al. Hyperhomocysteinemia and other thrombotic risk factors in women with placental vasculopathy. Br J Obstet Gynecol 2000; 107: 785–791.

Vollset SE, Refsum H, Irgens LM et al. Plasma total homocysteine, pregnancy complications, and adverse pregnancy outcomes: the Hordaland Homocysteine Study. Am J Clin Nutr 2000; 71: 962–968.

WHO Reg. 1. Make every mother and child count. 2005; http://www.who.int/whr/2005/download/en

Own Publication

I. Czeizel AE, Puhó HE, Ács N, Bánhidy F. Possible association of folic acid supplementation during pregnancy with reduction of preterm birth: a population-based study. Eur J Obstet Gynecol Reprod Biol 2010; 148: 135–140.

Closing Remarks

At present the leading causes of infant mortality and handicaps are PB and CAs. Out of 136 million total births per year worldwide, more than 4 million newborn infants die within the first days or weeks of life. The rate of CAs, depending on the definition of this pathological condition, is between 3 and 7% in different countries. The so-called true total (birth + fetal) prevalence of cases with CA is about 6.5% in Hungary; however, this high figure reflects the intensive research in this field and not an absolutely higher frequency. In agreement with this statement, the proportion of CAs within infant mortality is not higher in Hungary than in other European countries. However, the rate of PB is very high (about 9%) in Hungary compared with the rates of PB in other European countries. Our studies showed some adverse factors (e.g. very high rate of cervical incompetence due to the extremely high number of previous induced abortions by D + C method) in the background of this high PB rate. Advances in fetal and neonatal care have improved the survival chance for individuals with some CAs and PB, however, this progress may associate with the increase of handicapped persons.

Thus we stress the importance of old slogan: "prevention is better than cure." Preventive approaches are classified as primary (due to the avoidance of causes), secondary (early detection and medical treatment; previously elective termination of pregnancy after the prenatal diagnosis of fetal defects was also classified as secondary prevention, but now we do not use the term of prevention for this medical intervention) and tertiary (early surgical or other corrections of CA and the strong expert support for preterm babies) prevention.

There are several CAs with good chance for complete recovery (i.e. tertiary prevention), e.g. infants with congenital pyloric stenosis or ventricular septal defect have a healthy life after surgical correction. Similar progress has been achieved in the care and development of preterm babies. The secondary prevention is also very successful in some CAs. For example congenital dislocation of the hip was the most common CA in Hungary, but after the introduction of neonatal orthopedic screening followed by effective treatment, at present we cannot see children with this CA. There is a similar progress in the prevention of major part of hypothyroidism due to neonatal blood screening completed with appropriate treatment. The intensive case of preterm babies has improved significantly their survival rate. Nevertheless, the optimal solution would be the primary prevention of CAs and PB,

N. Ács et al., *Congenital Abnormalities and Preterm Birth Related to Maternal Illnesses During Pregnancy*, DOI 10.1007/978-90-481-8620-4, as the most effective and less problematic way of prevention. Now we have a good chance to prevent rubella MCA-syndrome or fetal varicella disease with vaccination. The appropriate use of antipyretic drugs in pregnant women with high fever related disorders can prevent the hyperthermia associated CAs. Last but not least the periconceptional folic acid and folic acid-containing multivitamin supplementation during the periconceptional period is a breakthrough in the primary prevention of CAs. This new primary preventive method is good for the prevention – beyond of neural-tube defects – of some cardiovascular and urinary tract's CAs, in addition some maternal disease/treatment related CAs such as antiepileptic drugs and high fever as well. In addition, recent data suggest that folic acid can reduce the rate of PB during the third trimester of pregnancy.

Our hope is that the data of the HCCSCA were able to show the public health importance of the population-based surveillance of cases with CAs and controls without CA. A surveillance data set as HCCSSCA effectively helps monitoring the change in the total prevalence of different CAs, to check the efficacy of medical care of pregnant women and to stimulate the introduction of preventive method.

Thus it is good to know that at present time major part of CAs and PB are preventable, and these adverse birth outcomes should not be considered as an irreducible component of fetal and infant life.

Appendix

List of own papers regarding the teratogenic/fetotoxic effect of drugs and prevention of CA by folic acid or folic acid-containing multivitamins mentioned in the book.

1. Studies Based on the HCCSCA

A. Antimicrobial Drugs

1. Czeizel AE, Rockenbauer M, Sorensen HT, Olsen J. A population-based case-control teratologic study of three *parenteral penicillin G*. Cong Anom 1999; 39: 37–42.
2. Czeizel AE, Rockenbauer M, Olsen J, Sorensen HT. Oral *phenoxymethylpenicillin* treatment during pregnancy. Arch Gynecol Obstet 2000; 263: 178–181.
3. Czeizel AE, Rockenbauer M, Sorensen HT, Olsen J. A population-based case-control teratologic study of penicillin V: oral *penamecillin* treatment during pregnancy. Cong Anom 1999; 39: 267–279.
4. Czeizel AE, Rockenbauer M, Sorensen HT, Olsen J. A population-based case-control teratologic study of *ampicillin* treatment during pregnancy. Am J Obstet Gynecol 2001; 185: 140–147.
5. Kazy Z, Puhó HE, Czeizel AE. The possible preterm birth preventive effect of *ampicillin* during pregnancy. Arch Gynecol Obstet 2006; 274: 215–221.
6. Czeizel AE, Rockenbauer M, Sorensen HT, Olsen J. *Augmentin* treatment during pregnancy and the prevalence of congenital abnormalities. A population-based case-control teratologic study. Eur J Obstet Gynecol Reprod Biol 2001; 97: 188–192.
7. Czeizel AE, Rockenbauer M, Sorensen HT, Olsen J. Teratogenic evaluation of *oxacillin*. Scand J Infect Dis 1999; 31: 311–312.
8. Czeizel AE, Rockenbauer M. A population-based case-control teratologic study of oral *oxytetracycline* treatment during pregnancy. Eur J Obstet Gynecol Reprod Biol 2000; 88: 27–33.
9. Czeizel AE, Rockenbauer M. Teratogenic study of *doxycycline*. Obstet Gynecol 1997; 89: 524–528.

10. Kazy Z, Puhó HE, Czeizel AE. Effect of *doxycycline* treatment during pregnancy for birth outcomes. Reprod Toxic 2007; 24: 279–280.
11. Czeizel AE, Rockenbauer M, Sorensen HT, Olsen J. Use of *cephalosporins* during pregnancy and congenital abnormalities. Am J Obstet Gynecol 2001; 184: 1289–1293.
12. Czeizel AE, Rockenbauer M, Sorensen HT, Olsen J. A population-based case-control teratologic study of oral *erythromycin* treatment during pregnancy. Reprod Toxicol 1999; 13: 531–536.
13. Czeizel AE, Rockenbauer M, Olsen J, Sorensen HT. A case-control teratological study of *spiramycin, roxithromycin, oleandomycin* and *josamycin.* Acta Obstet Gynecol Scand 2000; 79: 234–237.
14. Czeizel AE, Rockenbauer M, Sorensen HT, Olsen J. A teratological study of *lincosamides* (clindamycin and lincomycin). Scand J Infect Dis 2000; 32: 579–580.
15. Czeizel AE, Rockenbauer M, Olsen J, Sorensen HT. A teratological study of *aminoglycoside* antibiotic treatment during pregnancy. Scand J Infect Dis 2000; 32: 309–313.
16. Czeizel AE, Rockenbauer M, Sorensen HT, Olsen J. A population-based case-control teratologic study of oral *chloramphenicol* treatment during pregnancy. Eur J Epidemiol 2000; 16: 323–327.
17. Czeizel AE, Puhó E, Sørensen HT, Olsen J. A possible association between congenital abnormalities and the use of different *sulfonamides* during pregnancy. Cong Anom 2004; 44: 79–86.
18. Norgard B, Czeizel AE, Rockenbauer M, Olsen J, Sorensen HT. Population-based case-control study of the safety of *sulfasalazine* use during pregnancy. Aliment Pharmacol Ther 2001; 15: 483–486.
19. Czeizel AE. A case-control analysis of the teratogenic effects of *co-trimoxazole.* Reprod Toxicol 1990; 4: 305–313.
20. Czeizel AE, Rockenbauer M, Sorensen HT, Olsen J. The teratogenic risk of *trimethoprim-sulfonamides.* A population-based case-control study. Reprod Toxicol 2001; 15: 637–646.
21. Czeizel AE, Rockenbauer M, Olsen J, Sorensen HT. A population-based case-control study of the safety of oral *anti-tuberculosis drug* treatment during pregnancy. Int J Tuberc Lung Dis 2001; 5: 564–568.
22. Czeizel AE, Rockenbauer M, Sorensen HT, Olsen J. *Nitrofurantoin* and congenital abnormalities. Eur J Obstet Gynecol Reprod Biol 2001; 95: 119–126.
23. Czeizel AE, Rockenbauer M, Sorensen HT, Olsen J. A population-based case-control teratologic study of *furazidine,* a nitrofuran-derivative treatment during pregnancy. Clin Nephrol 2000; 53: 257–263.
24. Czeizel AE, Rockenbauer M, Sorensen HT, Olsen J. Risk of infantile pyloric stenosis in infants exposed to *nalidixid acid:* a population-based case-control study. Int J Gynecol Obstet 2001; 73: 221–228.
25. Czeizel AE, Kazy Z, Puhó E. Parenteral *polymyxin B* treatment during pregnancy. Reprod Toxicol 2005; 20: 181–182.

26. Dudás I, Puhó E, Czeizel AE. Population-based case-control study of *oxoline acid* use during pregnancy for birth outcomes. Cong Anom 2006; 46: 39–42.
27. Czeizel AE, Puhó E, Ács N, Bánhidy F. A population-based case-control study of oral *moroxydine*, an antiviral agent treatment during pregnancy. Int J Pharmacol 2006; 2: 188–192.
28. Czeizel AE, Tóth M, Rockenbauer M. No teratogenic effect after *clotrimazole* therapy during pregnancy. Epidemiology 1999; 10: 437–440.
29. Czeizel AE, Rockenbauer M. A lower rate of preterm birth after *clotrimazole* therapy during pregnancy. Paediatr Perinat Epidemiol 1999; 13: 58–64.
30. Czeizel AE, Fladung B, Vargha P. Preterm birth reduction after *clotrimazole* treatment during pregnancy. Eur J Obstet Gynecol Reprod Biol 2004; 116: 157–163.
31. Czeizel AE, Kazy Z, Vargha P. A case-control teratological study of vaginal *natamycin* treatment during pregnancy. Reprod Toxicol 2003; 17: 387–391.
32. Czeizel AE, Kazy Z. Puhó E. A population-based case-control teratologic study of oral *nystatin* treatment during pregnancy. Scan J Inf Dis 2003; 35: 830–835.
33. Métneki J, Czeizel AE. *Griseofulvin* teratology. Lancet 1987; i: 1042.
34. Czeizel AE, Metneki J, Kazy Z, Puhó E. A population-based case-control study of oral *griseofulvin* treatment during pregnancy. Acta Obstet Gynecol Scand 2004; 83: 827–831.
35. Czeizel AE, Kazy Z. Vargha P. A population-based case control teratological study of vaginal *econazole* treatment during pregnancy. Eur J Obstet Gynecol Reprod Biol 2003; 111: 135–140.
36. Czeizel AE, Kazy Z. Vargha P. Vaginal treatment with *povidone-iodine* suppositories during pregnancy. Int J Gynecol Obstet 2004; 84: 83–85.
37. Czeizel AE, Kazy Z, Puhó E. A population-based case-control teratologic study of topical *miconazole*. Cong Anom 2004; 44: 41–45.
38. Sorensen HT, Olesen C, Larsen H, Steffensen FH, Schonkeyder HC, Olsen J, Czeizel AE. Risk of malformation and other outcomes in children exposed to *fluconazole* in utero. Br J Clin Pharmacol 1999; 48: 234–238.
39. Czeizel AE, Kazy Z, Puhó E. *Tolfnaftate* spray treatment during pregnancy. Reprod Toxicol 2004; 18: 443–444.
40. Kazy Z, Puhó E, Czeizel AE. A case-control teratological study of local *ketoconazole* treatment during pregnancy. Cong Anom 2005; 45: 5–8.
41. Czeizel AE, Rockenbauer M. A population-based case-control teratologic study of oral *metronidazole* treatment during pregnancy. Br J Obstet Gynaecol 1998; 105: 322–327.
42. Sorensen HT, Larsen H, Nielsen GL, Jensen ES, Thulstrup AM, Schonkeyder HC, Nielsen GL, Czeizel AE and EUROMAP Study Group. Safety of *metronidazole* during pregnancy: cohort study of the risk of malformations preterm delivery and low birth weight in 124 women. J Antimicrob Chemother 1999; 44: 854–855.
43. Kazy Z, Puhó E, Czeizel AE. Teratogenic potential of vaginal *metronidazole* treatment during pregnancy. Eur J Obstet Gynecol Reprod Biol 2005; 123: 174–178.

44. Kazy Z, Puhó E, Czeizel AE. Gestational age and prevalence of preterm birth after vaginal *metronidazole* treatment during pregnancy. Int J Gynecol Obstet 2004; 87: 161–162.
45. Kazy Z, Puhó E, Czeizel AE. The possible association between the combination of *metronidazole and miconazole* treatment and poly/syndactyly in a population-based study. Reprod Toxicol 2005; 20: 89–94.
46. Kazy Z, Puhó E, Czeizel AE. Effect of vaginal *metronidazole* + *miconazole* treatment during pregnancy for gestational age and birth weight. Arch Gynecol Obstet 2005; 272: 294–297.
47. Kazy Z, Puhó E, Czeizel AE. *Levamisole* (Decaris) treatment during pregnacy. Reprod Toxicol 2004; 19: 3.
48. Ács N, Bánhidy F, Puhó E, Czeizel AE. A population-based study of *mebendazole* in pregnant women for pregnancy outcomes. Cong Anom 2005; 45: 85–88.
49. Czeizel AE, Kazy Z, Vargha P. Oral *tinidazole* treatment during pregnacy and teratogenesis. Int J Obstet Gynecol 2003; 83: 305–306.
50. Ács N, Bánhidy F, Puhó E, Czeizel AE. Teratogenic effect of vaginal *boric acid* treatment during pregnancy. Int J Obstet Gynecol 2006; 93: 55–56.

B. Other Drugs

51. Czeizel AE. *Diazepam*, phenytoin and aetiology of cleft lip and/or cleft papate. Lancet 1976; i: 810.
52. Czeizel AE, Lendvay A. In-utero exposure to *benzodiazepines*. Lancet 1987; i: 628.
53. Czeizel AE. Lack of evidence of teratogenicity of *benzodiazepine* drugs in Hungary. Reprod Toxicol 1988; I: 183–188.
54. Czeizel AE, Erõs E, Rockenbauer M, Sørensen HT, Olsen J. Shortterm oral *diazepam* treatment during pregnancy – a population-based teratological case-control study. Clin Drug Invest 2003; 23: 451–462.
55. Czeizel AE, Rockenbauer M, Sorensen HT, Olsen J. A population based case-control study of oral *chlordiazepoxide* use during pregnancy and risk of congenital abnormalities. Neurotox Terat 2004; 26: 593–598.
56. Erõs E, Czeizel AE, Rockenbauer M, Sorensen HT, Olsen J. A population-based case-control teratologic study of *nitrazepam, medazepam, tofisopam, alprazolum and clonazepam* treatment during pregnancy. Eur J Obstet Gynecol Reprod Biol 2002; 101: 147–154.
57. Lakos P, Czeizel AE. A teratological evaluation of *anticonvulsant* drugs. Acta Paediatr Acad Sci Hung 1977; 18: 145–153.
58. Czeizel AE, Bod M, Halász P. Evaluation of *anticonvulsant* drugs during pregnancy in a population-based Hungarian study. Eur J Epidemiol 1992; 8: 122–127.

59. Kjaer D, Puhó HE, Christensen J, Vestergaard M, Czeizel AE, Sorensen HT, Olsen J. *Antiepileptic* drugs, *folic acid* and congenital abnormalities – a Hungarian case-control study. Br J Obstet Gynecol 2008; 115: 98–103.
60. Kjaer D, Puhó HE, Christensen J, Vestergaard M, Czeizel AE, Sorensen HT, Olsen J. Use of *phenytoin, phenobarbitals*, or *diazepam* during pregnancy and risk of congenital abnormalities: a case-time-control study. Pharmacoepid Drug Safety 2007; 16: 181–188.
61. Czeizel AE, Vass J. Teratological surveillance of *oral contraceptive* use in early pregnancy. Adv Contracept Deliv Syst 1996; 12: 51–59.
62. Czeizel AE, Kodaj I. A changing pattern in the association of *oral contraceptives* and the different groups of congenital limb deficiencies. Contraception 1995; 51: 19–24.
63. Czeizel AE. Impact of recommendations against periconceptional *contraceptive pill* use. Contraception 1994; 49: 565–569.
64. Metneki J, Czeizel AE. *Contraceptive pills* and twins. Acta Genet Med Gamell 1980; 29: 233–236.
65. Wogelius P, Puhó HE, Pedersen L, Norgaard M, Czeizel AE, Sorensen HT. Maternal use of *oral contraceptives* and risk of hypospadias – a population-based case-control study. Eur J Epidemiol 2006; 21: 777–781.
66. Czeizel AE, Huiskes N. A case-control study to evaluate the risk of congenital anomalies as a result of *allylestrenol* therapy during pregnancy. Clin Therapeut 1988; 10: 725–739.
67. Dudás I, Gidai J, Czeizel AE. A population-based case-control teratogenic study of *hydroxyprogesteron* treatment during pregnancy. Cong Anom 2006; 46: 194–198.
68. Dudás I, Puhó E, Gidai J, Czeizel AE. A population-based case-control teratogenic study of *human chorionic gonadotropin* treatment during pregnancy. Cong Anom 2007; 47: 420–427.
69. Czeizel AE, Dudás I, Puhó E, Gidai J. No effect of *human chorionic gonadotropin* treatment during pregnancy for pregnancy outcomes. Cent Eur J Sci 2008; 3: 71–76.
70. Czeizel AE, Rockenbauer M. Population-based case-control study of teratogenic potential of *corticosteroids*. Teratology 1997; 56: 335–340.
71. Czeizel AE, Vargha P. A case-control study of congenital abnormality and *dimenhydrinate* usage during pregnancy. Arch Gynecol Obstet 2005; 271: 113–118.
72. Czeizel AE, Vargha P. Case-control study of *thiethylperazine,* an antiemetic drug. Br J Obstet Gynecol 2003; 110: 497–499.
73. Czeizel AE, Puhó E, Bánhidy F, Ács N. Oral *pyridoxine* during pregnancy. Potential protective effect for cardiovascular malformations. Clin Drug Invest 2004; 5: 259–269.
74. Bártfai Z, Kocsis J, Puhó HE, Czeizel AE. A population-based case-control study of *promethazine* use during pregnancy. Reprod Toxicol 2008; 25: 276–285.

75. Czeizel AE, Rockenbauer M, Mosonyi A. A population-based case-control teratologic study of *acetylsalicylic acid* treatments during pregnancy. Pharmacoepid Drug Safety 2000; 9: 193–205.
76. Norgard B, Puhó E, Czeizel AE, Skriver MV, Sorensen HT. *Aspirin* use during early pregnancy and the risk of congenital abnormalities: a population-based case-control study. Am J Obstet Gynecol 2005; 152: 922–923.
77. Rebordoso C, Kogerinas J, Horvath-Puhó E, Norgard B, Morales M, Czeizel AE, Viltsrup H, Sorensen HT, Olsen J. *Acetaminophen* use during pregnancy effects on risk for congenital abnormalities. Am J Obstet Gynecol 2008; 198: 178e1–178e7.
78. Czeizel AE, Dudás I, Puhó E. Shortterm *paracetamol* therapy during pregnancy and a lower rate of preterm birth. Paediatr Perinat Epidemiol 2005; 19: 106–111.
79. Czeizel AE, Tóth M, Mosonyi A. *Furosemide* as a fetal growth promoter. Clin Drug Invest 2000; 20: 53–58.
80. Czeizel AE, Rockenbauer M. A population-based case-control teratological study of *furosemide* treatment during pregnancy. Clin Drug Invest 1999; 18: 307–315.
81. Bánhidy F, Ács N, Puhó HE, Czeizel AE. A population-based case-control teratologic study of oral *dipyrone* treatment during pregnancy. Drug Safety 2006; 30: 1–13.
82. Kazy Z, Puhó E, Czeizel AE. A population-based case-control study of *Broncho-Vaxom* use during pregnancy. (Hungarian with English abstract) Orvosi Hetilap 2006; 146: 2359–2361.
83. Czeizel AE, Rockenbauer M. The evaluation of *drotaverin* intake during pregnancy on fetal development. Prenat Neonat Med 1996; 1: 137–145.
84. Czeizel AE. Teratogenicity of *ergotamine*. J Med Genet 1989; 26: 69–70.
85. Ács N, Bánhidy F, Puhó E, Czeizel AE. A possible dose-dependent teratogenic effect of *ergotamine*. Reprod Toxicol 2006; 22: 551–552.
86. Bánhidy F, Ács N, Puhó E, Czeizel AE. *Ergotamine* treatment during pregnancy and a higher rate of low birthweight and preterm birth. Br J Clin Pharmacol 2007; 1111: 2125–2132.
87. Czeizel AE. *Ovulation* induction and neural-tube defects. Lancet 1989; 2: 167.
88. Czeizel AE. *Reserpine* is not a human teratogen. J Med Genet 1988; 25: 787.
89. Sorensen HT, Czeizel AE, Rockenbauer M, Steffensen FH, Olsen J. The risk of limb deficiencies and other congenital abnormalities in children exposed in utero to *calcium channel blockers*. Acta Obstet Gynecol Scand 2001; 80: 397–401.
90. Czeizel AE, Puhó E, Bártfai Z, Somoskövi A. A possible association between oral *aminophylline* treatment during pregnancy and skeletal congenital abnormalities. Clin Drug Invest 2003; 2:. 803–816.
91. Bártfai Z, Somoskövi A, Puhó HE, Czeizel AE. No teratogenic effect of *prenoxdiazine*. A population-based case-control study. Cong Anom 2007; 47: 16–21.

92. Bánhidy F, Ács N, Puhó HE, Czeizel AE. *Phenolphthalein* treatment in pregnant women and congenital abnormalities in their offspring: a population-based case-control teratologic study. Drug Discover Therap 2008; 2: 357–367.
93. Ács N, Bánhidy F, Puhó HE, Czeizel AE. *Senna* treatment in pregnant women and congenital abnormalities in their offspring: a population-based case-control teratologic study. Reprod Toxic 2009; 28: 100–104.
94. Bánhidy F, Ács N, Puhó HE, Czeizel AE. Teratogenic potential of *pholedrine*, a sympathomimetic vasoconstritive drug: a population-based case-control study. Cong Anom 2010; 50: (in press).
95. Czeizel AE, Pataki T, Rockenbauer M. Reproductive outcome after exposure to *surgery under anaesthesia* during pregnancy. Arch Gynecol Obstet 1998; 261: 193–199.
96. Czeizel AE, Rockenbauer M. *Tetanus toxoid* and congenital abnormalities. Int J Gyn Obstet 1999; 64: 253–258.
97. Petik D, Puhó E, Czeizel AE. Evaluation of maternal *infusion* therapy during pregnancy for fetal development. Int J Med Sci 2005; 2: 129–134.

C. Pregnancy Supplements

98. Czeizel AE, Rockenbauer. Prevention of congenital abnormalities by *vitamin A*. Int J Vit Nutr Res 1998; 68: 219–231.
99. Czeizel AE, Tóth M, Rockenbauer M. Population-based case-control study of *folic acid* supplementation during pregancy. Teratology 1996, 53: 345–357.
100. Czeizel AE, Tímár L, Sárközi A. Dose-dependent effect of *folic acid* on the prevention of orofacial clefts. Pediatrics 1999; 104: e66.
101. Czeizel AE, Vargha P. Periconceptional *folic acid/multivitamin* supplementation and twin pregnancies. Am J Obstet Gynecol 2004; 191: 790–794.
102. Czeizel AE. Prevention of oral clefts through the use of *folic acid* and *multivitamin* supplements. Evidence and gaps. In: Wyszinnsky DF (ed.) Cleft Lip and Palate. From Origin to Treatment. Oxford University Press, New York, 2002. pp. 443–457.
103. Czeizel AE, Puhó HE, Bánhidy F. No association between periconceptional *multivitamin* supplementation and risk of multiple congenital abnormalities. A population-based case-control study. Am J Med Genet A. 2006; 140A: 2469–2477.
104. Czeizel AE, Puhó E. Maternal use of *nutritional supplement* during the first month of pregnancy and reduced risk of Down syndrome. A case-control study. Hum Nutr 2005; 21: 698–704.
105. Czeizel AE, Puhó HE, Langmar Z, Ács N, Bánhidy F. Possible association of *folic acid supplementation* during pregnancy with reduction of preterm birth – a population-based study. Eur J Obstet Gynecol Reprod Biol 2010; 148: 135–140.

2. Studies Based on the Budapest Monitoring System of Self-Poisoned Pregnant Women

106. Gidai J, Ács N, Bánhidy F, Czeizel AE. No association found between use of very large doses of *diazepam* by 112 pregnant women for a suicide attempt and congenital abnormalities in their offspring. Toxic Indust Health 2008; 24: 29–39.
107. Gidai J, Ács N, Bánhidy F, Czeizel AE. A study of the teratogenic and fetotoxic effects of large does of *chlordiazepoxide* used for self-poisoning by 35 pregnant women. Toxic Indust Health 2008; 24: 41–51.
108. Gidai J, Ács N, Bánhidy F, Czeizel AE. Congenital abnormalities in childen of 43 pregnant women who attempted suicide with large doses of *nitrazepam*. Pharmacoepid Drug Safety 2010; 19: 175–182.
109. Gidai J, Ács N, Bánhidy F, Czeizel AE. An evaluation of data for ten children born to mothers who attempted suicide by taking large doses of *alprazolam* during pregnancy. Toxic Indust Health 2008; 24: 53–60.
110. Gidai J, Ács N, Bánhidy F, Czeizel AE. A study of the effects of large dose of *medazepam* used for self-poisoning in ten pregnant women on fetal development. Toxic Indust Health 2008; 24: 61–68.
111. Petik D, Ács N, Bánhidy F, Czeizel AE. A study of the potential teratogenic effects of large doses of *promethazine* in 32 self-poisoned pregnant women. Toxic Indust Health 2008; 24: 87–96.
112. Petik D, Ács N, Bánhidy F, Czeizel AE. A study of the effects of large doses of *glutethimide* that were used fro self-poisoning during pregnancy on human fetuses. Toxic Indust Health 2008; 24: 69–78.
113. Petik D, Timmerman G, Czeizel AE, Ács N, Bánhidy F. A study of teratogenic and fetotoxic effect of large doses of *amobarbital* used for suicide attempt in 14 pregnant women. Toxic Indust Health 2008; 24: 79–85.
114. Petik D, Ács N, Bánhidy F, Czeizel AE. Fetal neurotoxic effect of drug interaction due to high doses of a *drug combination (amobarbital, glutethimide, promethazine)* used by pregnant women for sicide attempt. Pharmacoepid Drug Safety 2010 (in press).
115. Timmermann G, Ács N, Bánhidy F, Czeizel AE. Congenital abnormalities of 88 children born to mothers who attempted suicide with *phebobarbital* during pregnancy: the use of a disaster epidemiological model for the evaluation of drug teratogenicity. Pharmacoepid Drug Safety 2009; 18: 815–825.
116. Timmermann G, Ács N, Bánhidy F, Czeizel AE. A study of teratogenic and fetotoxic effects of large doses of *barbital, hexobarbital and butobarbital* used for self-poisoning by pregnant women. Toxic Indust Health 2008; 24: 109–119.
117. Timmermann G, Ács N, Bánhidy F, Czeizel AE. A study of teratogenic and fetotoxic effects of large doses of *meprobamate* used for self-poisoning in 42 pregnant women. Toxic Indust Health 2008; 24: 97–107.
118. Timmermann G, Ács N, Bánhidy F, Czeizel AE. A study of the potential teratogenic effects of large doses of *rarely used drugs* for suicide attempt by pregnant women. Toxic Indust Health 2008; 24: 121–131.

120. Czeizel AE, Tomcsik M. Acute toxicity of *folic acid* in pregnant women. Teratology 1999; 60: 3–4.

3. Intervention Trials of Folic Acid-Containing Multivitamin Supplementation Based on the Hungarian Periconceptional Service

121. Czeizel AE, Dobó M, Dudás I, Gasztonyi Z, Lantos I. The Hungarian Periconceptional Service as a model for community genetics. Commun Genet 1998; 1: 252–259.
122. Czeizel AE. Ten years experience in periconceptional care. Eur J Obstet Gynecol Reprod Biol 1999; 84. 43–49.
123. Czeizel AE. Periconceptional care: an experiment in community genetics. Commun Genet 2003; 3: 119–123.
124. Czeizel AE, Gasztonyi Z, Kuliev A. Periconceptional clinics: a medical healthcare infrastructure of new genetics. Fetal Diagn Ther 2005; 20: 515–518.
125. Czeizel AE, Dudás I. Prevention of the first occurrence of neural-tube defects by periconceptional vitamin supplementation. N Engl J Med 1992; 327: 1832–1835.
126. Czeizel AE. Prevention of congenital abnormalities by periconceptional multivitamin supplementation. Br Med J 1993; 306: 1645–1648.
127. Czeizel AE, Dudás I, Métneki J. Pregnancy outcomes in a randomised controlledtrial of periconceptional multivitamin supplementation. Final report. Arch Gynecol Obstet 1994; 255: 131–139.
128. Czeizel AE. Reduction of urinary tract and cardiovascular defects by periconceptional multivitamin supplementation. Am J Med Genet 1996; 62: 179–183.
129. Czeizel AE. Periconceptional folic acid containing multivitamin supplementation. Eur J Obstet Gynecol Reprod Biol 1998; 78: 151–161.
130. Hook EB, Czeizel AE. Can terathanasia explain the protective effect of folic acid supplementation on birth defects? Lancet 1997; 350: 513–515.
131. Czeizel AE, Dobó M, Vargha P. Hungarian cohort controlled trial of periconceptional multivitamin supplementation shows a reduction in certain congenital abnormalities. Birth Defects Res Part A 2004; 70: 853–861.
132. Czeizel AE, Medveczki E. Periconceptional multivitamin supplementation and multimalformed offspring. Obstet Gynecol 2003; 202: 1255–1261.
133. Czeizel AE. Randomized Control Trial of Multivitamin Supplementation on Birth Defects and Pregnancy Outcomes, 1984–1994. Complementary and Alternative Medicine. Data Archive, Data Set 16 October 2004. Sociometric Corporation, National Institute of Health, USA.
134. Czeizel AE. Periconceptional folic acid and multivitamin supplementation for the prevention of neural-tube defects and other congenital abnormalities. Birth Defects Res Part A 2009; 85: 260–268.

Index

C

U

V

W